T0207121

Exercise and Sport Pharmacology

Exercise and Sport Pharmacology is an essential book for teaching upper-level undergraduates or entry-level graduate students about how drugs can affect exercise and how exercise can affect the action of drugs. It leads students through the related pathology, exercise physiology, and drug action of many of today's chronically used medications, and discusses how drugs can affect exercise performance.

This new second edition of the book is divided into four parts: Section I provides the basics of pharmacology, exercise physiology, autonomic pharmacology, and the stress response; Section II presents chapters on major cardiovascular and respiratory drug classes; Section III describes frequently prescribed medications for such common conditions as diabetes, depression, pain, fever, inflammation, and obesity; and Section IV includes discussions of nutritional supplements and commonly used drugs such as caffeine, nicotine, cannabis, and performance-enhancing drugs. The second edition offers many updates, enhances muscle cell physiology, includes the involvement of the gut microbiome, and each chapter has a new section on the effects of aging.

In Sections II and III, chapters include an overview of the pathology that therapeutic drugs are designed to treat and how the drugs work in the human body. In contrast to standard pharmacology texts, *Exercise and Sport Pharmacology* also includes the effect of exercise on the pathology of the condition and the effect of exercise on how the body responds to a drug. Each chapter has a section on whether the drugs under discussion have performance-enhancing potential. Section IV is concerned with self-medication and drugs or supplements taken without a prescription or with limited medical supervision.

Throughout, figures and tables as well as data from experiments in exercise pharmacology help to illustrate and summarize content. Each chapter opens with an on-going case example to preview and apply chapter content. In the text, boldface terms indicate which concepts are contained in the book's Glossary. Chapters conclude with a Key Concepts Review and Review Questions.

Mark D. Mamrack Ph.D. is an emeritus faculty member and former Associate Dean at Wright State University in Dayton, Ohio. In over three decades at Wright State University, his research focused on cell signaling and growth control. He taught classes in cell and molecular biology and began teaching exercise pharmacology in 2002. That experience led to the creation of this text, *Exercise and Sport Pharmacology*, first published in 2015. This second edition expands and enhances content while maintaining the overall structure of the first edition.

Exercise and Sport Pharmacology

Mark D. Mamrack

Second Edition

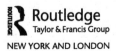

NEW YORK AND LONDON

Second edition published 2021
by Routledge
52 Vanderbilt Avenue, New York, NY 10017

and by Routledge
2 Park Square, Milton Park, Abingdon, Oxon, OX14 4RN

Routledge is an imprint of the Taylor & Francis Group, an informa business

First edition published by Holcomb Hathaway, Publishers, Inc. 2015

Library of Congress Cataloging-in-Publication Data
Names: Mamrack, Mark D, author.
Title: Exercise and sport pharmacology / Mark D. Mamrack.
Description: Second edition. | New York, NY: Routledge, 2020. | Includes
bibliographical references and index. | Identifiers: LCCN 2019044604 (print) |
LCCN 2019044605 (ebook) | ISBN 9781138613218 (hardback) |
ISBN 9781138613232 (paperback) | ISBN 9781315213071 (ebook)
Subjects: LCSH: Exercise—Physiological aspects. | Drugs—Physiological
effect. | Doping in sports. | Sports—Physiological aspects.
Classification: LCC RM301.15 .M36 2020 (print) | LCC RM301.15 (ebook) |
DDC 613.7/1—dc23
LC record available at https://lccn.loc.gov/2019044604
LC ebook record available at https://lccn.loc.gov/2019044605

ISBN: 978-1-138-61321-8 (hbk)
ISBN: 978-1-138-61323-2 (pbk)
ISBN: 978-1-003-03538-1 (ebk)

Typeset in Times New Roman
by codeMantra

Visit the eResource: www.routledge.com/9781138613232

Contents

Figures

Tables

Preface

The second edition of *Exercise and Sport Pharmacology* updates and enhances features of the first edition. It remains an accessible book useful for teaching advanced undergraduates or entry-level graduate students about common human afflictions and the drugs used to treat them. Importantly, it integrates the role of exercise into prevention, treatment, and recovery of these common diseases. Exercise prescription, when integrated with drug treatment, leads to the discussion of how drugs can affect exercise and how exercise can affect the action of the drugs. This book is intended to give students, in human performance and exercise-related majors, the specific pharmacology they need at the appropriate level using relevant examples. The book is also helpful to those interested in how exercise contributes to a healthy lifestyle.

The need for this book evolved several years ago when I was asked to teach pharmacology to majors in our exercise biology concentration. These students had previously been taking Pharmacology for Nurses, a course that did not meet their requirements because it gave them information they didn't need (for example, these students didn't need to memorize drug names, indications, and side effects), and it failed to give them the needed sport and exercise context for the information they did learn. The faculty in our exercise biology program believed that their students needed the basics of pharmacology and coverage of cardiovascular drugs since many of them worked in cardiac rehabilitation centers. They also suggested covering drugs banned by the National Collegiate Athletic Association (NCAA) and United States Olympic Committee (USOC) that act as performance-enhancing substances (PES). I agreed to teach the course but quickly found that none of the available textbooks were right for this new course. I began to provide the students with my lecture notes, and each year, the notes became more detailed. This book is the natural evolution of that ongoing effort.

At our university, the course has succeeded for upper-level human performance undergraduates because it draws on many other classes (Exercise Physiology, Cell Biology, Biochemistry, Psychology, Nutrition, and so on). The very nature of the topic, the interaction between exercise and drugs, requires the integration of information from the chemical level, the cellular and physiological level, and even a societal level. Exercise science students enjoy the material because they see how their training fits with real-world scenarios. Pre-med students love it because it involves treating sick people. And most students are intrigued by the ongoing saga of our sports heroes succumbing to the temptation of performance-enhancing substances and the question of whether these substances have any positive effect. I suspect that many undergraduate programs have or will identify a need for a course such as this one, integrating requisite levels of biology with an emphasis on human performance. Graduate students entering programs in exercise physiology and sports science can also benefit from the information provided on underlying mechanisms and the research studies that provide the basis of the information presented.

The Book's Organization

The second edition adds discussion of the role of the microbiome in health and drug action. Skeletal muscle biology is expanded, with information added on recovery and adaptation. In response to reviewers, each chapter now addresses the aging process and its effect on health, disease, and physical activity. *Exercise and Sport Pharmacology* is divided into four parts. Section I encompasses the basics of pharmacology, exercise physiology, and autonomic pharmacology and stress. Part I provides foundational information needed to understand concepts discussed in later chapters and build background knowledge to minimize redundancy. Sections II and III cover many of the widely prescribed drugs for common chronic conditions that human performance majors are likely to encounter in their careers. Section II covers cardiovascular and respiratory drugs, with an emphasis on hypertension. Section III presents other frequently prescribed medications, including psychotherapeutic agents, lipid-modifying agents, analgesics and anti-inflammatory drugs, and antidiabetic and antiobesity drugs.

Section IV discusses self-medication. Chapters cover supplements and commonly used drugs, such as caffeine, ethanol, nicotine, and cannabis. The book's final chapter discusses performance-enhancing substances with a focus on how they work and the evidence that supports their effect or lack of effect on athletic performance.

The Book's Pedagogy

Throughout, figures and tables help to illustrate and summarize content. Most chapters open with an ongoing case example to apply and preview chapter content. In the text, boldface terms indicate which concepts can be found in the book's glossary for easy reference. Chapters conclude with a list of Review Questions and Key Concepts Review.

It is my hope that this book will fill a specific need for your department and your students. My goal was to provide the right mix of science, application, and real-world examples to bring this information to life for student readers. My own classes have enjoyed using the book, and I look forward to hearing from instructors and students from other universities regarding how this text succeeds in their program.

About the Author

After finishing his BS in Biochemistry at Purdue University, Mark D. Mamrack entered the PhD program in the Pharmacology Department at Baylor College of Medicine. He became interested in protein phosphorylation as a mechanism for regulating protein function, particularly proteins found in the cell nucleolus. He continued to study protein phosphorylation and its role in cancer during his post-doctoral work at Oak Ridge National Lab (Oak Ridge, Tennessee). While at Oak Ridge, Mark was recruited by the University of Tennessee Graduate School of Biomedical Sciences to teach cell biology to first-year PhD students. It was that experience that resulted in his taking a faculty position at Wright State University in Dayton, Ohio, where he continued his research into cell signaling and growth control. He has taught exercise and sport pharmacology since 2002. His experience in teaching the class led to the creation of this text, *Exercise and Sport Pharmacology*.

Acknowledgments

I would like to thank my wife Irene for her patience and support in what continues to be an all-encompassing project. I would also like to thank the reviewers who offered constructive feedback at various stages of the writing process. The book is better as a result of their suggestions, and I appreciate their help. I want to acknowledge the wonderful and professional editorial support I received during the first edition as their efforts at Holcomb and Hathaway Publishing, especially those of Colette Kelly and Gay Pauley, provided the strong foundation that facilitated this second edition.

Mark D. Mamrack

Section I

Introduction

1 Basic Pharmacology

Abstract

Exercise and sport pharmacology pertain to the interaction of exercise and the physiological responses to drugs. Pharmacokinetics concerns the fate of the drug in the body. Pharmacodynamics concerns the response of the body to drugs. Both pharmacokinetics and pharmacodynamics are affected by exercise, usually in an intensity-dependent manner.

When a drug enters the body, only a fraction of it reaches its target. That fraction can vary, as many properly working organ systems come into play, providing a large degree of variation in drug responsiveness in the human population. Many factors contribute to the bioavailability of the drug, such as genetic background, age, percent body fat, and degree of physical fitness. Most drugs are chemically altered and eliminated from the body by diverse mechanisms, which also contribute to the variability seen in human populations. The dose of a drug has to be sufficient to allow enough drug to reach an effective concentration at the site of action. Drugs alter existing physiological pathways, usually by interacting with specific protein receptors. Exercise can change the fate of the drug in the body. As exercise intensity increases, blood is redirected, and rates of metabolism and elimination can change. Since the bioavailability of the drug can change with exercise, the primary or desirable response to the drug can change. The possibility of unwanted side effects can also change. Drugs that have a narrow therapeutic index and are flow-limited during exercise should be monitored closely. In the future, pharmacogenomics may help health providers match subsets of the population with the most effective and safest drug option. The gut microbiome influences human health and is affected by drug treatment and physical activity.

Learning Objectives

1 Distinguish pharmacokinetics from pharmacodynamics.
2 Understand how exercise may affect pharmacokinetics and pharmacodynamics.
3 Understand the concept of bioavailability and factors that affect it, including absorption, distribution, metabolism, and clearance.
4 Understand drug receptors and how drugs cause their biological effects.
5 Appreciate the future role for pharmacogenomics.
6 Appreciate the importance of the gut microbiome.

Introduction

Pharmacology is the study of drug action, including the chemistry, effects, and uses of drugs. **Exercise and sport pharmacology** is a specialized branch of pharmacology that studies the interaction between the physiological changes caused by drugs and the physiological changes caused by physical activity. It is concerned with how drugs might affect people engaged in sports or exercise programs, including athletes and those who are overweight, unfit, disabled, or elderly. Exercise and sport pharmacology is an emerging field. Its scope ranges from studying the effects of drugs on athletes in competition to examining drugs' effects on patients in cardiac rehabilitation (Reents 2000). Questions related to exercise and sport pharmacology include:

- Does physical activity affect the distribution, metabolism, excretion, and duration of drugs? Does exercise affect how tissues respond to a drug?
- Does physical activity affect drug interactions, tolerance, or side effects?
- What drugs can interfere with regular exercise, training, or performance?
- What drugs are illegal, and what drugs are banned by sport organizations?

Very little is known about the interaction between drugs and many forms of physical activity. Many drugs come to market without testing related to exercise or sport performance. For example, NSAIDs (non-steroidal anti-inflammatory drugs) can cause bleeding in the gastro-intestinal tract (GI-tract). Marathon runners often have GI-tract issues. Are these issues compounded when athletes use drugs like ibuprofen, an NSAID? Statins are widely prescribed for lowering blood cholesterol, and one side effect of statins involves muscle damage. Many of the patients who use statins also engage in exercise programs. Is the pain that some of these patients experience normal soreness following exercise, or is it a more serious problem, a result of the statin? Diuretics are effective as a treatment for high blood pressure and fluid retention. If a person taking a diuretic experiences dizziness and cramping after playing tennis on a hot Florida afternoon, are the dizziness and cramping due to a sodium or potassium imbalance from taking the diuretic? Exercise and sport pharmacology seeks to answer these questions and more.

Overall, taking a lot of pills is part of our culture. Prescription drugs (**pharmaceuticals**) accounted for about $450 billion in sales in the United States alone during 2016. Globally, spending on pharmaceuticals is expected to reach $1.5 trillion in 2021 (www.reuters.com/article/us-health-pharmaceuticals-spending/global-prescription-drug-spend-seen-at-1-5-trillion-in-2021-report-idUSKBN13V0CB). An estimate for retail prescriptions in 2019 suggests nearly 4.25 billion in just the United States, an average of more than 10 prescriptions per person (www.statista.com/statistics/261303/total-number-of-retail-prescriptions-filled-annually-in-the-us/). Over-the-counter (**OTC**) drugs, such as Tylenol and aspirin, are drugs (or drug combinations) that do not require a prescription by a doctor or other appropriate health-care practitioner. Retail sales of these drugs might exceed $30 billion annually in the United States, though what constitutes an OTC drug can vary when researchers make these broad groupings. Nutritional supplements (**nutraceuticals**), discussed in Chapter 13, may total another $50 billion in sales, depending on what is included in this category. The point is that this is big business—for the drug companies, the governments that regulate (and tax) it, the insurance and health maintenance organization (HMO) industry, and the public. There are more than 100,000 different drug-related products on the market. Consider the following statements about exercise and drug-related product use in the United States:

- As much as one-third of the population has high blood pressure (hypertension) and should be exercising, but a percentage of these individuals will probably also require anti-hypertensive drugs.
- Although exercise helps one maintain healthy blood lipids, many individuals still require lipid-lowering drugs.
- The number of individuals diagnosed with major depressive disorder is increasing. They may require anti-depressant drugs, with exercise recommended as an adjunct therapy.
- The aging of our population will, in all likelihood, account partially for an increase in drug use.
- Nutraceuticals are regulated differently from pharmaceuticals, and consumers spend large amounts of money on supplements that often have no documented benefit. These products can enter the market without the same requirements for safety and labeling of contents as pharmaceuticals. They can contain many compounds, some of which may affect people's ability to participate in sport or physical activity, or result in their being banned from competition.
- Therapeutic agents taken to enhance performance continue to plague amateur and professional sport as our society tries to enforce anti-doping policies and encourage drug-free competition. Performance-enhancing substances (PES) used within recreational and sub-elite athletic groups indicate the scope of the problem and the difficulty in attaining this goal.

These trends are similar for most of the world's developed countries. Cholesterol-lowering drugs, anti-depressants, drugs for hypertension, pain-killers, and herbal remedies for the common cold are widely used throughout the world.

Drugs with high abuse potential are bought and sold illegally on the black market. The Controlled Substances Act (CSA), passed in 1970, regulates the manufacture, importation, possession, use, and distribution of certain substances. Five Schedules (i.e., classifications) were created to list these drugs based on criteria related to their potential for abuse, their usefulness as a medical treatment, and agreements with other countries. For example, heroin is listed under Schedule I, cocaine and methamphetamine are under Schedule II, and anabolic steroids are under Schedule III. The Food and Drug Administration (FDA) and the Drug Enforcement Administration (DEA) make changes to the list of drugs under each Schedule. The FDA is responsible for the regulation and supervision of food safety, pharmaceuticals, and OTC drugs, as well as for ensuring safety and accurate labeling of many additional therapeutic agents. The Controlled Substance Schedules are available online at www.deadiversion.usdoj.gov/schedules/.

Since most drugs come to market without having been tested for their effects on exercise and sport, research that combines drugs and exercise (if done at all) is done after drugs are on the market. Moreover, many long-term side effects of drugs are not known until the drug has been on the market for several years. As an example, Vioxx, a drug prescribed for arthritis pain, was removed from the market after reports of serious cardiovascular complications, and many lawsuits have resulted.

Brief Background Concerning Physical Activity and Exercise

As this book concerns pharmacology *and* exercise, before we delve into principles of drug action in this chapter, we need to first cover some basic concepts and definitions for exercise, which will be detailed in Chapter 2. Basically, modern humans either sit, stand and possibly move, or lay down. Laying down is related to sleeping and the importance of sleeping for overall health will be discussed in Chapter 3. Our first distinction then is between sitting and physical activity. We will define physical activity shortly. We need to distinguish two interrelated health problems—too much time sitting and too little exercise. Too much time sitting is referred to as sedentary behavior and constitutes a risk to health, such as cardiovascular disease, obesity, metabolic syndrome, and diabetes. Regular exercise provides improved health outcomes; too little exercise is also associated with poor health.

The observation that sedentary behavior is deleterious to health has been around for centuries. Around 1700, Ramazzini distinguished "chair workers" from healthier "messengers." In the late 1940s, an English study began that compared the rates of coronary heart disease between conductors/ticket agents and drivers on the double-decker buses in London. The physically active conductors had a lower incidence of coronary heart disease than the drivers (Morris, Heady, Raffle, et al. 1953). In 1960, Paffenbarger devised a questionnaire to create a Physical Activity Index. It, and numerous modified versions since, computed distance walked and flights of stairs climbed, as well as sports and recreation time (Paffenbarger, Wing, & Hyde 1978). What has become clearer in recent years is the diverse negative health consequence of sitting too much. Physiological change/compensation occurs with extensive sitting. What constitutes *extensive* sitting? It varies with the individual's age, health status, fitness level, and possibly gender—but more than eight hours per day can be bad and more than 14 hours is very bad for your health.

One of the first statistical studies on sitting found that sedentary time was a stronger predictor for cardiovascular and metabolic (cardiometabolic) health than the amount of moderate-vigorous activity undertaken (Henson, Yates, Biddle, et al. 2013). Analysis involving close to 900 participants showed that the upper third of sedentary time (with a mean of 11.7 hours) had significantly poorer measures of cardiometabolic health. Sedentary behavior of modern humans has created a mismatch with our evolutionary history and how our ancestors survived. Many adults now spend up to 70% of their waking hours sedentary, a figure drastically higher than that of our ancestors. Sedentary time correlates with markers of diabetes risk, independent of the amount of moderate-to-vigorous physical activity undertaken (Henson, Edwardson, Morgan, et al. 2015). These markers were significantly elevated after subjects maintained a sedentary condition for seven days, showing that sitting negatively impacts cardiometabolic health (Lyden, Keadle, Staudenmayer, et al. 2015). Magnetic resonance images and individual accelerometer data was gathered from 66 participants in diabetes prevention programs. Each 30 minutes of sedentary time was associated with an increase in heart fat, liver fat, and visceral fat (Henson et al. 2015). In a study of 11,000 adults over 12 years, those who reduced their moderate-vigorous activity and increased their TV time had a 6.7 cm average increase in waist circumference (Shibata, Oka, Sugiyama, et al. 2016).

The effect is worldwide. Using 358 population-based surveys across 168 countries, the prevalence of insufficient physical activity for 1.9 million participants was determined. Globally, the prevalence of insufficient physical activity in 2016 was 23.4% in men and 31.7% in women. In 2016, the highest levels were observed in women in Latin America (43.7%), south Asia (43.0%), and high-income Western countries (42.3%). Lowest levels were in men from Asia (17.6%), and sub-Saharan Africa (17.9%). High-income countries (36.8%) had twice the incidence of low-income countries (16.2%), steadily increasing since first measured in 2001 (Guthold, Stevens, Riley, & Bull 2018). Another study examined the relationship between total sitting-time and all-cause mortality in older women. Six thousand six hundred fifty-six participants were followed for up to nine years and self-reported total sitting-time was linked to all-cause mortality data. After six years, about 30% of the participants had died. Compared to those that sat less than four hours a day, those who sat 8 to 11 h/day had a 1.45 times higher risk of death; those who sat more than 11 h/day had a 1.65 times higher risk of death. Prolonged sitting-time was positively associated with all-cause mortality (Pavey, Peeters, & Brown, 2015). Interestingly, the increased mortality risk for prolonged sitting was only among participants not meeting physical activity guidelines. Physical inactivity has a deleterious effect on health that is comparable to smoking and obesity. Close to 10% of all deaths worldwide can be attributed to physical inactivity. The less time spent sitting, a higher daily amount of physical activity, and overall cardiorespiratory fitness are associated with lower mortality rates and lower risks of obesity, diabetes, hypertension, cardiovascular disease, cancer, and aging-associated frailty. The public health message for disease prevention, successful aging, and reduction of premature mortality is for less sitting and higher cardiorespiratory fitness resulting from exercise (Bouchard, Blair, & Katzmarzyk 2015).

To avoid the dire consequences of sitting too much, we need to stand up and move around. Physical activity can be anything from mowing the lawn, waiting tables, or training for a marathon. For clarity purposes and this book, we will loosely make the following distinctions, acknowledging that there is considerable overlap. One main distinction is the one based on *intent*—what the individual wants to get out of the experience. For instance, some jobs or lifestyles require large amounts of *physical activity*. Physical activity is basically not sitting. Many people need to reserve time to *exercise*, at least that is their intent. Exercise can be moderate to vigorous as we will explore in the next chapter. To reap the health benefits of regular exercise, the weekly recommendation is 150 minutes of moderate-intensity activity or 75 minutes of vigorous-intensity activity (or some combination), with two days of resistance exercise. *Training* refers to a lifestyle where improvement in body composition, endurance, and strength are the desired outcome. *Competition or performance* involves levels of focus and sacrifice that a relatively small fraction of the population engages in, and usually only for a portion of their life—though many compete as long as they are able. Therefore, when we discuss exercise pharmacology, we need to distinguish the population—the difference between a couch potato, a regular jogger, a weekend warrior, or a competitive / professional athlete.

After the introductory section of the book, each chapter examines common human afflictions and the drugs used to treat them. We also look at the effect of exercise on the affliction and whether exercise changes how the drugs work. We will see how exercise affects blood pressure and cardiovascular health, lung function, blood lipids, mental health, and so forth. How is it that exercise can affect the body so profoundly? Let's think simply about this for now. When we get up and go for a walk, our brain has to get busy. Where are we going? Is it safe? Have I been there before? Will I remember how to get home (or find my car)? What is that noise—have I heard it before? Maybe I should have brought food and water! Physical activity stimulates learning and memory in portions of the brain—it is necessary for our survival. Our heart has to increase cardiac output now that we are moving. Our vasculature needs to redirect blood to working muscles. The lungs need to increase flow for increased gas exchange. Gut and kidney function can slow down and be dealt with later. The liver needs to alter metabolic processes to make sugar and fat available for muscle. Muscle needs to efficiently use oxygen to supply the contraction machinery with sufficient energy (ATP). The entire body takes part in surviving the physical activity it is undertaking. We return to exercise physiology and muscle function in Chapter 2, after we cover the principles of drug action.

Fundamentals of Pharmacology

A **drug**, in pharmacological terms, is a chemical used to prevent, treat, or cure disease. Drugs can alter normal bodily functions or enhance mental or physical well-being. Usually, a new drug is first given a chemical name, then is assigned a generic name, and finally receives a brand name. The naming of drugs is referred to as drug nomenclature. The chemical name is based on the molecular structure of the drug and can be very long and complex. When approved by the FDA, the drug then is given a generic name, often a shorthand version of the chemical name. The pharmaceutical company that develops and patents the drug is the source of its brand name, which is its trademarked proprietary name. For example, N-(4-hydroxyphenyl) acetamide (also known as *para*-acetylaminophenol) is the chemical name for a drug used for pain relief and as a fever reducer. It became known generically as paracetamol or acetaminophen, and its brand names include Tylenol (*para*-ace<u>t</u>ylaminoph<u>enol</u>) and Panadol. Another example is 2-[4-(2-methylpropyl)phenyl]propanoic acid, also known as ibuprofen, the active ingredient in the pain relievers with the brand names Advil and Motrin.

Drug classification can vary greatly. Classifications can be based on chemical similarity, the drug's mechanism, its **site of action** (the place where the drug will exert its primary effect), and/or its primary effect. Names of drug classes also change over time. Therefore, drug nomenclature and classification are somewhat fluid, and care should be taken not to overgeneralize when classifying drugs. New drugs to the market are usually protected by patent laws. Once the patent expires, generic versions can become available often at a reduced price to the consumer. Off-label use of a drug is possible (the drug is prescribed for reasons other than original approval), but may not be covered by insurance for that indication. When warranted, drugs approved for one use can go through the process a second time and be approved for another indication.

Pharmacology is the study of how drugs interact with an organism and cause a change in function. Pharmacology can be divided conceptually into **pharmacokinetics**, the study of what happens to the drug after it enters the body, and **pharmacodynamics**, the study of what happens to the body in response to the drug at the physiological, cellular, metabolic, and receptor levels. **Therapeutics** refers to the medical aspects of treatment and care of patients, with the intent of relieving injury and pain or preventing and treating disease.

Exercise and sport pharmacology studies issues such as:

1   The way in which (strenuous) physical activity changes the pharmacokinetics of certain drugs, including whether the drug's distribution in the body will change,

whether the drug will be cleared from the body faster or slower, and whether physical activity compromises the drug's therapeutic effect.

2   How the body will respond, including whether the drug will affect certain physical activities and whether the drug's action will affect performance, such as strength or endurance.

In many cases, individuals want to know whether the drug or supplement they are taking will affect their physical activity participation or performance. Sport and exercise performance depend on the body's ability to mobilize and utilize energy, as well as the work capacity of muscles, among other factors discussed in Chapter 2. Drugs can enhance or interfere with energy availability and work capacity. When we consider whether a drug can affect performance, we can generally classify drugs as either:

*   **Ergogenic drugs:** drugs that increase work capacity; these are usually illegal for most sports and competitions. Examples include anabolic steroids and growth hormone.
*   **Ergolytic drugs:** drugs that decrease work capacity. Athletes and other physically active individuals would prefer to avoid ergolytic drugs, such as beta-blockers and diuretics.

The next sections discuss what happens to drugs when they enter the body, how the body responds, and how these processes might be altered when a person is exercising.

Pharmacokinetics

Pharmacokinetics is the study of what happens to a drug when it enters the body. For the drug treatment to be effective, the drug must reach its site of action in sufficient quantity. As we will see, this can be a complicated process for many drugs. The term **bioavailability** is used to encompass the many fates of the drug and whether sufficient drug is available at its site of action. The route of drug administration is important; the number of cell membranes the drug needs to cross and the different organ systems the drug passes through before it reaches its site of action are also relevant. The fate of a drug is usually broken down into four main processes: **drug absorption**, **drug distribution**, **drug metabolism**, and **drug elimination**. We will look at each of these processes in some detail and then consider what happens during physical activity.

Drug Absorption

The process of drug entry or uptake is called drug absorption. When drugs enter the body, they get distributed to their site of action or the body compartment (e.g., organs, tissues, cells) where they will exert their primary effect.

Drugs are delivered through many different routes. The most common delivery route is oral (abbreviated as **PO**, from the Latin *per os*, meaning by mouth). This type of administration is also called *enteral* and includes drugs absorbed in the gastro-intestinal tract, including rectally in the form of suppositories. *Parenteral* (or injection) routes include injection under the skin (subcutaneous, **SC**), injection into muscle (intramuscular, **IM**), or injection directly into a vein (intravenous, **IV**). Several other injection sites are used, including directly into the heart or bone marrow. *Topical* routes include direct application of a cream to the skin, inhalation into the lungs, or eye and nose drops.

To reach the site of action, drugs need to pass barriers the body uses to limit exposure to possible toxic or infectious agents. The drug's bioavailability is dependent on the portion of active drug that actually makes it through the barriers to its site of action. Many factors contribute to bioavailability. For most drugs that act systemically, the blood level—amount of drug in the blood—is related to the drug's bioavailability. We sometimes use other terms instead of "blood levels" when referring to the levels of drugs in the blood. **Serum** is the soluble portion of blood that remains after it is allowed to coagulate and the solid portion is removed by centrifugation. **Plasma** is the soluble portion of uncoagulated blood that remains after centrifugation to remove blood cells. Hence, levels of the drug in the blood are calculated as the concentration of free (unbound, discussed below) drug in a preparation of serum or plasma. Though technically distinguishable, the terms 'blood level,' 'serum level,' or 'plasma level' are often used interchangeably.

The blood level of a drug is dependent on the route of administration, especially when the route requires the drug to be adsorbed across cell membranes, such as with PO or topical routes. With IV administration, serum levels are instantaneous and generally higher than with IM or SC. Additional routes of administration are useful for certain drugs. For example, **buccal administration** refers to placing the drug inside the mouth between the lining of the cheek and the gums. **Sublingual administration** is placement under the tongue. In these cases, the drug diffuses into the underlying capillary bed and enters the venous circulation relatively rapidly. With buccal and sublingual administration, the medication avoids the digestive system. New formulations of certain drugs, such as morphine and insulin, are being developed that can be given buccally.

The drug delivery method has an impact on drug absorption. Drugs taken PO (orally) can vary widely in their absorption rates. These drugs pass through the gastric/intestinal system, then through the portal system to the liver, and finally into circulation (Figure 1.1). They are subject to first-pass metabolism in the liver, which is the primary site for drug metabolism, as we will discuss below. **First-pass metabolism** means that a certain percentage of the absorbed drug may be chemically altered in the liver before it enters the bloodstream and reaches its site of action. The metabolism of this "first pass" through the liver may, therefore, alter the drug's bioavailability.

Drugs taken PO are also subject to dissolution (the dissolving of the drug so that individual molecules can be absorbed), binding to foods, and low pH. Low pH can have a positive or negative effect on drug delivery. Drugs that are weak acids are often well absorbed in the stomach because of the low pH in the stomach. Other drugs can break down at low pH and require special compounding (addition of inert solids) to help them survive passage to the intestines.

A drug's relative lipid solubility is also important in PO and topical administration delivery, because drugs with more lipid solubility more easily pass through the phospholipid bilayer of cell membranes. Thus, lipid-soluble drugs are generally taken up faster from the gut than water-soluble drugs. Lipid solubility matters less for reaching peak blood levels when drugs are administered into a vein, under the skin, and into muscle.

Our knowledge of drug absorption affects the very makeup of drugs. Innovations in oral solid drug delivery systems (OSDDS) and nanoformulations, which use nano particles, are examples of how strategically designed processes can improve drug delivery. Goals of these new formulations, for existing drugs or drugs in development, are to improve water solubility, bioavailability, effectiveness, and efficiency. These new delivery

Figure 1.1 Overview of drug absorption.

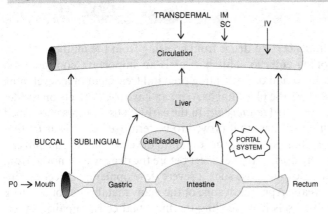

Legend: A general scheme is shown indicating the pathways drugs use to enter the circulation. Drugs taken orally are subject to first-pass influences, such as biotransformation, because they must pass through the liver before entering the circulation. The enterohepatic cycle is also illustrated, wherein material flows from the intestine to the liver and back to the intestine via the portal system.

systems improve the oral delivery of peptides and proteins, which previously needed to be injected (to avoid their being digested in the GI-tract). Development of drug therapies for diseases in our aging population is taking advantage of this technology, as OSDDS can provide advantages in dosing and duration of action, where the elderly often have issues. OSDDS also helps with drug delivery when problems exist that are related to low solubility, poor stability, unpleasant taste, short duration of action, or highly variable absorption rates in patients. A common example would be new formulations of older drugs that provide time release for up to 12 hours' duration of action. Nanoformulated versions of non-steroidal anti-inflammatory drugs are now on the market (e.g., Zorvolex), which are given at lower dosages because of improved absorption.

Drug Distribution

Once inside the body, drugs will distribute and potentially concentrate in a variety of compartments based on their chemical properties. Though serum concentration is a useful measure that relates to bioavailability, other factors come into play when we consider the distribution of drugs throughout the body. Tissues differ in their blood supply or perfusion rate (the rate that blood flows through a tissue), which affects distribution. For instance, levels of a drug in bone may differ from levels in the liver or kidney due to differences in blood supply (less blood supply to bone as opposed to more to liver and kidneys). In the central nervous system (CNS), the vasculature can form tight seals and limit "leakage" into tissues. The blood–brain barrier, as it is referred to, restricts the bioavailability of certain drugs to brain tissue. Certain antibiotics (not recommended for types of meningitis) and peripherally acting stimulants (sympathomimetics such as pseudoephedrine; see Chapter 8) poorly cross the blood–brain barrier under normal circumstances. Cells in the blood vessel walls called pericytes help maintain the barrier function, in part by interacting with extensions from specialized cells in the brain called astrocytes.

Teratogenesis and the Placental Barrier

A "placental barrier" limits certain drugs from crossing from the mother's bloodstream into her developing embryo. This barrier is an important consideration when treating a pregnant woman or attempting prenatal treatment of a developing infant. Some drugs that cross the placental barrier can have toxic effects on the developing embryo; these are called *teratogenic*. In the early 1960s, doctors prescribed a drug to prevent morning sickness that proved to be teratogenic. This drug, thalidomide, caused the long bones of the arms to fail to develop, but not the fingers. About 10,000 children were born with the defect before the drug was removed from the market. How this drug could cause such a severe developmental defect has interested researchers for years. Apparently, one of the many metabolites of the drug blocks developing blood vessels from feeding the limb bud cells, impairing their growth and development. Interestingly, thalidomide is now part of an anti-cancer treatment for multiple myeloma. It is also effective in treating leprosy.

Other factors that affect a drug's distribution and its bioavailability include non-specific binding to serum proteins. Only "free" drug passes from blood into cells, so if drugs bind to non-target proteins in the blood, their distribution is slowed. In humans, the major serum proteins responsible for non-specific binding are albumin and orosomucoid. Serum proteins such as these help transport a variety of substances in the blood, including fatty acids. Drugs vary greatly in their ability to bind these proteins and other components found in blood. There are well-documented cases, dating back to studies done in the 1950s and 1960s, of unexpected drug interactions resulting from relative affinities of different drugs for the non-specific binding sites on serum proteins. If a second drug is taken that has a higher affinity for one of these binding sites, the first drug will be displaced into the bloodstream as free (unbound) drug, and its effective concentration in the blood will spike, possibly causing unwanted effects. The classic example involves the diuretic furosemide and the anti-coagulant warfarin. Patients susceptible to stroke often take warfarin as a blood thinner. They also may need a diuretic for controlling blood pressure or fluid retention resulting from congestive heart failure. Furosemide has a higher affinity for the non-specific sites and displaces warfarin, dangerously increasing warfarin's free level in the blood and leading to extended clotting times. These patients have cuts that don't heal and can suffer significant blood loss in their GI-tract. Another example explains why it is not recommended to take aspirin after taking ibuprofen. Aspirin displaces ibuprofen from its binding sites on serum proteins and causes a spike in free ibuprofen levels, increasing the chance of ibuprofen-related toxic side effects.

The **volume of distribution** (V_d) is a theoretical measure of volume (sometimes called an "apparent volume"). It is not an actual volume of fluid occupying compartments in the body but rather a calculation of the apparent volume into which a drug would need to distribute to achieve the desired concentration in the plasma. The volume of distribution depends on the drug's chemical and physiological properties, including size, charge, and solubility. Drugs that tend to remain in the circulation have a low volume of distribution. Other drugs are highly lipid soluble and partition to fatty tissue; they have a high volume of distribution. Under these conditions, less drug remains in the circulation, creating a low plasma concentration because a lot of the drug is in fat cells.

We calculate the volume of distribution by dividing the amount of drug given (A) by the concentration of the drug in the blood (C): $V_d = A/C$. If a 20 mg dose of a drug is administered, and the blood concentration is 0.1 mg/L, then $V_d = 20$ mg/0.1 mg/L = 200 L. For example, aspirin (salicylic acid) is charged and binds serum proteins, properties that help it stay in the circulation. It has a low V_d of around 10 L. An anti-depressant called desipramine is more lipid soluble and has a high V_d of over 2,000 L. The volume of distribution has clinical significance, as we can rearrange the above relationship to help determine an appropriate dose of the drug. The amount (A) of drug needed as a dose is calculated from the desired blood concentration (C) multiplied by the known V_d for that drug: $A = V_d \times C$ or 200 L × 0.1 mg/L = 20 mg dose. The volume of distribution varies with an individual's height and weight, with the most variation related to percent body fat, an issue in overweight and obese patients. It can also vary with age, as the proportion of each body compartment changes with the aging process. Therefore, dosage may need to be modified in obese or elderly patients.

As stated above, a factor that affects a drug's volume of distribution is the percent body fat of an individual. The volume of distribution depends on whether the drug enters and is retained in fat (adipose) tissue. If the drug does enter and persist in fat tissue, then its effective volume of distribution increases, whereas if it does not, its V_d decreases. Since many dosing strategies are based on the individual's weight (i.e., mg per kg body weight), a modified dosing strategy may be needed when prescribing a drug that is excluded from fat tissue if the patient is obese. Because the drug does not distribute to a significant portion of the mass of a person who is obese, the blood concentration will be higher, which could possibly cause unwanted side effects. Therefore, a dose based on body weight alone could be too high. If the drug does partition to fat tissue, then fat tissue can act as a non-target reservoir, and there would be an increase in the volume of distribution in a patient who is obese. The drug will tend to concentrate in this non-target tissue, decreasing the amount of drug available at its site of action. Higher doses will be necessary. Moreover, the drug may persist in these individuals much longer than in a leaner person. When administration of the drug ends, it will slowly diffuse from its reservoir in the fat tissue. For example, anabolic steroids and the active ingredients in marijuana are fat-soluble and can persist in the body for considerable time after cessation of the drug. This property means that users are at risk of detection days to weeks after taking their last dose.

The age, physical condition, and hydration state of the individual can also be important for blood flow and drug distribution. In healthy individuals, almost half of the blood flow is directed to the kidneys and liver when at rest. The elderly can have decreased renal and liver perfusion rates, as do those with impaired hepatic and kidney function. The decreased blood flow to the kidneys and liver slows the ability of those organs to do their usual job of eliminating drugs and decreasing the drug's bioavailability. The resulting increase in bioavailability can increase blood levels and alter drug distribution. Deconditioned individuals may also have decreased liver and kidney function and show a similar effect. Dehydration and hypovolemia (decreased volume of the blood plasma) also cause changes in drug distribution and bioavailability as the body undergoes compensatory mechanisms. Dehydration can decrease the volume of distribution and cause an elevated drug concentration in the blood. Therefore, drug distribution is dependent on many variables that affect the concentration of drug in the blood, which affects the overall volume of distribution in the body. For drug safety, the goal is to keep the concentration of drug in the blood within a range considered safe, while allowing enough of the drug to reach its site of action to be effective.

Drug Metabolism

When most drugs enter the body, they are chemically converted by enzymatic reactions, collectively referred to as drug metabolism. These processes are also called **biotransformation** because, in some cases, the drug's biological activity changes after it has been chemically modified. Although enzymes found in the blood metabolize some drugs, most biotransformation of drugs occurs inside cells by the action of microsomal enzymes, associated primarily with the surface of the smooth endoplasmic reticulum of the liver. Biochemists call these microsomal enzymes because they were originally found in a subcellular ("microsomal") fraction generated after breaking cells apart and separating the parts by centrifugation. These microsomal enzymes can inactivate, activate, or generate toxic metabolites depending on the drug and the individual.

Drug-metabolizing enzymes include a family of enzymes called the cytochrome P450 proteins, which are members of a larger group of enzymes called mixed function oxidases. The cytochrome P450 enzymes are ubiquitous in nature. The cytochrome P450 portion of these enzymes are members of a class of molecules called hemes. Hemes often are involved in binding gas molecules like hemoglobin and myoglobin bind oxygen. These cytochrome P450 proteins also bind oxygen and use both oxygen atoms in O_2 during the chemical reaction. They attach one oxygen atom to the organic substrate and the other oxygen atom to produce H_2O as a byproduct. The oxidized drugs become more polar as a result of the added oxygen and are easier to eliminate by the kidneys. Although these cytochrome P450 proteins are found in most cells, the liver has very high levels of them and, therefore, high levels of drug-metabolizing activity. Since drugs taken orally pass though the liver on their way to the circulation, they are subject to first-pass metabolism, as mentioned above.

The human genome contains 57 genes that code for the different cytochrome P450 proteins. Many of these enzymes recognize multiple substrates and can catalyze multiple reactions; thousands of endogenous and exogenous compounds are metabolized as a result. Humans and most living things on this planet use these enzymes to modify and eliminate unwanted chemicals, and their capacity is enormous. The result is a complex metabolic pathway for most drugs that can vary widely in the population. The complexity and variance of drug metabolic pathways in the human population, which result from the genetic variation observed in this large gene family with 57 members, are very significant for a variety of reasons. This variation helps describe why drugs work in some individuals and not others, and why some experience toxic side effects while others do not. This variation is discussed further in the section on pharmacogenomics below.

Metabolism does not always mean detoxification or inactivation of a drug. Some drugs are given as a pro-drug that requires conversion to active metabolites. An example is enalapril, a drug used to treat hypertension, which is metabolized to the active form enalaprilat. Enalaprilat, however, has a net charge and is not well absorbed in the gut, so it is chemically modified to enalapril to negate the charge and improve its absorption. After enalapril is absorbed from the gut and transported to the liver, it is subjected to first-pass metabolism, and the chemical modification is removed by liver enzymes, producing the active form enalaprilat. For some drugs, however, toxic effects can result from metabolites. Genetic diversity within the human population and the complexity of biochemical reactions performed by the mixture of cytochrome P450 enzymes creates diverse metabolic profiles for most drugs. The result is great variability in the biotransformation and metabolic byproducts of most drugs. The metabolic rates and variability of biotransformation can also change with age, disease status, and the level of physical fitness of the patient.

Drug combinations can also influence metabolic rate and product formation. Some drugs are very potent inducers of metabolizing enzymes, such as phenobarbital. Ethanol also induces liver enzymes. One of the metabolites of acetaminophen (found in Tylenol, also called paracetamol) is hepatotoxic. Alcohol consumption can alter the metabolic profile and increase the rate of formation of the toxic metabolite of acetaminophen. Liver problems are seen in patients who drink alcohol and take high doses of acetaminophen. Liver toxicity is also observed in those who drink excessively and abuse prescription pain medications that contain acetaminophen in combination with a narcotic analgesic (e.g., Percocet or Darvocet).

Clearance or Elimination

Drug elimination is the irreversible loss of drug from the body. Drug excretion is the process by which unchanged drug or metabolites are removed, mainly via urine formation in the kidneys or feces formation in the hepatobiliary system. The rate of drug elimination is the drug amount (i.e., milligrams) removed from the body per unit of time (mg/h). Clearance is defined as the ratio between the rate of drug elimination and the drug's plasma concentration. Clearance is a useful term because it normalizes drug excretion rate to plasma concentration. Drug clearance is used to calculate the maintenance dose needed to achieve a desired steady-state concentration of the drug in the blood.

Clearance will depend on bioavailability (the drug needs to get into the bloodstream), protein binding (only "free" drug will clear the kidneys), bile flow, and the state of hydration. Clearance can also vary with age and disease state. Renal excretion is the most common form of elimination from the body. When the kidneys filter blood, unbound drug enters the filtrate and is usually excreted during urine formation. In some rare cases, the drug can use existing transporters and get taken back into the blood. Due to the central role of the kidneys in this process, physiological conditions that decrease kidney function (e.g., dehydration, renal disease, old age) potentially can lead to slower clearance rates.

Another form of clearance occurs during bile formation in the liver. Some drugs, particularly larger drugs containing both polar and lipophilic groups, are extensively excreted in this way, along with their metabolites. Drugs joined together with glucuronic acid (an acid derived from glucose) are also targeted for biliary excretion. Bile, which may contain excreted drugs, is stored in the gallbladder. After bile transport to the intestine, drugs secreted in bile can be reabsorbed and returned to the liver (Figure 1.1). This cycle of liver to intestine and back to liver can prolong the time the drug remains in the body. When some of the secreted drug is not reabsorbed from the intestine, the drug can be eliminated from the body during stool formation. Other minor pathways of excretion include sweat, expired air, breast milk, and seminal fluid.

Figure 1.2 Drug clearance and dosing.

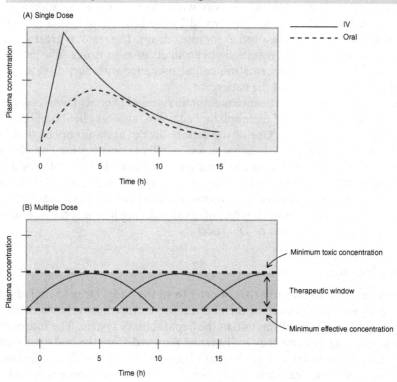

Legend: Drug clearance and dosing half-life can be determined from (A). Doses given at specified time intervals create the therapeutic window, as shown in (B).

The half-life ($T_{1/2}$) of a drug is the time necessary to decrease the drug's serum concentration by 50%. The half-life is dependent on plasma concentration and clearance of the drug; it can be determined graphically from plots similar to Figure 1.2(A). A drug given IV will have peak concentrations in the blood much faster than a drug taken PO, but both have a similar clearance rate. Drugs are often given in multiple doses at time intervals related to the drug's half-life, to maintain serum concentration in a steady state. The **therapeutic window**, illustrated in Figure 1.2(B), shows the minimum toxic concentration and the minimum effective concentration for a drug given in repeated doses. The minimum toxic concentration and the minimum effective concentration are determined from studies where subjects receive increasing doses of the drug, and the blood level of the drug is monitored. This type of data is generated using **dose–response curves** (discussed below).

Effect of Exercise on Pharmacokinetics

Exercise can affect drug bioavailability and clearance. For example, relative blood flow to the liver and kidneys decreases as intensity of exercise increases. Since the liver and kidneys play a major role in metabolizing and eliminating drugs, decreased blood flow to these organs means that drug metabolism and elimination rates will be altered during exercise and for a period of time following exercise. Clearance of drugs from the body will be slowed significantly for drugs that depend on the kidneys for elimination. At even moderate levels of exercise, blood flow to the kidneys is significantly decreased, and the clearance rate will similarly decrease. The data in Table 1.1 show the significance of this shift in blood flow (Lenz 2010). At rest, almost 50% of the blood is distributed to the liver and kidneys. At moderate exercise levels, the flow decreases to only about 6% of total blood flow to these organs, while blood flow to muscle increases to 47%. Redistribution of blood flow during exercise can affect drug absorption, as shown in Table 1.1. For example, the increased blood flow to muscle and the skin during exercise could increase absorption following IM or SC injection, such as with insulin or a nicotine patch (Lenz). At low exercise intensity, the time a drug spends in the stomach can decrease; with increasing exercise intensity, emptying of the stomach slows significantly and the drug will be delayed getting to the intestine.

Drugs whose pharmacokinetic properties are influenced by exercise are said to be **flow-limited.** The blood levels of flow-limited drugs are altered during exercise, primarily due to redistribution of blood flow that accompanies physical exertion. Many drugs with a short half-life (generally several hours or less) may have flow-limited effects, especially during aerobic activities of long duration. The decrease in blood flow to the kidneys during prolonged exercise will slow the clearance and extend the drug's half-life. For many long-acting drugs (roughly eight hours or longer), major changes in pharmacokinetics (i.e., major effects on drug distribution and clearance) are not expected with a mild exercise program.

An individual's level of physical fitness also has an impact on a drug's pharmacokinetic properties. The cardiac output of a trained individual is greater during exercise (discussed in Chapter 2) than an untrained individual's. Differences in pharmacokinetic properties during exercise may, therefore, vary because of the greater cardiac output. As another example, drug metabolic capacity in the liver is known to increase with overall fitness level, which may increase the clearance rate and shorten the drug's half-life for certain drugs. Fit individuals tend to have a lower body fat percentage, minimizing the contribution of fat tissue discussed previously.

Table 1.1 Redistribution of blood following exercise

	Rest	*Light Exercise*	*Moderate Exercise*	*Vigorous Exercise*
Muscle	20	47	71	88
Skin	6	15	12	2
Liver	27	12	3	1
Kidney	22	10	3	1
Brain	14	8	4	3
Heart	4	4	4	4
Other	7	4	3	1

Legend: The percentage of blood flow to different organs changes compared to resting conditions with exercise at different intensities. Data modified from Lenz (2010).

Pharmacodynamics

Whereas pharmacokinetics is concerned with what happens to a drug upon entering the body, pharmacodynamics is concerned with how the body responds to the drug. Drugs generally alter existing physiological processes. Since drugs can cause many different changes in the body, clearly pharmacodynamics has a very wide scope.

Measuring Drug Effects

The effect of a drug can be monitored at the whole animal or patient level. For instance, a change in body temperature or blood pressure can be measured following drug treatment. We can also establish model systems to study drug action at the organ, tissue, cellular, or molecular level. Modern drug design often targets a particular enzyme or a specific protein–protein interaction in a relevant physiological pathway. Analysis of drug effects on human organs can be performed with sophisticated instrumentation, such as ultrasound or other imaging techniques (i.e., CT scan). With experimental animals, we can use isolated organs or tissues. Cells grown in tissue culture can be treated with drugs to determine effects at the cellular level. Drugs can be tested in cell-free extracts, subcellular fractions, or with pure proteins. Some drugs are known to cause changes in gene expression in target cells. Studying drug action can, therefore, involve the study of physiological changes, cellular responses, and interactions at the molecular level.

During drug testing, volunteers or research animals are given a series of increasing doses of the drug, and the response is quantified at each dose. Secondary or unwanted effects can also be measured. In some studies, researchers will monitor blood levels over time at the different doses and make estimates of bioavailability and clearance. Initial studies may be needed to determine the basic pharmacokinetic properties of the drug to optimize the best time to measure the response, or whether multiple doses are required. In some cases, the drug response is measured versus a placebo (an identical appearing inactive pill) administered 'blindly' where the participant and the staff person do not know the pill's identity. The same subjects are repeatedly tested (i.e., a crossover study) with different doses or placebo and the results are decoded at the end of the trial. Experimental design for exercise pharmacology studies are discussed more in Chapter 2. For subjects with a particular disease, a fixed dose for treatment is the starting point. A dilution series is then created to determine the lowest effective dose.

The response dependent on the dose creates a very useful data set that can be plotted in a variety of ways. Dose–response curves plot the measurable effect (response) on the Y-axis versus dose or blood concentration on the X-axis. Since the dose can vary over a very wide range, sometimes the X-axis shows the log of the dose. From this curve, a ceiling or maximum effect is determined (Figure 1.3), as the response no longer increases with increasing dose. If blood concentration is determined during the trial, the resulting curve is more properly referred to as a concentration-response curve.

A drug's **efficacy** is the maximum *response* for the drug's primary effect. The drug's **potency** is the *quantity* of drug required to produce a designated intensity of effect. Potency and efficacy are not synonyms, though they are often misused that way. The amount of drug needed to achieve the maximum effect is determined from a dose–response curve. By comparing the dose–response curves for related drugs, we can compare their relative efficacy and potency. The relative efficacy is determined from the Y-axis. Preference is given to drugs of greater efficacy, if cost and safety are similar. In

Figure 1.3 Graded dose–response curves.

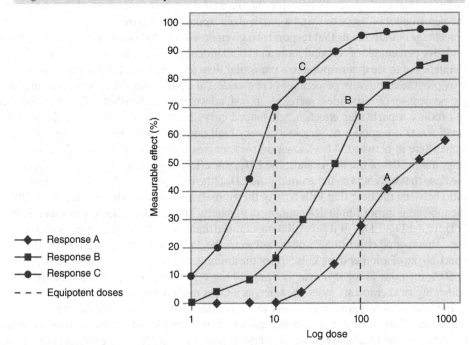

Legend: Three different drugs are shown. Note the different maximal efficacies and the different pharmacologic potencies.

Figure 1.3, drug C has the greatest efficacy. The potency of drugs, on the other hand, can be determined from the X-axis. In Figure 1.3, drug A is clearly less potent than either drug B or drug C, since it takes a much higher dose of A to produce a similar level of response.

We can use these curves to calculate equipotent doses. Equipotent doses for drugs of the same class are the doses that give the same efficacy. In Figure 1.3, the dashed lines indicate that the equipotent doses are 10 mg for drug C and 100 mg for drug B, for an efficacy of 70%. Knowing equipotent doses for drugs is helpful when prescribing medications. For example, bumetanide is more potent than furosemide as a diuretic for treating hypertension, but they are similar in efficacy. If given by same route in equipotent doses (1 mg bumetanide and 40 mg furosemide), they have similar diuretic efficacy and side effect profiles. Some patients will require several different prescriptions before they find the drug that works for them with the fewest unwanted effects. Also, sometimes doctors are limited in the drugs they prescribe by which drugs are covered by the patient's insurance, so having the equipotent doses available for the many possible drug products can be very useful.

Determining Drug Safety

During research and development (R&D) for drugs, the ED (effective dose) and LD (lethal dose) for experimental animals are determined. These data are also plotted as a dose–response curve, often with log of the dose of drug on the X-axis to cover a wide range of doses. Data from large experimental trials can be plotted in a variety of ways to illustrate different relationships. Let's examine the quantal dose–response curves (curves that plot the percentages of users showing a particular response) in Figure 1.4. In this example, the percentage of individuals that respond at a given dose is plotted two ways: (1) plotting the cumulative percentage of responders at a particular dose (curves A and C) and (2) plotting the frequency of those that respond to a particular dose (curves B and D). Figure 1.3 shows that if we plot the cumulative percentage of responders at a particular dose, as the dose increases the percentage of responders increases. If instead we plot the distribution of doses required to produce a particular effect, a bell-shaped curve is generated. This curve shows that a small fraction responds at very low or very high doses, with the majority requiring doses somewhere in between. Also shown on these curves is the dose that gives the therapeutic response in 50% of the individuals, the **ED_{50}** (the effective dose in 50% of the subjects), and the dose that kills 50% of the animals, the **LD_{50}** (the lethal dose in 50% of the animals). The ratio between the dose that kills 50% of the animals and the dose that is effective in 50% of the subjects is important in determining drug safety. This ratio is called the **therapeutic index (TI)**: TI = LD_{50}/ED_{50}. If it takes 100 mg of one drug to kill 50% of the animals and 5 mg to see a therapeutic effect in 50% of the subjects, the TI is 100 mg/5 mg = 20. If, on the other hand, 50 mg of another drug kills 50% of the animals and 10 mg gives a therapeutic response in 50%, then the TI for this drug is 50 mg/10 mg = 5. These examples illustrate that drugs with a higher therapeutic index are safer, as it takes more of the drug to be lethal.

In the case of humans, we modify the definition of TI by substituting the lethal dose with doses that cause unwanted side effects. For example, TI can be defined as the ratio between the toxic (unwanted side effect) dose (TD) in 1% of the subjects (TD_1) and the effective dose in 90% (ED_{90}): TI = TD_1/ED_{90}. This ratio skews the value in terms of drug safety, with a larger value for the TI being safer. Suppose drug A has a TD_1 of

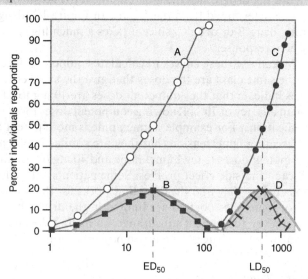

Figure 1.4 Quantal dose–response curves.

A –○– Therapeutic effect
B –■– Percent effect
C –●– Lethal effect
D –✕– Percent effect

Legend: Ascending curves (diamond, triangle) represent the cumulative percent of subjects exhibiting the therapeutic or lethal effect. Bell-shaped curves (squares, Xs) show the distribution of doses of drug required to produce a specified effect. The dose that gives a therapeutic effect in 50% of the subjects is the ED_{50}. The dose that causes the lethal effect in 50% of the animals is the LD_{50}.

100 mg and an ED_{90} of 10 mg, giving a TI of 10. In contrast, drug B has a TD_1 of 100 mg and an ED_{90} of 50 mg, with a TI of 2. Drug A is the safer of the two drugs. For perspective, valium (used to treat anxiety) has a TI over 100, while the TI for digitalis (a cardiac glycoside used for congestive heart failure) is only about 2 to 3. If a patient misses his dose of digitalis, he should not double the dose the next day. He could experience a toxic effect. We can make the TI more exact by comparing the serum concentration (rather than the administered dose) that causes toxicity relative to the serum concentration that produces efficacy.

Effect of Exercise on Pharmacodynamics

When drugs with a long half-life and duration of action are combined with a mild exercise program, major changes in pharmacodynamics are not expected. The small changes in blood flow to the liver and kidneys will not have a major effect on drug clearance or bioavailability. However, as intensity of exercise increases and blood flow is redirected (see Table 1.1), some drug actions could be altered. The effect of exercise is greatest on drugs with a steep dose–response curve and/or a narrow therapeutic index (where the ED_{90} and TD_1 are relatively close, giving a low TI value). A steep dose–response curve indicates that slight changes in blood concentration can cause a relatively large difference in response; small changes along the x-axis translate to large changes in response on the y-axis. With a narrow TI, the change in blood concentration from exercise could increase the chance of an unwanted side effect. Refer back to the therapeutic window in Figure 1.1B, and recall that it is based on the rates of absorption and clearance. Deceased blood flow to the gut, liver, and kidneys during exercise could ultimately affect levels of the drug in the blood. The need for continuity of a drug blood level for therapeutic effectiveness may be disrupted by intense exercise of long duration. Drugs that require monitoring in patients, such as insulin, theophylline, lithium, or digoxin, may be most susceptible to these types of effects.

Drug Properties

Binding to Receptors

Researchers for many years have studied the question of how drugs exert their biological effect. Since most drugs appear to affect already existing biological processes, drugs were predicted to modify those same processes somehow. The supposition was that drugs bind to some type of a **drug receptor**, probably a protein, that was involved in the process. These specific protein receptors were the mediators of the drug's action. One of the first drug receptors identified was the receptor for the cardiac glycosides, potent drugs used to treat congestive heart failure (Matsui & Schwartz 1968). These drugs were shown to bind the Na^+/K^+ ATPase (pump) in heart cell membranes, a protein essential in maintaining the sodium and potassium gradients in heart muscle and most other cell types.

For many other drugs, the protein receptor has also been identified; in some cases, the receptor's affinity for the drug and the number of receptors per cell have been quantified. We can determine the affinity of the drug for the receptor biochemically, often by using a version of the drug that has been made radioactive with isotopes of carbon or hydrogen. The strength of the interaction between the drug and the protein can have important consequences to the drug's activity. Since drugs often mimic

Table 1.2 Three ways drugs are synthesized to interact with receptors

1 **Agonists** bind receptor with a certain affinity and initiate a response.
Produce "intrinsic activity" by mimicking the endogenous ligand and causing a similar response.

2 **Antagonists** bind receptor with a certain affinity but do not initiate response.
Act as "blockers" for the endogenous ligand. Most blockers act competitively, so more potent antagonists have greater affinity for the receptor and compete more effectively with the endogenous ligand.

3 **Inverse agonists** bind receptor at the same site as an agonist.
Produce opposite pharmacological response of an agonist, decreasing the intrinsic activity. They are effective for receptors that have constitutive activity (continuous intrinsic activity). An agonist increases receptor activity above basal (minimal) level, whereas an inverse agonist decreases receptor activity below basal level.

normal cell constituents that interact with the same proteins, the relative affinities of the drug or the cellular constituent for the same protein can affect the drug's activity. Molecules, including drugs, hormones, and neurotransmitters, that bind to a receptor are called **ligands**, and the molecule that normally binds the target protein is often referred to as the **endogenous ligand**. Examples of endogenous ligands include hormones and neurotransmitters. The result is that many drugs work by altering existing physiological pathways, by competing with endogenous ligands at binding sites on the target proteins involved in the process. Drugs are synthesized to interact with receptors in the three main ways shown in Table 1.2.

Using Drugs to Discover the Endogenous Ligand: Endorphins

In some cases, studying the effect of drugs on a physiological process has led to the discovery of the cellular molecules that the drugs are mimicking. Since protein receptors bind the endogenous molecule referred to as a ligand, pharmacological approaches (using agonist and antagonist drugs) have helped identify the physiologically relevant molecule. For example, researchers discovered endorphins (endogenous morphine) while looking for endogenous "opiates" (Hughes 1975). Opiates are the active ingredients (e.g., morphine and codeine) derived from opium, a product of the poppy plant *Papaver somniferum*. Opiates (and endorphins) relieve pain, slow the GI-tract, depress respiratory activity, and elevate mood. The availability of powerful narcotic antagonists (receptor blockers, such as naloxone) made it possible to screen for the endogenous opiates in animal and human studies. Since, as an antagonist, naloxone binds and blocks opiate receptors, researchers were able to observe a measurable decrease in endorphin activity in their experiments. They tested different brain extracts for the presence of endorphins, eventually isolating the peptide endorphin, whose activity was blocked by naloxone (Pert & Snyder 1973). The identification of endogenous cannabinoids, the active ingredients in marijuana, was hampered by the lack of a strong antagonist, but rapidly evolving molecular techniques at the time helped identify the cannabinoid receptor and eventually the endogenous cannabinoids (Martin, Mechoulam, & Razdan 1999).

Receptors can show **down-regulation**—the process that reduces the responses of a cell to a stimulus—following repeated agonist stimulation by a drug. Many molecular mechanisms have been reported as causing down-regulation. Common mechanisms involve reduced activity of the receptor following chemical modification (e.g., phosphorylation), a decrease in receptor number due to sequestration (internalization from the cell membrane), or degradation (receptor proteins are specifically degraded in lysosomes or proteosomes). In contrast, drugs that act as antagonists can sometimes cause **up-regulation,** usually by increasing receptor number as the cell responds to the suppression of the activity caused by the drug. Drug receptors that have enzyme activity can be targeted with substrate analogs. Competitive inhibitors compete for the substrate-binding site on the enzyme. Under some circumstances, the cell can respond by increasing the concentration of the endogenous substrate to out-compete the drug. Noncompetitive inhibitors bind enzymes at sites other than the active site and generally are less sensitive than competitive inhibitors to the concentration of endogenous substrate. For example, drugs can be designed to target allosteric regulatory sites on enzymes.

Tolerance and Withdrawal

Other properties of drugs can be partially explained at the molecular or receptor level. For instance, **tolerance** is defined by the need to increase dose over time to maintain the desired response. Sometimes the body becomes more efficient at metabolizing the drug to an inactive form. Cells may decrease the uptake of the drug. Cells may also respond by increasing the amount of endogenous ligand or the number of enzyme/receptor molecules. **Withdrawal syndrome** is the physiological response that occurs following the abrupt cessation of drug treatment. Mechanistically, very little is known about withdrawal. The rapid increase in unoccupied receptors, whose numbers likely changed as a result of prolonged use of the drug, apparently can trigger powerful physiological (and psychological) changes. The normal physiological pathway, with its associated feedback loops, may also be altered due to the prolonged presence of the drug and require considerable time to return to normal following drug withdrawal. Stepping down the dose over time can reduce the severity of the withdrawal syndrome in some cases. The physiological changes resulting from drug cessation can vary from mild to severe and life-threatening. Individuals who abruptly stop taking caffeine may experience headaches and sleep disorders for several days. Those who drink excessively and go "cold turkey" can have life-threatening seizures. Valium withdrawal can also cause seizures with life-threatening consequences.

Dependence and Addiction

Drug **dependence** can be both physical and psychological. Dependence often occurs with drugs that have a withdrawal syndrome. The dependent individual continues drug use to avoid the discomfort of withdrawal. Physical drug dependence occurs when the drug is needed for normal functioning. Drug **addiction** is defined by the presence of physical or psychological dependence and a withdrawal syndrome. Addiction is the compulsive use of a drug despite the harmful effects; addiction results from dependence, tolerance, and withdrawal. People addicted to heroin, for example, will continue the habit to avoid the extreme discomfort of going through withdrawal. They continue to use the drug for the pleasure, release, or escape the drug provides, but the extreme discomfort associated with cessation makes it even harder to quit—even if they know they should. They need to keep taking the drug to function and may require more drug over time to get their desired effect. Addicts often need psychological support in addition to medical attention for dealing with withdrawal. Reconnection to family and friends to create the necessary support system is critical in successfully recovering from addiction, as is resolving the mental and physical issues that led to the initial use of the addicting drugs.

Drug Interactions

Taking two or more drugs concurrently can result in interactions that may enhance or diminish any of the drugs' effects. Drug interactions can also generate adverse effects. Problems occur when patients take over-the-counter medications, such as pain medications, antihistamines, decongestants, or cough medicines, while also taking prescription medications.

Enhanced effects of drug combinations include:

- *Summation* (additive effect)
- *Potentiation* (one drug causes an increased response to another drug)
- *Synergism* (super-additive, more than the sum of the parts; two drugs together produce more response than the sum of the effects of taking each alone).

Other types of interactions can be summarized as:

- *Pharmaceutical* (the two drugs do not mix well in solution, for example)
- *Pharmacokinetic* (interference with metabolism, elimination, etc.)
- *Pharmacodynamic* (altered drug actions).

There are many examples of drug interactions. The use of NSAIDs for pain can cause issues for patients on blood pressure drugs, blood thinners, and other medications. The herbal supplement St. John's Wort can interact with a wide variety of medications. In some cases, the effectiveness of the prescribed medication is diminished; in other cases, the chance of a toxic side effect increases. Negative drug–drug interactions often involve overlapping drug-metabolizing enzymes or drug transporters that help move drugs across membranes (Obach 2003). Websites are available that allow one to enter different drugs and OTC medications to see if there are documented interactions. Another very common example involves the consumption of alcohol while taking medications, such as increasing the sedative effect of certain antihistamines. Most prescription and OTC drugs come with warning labels concerning known negative drug interactions.

Pharmacogenomics

Personalized medicine is rapidly becoming a possibility. It is now possible to link a patient's genotype and gene expression profile to the health condition and needed treatment. The goal of this personalized medicine is to diagnose accurately the patient's disease and to predict which choice of drugs will be the most safe and effective.

Adverse drug reactions lead to more than 100,000 deaths per year and 5% to 7% of hospital admissions. **Pharmacogenomics** is the study of a patient's genetic makeup to serve as a basis for predicting responses to drugs, choosing among different medications, optimizing dose, minimizing secondary effects, and determining preventative measures to support the patient's treatment regime.

Most drugs work in only 30% to 50% of the population. Though health maintenance organizations and insurance companies might prefer to use a single drug for all patients so that they can negotiate the best price, the reality is that few drugs work the same in everybody. The complexity in the family of drug-metabolizing enzymes (recall that there are 57 different cytochrome P450 genes in humans, and one cytochrome P450 family member has 75 different alleles!) suggests that most individuals will vary greatly in the way they metabolize a particular drug. Bioavailability and clearance will likely vary, as well. The fact that quantal dose–response curves (Figure 1.4) that plot the percentages of users registering a particular response produce bell-shaped curves indicates that a certain percentage of a population will be sensitive or relatively resistant to the action of the drug. The bell-shaped curve also suggests a polygenetic response, meaning that many gene products contribute to the drug response. As discussed earlier in this chapter, many different gene products are involved in the response to a drug. These include gene products that affect: absorption, distribution, metabolism, clearance, binding to proteins (specific, non-specific), and response (receptor subtypes, secondary/side effects).

The current gold standard for clinical trials is the double-blind study, where neither patients nor doctors know who is receiving the drug or the placebo at the time of the trial. After completion of the trial, the identity of the different treatment groups is decoded and the results quantified. In rare cases, a trial may be stopped if serious side effects are noticed and the trial groups must be decoded. Double-blind testing can result in the loss of new drugs from the drug pipeline if a low percentage of the study participants respond significantly or if side effects occur too frequently. If the responders could be identified genetically, or the ones with the unwanted effects could be identified without discontinuing the trial, then the drug could still have market potential. Since most drugs require the investment of many millions of dollars to get them to the clinical trial stage, drug companies could salvage their investment if they could identify their target group. Therefore, a genetic approach could be used to:

- Diagnose disease and genetic predisposition to disease.
- Identify a therapeutic approach and preventative measures.
- Choose the best therapeutic agent.
- Minimize side effects.

Ideally, pharmacogenomics will be integrated into drug design and delivery. A first step is to develop a biomarker profile so that responders and non-responders can be screened. Biomarker profile development involves many approaches, including mapping single nucleotide polymorphisms, gene expression, or display technologies and, as the cost of personalized DNA sequencing comes down, probably actual DNA sequencing of relevant portions of an individual's genome.

Once biomarker profiles have been developed, one approach to screening the profiles will probably use metabolic markers, because of the diversity of drug metabolism in the population. Blood samples from clinical trials would be banked to allow researchers to test responders, non-responders, and those with unwanted side effects. Drug companies would submit data for biomarkers when requesting approval from the FDA. Over time, a large database would be created to profile drug responses with biomarkers.

In the future, the goal would be for doctors and health providers to choose from a selection of three drugs, each with greater than 35% coverage of the population. A screen or test for the side effect profile would be done. The provider would make a tailored recommendation for the patient that matches the individual's genetic profile.

Possible Role for Microbiome in Exercise Pharmacology

The hundred trillion microbes that reside in our gut outnumber the cells in our body by a ten-to-one ratio. This **microbiome** consists of thousands of species and strains; the microbial composition varies from individual to individual and is sensitive to environmental factors such as diet, activity level, and drug use. The microbes help digest food and provide many vitamins and nutrients important for our health. Advances in DNA sequencing technology have made the detailed analysis of the microbiome possible. These microbes are hard to grow in petri dishes, so little was known previously. DNA technology can identify the different species and strains present and their relative frequency. Therefore, people or experimental animals can have their microbiome analyzed under various conditions. The increased prominence (or disappearance) of different microbial species is now indicative of certain pathological conditions.

Experimentally, existing microbes can be eliminated (e.g., antibiotics) and replaced with test microbes (fecal transplantation) in humans or test animals. This powerful experimental design can test many diverse hypotheses. For example, mice fed a high fat diet had a dramatic loss in microbial diversity and early physiological signs of diabetes. Transfer of gut microbes from these animals conferred the health problems to previously normal mice. Transfer from normal mice to the prediabetic mice returned their physiology to normal, as did reversion to a normal diet—albeit slowly. Many of these initial studies showed that the gut microbiome influenced weight gain, diabetes, cardiovascular health, and response to junk food or artificial sweeteners. More recent studies show its involvement in mood and mental health, including autism, Alzheimer's, and possibly Parkinson's disease. The gut microbes produce many molecules, including neurotransmitters, that stimulate the Vagus nerve endings and other cells in the gut, or are released into the blood stream to act elsewhere in the body, including the brain.

A large-scale study with 1,046 participants showed that host genetics play a very minor role in determining microbiome composition. The variability of the microbiomes of genetically unrelated individuals who share a household was significantly associated with diet, drug treatment and body shape measurement (Kosower et al., 2018). Microbiome data improve the prediction accuracy for diabetes and obesity measures. Diet and lifestyle are the most dominant factors shaping our microbiome composition, and can be captured by fecal analysis. Exercise training directly opposes some of the obesity-related changes of gut microbiota in mice and hypertensive obese rats. Exercise-responsive taxa have been identified in rodents and humans. Exercise training induces changes in the human gut microbiota that are contingent on the sustainment of exercise (Rothschild et al., 2018). We cannot change our genes, but we can reshape the composition of the different kinds of bacteria we host in our bodies, with diet and exercise as the most effective ways.

We are in the early stages of understanding and appreciating the complex interactions between our gut microbiome and human health. Certain drugs, such as the ones used for acid-reflux disease, can affect the microbe population and possibly explain some of the drug's side effects. Antibiotic therapy can severely cause changes in the gut ecosystem. In extreme cases, fecal transplantation—capsules of treated feces from screened healthy donors, have been given to patients to restore their microbiome. There are drugs that work in the gut to decrease dietary fat or cholesterol which we will discuss in later chapters. For the purposes of this text, we need to be cognizant of the importance of the gut microbiome in human health, though the direct effect on the microbiome is not known for most of the drugs we cover. However, the positive effect of exercise on the microbiome has been established and could be a contributor to the overall benefits of exercise on human health.

Elder Concerns

Proper dosage for many drugs is difficult in the aging population, where there is a large interindividual variability in drug response. There are many reasons, and the effects of aging vary greatly across this population—we all age differently. The elderly often take several drugs to treat multiple diseases. **Polypharmacy** and possible drug interactions are problematic in the young and more so in the elderly. Aging involves progressive impairment of multiple organs, decreasing the body's overall functional capacity. This decrease in functional capacity of many organs will affect pharmacokinetics and pharmacodynamics.

Intestinal absorption of most drugs is not altered in the elderly (Turnheim 2004). However, with aging, total body water and lean body mass tend to decrease, with an increase in total body fat. As discussed previously in this chapter, the decrease in total body water will decrease the volume of distribution for hydrophilic drugs, resulting in increased plasma concentrations. In contrast, the distribution volume of lipophilic drugs increases, their plasma concentrations will decrease, and they may have a prolonged half-life (Shi & Klotz 2011).

As we age, liver mass and perfusion decrease. For drugs that experience a significant hepatic first-pass effect, the reduction in liver function will increase their bioavailability. The progressive loss of liver function with age will decrease the rate for drugs normally cleared by the liver. However, metabolic reactions in liver microsomes are similar in young and old populations (Shi & Klotz 2011). The genetic influence on activities of cytochrome P450 enzymes is much more striking than age effects.

About one-third of the elderly have normal renal filtration rates, but renal excretion is decreased as much as 50% in about two-thirds of elderly subjects. Moreover, many of these subjects have confounding factors such as hypertension and coronary heart disease, possible contributors to a decline in kidney function. These elderly patients should be treated as renally insufficient patients.

From a pharmacodynamic perspective, one of the characteristics of old age is a progressive decline in homeostatic mechanisms. The body does not rebound as quickly or as thoroughly to many medications. The result is that drug effects persist longer, with stronger drug responses in the elderly than in younger subjects. Additionally, the rate and intensity of adverse effects are higher. Examples include dizziness with agents that lower blood pressure, dehydration, and electrolyte imbalance in response to diuretics, low blood sugar with drugs that treat diabetes, and gastrointestinal irritation with non-steroidal anti-inflammatory drugs. The brain is especially sensitive to the aging effects on drug pharmacokinetics and pharmacodynamics. Centrally acting drugs may impair intellectual function and motor coordination (Turnheim 2004).

The complexity of interactions between multiple diseases, polypharmacy, and age-related changes in pharmacokinetics and pharmacodynamics suggests that drugs should be used restrictively in geriatric patients. These effects are especially pronounced in malnourished or frail patients. When determining the proper dosage for the elderly, the recommendation is "start low, go slow" (Turnheim 2004).

Conclusion

Exercise and sport pharmacology pertain to the interaction of exercise and the physiological responses to drugs. Both pharmacokinetics and pharmacodynamics are affected by exercise, usually in an intensity-dependent manner. Many factors contribute to the bioavailability of the drug, and the dose of a drug has to be sufficient to allow enough drug to reach an effective concentration at the site of action. The gut microbiome influences human health and is affected by drug treatment and physical activity. Pharmacogenomics may help health providers match subsets of the population with the most effective and safest drug option. Proper dosing of drugs in the elderly population is difficult and needs to be closely monitored.

Key Concepts Review

addiction	ligand
agonist	microbiome
antagonist	nutraceutical
bioavailability	OTC drug
biotransformation	pharmaceuticals
buccal administration	pharmacodynamics
dependence	pharmacogenomics
dose–response curve	pharmacokinetics
down-regulation	pharmacology
drug	plasma
drug absorption	PO
drug distribution	potency
drug elimination	SC
drug metabolism	serum
drug receptor	site of action
efficacy	sublingual administration
endogenous ligand	$T_{1/2}$
ergogenic drug	therapeutic index (TI)
ergolytic drug	therapeutic window
exercise and sport pharmacology	therapeutics
first-pass metabolism	tolerance
flow-limited	up-regulation
IM	volume of distribution
inverse agonist	withdrawal syndrome
IV	

Review Questions

1 Distinguish between pharmacokinetics, pharmacodynamics, and pharmacology.
2 How might you design a study to determine the effect of a certain class of drugs on exercise performance? What factors must you be concerned with, and which do you need to control?
3 How would you determine a drug's dose–response curve?
4 What is meant by drug efficacy? Potency?
5 How would you determine equipotent doses for two drugs of the same class?
6 What features of a drug's action may make its pharmacokinetic properties more sensitive to exercise?
7 How might a drug's volume of distribution be altered in the case of a person who is obese? A person who is elderly?
8 How might you explain an antagonist with partial agonist activity?
9 What are some of the ways that taking a second drug can affect the activity of the first drug—or either drug?
10 Quantal dose–response curves often show a characteristic bell shape. Why is this important when developing dosing strategies for patients?

References

Bouchard C, Blair SN, Katzmarzyk PT (2015) Less sitting, more physical activity, or higher fitness? *Mayo Clin Proc* 90:1533–1540

Drug Enforcement Administration, Office of Diversion Control (nd) Controlled substances schedule.   www.deadiversion.usdoj.gov/schedules/;   www.imshealth.com/cds/imshealth/Global/Content/Corporate/IMS%20Health%20Institute/Reports/Secure/IIHI_US_Use_of_Meds_for_2013.pdf

Guthold R, Stevens GA, Riley LM, Bull FC (2018) Worldwide trends in insufficient physical activity from 2001 to 2016: a pooled analysis of 358 population-based surveys with 1.9 million participants. *Lancet* 6:e1077–e1086

Henson J, Yates T, Biddle SJH, Edwardson CL, Khunti K, Wilmot EG, Gray LJ, Gorely T, Nimmo MA, Davies MJ (2013) Associations of the objectively measured sedentary behaviour and physical activity with the markers of cardiometabolic health. *Diabetologia* 56:1012–1020

Henson J, Edwardson CL, Morgan B, Horsfield MA, Bodicoat DH, Biddle SJH, Gorely T, Nimmo MA, Mccann GP, Khunti K, Davies MJ, Yates T (2015) Associations of sedentary time with fat distribution in a high-risk population. *MSSE* 47:1727–1734

Hughes, J (1975). Isolation of an endogenous compound from the brain with pharmacological properties similar to morphine. *Brain Res* 88:295–308

Lenz, TL (2010). Pharmacokinetic drug interactions with physical activity. *Amer J Lifestyle Med* 4:226–229

Kosower N, Malka Gl, Wolf BC, Avnit-Sagi T, Lotan-Pompan M, Weinberger A, Halpern Z, Carmi S, Fu J, Wijmenga C, Zhernakova A, Elinav E, Segal E (2018) Environment dominates over host genetics in shaping human gut microbiota. *Nature* 555(7695):210–215

Lyden K, Keadle SK, Staudenmayer J, Braun B, Freedson PS (2015) Discrete features of sedentary behavior impact cardiometabolic risk factors. *MSSE* 47:1079–1086

Martin BR, Mechoulam R, Razdan RK (1999) Discovery and characterization of endogenous cannabinoids. *Life Sci* 65:573–595

Matsui H, Schwartz A (1968). Mechanism of cardiac glycoside inhibition of the (Na+-K+)–dependent ATPase from cardiac tissue. *Biochim Biophys Acta Enzymology* 151:655–663

Morris JN, Heady JA, Raffle PAB, Roberts CG, Parks JW (1953) Coronary heart disease and physical activity of work. *Lancet* 265:1053–1057

Obach RS (2003) Drug-drug interactions: an important negative attribute in drugs. *Drugs Today* 39:301–338

Paffenbarger RS, Wing AL, Hyde RT (1978) Physical activity as an index of heart attack risk in college alumni. *Am J Epidemiol* 108:161–175

Pavey TG, Peeters GG, Brown WJ (2015) Sitting-time and 9-year all-cause mortality in older women. *Br J Sports Med* 49:95–99

Pert CB, Snyder SH (1973) Opiate receptor: demonstration in nervous tissue. *Science* 179:1011–1014

Reents S (2000) *Sport and Exercise Pharmacology.* Champaign, IL: Human Kinetics

Rothschild D, Weissbrod O, Barkan E, Kurilshikov A, Korem T, Zeevi D, Costea PI, Godneva A, Kalka IN, Bar N, Shilo S, Lador D, Vila AV, Zmora N, Pevsner-Fischer M, Israeli D, Allen JM, Mailing LJ, Niemiro GM, Moore R, Cook MD, White BA, Holscher HD, Woods JA (2018) Exercise alters gut microbiota composition and function in lean and obese humans. *Med Sci Sports Exerc* 50:747–757

Shi S, Klotz U (2011) Age-related changes in pharmacokinetics. *Curr Drug Metab* 12:601–610.

Shibata A, Oka K, Sugiyama T, Salmon J, Dunstan DW, Owen N (2016) Physical activity, television viewing time, and 12-year changes in waist circumference. *MSSE* 48:633–640

Turnheim K (2004) Drug therapy in the elderly. *Exp Gerontol* 39:1731–1738.

2 Basics of Exercise Performance

Abstract

For improved health and to slow aging, experts recommend daily cardiovascular exercise and regular resistance training. An evaluation of fitness is based on oxygen distribution and utilization, which can be quantified with VO_2max. VO_2max is directly related to heart rate, so exercise heart rate provides a relative measure of exercise intensity. With regular exercise, we see an increase in VO_2max, which is primarily reflected by an increase in stroke volume. Exercise causes changes in metabolism, and regular cardiovascular exercise can influence the distribution of muscle fiber type. Increasing the amount of slow-twitch oxidative muscle improves blood sugar control and insulin sensitivity. Muscle mass decreases with aging, part of a process called sarcopenia. Regular exercise helps slow this aging process.

The effect of drugs or supplements on exercise can be studied experimentally. It is important that researchers control for both the drug/supplement effect and the exercise effect when designing studies. A double-blind approach helps to eliminate a placebo effect.

As the policies and testing for drug use have become more complex, knowledge in these areas has become more important for athletes and coaches. Urine samples are tested for banned substances both in season and year-round for most competitive athletes. The detection of some drugs may require blood testing.

Learning Objectives

1 Understand the role for exercise in maintaining good health.
2 Learn the components of an exercise prescription.
3 Learn what being fit means and how to become fit.
4 Understand where the energy to exercise comes from.
5 Distinguish between the different muscle fiber types and their roles.
6 Understand concepts involved in research in exercise pharmacology.
7 Describe the evidence pyramid.
8 Describe some of the issues involved in drug testing and what can happen if someone fails a drug test.

Introduction

Worldwide, physical inactivity is responsible for 9% of premature deaths, or more than five million people. Inactivity significantly leads to coronary heart disease, Type 2 diabetes, and breast and colon cancer. More than half of U.S. adults do not meet the recommendations for sufficient physical activity. Adolescents and adults spend almost eight hours a day in sedentary behaviors, and about a third of all adults engage in no leisure time physical activity. Obesity rates for children and adults have grown steadily during the last two decades. The percentage of obese individuals in the United States is around 35%. The combined percentage of the U.S. population that is overweight and obese approaches 70%. Obesity is associated with significant morbidity and mortality. It is linked to elevated rates of diabetes, dyslipidemia (e.g., high blood levels of total cholesterol or triglycerides), and liver and gallbladder disease. It is also associated with high blood pressure, coronary heart disease, an increased risk for stroke, and a host of other problems (see Chapter 12 for more details).

The disorder called **metabolic syndrome** is a cluster of risk factors associated with an increased risk for cardiovascular disease and Type 2 diabetes. It involves a complex interaction between genetic, metabolic, and environmental factors. Major environmental factors include diet, a sedentary lifestyle, and smoking. The numbers in the United States are significant, as 24% of adults may have metabolic syndrome. Regular exercise improved the status of patients with metabolic syndrome and diabetes, often in conjunction with reductions in blood pressure. These improvements in health can decrease prescription drug use compared to sedentary individuals. The implication of maintaining or lowering medicine use by exercise training is very important. Regular exercise could reduce health-care costs—such as fewer trips to the doctor, less lab work for blood tests, or prescriptions from the pharmacy. It can reduce the side effects associated with taking multiple drugs and improve physical and psychological health (Nystoriak & Bhatnagar 2018).

Frequent exercise lowers blood pressure, increases insulin sensitivity, creates a more favorable plasma lipoprotein profile, and decreases the risk of cardiovascular disease. It suppresses atherogenesis, increases the availability of vasodilatory mediators such as nitric oxide, and has beneficial effects on the heart (discussed in Chapters 4 and 5). Regular exercise reduces mortality and the risk of recurrent breast cancer by approximately 50%. There is a lower risk of cancer-specific mortality in adults with higher levels of muscle strength. Regular exercise reduces the risk of developing Alzheimer's disease and leads to higher academic performance in children and adults. Physical training improves exercise capacity, endothelial function, autonomic function and dealing with stress, as well as a reduction of adverse psychosocial and inflammatory parameters. In addition, regular exercise promotes quality sleep, slows the aging process, and contributes to good mental health.

Medication and exercise are beneficial tools for chronic-disease management, but "exercise as medicine" is seldom applied with sufficient detail. When a doctor prescribes a drug, there is a specific dose, administration, frequency, and duration to the treatment. When it comes to exercise prescription, a similar strategy should be adopted. For example, how hard and for how long should one exercise to gain these benefits? What does being in "good shape" actually mean, and can this be quantified and studied? Related to exercise pharmacology, questions include: what effects does exercise have on individuals who are taking medications, and what effects do drugs have on those who exercise? In order to start to answer these exercise pharmacology–related questions, it is important to understand the basics of exercise physiology, particularly the physiological changes observed during exercise.

This next section will cover some of these basics related to the cardiovascular, metabolic, and muscular systems. This chapter will also cover exercise prescription for health, the need for and complexity of exercise pharmacology research, and the methods of testing for drugs that may enhance or affect performance.

Cardiovascular Fitness

The limiting factor to performing physical work is the person's level of **cardiovascular fitness**. Cardiovascular (sometimes called aerobic) fitness depends on: (1) the ability of the heart to pump oxygen-rich blood to the tissues, and (2) the ability of tissues to use oxygen to produce adenosine triphosphate (ATP). The oxygen we breathe must pass from the lungs through the heart and get distributed to the tissues. Cells that make up the body's tissues require oxygen to make ATP, as the body uses this energy-rich molecule to do cellular work (more information below). Cells can cope with limited amounts of oxygen and produce significantly smaller amounts of ATP, but only for brief periods of time. We measure the volume of oxygen consumed, VO_2, as the rate of oxygen consumption standardized relative to body weight:

the volume of oxygen consumed (*milliliters*)
per *kilogram* body weight
per *minute* of exercise.

Hence the units of VO_2 are ml O_2/kg/min. We can measure VO_2 by using an apparatus called a metabolic cart, which contains both oxygen and carbon dioxide analyzers. This device uses a mask to measure the different oxygen levels in inspired and expired air. It determines the amount of oxygen consumed over time during exercise.

In the body, VO_2 depends on cardiac output (Q) and the difference in O_2 content (C) between arterial and venous circulation, based on the equation:

$$VO_2 = Q(C_aO_2 - C_vO_2)$$

Cardiac output depends on the stroke volume (SV), the amount of blood that passes through the heart in one contraction, and heart rate (HR):

$$Q = SV \times HR$$

Therefore, heart rate and stroke volume are variables that help us determine how the body uses O_2 (VO_2) during exercise.

VO_2max is the maximum oxygen consumption that a person can achieve. This is a measure of the person's cardiorespiratory fitness level that often serves as the basis for exercise prescriptions. Exercise training improves VO_2max. Improvement in VO_2max is a direct function of increased stroke volume at maximal workload. The consequences of an increased stroke volume are shown in this example:

At *rest*:

$$Q = SV \times HR$$

Trained: 5,000 ml = 100 ml × 50 beats/min
Untrained: 5,000 ml = 71 ml × 70 beats/min

The example shows that for a comparable total output (5,000 ml), the trained individual pushes more blood per stroke and has a lower resting heart rate than an untrained individual.

At **maximum heart rate**, or the highest heart rate attainable when exercising,

Trained: 35,000 ml = 179 ml × 195 beats/min
Untrained: 22,000 ml = 113 ml × 195 beats/min

When the two individuals reach the same maximum heart rate, the trained individual (with an increased SV) distributes considerably more blood than the untrained individual. Therefore, the trained individual will have a higher VO_2max and a higher fitness level.

Exercise intensity, or the degree of physiological strain, can be measured with VO_2. Exercise intensity can also be measured in watts, as external work on a cycle ergometer, for example. When a subject exercises with escalation of the intensity (or "workload") at fixed intervals, the interval of exercise where the subject fails to continue exercising provides an estimate of **exercise capacity**. Exercise capacity is based on an individual's VO_2max. It is the maximum amount of exertion an individual can sustain. Maximum exertion depends on the intensity and duration of effort. See Table 2.1. An evaluation of the person's fitness level then can be based on the estimate of his or her exercise capacity (Table 2.1).

The Wingate Test is standardized test for exercise capacity. It is commonly performed on a cycle ergometer to measure an individual's anaerobic power and capacity output. The test requires the participant to cycle at maximal effort for 30 seconds. It can also be performed on an arm-crank ergometer. The test is a useful assessment tool for athletes in sports which demand short-duration maximal efforts.

The intensity of exercise is expressed as a percent of VO_2max, when a metabolic cart is available to measure oxygen consumption. Since VO_2max depends on the maximum

Table 2.1 Relationship between measures of VO_2 and exercise capacity

VO_2 Value	Exercise Capacity
3–5 ml/kg/min	Resting value
<20 ml/kg/min	Poor health (cardiovascular disease)
30 ml/kg/min	Below average to average
40 ml/kg/min	Better than average fitness level
50 ml/kg/min	Trained individual on exercise program
60 ml/kg/min or greater	Highly trained athlete

Legend: An individual's exercise capacity is determined at the point when he or she terminates an exercise with escalating fixed intervals of workload. Exercise capacity can vary with age and gender. These values are applicable to young adults.

heart rate (discussed earlier), the intensity of exercise can also be expressed as a percent of maximum heart rate. The maximum heart rate depends on age, and for years it has been calculated with a simple formula:

220 – age = maximum heart rate

However, there is a newer refinement of this calculation (Nes, Janszky, Wisloff, et al. 2013). The HUNT Fitness Study (Nes) used 3,320 healthy men and women to determine the effect of age on maximum heart rate. The data showed that three former prediction formulas, including the one mentioned above, underestimated maximum heart rate in individuals over 30 years old. The results did not show evidence of interaction with gender, physical activity, or BMI, though the standard error of close to 11 beats per minute was taken into account (Nes). Improving the accuracy of calculations for maximum heart rate as we age is important because the benefits of exercise are intensity dependent. To gain many of the potential benefits, exercisers must monitor intensity, and many people tend to overestimate their exercise intensity (Canning et al. 2014). The new formula uses 64% of age:

211 – 0.64 × age = maximum heart rate

We can approximate target heart rates for different intensities of exercise by multiplying maximum heart rate by a percentage of maximum effort. For working out at 55% VO_2max, we would multiply the calculated target heart rate by 0.55. For example, for a 60-year-old woman working out at 55% VO_2max:

211 – (0.64 × 60) = 172.6

172.6 × 0.55 = 95 beats per minute

The exerciser in our example will be working at 55% VO_2max if she maintains her heart rate at 95 beats per minute. As people begin (or maintain) exercise programs, it is important that they hit their target intensity level of exercise, since many people tend to overestimate their level of intensity (Canning). Fortunately, many exercise machines provide heart rate detection, and exercisers can use heart rate monitors or take their pulse when exercising. Using one of these methods, individuals can more accurately determine the level of their exercise intensity.

The metabolic equivalent of task (MET) is the ratio of energy expended performing physical activity divided by the energy expended when sitting at rest. This reference point of sitting at rest is set by convention at 3.5 ml of oxygen per kilogram per minute. It is not the basal metabolic rate, which is the minimum metabolic rate obtained under specified conditions for the person and can vary with the individual's body composition and fitness level. MET is an index of the intensity of activities relative to the one MET set at rest for an "average" individual. Walking at a slow pace has a MET value of 2, thereby requiring twice the energy expenditure than at rest. MET values range from 0.9 (sleeping) to 23 (running at competitive pace). Energy expenditure (e.g., in calories or joules) during an activity depends on the person's body mass—the energy cost increases with weight. However, when calculating MET, the ratio (active energy spent/

resting energy spent) becomes unitless and thus independent of the person's weight. MET is useful as a means of expressing the intensity and energy expenditure among persons of different weights.

Besides monitoring your heart rate, exercise intensity can be estimated by the level of perceived exertion. Similar to the talk test where exercise intensity is related to how hard it is to converse, the **Borg Rating of Perceived Exertion (RPE)** is another way to determine work level. Perceived exertion is rated on a scale between six (no effort) and twenty (maximum effort). Level nine is the effort needed to walk at an easy pace. Levels 12–14 are moderate-intensity, such as walking briskly or jogging at an easy pace. Above level 15, talking is a hassle; levels 19 and 20 cannot be maintained for very long. RPE is often used in research studies to document how hard the subject feels they are working, compared to the actual amount of work measured with an ergometer or other device. The scale starts at six because for an average healthy adult, the RPE times ten gives an approximate heart rate ($14 \times 10 = 140$ bpm), though this can be affected by age and health condition.

Exercise Metabolism

In addition to the cardiovascular system, exercise also affects the body's metabolic system. When we eat, our cells convert the energy from fat, carbohydrates (e.g., the sugar glucose), and protein into **adenosine triphosphate (ATP)**, and our cells use the energy in ATP to perform functions necessary for life. The organic molecules we consume are oxidized in discrete stepwise reactions; the final step requires oxygen. The energy that is released during these oxidation reactions is used to make ATP or given off as heat.

ATP is the energy currency in cells (see Figure 2.1). The energy released when ATP is broken down is, in turn, used by energy-requiring reactions. The intracellular concentration of ATP is maintained at a steady-state level, so that rates of synthesis roughly match rates of utilization. This is especially important when exercise increases the demand for energy. During exercise, contraction of muscle proteins, along with many other ATP-utilizing enzymes, markedly increases ATP utilization (as much as 100 times use at rest), and ATP synthesis must keep pace. The demand for ATP production is proportional to power output during exercise: the harder the effort, the more ATP is needed.

Intracellular stores of fat and carbohydrate are used to maintain ATP levels in muscle cells during exercise. Additionally, fatty acids and glucose are also taken up from the blood through membrane transporters in muscle cells. Adipocytes (fat cells) and the liver help maintain blood levels of fatty acids; the liver is also largely responsible for maintaining blood glucose levels. Regulation of these processes is complex, involving hormonal and neuronal control mechanisms that maintain blood levels of glucose and free fatty acids. These specific transporters in muscle cell membranes use the concentration gradient (high concentration in blood, low in muscle) for the uptake of glucose and other nutrients by the process called facilitated diffusion. Hormonal and neuronal input also increases the rate of uptake of fatty acids or glucose.

Aerobic Metabolism

A small amount of ATP is made in the cytoplasm through the glycolytic pathway. In the glycolytic pathway, glucose is converted to two molecules of pyruvate, a three-carbon intermediate. This series of reactions does not require oxygen and produces a

Figure 2.1 ATP: the energy currency inside cells.

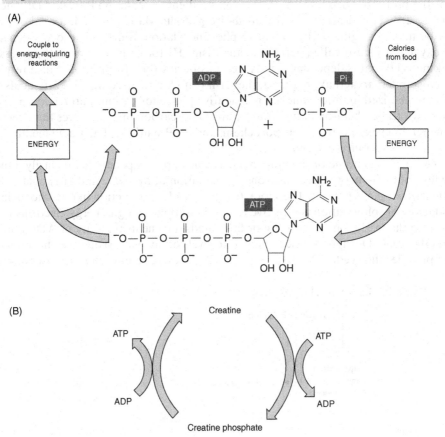

Legend: (A) Adenosine triphosphate (ATP) is made from adenosine diphosphate (ADP) and inorganic phosphate (Pi), with energy supplied by the oxidation of organic molecules (sugar, fat, or protein). When ATP is hydrolyzed back to ADP and Pi, energy is released and is used by cells to make unfavorable reactions favorable, with some energy also released as heat. (B) In muscle cells, the energy stored in ATP can be transferred and stored in phosphocreatine. At times of low demand on ATP use, creatine is converted to creatine phosphate (also called phosphocreatine) at the expense of an ATP. Muscle cells then have a very fast way of generating ATP during short bursts of peak demand, by using phosphocreatine to supply the high-energy phosphate to make ATP from ADP.

net gain of two ATP per glucose. Pyruvate contains considerable energy. When sufficient oxygen is present, pyruvate enters mitochondria and is completely oxidized to CO_2. Aerobic means "with oxygen"; therefore, **aerobic metabolism** refers to the production of ATP by a process that requires oxygen. In mitochondria, pyruvate is converted to a two-carbon intermediate that feeds the Krebs cycle of reactions, becoming completely oxidized to CO_2. High-energy electrons released during the oxidation reactions are bound to intermediate electron carriers. These electron carriers feed an electron-transport chain that uses the energy released during electron transfer (proton-motive force) to generate a proton gradient across the inner membrane of a mitochondrion. The electrons ultimately bind and reduce oxygen (O_2), forming water molecules (H_2O) with readily available protons (H^+).

The enzyme ATP synthase is localized in the inner membrane of mitochondria and uses the proton-motive force in the proton gradient to make ATP from ADP and Pi (Figure 2.1). This process is called **oxidative phosphorylation**. An additional 32 ATP can be made per glucose by oxidative phosphorylation. Since this process depends on oxygen, it is also called aerobic metabolism. Historically, this overall process of making ATP that is dependent on oxygen has been called respiration. Since respiration also refers to actual breathing, the term is no longer used much. Fatty acids are also metabolized in mitochondria by oxidative phosphorylation. Fatty acids are broken down (called beta-oxidation) into similar two-carbon intermediates that feed the same Krebs cycle, electron transport chain, and ATP synthase. Fatty acid metabolism therefore also requires oxygen.

The inner membrane of the mitochondrion has great capacity. It can easily handle the flow of high-energy electrons from the oxidation of pyruvate and fatty acids when sufficient oxygen is present. Therefore, the rate of ATP production in mitochondria by oxidative phosphorylation is sensitive to: (1) the supply of high-energy electrons coming from the oxidation of pyruvate or fatty acids, (2) the availability of ADP and Pi, and (3) oxygen. During exercise at moderate levels of intensity, oxidative phosphorylation provides the needed ATP (see Figure 2.2). As exercise intensity increases above a

Figure 2.2 Basics of ATP production.

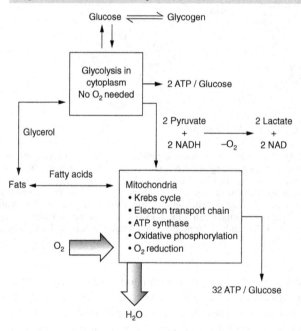

Legend: The major components of ATP production are shown. Glucose, either from breakdown of muscle cell glycogen or uptake from the blood, is metabolized in the cytoplasm in a series of steps called glycolysis. Two ATP are produced per glucose, as well as three-carbon intermediates called pyruvate. When oxygen is present, pyruvate enters the mitochondria, where it is completely oxidized. The energy that is released drives the process of oxidative phosphorylation, making an additional 32 ATP per glucose. If oxygen is limiting or the demand for ATP is very high, pyruvate is converted to lactate in the cytoplasm in order to maintain glycolysis and its limited ATP production. Lactate is dumped into the bloodstream over time. Note that fatty acids feed directly into mitochondria, where they undergo beta-oxidation, so that ATP production from fatty acids requires oxygen.

certain threshold and the demand for ATP rises, pyruvate and ADP entry into mitochondria cannot keep up, and the oxygen demand for oxidative phosphorylation cannot be met. Fatty acid utilization similarly fails to keep up as exercise intensity increases.

Anaerobic Metabolism

Short-term bursts of exercise put intense demand on the ATP supply to support muscle activity. Oxidative ATP production is too slow to meet the high demand for ATP. As a result, glycolysis in the cytoplasm is stimulated to meet the demand. ATP is also produced from creatine phosphate (Figure 2.1B). These mechanisms for ATP production are called **substrate-level phosphorylation** (the enzymatic transfer of high-energy phosphate intermediates to ADP making ATP). ATP production can be six times faster than oxidative phosphorylation in mitochondria, but can only be maintained for 10 to 20 seconds. The three-carbon product of glycolysis, pyruvate, begins to build up in the cytoplasm faster than mitochondria can import and oxidize it. The excess pyruvate is reduced to lactate by a process called **fermentation**. The formation of lactate maintains glycolysis and ATP production (Figure 2.2). Since this process does not require oxygen, it is sometimes referred to as **anaerobic metabolism**. This fast generation of ATP in the cytoplasm can be maintained briefly as sources of creatine phosphate and glucose become limiting and lactate begins to build up. Under heavy workloads and high levels of anaerobic metabolism in muscle, lactate released by muscle cells is taken up by tissues that maintain oxidative metabolism, including liver, heart, and Type I muscle fibers (defined in next section). Lactate can be completely oxidized in the liver and other tissues to yield its ATP-generating potential.

Blood levels of lactate are a good indicator of exercise intensity and training adaptations (less lactate production as an individual becomes more fit). Exercise at lower intensity can be met by oxidative phosphorylation in muscle cell mitochondria. Increasing exercise intensity generates more lactate that makes its way into the bloodstream. As physical training continues and muscle tissue adapts, oxidative capacity and mitochondrial function improve to better meet the demand for ATP, contributing to an improved VO_2max and less lactate production.

Lipolysis

Energy available from lipid reserves (i.e., fat) dwarfs the relatively finite amount of energy available from stored glycogen (i.e., carbohydrates or sugars). The primary storage form of fat are molecules called triglycerides (Figure 2.3). Adipose tissue, composed of adipocytes (fat cells), is the major storage site for triglycerides, although the liver and other tissues have some limited storage capacity. Healthy humans tend to range from 10% to 25% fat by weight. **Lipolysis**, the enzymatic breakdown of triglycerides by lipases, releases fatty acids and produces glycerol; the free fatty acids can produce ATP in mitochondria and glycerol can feed into glycolysis. Lipolysis is stimulated by epinephrine/adrenaline. Epinephrine/adrenaline is discussed in greater detail in Chapter 3. Hormones such as thyroid-stimulating hormone also regulate lipid breakdown. Insulin inhibits lipolysis. As exercise continues, fat reserves are mobilized. We can determine the extent of lipolysis during exercise by measuring the concentration of free fatty acids (FFA) and glycerol in the serum. Serum concentration of glycerol serves as a measure of the contribution from adipocyte lipolysis.

Figure 2.3 Structure of a triacylglycerol—a storage form of fat.

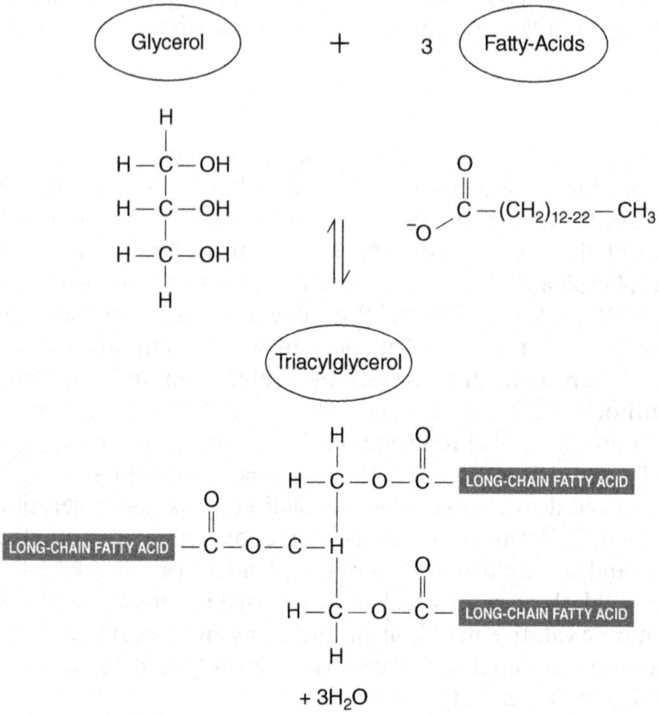

Legend: Glycerol has three carbons that each bond to a long-chain fatty acid. Fatty acids can range in length from 12 to 24 carbons or longer. Fatty acids also differ in their level of saturation, meaning they can have zero (saturated), one (monosaturated), or more carbon–carbon double bonds (polyunsaturated). During exercise, lipases release the fatty acids from glycerol in adipocytes or the vasculature, and muscle cells take up the free fatty acids to fuel ATP production.

Lipid breakdown also occurs in muscle, liver, and the vasculature. Since fatty acids feed oxidative phosphorylation in mitochondria, ATP production from fat is dependent on oxygen. Therefore, as power output or exercise intensity increases, fats contribute less and cytoplasmic carbohydrates more for ATP production (Table 2.2). During rest or after eating, fatty acids combine with glycerol to reform triglycerides for energy storage.

A "metabolomic" approach helped create metabolic signatures for individuals who differed in their training level or cardiovascular disease susceptibility (Lewis, Farrell, Wood, et al. 2010). Mass spectroscopy was used to quantify more than 200 metabolites in human plasma before and after exercise. Subjects ranged in fitness level from marathon runners to those with heart disease. Each subject exercised maximally for ten minutes on a cycle ergometer. Many metabolites increased (and some decreased) following exercise. Glycerol levels in the blood, reflective of lipolysis in adipocytes, correlated with fitness level. Fitter individuals had higher glycerol levels during and post exercise, suggesting they had better rates of fat mobilization in adipocytes. They also had increased levels of markers of mitochondrial oxidation of fatty acids, consistent with their ability to meet the demand for ATP. At rest, unfit individuals had higher blood levels of glycerol and a higher resting heart rate. These resting levels may reflect adipose mass or resistance to insulin. The wide variety of changes in many plasma indicators confirms the complex physiological and

Table 2.2 Percentage contributions of different energy sources at different workloads

Energy Substrates	44% VO_2max	57% VO_2max	72% VO_2max
Free fatty acids	31%	25%	15%
Other fat sources (e.g., muscle triglycerides)	24%	24%	9%
Plasma glucose	10%	13%	18%
Muscle glycogen	35%	38%	58%

Legend: Oxidation rates were calculated for different energy sources by using stable isotope methodologies. Eight cyclists were studied at rest and at three 30-minute stages of exercise at different workloads. Source: Data modified from Van Loon, Greenhaff, Constantin-Teodosiu, et al. (2001).

biochemical response to exercise and helps identify possible molecular pathways involved in the response (Lewis et al.).

To summarize the key points, low-intensity and endurance exercise draw heavily on fat reserves. Fat metabolism is aerobic (requires oxygen). Fat continues to serve as a major source to sustain energy production to about 55% to 60% of maximum workload. Depending on the individual and conditions, this intensity is considered the anaerobic threshold. As exercise intensity increases, glycogen in muscle is converted to glucose (referred to as **glycogenolysis)** and carbohydrates increasingly contribute to ATP production (Table 2.2). Increasing exercise intensity also increases epinephrine release, and epinephrine stimulates receptors in skeletal muscle to increase glycogenolysis. As muscle becomes more dependent on anaerobic metabolism at high workloads, fat oxidation and oxidative phosphorylation (respiration) contribute a lower percentage of total energy demand. At high exercise intensity and workloads, muscle cells become more dependent on anaerobic metabolism and ferment pyruvate to lactate while continuing to make ATP. Blood lactate levels correspond to the higher workloads and glycogenolysis as the primary energy source. With training, the anaerobic threshold (where lactate production starts to increase) shifts to higher workloads.

Muscle Fiber Types

Exercise burns calories and helps maintain muscle mass. Muscle mass contributes to the resting or basal metabolic rate and the amount of energy burned at rest. There are three major muscle fiber types, and they differ in their preferred energy source and their role in exercise performance. They also can be distinguished by the expression of different isoforms of myosin heavy chain—the muscle fiber protein involved in contraction. Interestingly, there is considerable debate whether the relative amounts of different fiber types may be influenced by exercise or diet or may correlate with diseases such as diabetes. After a brief description of the three muscle fiber types, we will examine whether muscle fiber types can functionally change or whether our muscle fiber makeup is genetically predetermined.

Slow Twitch (Oxidative) or Type I

Slow-twitch oxidative muscle fibers are rich in mitochondria and are efficient at aerobic metabolism, including beta-oxidation of fatty acids as an energy source. Type I fibers are highly oxidative, allowing them to be relatively fatigue resistant, but have slower contraction rates. They store little glycogen. Type I fibers play an important role in endurance exercise. Type I fibers are also referred to as red muscle fibers, because they have high myoglobin content, which gives them extra oxygen-binding capacity. Myoglobin is a heme-binding protein closely related to hemoglobin (see Figure 2.4). The heme group contains iron and binds oxygen, producing the red color.

Fast Twitch (Oxidative) or Type IIa

Fast-twitch oxidative muscle fibers are intermediate in their amount of glycogen and mitochondria compared to the Type I and the Type IIx (see below); hence, they are also known as oxidative-glycolytic fibers. Type IIa fibers are intermediate in their level of fatigue resistance. They have available energy stored in glycogen, but in limited amounts. These fibers are also red, because myoglobin is present.

Fast Twitch (Glycolytic) or Type IIx

Fast-twitch glycolytic fibers have a fast contraction speed but low fatigue resistance. They have the highest capacity to perform glycolysis and the most stored glycogen. Athletes use Type IIx fibers for power when sprinting and weight lifting. They are also referred to as white fibers, because they lack myoglobin and have relatively few mitochondria.

Endurance runners have a higher proportion of Type I fibers relative to sprinters, who have a higher proportion of Type IIx fibers. Type I fibers are more sensitive to insulin. Type 2 diabetics have a higher proportion of Type IIx fibers (Tanner, Barakat, Dohm, et al. 2002), which tend to be insulin resistant (Gaster, Staehr, Beck-Nielsen, et al. 2001). Animal studies show a decrease in the proportion of slow-twitch fibers

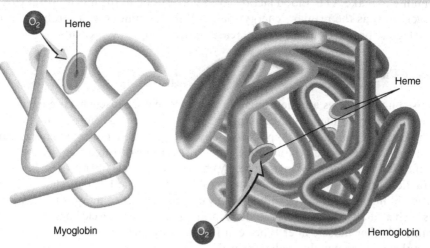

Figure 2.4 Comparison of the heme-containing proteins myoglobin and hemoglobin, which bind oxygen.

O$_2$

Heme

Heme

Myoglobin

O$_2$

Hemoglobin

Legend: The structure of the monomer myoglobin is compared to the subunits of the tetramer hemoglobin. Note the presence of the heme (only two of four shown for hemoglobin), which contains the iron necessary for binding oxygen.

that precedes changes observed in the onset of diabetes. The conclusion? Exercise with an endurance component helps maintain slow-twitch fibers and can lower the risk of diabetes, heart disease, and obesity (Yan, Okutsu, Akhtar, & Lira 2011).

Extensive research has examined how exercise contributes muscle fiber remodeling. Animal studies show significant remodeling, but experiments in humans have not been as conclusive. Are humans more dependent on their genetic makeup, or are the changes more subtle and harder to detect? What mechanisms might be involved in causing muscle fiber remodeling following training? Nerve input causes muscle contraction stimulated by calcium release within muscle cells. As workload increases, the free calcium may trigger other processes. For example, calcium binds and activates calmodulin, the universal regulator of calcium signaling. Activated calmodulin binds and stimulates a host of potential target enzymes. Among those enzymes are some that perpetuate the calcium signal, resulting in changes that persist hours or days after the original spike in intracellular calcium. There is a calcium–calmodulin-dependent protein phosphatase called calcineurin (or PP2B), as well as several calmodulin-dependent protein kinases (Figure 2.5). The calcium-dependent signal can activate transcription factors that increase expression of specific genes, resulting in production of RNA, leading to new protein synthesis. These activated genes include those involved in conversion of muscle fiber type (Basal-Duby & Olson 2006). In humans, endurance training, including strength training, causes Type IIa and Type IIx inter-conversions; shifts from Type II to Type I fibers are less well substantiated (Wilson, Loenneke, Jo, et al. 2012).

Other families of transcription factors are activated by signals generated by exercise. An important one is a member of the family of regulatory proteins called peroxisome proliferator-activated receptors (PPARs). The PPAR family members are important in regulation of metabolic processes, including mitochondrial genes involved in oxidative metabolism. (Regulation of PPAR activity will appear again in several later chapters.) One PPAR subtype regulates transcriptional pathways that coordinate increases in mitochondrial activity and associated changes in slow-twitch fibers (Figure 2.5). The activated genes increase production of proteins that increase the oxidative metabolic capacity of these cells. Training, diet, and underlying genetics produce outcomes that are based, in part, on the composition and adaptability of skeletal muscle fibers.

Recovery and Adaptation

Training can cause muscle damage, glycogen depletion, hyperthermia, and dehydration. Sufficient recovery is needed to avoid sub-optimal performance during subsequent training sessions and for muscle adaptation to succeed. Muscle will adapt to repeated bouts of exercise by growing in size (hypertrophy) and improving its oxidative capacity to produce ATP. Without sufficient recovery time, a resulting chronic imbalance might lead to an overtraining syndrome. This syndrome includes muscle damage, poorer neuromuscular contractile properties, stiffness, loss of range of motion, unbalanced hormonal responses, insufficient muscle glycogen synthesis, and psychological fatigue.

For recovery, the most important thing is to rehydrate, replacing the fluids and salts lost during exercise. Sufficient water content is needed for nearly every bodily function. Also important is to replenish energy stores with high-quality protein and

Figure 2.5 Role for calcium signaling in muscle cell remodeling.

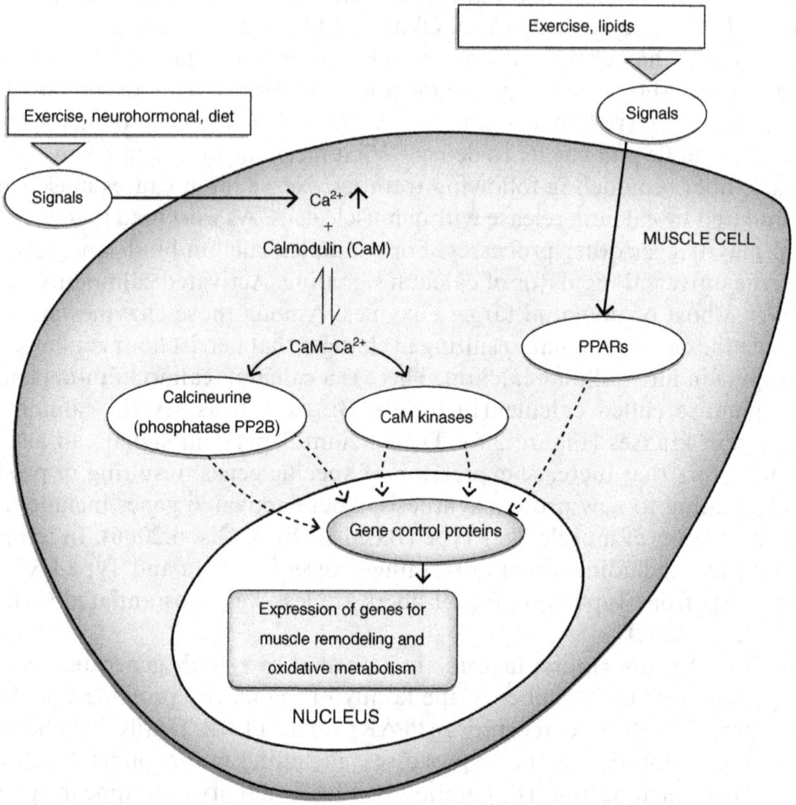

Legend: A simplified model shows an overview of the key events in how calcium signaling and PPARs cause changes in gene expression. Altered gene expression causes the production of proteins that help increase the oxidative capacity of the muscle cells and drives the remodeling of fibers to a slow-twitch phenotype. The dashed lines simplify the complex pathways of how signals in the cytoplasm are relayed to the nucleus. More details on calcium signaling can be found in Basal-Duby and Olson (2006).

complex carbohydrate. Proper nutrition helps recovery, tissue repair, build muscle, and be ready for the next challenge. Rest is needed—allow time for the repair and recovery process to occur at a natural pace. Gentle stretching and movement improve circulation, which helps promote nutrient and waste product transport. One of the best practices for recovery after strenuous activity is massage therapy (Dupuy et al. 2018). It not only feels good but increases circulation and helps relaxation. Other techniques for recovery and to decrease delayed onset muscle soreness (DOMS) utilize ice baths or heat—there are proponents for either. There are also techniques that alternate cold and hot called contrast water therapy. For successful recovery, sufficient quality sleep is essential (more details in Chapter 3). While sleeping, your body produces growth hormone, which is important for tissue growth and repair. It is also very important to not overdo it. Excessive training with a lack of rest days can limit fitness gains. To recover faster, design a smart workout routine that includes cross-training and a variety of complimentary exercises with sufficient time in between (Dupuy).

Adaptation

Exercise training improves overall mitochondrial quantity and quality through coordinated adaptive processes. Mitochondrial adaptation includes mitochondrial biogenesis and mitochondrial dynamics. Biogenesis of mitochondria involves synthesis and incorporation of new proteins and mitochondrial DNA into the existing mitochondria. Mitochondria are dynamic, undergoing fusion and fission rapidly—in less than a minute (Song, Ghochani, McCaffery, et al. 2009). Mitochondrial fusion is the process where individual mitochondria combine (fuse) into an elongated reticular structure. Fusion creates the mitochondrial reticulum and is dominant in metabolically active cells. It allows the spreading of metabolites, enzymes, and mitochondrial gene products throughout the entire mitochondrial reticulum. Fusion allows the mitochondrial membrane potential to equilibrate from oxygen-rich areas along the reticulum to remote, low-oxygen areas, driving ATP synthesis. Fusion is balanced by fission, where portions of the reticulum pinch off into smaller structures. The resulting individual mitochondrial fragments can be transported to cell locations along the cytoskeleton to where greater energy production is needed. Moreover, mitochondrial fragments produced by fission allows for degradation of damaged and dysfunctional mitochondria by a specialized type of autophagy called mitophagy. These dynamic, exercise-inducible processes underlie enhanced physical performance, as well as other health benefits, as a result of exercise training.

In skeletal muscle, the mitochondrial reticulum clusters underneath the sarcoplasm with individual mitochondria located between myofibrils on either side of the Z-line. Both acute exercise and exercise training increase the synthesis of mitochondrial proteins in human skeletal muscle, indicating mitochondrial biosynthesis (reviewed in Drake). Newly synthesized proteins, lipids, and mitochondrial DNA assemble into pre-existing mitochondria, expanding the mitochondrial reticulum. By increasing mitochondrial quantity and efficiency, oxygen utilization improves so that oxidation of fat and carbohydrate increases, contributing to the improved aerobic capacity and VO_2max observed with training.

Following acute exercise, mitochondria undergo fission into smaller fragments. The generation of reactive oxygen species (ROS) is intrinsically linked to respiratory activity and occurs at many sites during the redox reactions of the electron transport chain and ATP synthesis (Trewin, Berry, & Wojtovich 2018). Most of the oxygen we inhale is concentrated in mitochondria and used to accept electrons during the last step of the electron transport chain, becoming reduced and forming water—H_2O. The high levels of oxygen in mitochondria promote ROS generation. Acute exercise increases oxygen utilization and ROS generation; ROS initiate damage control mechanisms, mitochondrial fragmentation by fission, and components of inflammation. During recovery following the high rate of ATP (and ROS) production, recycling of damaged mitochondrial components stimulates new mitochondrial biosynthesis. Fission facilitates mitophagy, segregating damaged mitochondrial subdomains for elimination. These damaged regions of mitochondria divide into fragments amenable to autophagosome engulfment, fusion with lysosomes, and degradation via mitophagy. The clearance of damaged mitochondria after exercise makes way for the incorporation of newly synthesized mitochondria during recovery, facilitating improvement of mitochondrial quality (Drake, Wilson, & Yan 2016). There is also an upregulation of cellular antioxidant defense systems and anti-inflammatory responses during recovery, providing additional benefits when training.

Aging and Sarcopenia

The sedentary lifestyle of older people promotes and contributes the loss of muscle mass, a process called sarcopenia. Sarcopenia affects almost 50 million people worldwide. As we age, skeletal muscle suffers a decrease in myofiber size and number. There

Endocrine Functions of Muscle

Skeletal muscle is a primary regulator of energy homeostasis and a potent coordinator of exercise-induced adaptations in other organs, including the liver, fat tissue (adipocytes), and brain. Contraction of skeletal muscles during exercise releases proteins and vesicles (more information below) that regulate whole-body metabolism. Indeed, the release or uptake of metabolites by contracting muscle cells can mediate many tissue interactions, including the central nervous system. The protein hormones released by muscle cells are called myokines (or a new term 'exerkines'), and can exert local and long-distance hormonal effects (Safdar & Tarnopolsky 2018). One example is how exercise improves a broad range of brain functions related to vascularization, neuroplasticity, memory, sleep, and mood. Cathepsin B is secreted from skeletal muscles and upregulates brain-derived neurotrophic factor following exercise (Moon, Becke, Berron, et al. 2016). Brain-derived neurotrophic factor regulates adult neurogenesis and synaptic plasticity, providing a possible mechanism how exercise improves brain functions, including cognition, memory, and motor coordination (discussed in more detail in Chapter 9). Another example is Irisin, which is released from muscle after exercise and may be involved in energy expenditure, thermogenesis, and provide neuroprotection (reviewed by Fatouros 2018).

The secretion of extracellular vesicles from cells into the blood stream is an evolutionary conserved process that is an essential component of intercellular communication. The term extracellular vesicles is a collective term for a mixture of different types of structures surrounded by a lipid bilayer. Healthy cells shed microvesicles of varying size from their plasma membranes. In addition, exosomes are generated within the cell, fuse with the cell membrane, and are released into the extracellular environment. Extracellular vesicles in the blood are heterogeneous and contain unique proteins, lipids, and nucleic acids. The nucleic acid component can be complex and contain microRNAs (defined below), messenger RNA, and mitochondrial DNA. A majority of myokines/exerkines released after exercise are found in extracellular vesicles (Safdar & Tarnopolsky 2018). They transfer their cargo to recipient cells initiating cell-specific responses. Moreover, circulatory extracellular vesicle content increases in an intensity-dependent manner in response to endurance exercise. Skeletal muscle, liver, adipose tissue, brain, and bone secrete proteins and extracellular vesicles during exercise, providing a powerful mechanism to mediate and coordinate the response to physical activity.

Proteomic analysis of extracellular vesicles demonstrated a robust exercise-induced increase in several classes of proteins associated with microvesicles and exosomes. A one-hour bout of cycling exercise in healthy humans increased over 300 proteins in the circulation, including those that compose exosomes and small vesicles. Many of these vesicles localized to the liver to transfer their protein cargo. The target specificity of extracellular vesicles is mediated by adhesion proteins on the surface of the vesicles and a significant increase in a wide range of adhesion proteins followed exercise (Whithan 2018). The release of exosomes is generally associated with increases in intracellular calcium. Since motor neuron stimulation of skeletal muscle fibers leads to a rapid release of calcium from the sarcoplasmic reticulum, muscle has the capacity to release small vesicles rapidly into circulation and coordinate signaling between important metabolic tissues (Figure 2.5).

Small non-coding microRNAs regulate gene expression by causing mRNA degradation or inhibiting translation. They play a crucial role in cell differentiation, proliferation, and apoptosis, and help maintain homeostasis (Denham, Gray, Scott-Hamilton, et al. 2018). Circulating microRNAs vary with disease state, pregnancy, or physical exercise. They are a novel class of biomarkers of aerobic capacity and training adaptation and are promising candidates for biomarkers of sarcopenia (more details below). Many microRNAs are modulated by exercise training and could control signaling pathways responsible for health benefits achieved from exercise. They provide targets for interventions to slow muscle aging.

Though in its infancy, the study of molecules involved in coordinating the response to exercise are future targets for therapeutic manipulation of the positive benefits of exercise. For example, adipose tissue secretes exosomes containing microRNAs capable of regulating gene expression in the liver and other tissues (Thomou, Mori, Dreyfuss, et al. 2017). Exercise exerts metabolic demands on the body that are unequal among tissues. Since new protein synthesis and protein degradation cost energy, vesicle trafficking of metabolic mediators might be a process by which tissues share resources during the high-energy demands of physical exertion. It will be possible to isolate exosomes from athletes following exercise or create exosomes bioengineered to incorporate one or many of known exerkines to treat obesity, Type 2 diabetes, and other aging-associated metabolic disorders such as sarcopenia (Safdar & Tarnopolsky 2018).

In summary, contracting skeletal muscle during exercise causes a significant perturbation of homeostasis throughout the body. The integrated response of diverse tissues restores homeostasis in the short term, and produces adaptations during training. Many of these signals are mediated by extracellular vesicles, allowing very specific targeted responses. These vesicles have great therapeutic and diagnostic potential.

is a diminished ability of satellite cells (muscle stem cells) to activate and proliferate upon injury leading to impaired muscle remodeling. Sarcopenia represents a major healthcare challenge for older adults. A large percentage of older adults experience functional limitations with everyday tasks and suffer a high incidence of injuries, which result in a significant economic burden. The loss of muscle mass, strength, and physical function is characteristic of aging. Progression of sarcopenia is gradual but may be accelerated by periods of physical inactivity following injury or illness. Structural and functional decline of skeletal muscle is linked to a decline in mitochondrial function. Abnormal mitochondria can cause maladaptive changes within motor neurons and muscle fibers, impacting the neuromuscular junction. Mechanisms involve accumulation of mitochondrial DNA damage, reduced mitochondrial biogenesis, oxidative stress and respiratory chain defects, and loss of quality control via fission and mitophagy. Sarcopenia may also result from impaired protein turnover—the continual process where aged proteins are regularly replaced with new ones.

Causative agents for sarcopenia include physical inactivity and poor diet, which contribute to loss of muscle mass and strength regardless of age. Aging leads to a decline in different hormones (e.g., estrogens, androgens, and growth hormone) and vitamin D. A decreased sensitivity to insulin is common in the elderly and can lead to an imbalance in protein turnover in muscle, favoring protein degradation. Fiber wasting can result, with preferential decrease of fast twitch (Type II) fibers. Chronic drug treatment in the elderly may affect muscle tissue over time. Loss of muscle mass can also modify the pharmacokinetic properties of drugs, thereby increasing the risk of undesirable outcomes. Furthermore, pro-inflammatory cytokines (e.g., Il-6 and Il-1) increase with age and chronic disease and have detrimental effects on muscle.

Lifelong physical activity, which promotes mitochondrial health across tissues, is an effective countermeasure for sarcopenia. Furthermore, exercise is currently the only effective option to treat sarcopenia. Endurance exercise is the traditional form of training to improve mitochondrial function, protein turnover, and oxidative capacity. Short-term resistance exercise training is also effective and can increase mitochondrial content of muscle. In a study with 65- to 80-year-old males and females, short-term resistance training provided improved strength, power, rate of force development, muscle aerobic capacity, glucose tolerance, and plasma lipid profile (Frank, Andersson, Pontén, et al. 2016). The compliance to resistance training was very high in this study, suggesting that resistance training can be recommended as a complement or alternative to endurance exercise. These improvements are important for quality of life and independence and to reduce the incidence of fall injuries.

Telomeres and Aging

Vascular aging is associated with endothelial dysfunction and atherogenesis. A key cellular process of aging is the shortening of telomeres, the DNA sequences that protect the ends of chromosomes. Telomeres shorten as we age until they reach a critical length that causes cells to stop dividing (replicative senescence) or undergo programmed cell death (apoptosis). Telomere length is maintained by a highly regulated enzyme called telomerase. Telomere shortening in circulating leukocytes is associated with cardiovascular morbidity. The regulation of telomerase activity in leukocytes is similar to cells in the vessel wall and most other cells in the adult body.

Long-term endurance training is associated with higher telomerase activity compared with inactive control subjects. Twins with a higher level of physical activity exhibit longer telomeres in middle age compared with inactive siblings (Cherkas, Hunkin, Kato, et al. 2008). Moderate levels of physical activity may reduce telomere shortening, an important cellular adaptation that may prevent age-related diseases. A randomized controlled trial showed that endurance training and interval training increased telomerase activity and telomere length in leukocytes, whereas resistance training did not (Werner, Hecksteden, Morsch, et al. 2019). However, another study found improvement in endothelial function with resistance training when done with greater frequency, rather than intensity (Ashor, Lara, Siervo, et al. 2015), so the type of resistance exercise protocol may be important. Clearly though, sustained physical activity as we age can slow cellular senescence, improve regenerative capacity, and provide healthy aging (Werner).

Prescribing Exercise Health

Physiological capacity for exercise peaks around 30 years old and declines with increasing age; however, regular exercise training can slow the decline in fitness as we age. Remember that fitness depends on the capacity of lungs and heart to pump oxygen to muscles and organs and the ability of tissues to utilize oxygen to form ATP. Therefore, the goals of training/exercise are to: (1) develop the capacity of the central circulation system and (2) enhance the aerobic capacity of specific muscles. An exercise plan to improve or maintain cardiovascular fitness requires an increase in heart rate to 60% to 80% of maximum heart rate for approximately 30 minutes. To gain the most benefit, the individual should perform this cardiovascular type of exercise up to five times per week for a total of 150 minutes (Garber, Blissmer, Deschenes, et al. 2011). However, benefits are observed at lower levels of activity. As stated previously, many exercise machines monitor heart rate, and some provide a "training zone" chart that shows the age and heart rate relationship discussed above so that the exerciser can achieve a target heart rate. However, these charts are based on a limited set of parameters for "average" adults. The human population varies greatly in terms of fitness and cardiovascular health, so these charts provide only a rough (ballpark) estimate for target heart rate. Strength (e.g., resistance training with weights) and aerobic programs can be done on alternate days. Following strenuous strength/weight training, a 48-hour rest is recommended to allow those muscle groups to recover. Table 2.3 presents possible components of a training program.

Table 2.3 Components of training program

Component	Activity	Time (minutes)
Warm-up	Stretching, walking	10
Strength training	Weights, resistance	10–20
Aerobic training	Vigorous activity (60%–80% max)	20–40
Cool-down	Walking, stretching, floor exercise	5–10

Legend: A common training recommendation includes aerobic training three to five times a week and weight training twice a week.

Table 2.4 A basic exercise prescription

Parameter	Recommendation
Frequency	3–5 days per week aerobic exercise (150 minutes per week)
	2 days per week strength and resistance training
Intensity	50%–60% (brisk walk but easy to converse)
	60%–85% max heart rate or VO_2max (harder to converse)
Duration	15–60 minutes (continuous)
	Note: 10–15 minutes several times a day is also beneficial
Mode	All kinds of activities, endurance sports
Level of fitness	Beginners: start with walking
	Higher level: increase workload (pace, duration, distance)

Legend: The key components of an exercise prescription—frequency, intensity, duration (time), and type of physical activity—are shown, with recommended targets.

An **exercise prescription** is given to individuals who need to improve their cardiovascular health and fitness level. The components of a prescription include the *frequency, intensity, and duration* of the activities. The current guidelines call for a minimum of 150 minutes of aerobic exercise and two sessions of strength training per week. For most people, it is important to start at a comfortable level. As one's fitness level improves, the workload or intensity can be increased. Changing routines and doing a variety of exercises and activities can help reduce boredom. Cross training also provides benefits, as the body becomes accustomed to repetitive activities and the level of physical benefit may decrease. Cross training also enlists more muscle groups for all around fitness improvement. A workout partner can help with motivation, as can keeping a journal or digital exercise log. An occasional day of rest is also beneficial. Table 2.4 gives a possible exercise prescription.

A Dose–Response Curve for Exercise

Many studies confirm the increase in stroke volume and improved VO_2max that result from training. For example, Church, Earnest, Skinner, and Blair (2007) found an increase in fitness with increasing levels of exercise training—an exercise dose–response curve. In this study, 464 post-menopausal women with sedentary lifestyles were recruited. They ranged in age from 45 to 75 years old and were overweight to obese, with BMI ranging from 25 to 43. They were split into four groups, with the control group maintaining its sedentary lifestyle. The other three groups exercised in controlled, supervised conditions for six months at different levels of intensity, alternating between cycle ergometry and a treadmill. The results showed a graded dose–response in oxygen uptake and power output with increasing exercise intensity (see Table 2.5). Even at the lowest level of activity, a significant increase in fitness was observed. These results suggest that even a moderate level of activity can have a positive outcome in overweight post-menopausal women.

Table 2.5 Results of a study showing an increase in fitness with increasing levels of exercise training

Measure	Exercise Intensity over Six Months		
	4 kcal/kg	8 kcal/kg	12 kcal/kg
VO$_2$ abs (%)	4.2	6.0	8.2
VO$_2$ rel (%)	4.7	7.0	8.5
W peak (%)	7.6	10.7	12.9
Number of subjects	155	104	103

Legend: Figures are percent change in fitness measure. Previously sedentary, overweight, or obese post-menopausal women experienced a graded dose–response change in fitness with increasing levels of exercise training.
Note: VO$_2$ abs: peak absolute oxygen consumption (L/min); VO$_2$ rel: peak relative oxygen consumption (L/min/kg); W peak: peak power output (watts). Values are % increase over control ($n = 102$); $p < 0.001$ for pairwise comparison of control with each treatment group (adapted from Church et al.).

Interval training, where one does short bursts at maximal intensity interspersed with traditional aerobic activity, also offers benefits. It can improve fitness level and stamina. High-Intensity Interval Training (HIIT) is an off-shoot. HIIT involves burst activity with short intervals of rest. There is considerable variation, but one example would be 20 seconds of maximal activity followed by 10 seconds of rest. The entire workout can be done in 15 minutes, providing time savings to those on tight schedules. Both HIIT and endurance training improved cardiorespiratory fitness similarly (i.e., VO$_2$ peak and submaximal ventilation thresholds). HIIT and endurance training show specific neuromuscular adaptations, possibly related to differences in exercise load intensity and training volume. Adherence to an exercise program is difficult for many people and adherence to HIIT may be more difficult, despite being more time-efficient. Ongoing support and structured HIIT programs can help people maintain the program and reap the benefits.

Research in Exercise Pharmacology

When a drug becomes popular as a performance-enhancing substance, considerable research is done to quantify its effectiveness and the limits of its detection, so that its use may be regulated. For many common drugs used by millions of patients, however, little research exists on the effects of exercise on the drugs' pharmacokinetics and pharmacodynamics. More research is necessary to learn how these drugs affect exercise performance and participation, as well as how exercise influences the pharmacokinetic and pharmacodynamic properties of the drugs.

As discussed above, exercise involves complex physiological processes. Drugs also involve complex physiological changes. Thus, the study of interactions of exercise and drugs is complex. This section presents several issues involved in exercise pharmacology research.

Research Approaches and Experimental Design

Although some experimentation can be done in animals, primarily rodents, most pharmacology studies require human participants. Using human participants in research studies requires approval from oversight committees. Sample size can also be an issue, as determining statistical significance depends on sample size. Sample sizes for "pilot" studies may be relatively low (involving perhaps five to eight subjects, depending on what is being measured). A larger n (the number of participants or data points) allows for stronger statistical conclusions.

In exercise pharmacology research, most experimental designs will have at least four groups. In some cases, the same set of test subjects can be used for all four conditions (referred to as a **cross-over study**). The subjects should be randomly assigned to the different groups. The four groups are:

1   Drug-treated / no exercise
2   Drug-treated / exercise
3   Placebo / no exercise
4   Placebo / exercise

This basic design helps distinguish the contribution of either exercise or the drug in the outcome. The placebo should appear like the drug and should be part of a blind or double-blind protocol.

Blind versus Double-Blind Studies

In a **blind study**, participants do not know whether they are receiving the drug or the placebo; in a **double-blind study**, neither the administrator nor the subject knows whether the subject is receiving the drug or the placebo until after the study, when the identity key is accessed. The placebo effect is well documented. Subjects may respond to a sugar pill if they think they are receiving a drug. The person delivering the drug can also affect the outcome; we see a similar phenomenon in studies that show how a doctor's bedside matter can influence outcome. Therefore, the double-blind protocol is preferred in order to minimize the placebo effect or bias. For the strongest possible study, it should be a *randomized, cross-over, double-blind* study.

Choosing Subjects

The choice of study subjects can also impact results. Many studies are done on college-age males, as this group tends to "volunteer" (sometimes receiving a small payment) readily. However, such factors as age, gender, race, and fitness level are important. Larger sample sizes can handle less homogeneity in the subjects. For small-scale studies, it may be necessary to have a relatively homogeneous group, to minimize variation (i.e., 20- to 24-year-old, fit males). Some studies will use test subjects with a defined condition (e.g., diabetes, hypertension, hyperlipidemia), but using them raises additional safety concerns and doubles the scope of the project, since the research design outlined above should be duplicated for the disease group (four groups of healthy volunteers and four groups of those with the condition). This experimental design allows the researcher to compare the patient group to healthy subjects.

The Protocol

The drug portion of the study is also potentially complicated. For some drugs, the protocol may simply be to give pills (with the dosage based on body weight), wait one hour, and do the exercise test. However, many drugs vary in terms of absorption rates and the timing of peak blood values. Some drugs' primary effect may not occur until several hours after peak blood levels (e.g., caffeine). Dosage and mode of administration are usually based on best practice, but some research projects may use newer drugs or drugs being tested for another application. Under these conditions, preliminary studies may be needed to define proper conditions for dosage, duration of action, and timing for the exercise test.

Length of the Study

Many drugs are given for chronic conditions over extended periods of time, such as months or years. Many patients are resigned to the fact that they will be on a drug for the rest of their lives. Often, tolerance develops to some of the drug's effects, which is helpful for the undesired effects but not helpful for the therapeutic effect. Sometimes, higher doses or a change to another member of the same drug class is needed. For an experimental design, the exercise test may be best suited for individuals who have had exposure to the drug for an extended time. For example, a single dose given to a fit, college-age male may not be the best experimental design to test a drug that is commonly used by middle-aged, deconditioned females who are also taking a cholesterol-lowering drug that may affect muscle tissue. Some drugs require multiple doses to generate their effect, so test subjects may need to follow a similar protocol.

Exercise Component

Research in exercise pharmacology seeks to determine whether a drug treatment and exercise interact, and, if so, what the effects may be. The hypothesis could be that drug treatment is either ergogenic (the drug increases work capacity) or ergolytic (the drug decreases work capacity). The hypothesis could also be that exercise alters the drug's effectiveness. Since exercise is a critical part of any of these types of studies, the exercise component needs careful thought and planning. For example, should the exercise component test power output or endurance? In the case of anabolic steroids, they may increase muscle strength but have little direct effect on aerobic performance; hence, a muscle strength exercise would be the logical choice. Alternatively, an effect of caffeine may show up only with sustained exercise, so the exercise protocol might determine the time to exhaustion on a cycle ergometer.

Another variable to consider is the intensity of exercise: whether the exercise is performed at maximal or submaximal levels of intensity. Renal responses are intensity dependent, which is important if we wish to determine whether a drug is flow-limited (see Chapter 1). Drugs with a short half-life may have an elongated duration of action during high-intensity exercise that decreases the renal perfusion rate. Some ergolytic or ergogenic effects may require maximal level of exercise, while other effects may be masked at maximal exercise, such as those of certain weak stimulants.

The purpose of the study needs to be clear, as the design may differ if, for example, the purpose is to determine whether a drug improves performance of elite athletes versus whether it affects the exercise regimen of middle-aged patients with cardiovascular disease. How many people really exercise at maximal intensity levels? And with so many deconditioned people taking drugs and not exercising, how can conclusions be extrapolated to them if all of the study subjects are fit and exercising at VO_2max? A good study design can help with the interpretation of results, and a poor design can create problems.

Examples of common lab-based exercise protocols include:

1   Steady-state submaximal exercise
2   Exercise to exhaustion at fixed heart rate (or fixed VO_2max)
3   Graded intervals to reach a specified limit
4   Combination of graded and steady-state exercise to exhaustion.

Lab-based protocols (e.g., heart rate, power output, variable resistance on a cycle er-gometer or grade on a treadmill) are usually easier to monitor than field-based protocols. Field-based studies (e.g., running, swimming, team sports) are technically challenging—it is difficult to monitor them and to do blood draws—but they can pro-vide outcomes that more closely resemble "real world" lifestyles.

More drug and exercise studies are needed for most therapeutic agents, especially drugs that affect the cardiovascular system and are taken by millions of people. Avail-able data must be analyzed critically. It is difficult to extrapolate from one group of individuals to another group. It is also difficult to extrapolate from one member of a class of drugs to another. For example, does it matter which of the many statins (cholesterol-lowering drugs) is used for the study? As with most experimental research, careful evaluation of published reports is necessary to draw valid conclusions on the safety, effectiveness, or performance-changing properties of drugs. When reading re-search articles, ask yourself questions as to the appropriateness of the study subjects, the drug treatment, and the type of exercise performed, to determine whether the re-sults are valid.

Hierarchy of Evidence in Research

Before a drug comes to market, extensive research is conducted on its effectiveness and safety. Research on the impact of drugs or nutritional supplements on exercise phys-iology is performed in laboratories around the world. How does this vast amount of research provide the basis for treatment and guidelines for safe use? The **evidence pyr-amid** is meant to serve as a guideline to using the hierarchy of evidence for researching and defending a hypothesis or developing a protocol (see Figure 2.6).

The base of the pyramid is ideas supported by laboratory research and published in peer-reviewed journals. Sometimes referred to as the "primary literature," these publications provide the underpinnings for the generation of new knowledge. These studies are often conducted on experimental animals or cells grown in culture. As pub-lications accumulate in certain areas of research, investigators write review articles that combine results from many primary research articles. These reviews can point out inconsistencies in the published data or help advance our understanding based on conclusions supported by the published research.

In a clinical setting, experimental results can form the basis for **case reports**, collec-tions of reports on the treatment of a single patient or a small group of patients. Ob-servations and case reports can provide evidence suggesting that additional research should be performed. Because there are no control groups in case reports, outcomes cannot be compared and statistics cannot be used.

The next step up the evidence pyramid involves **case-control studies**. Case-control studies compare patients who have a specific condition with people who do not, and

Figure 2.6 A modified version of the evidence pyramid.

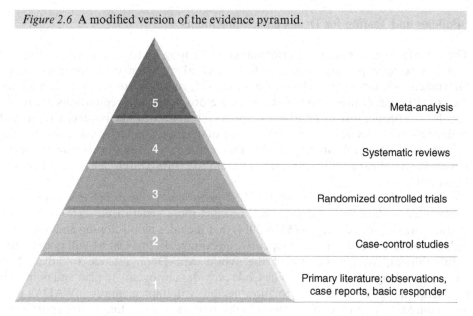

the researchers use a finding of statistical significance to confirm a difference between the groups. **Cohort studies** are the next step toward strengthening a conclusion. In a cohort study, the investigators observe a large population of patients over time and compare them with a matched control group that does not have the condition or has not undergone the treatment being studied.

If cohort studies support a conclusion (or hypothesis), then **randomized controlled trials** are undertaken. In these trials, subjects are randomly assigned to the different treatment groups, often under a double-blind protocol. Though these studies may have relatively small sample sizes, good experimental design and use of statistics can provide sound evidence of cause and effect. After many of these types of studies are published, **systematic reviews** are written that summarize the conclusions supported by the experimental evidence.

Finally, at the top of the evidence pyramid is the **meta-analysis**, in which the researcher uses a quantitative approach for increasing the statistical power for specified endpoints (or subgroups, such as "middle-aged obese women"). Such methodology pools results from published studies that meet appropriate inclusion criteria. An inclusion criterion might restrict the meta-analysis to placebo-controlled studies or studies with sufficient data to allow statistical analysis. Meta-analyses are becoming more frequent, as scientific literature is now digital and searchable. Improvements in data storage and the processing speed of computers aid researchers in performing this type of analysis. A benefit of a meta-analysis is that questions not posed at the start of the individual studies can be addressed with this retrospective approach. For example, does this drug, when combined with resistance training, improve some measure of fitness? Since a meta-analysis can greatly increase the sample size (i.e., provide a large increase in n), stronger statistically based conclusions can be made. The increase in sample size from the combined independent studies can sometimes help resolve uncertainty when studies disagree.

Policies and Testing for Drugs and Supplements

The use of drugs to enhance performance has a long history, and how a drug can improve exercise performance is a fundamental question in exercise and sport pharmacology. Drugs that clearly improve performance provide an unfair advantage to the competitors who use them. Therefore, rules and regulations are necessary for the proper testing of athletes, and a system needs to be in place to deal with violations. This section covers the basics of testing for performance-enhancing substances (PES), and subsequent chapters include a section that evaluates the different classes of drugs for their doping potential ("PES Watch"). Chapter 16 covers PES in detail.

Drugs used for doping are often called *performance-enhancing drugs*, or PEDs. *Performance-enhancing substances*, or PES, is a more generalized term used by the World Anti-Doping Agency (WADA 2014) that includes blood-doping and other procedures that are used to gain a competitive advantage. In this text we will refer to PES.

In athletics, WADA developed the World Anti-Doping Code to advance its anti-doping program worldwide. The Code provides uniformity in plan and policy but is general enough in some areas to allow flexibility in implementation. WADA's goals are two-fold: (1) to protect the athletes' right to participate in doping-free sport, while promoting fairness and good health, and (2) to ensure coordinated anti-doping programs at the national and international levels. National and international sports governing bodies often link their testing procedures and policies to those established in the WADA Code. This is the case for the United States Olympic Committee (USOC), for example. The Code defines doping, specifies what constitutes a violation, and provides standards for testing. It describes in detail the management of test results and sanctions on individuals, teams, or sporting bodies. WADA maintains the Prohibited List. Athletes are responsible for knowing what constitutes a violation and what substances and methods are on the list.

A Quick Glance at the History of Performance-Enhancing Substances

Competitors have always looked for ways to gain an advantage. This practice dates back to the early Olympic Games in Greece, where consumption of organ meat, such as bull testicles, and extracts from opium was thought to have a positive effect on performance. In the late 19th century, an extract from coca leaves mixed with wine was popular. Amphetamine use, both in athletics and in the military, dates back to the mid-1900s. Early Tour de France riders thought smoking cigarettes improved pulmonary function. During international competitions in the 1950s, it was clear that athletes were experimenting with anabolic steroids (i.e., to increase testosterone activity). The 1968 Summer Olympics in Mexico City were the first games in which competitors were tested for performance-enhancing substances. Since then, the list of drugs and their illicit uses has grown, leading to the creation of the World Anti-Doping Agency (WADA), which regulates and monitors doping in sport.

The National Collegiate Athletic Association (NCAA) has drafted its own policies, and it partners with the National Center for Drug Free Sport ("Drug Free Sport") to administer the program. The NCAA's program is similar to the WADA program in terms of the basic process. For example, athletes can be tested before, during, or after their competitive season. For the NCAA, competitors at championship events or in post-season football should expect to be tested. NCAA member institutions can expect a minimum of one visit per year for drug testing. Athletes must sign a consent form, and an institution or governing body representative must be present at the time of the sampling.

Most sports governing bodies follow a similar protocol. Athletes are generally notified a day in advance for a year-around random drug test. Urine samples are collected in the presence of a certified collector. The sample must be of sufficient volume, specific gravity (i.e., not too dilute), and pH (between 4.5 and 7.5). The sample is split, with at least 60 ml making the "A" sample and 25 ml making the "B" sample. The samples are sealed and given a unique number (no names are used), and everyone involved signs to certify the process. The samples are delivered to a certified testing lab. The "A" sample is used for testing for banned drugs, related compounds, metabolites, and/ or other markers. The lab separates the components by gas or liquid chromatography and identifies them through mass spectrometry. If a test is positive for a banned substance, the institution or regulatory body is notified. The "B" sample is then tested, and if it supports the previous result, the institution is notified and the athlete declared ineligible. Rules for restoration of eligibility vary depending on the governing body. An athlete can be declared ineligible if he or she fails to show up for the test, fails to complete the test, or in any way attempts to alter the validity of the test.

Most drug testing is currently done with urine samples. The sensitivity of the detection techniques is such that some drugs can be detected days to weeks after use. Some anabolic steroids can be detected months after the last dose. This ability to detect low levels of steroids has caused many athletes to switch to human growth hormone in their attempts to gain a competitive edge. Human growth hormone is the most important banned substance that is not currently detectable in urine (more details in Chapter 16). Its detection requires analysis of a blood sample, which increases the complexity and cost of the testing protocol. Human growth hormone is expensive and probably is a greater factor in professional sports than in amateur sports. The labor agreements reached in 2011 for the National Football League (NFL) and Major League Baseball (MLB) allow for the blood testing of human growth hormone. However, implementation was delayed as a result of concerns over a valid protocol for the blood test. WADA developed a validated protocol called the Isoforms Test. The Isoforms Test, performed by all WADA accredited laboratories, was first applied at the 2006 Winter Olympic Games and the 2008 Summer Olympic Games. The NFL has used the Isoforms Test since the 2014 season. The first season had no positive tests though positive tests were reported in 2017. Testing must occur within a day or so of taking human growth hormone for a positive test result. If caught, players are subject to a minimum four-game suspension.

It is currently legal to randomly drug test student athletes in college and high school. About 20% of high schools in the United States have drug testing policies, though many schools use it as a way to discourage students from abusing drugs and alcohol. The availability of PES has increased with access to Internet suppliers, marketing of stimulant-containing beverages, and increasing use of topically applied anabolic androgenic steroids. Multiple studies have prompted concern that the onset of use may be increasing in high school students or younger (LaBotz & Griesemer 2016).

The NCAA and WADA maintain websites that list banned drugs, banned methods or procedures, and exemptions. The classes of banned drugs include stimulants, anabolic agents, diuretics and masking agents, peptide hormones and analogs, anti-estrogens, beta-2 agonists, street drugs, and, for certain sports, alcohol and beta-blockers. Some drugs have a defined concentration limit. For the NCAA, a urine test for caffeine is positive if it is over 15 µg/ml, marijuana is over 15 ng/ml, and testosterone use if the ratio of testosterone to epitestosterone is greater than 6:1. Some compounds are on the WADA Watch List, rather than the Prohibited List. WADA is tracking the levels of these substances among competitors. Testing positive for these substances does not cause disqualification.

Elder Concerns

Earlier in this chapter, there was discussion of sarcopenia and aging as it relates to telomere length. Regular exercise provides the strongest anti-aging remedy known. As we will see in subsequent chapters, exercise also improves outcomes in most chronic diseases. This point should actually be pretty obvious, as anti-aging mechanisms will certainly overlap with the mechanisms that allow exercise to improve health and treat or prevent disease.

Conclusion

Daily cardiovascular exercise and regular resistance training improve health and slow aging. Fitness is based on oxygen distribution and utilization, quantified as VO_2max. Since VO_2max is directly related to heart rate, exercise heart rate provides a relative measure of exercise intensity. Regular exercise causes an increase in stroke volume, improved oxygen utilization, and an increase in VO_2max. Over time, regular exercise causes muscle tissue to adapt. Aging results in loss of muscle tissue called sarcopenia. However, regular exercise can slow the progression of sarcopenia.

When measuring the effect of drugs or supplements on exercise, a double-blind approach helps to eliminate a placebo effect. Urine samples are tested for banned substances both in season and year-round for most competitive athletes. The detection of some drugs may require blood testing.

Key Concepts Review

adenosine triphosphate (ATP)
aerobic metabolism
anaerobic metabolism
blind study
cardiovascular fitness
case-control study
case report
cohort study
double-blind study
evidence pyramid
exercise capacity
exercise intensity
exercise prescription
fast-twitch glycolytic fibers

fast-twitch oxidative fibers
fermentation
glycogenolysis
lipolysis
maximum heart rate
meta-analysis
metabolic syndrome
oxidative phosphorylation
randomized controlled trial
slow-twitch oxidative fibers
substrate-level phosphorylation
systematic review
VO2max

Review Questions

1   Bill is 60 years old and in reasonable shape. Working out on an elliptical machine, Bill sees that his heart rate is 135 bpm. Can you determine his approximate exercise intensity without hooking him to a metabolic cart? What is he burning for energy, primarily?

2   Your mother asks your advice about starting an exercise program. She is in pretty good health, but wants to drop some weight besides improving her cardiovascular health. What kind of exercise plan would you recommend to get started? How would you explain to her the benefits of such a plan? After the initial couple of weeks, would you recommend any changes that might help her with her long-term fitness goals?

3   Compare and contrast the three major muscle fiber types in terms of their metabolism and fuel preference.

4   You are a graduate student working in an exercise physiology lab. You see a claim in a bodybuilding magazine about a supplement that rapidly increases power, strength, and muscle mass. How would you set up an experiment to test whether these claims are true?

5   Obesity is now considered by some to be reaching epidemic proportions. What is contributing to this trend, and what can be done?

References

Ashor AW, Lara J, Siervo M, Celis-Morales C, Oggioni C, Jakovljevic DG, Mathers JC (2015) Exercise modalities and endothelial function: a systematic review and dose-response meta-analysis of randomized controlled trials. *Sports Med* 45:279–296

Basal-Duby RB, Olson EN (2006) Signaling pathways in skeletal muscle remodeling. *Annu Rev Biochem* 75:19–37

Canning KL, Brown RE, Jamnik VK, Salmon A, Ardern CI, Kuk JL (2014) Individuals underestimate moderate and vigorous intensity physical activity. *PLoS One* 9(5):e97927

Cherkas LF, Hunkin JL, Kato BS, Richards JB, Gardner JP, Surdulescu GL, Kimura M, Lu X, Spector TD, Aviv A (2008) The association between physical activity in leisure time and leukocyte telomere length. *Arch Intern Med* 168:154–158

Church TS, Earnest CP, Skinner JS, Blair SN (2007) Effects of different doses of physical activity on cardiorespiratory fitness among sedentary, overweight or obese postmenopausal women with elevated blood pressure. *JAMA* 297:2081–2091

Denham J, Gray AJ, Scott-Hamilton J, Hagstrom AD, Murphy AJ. (2018) Small non-coding RNAs are altered by short-term sprint interval training in men. *Physiol Rep* 6:e13653

Drake JC, Wilson RJ, Yan Z (2016) Molecular mechanisms for mitochondrial adaptation to exercise training in skeletal muscle. *FASEB J* 30:13–22

Dupuy O, Douzi W, Theurot D, Bosquet L, Dugué B (2018) An evidence-based approach for choosing post-exercise recovery techniques to reduce markers of muscle damage, soreness, fatigue, and inflammation: a systematic review with meta-analysis. *Front Physiol* 9:403–418

Fatouros IG (2018) Is irisin the new player in exercise-induced adaptations or not? A 2017 update. *Clin Chem Lab Med* 56: 525–548

Frank P, Andersson E, Pontén M, Ekblom B, Ekblom M, Sahlin K (2016) Strength training improves muscle aerobic capacity and glucose tolerance in elderly. *Scand J Med Sci Sports* 26:764–773

Garber CE, Blissmer B, Deschenes MR, Franklin BA, Lamonte MJ, Lee IM, … Swain DP, American College of Sports Medicine (2011). American College of Sports Medicine position stand. Quantity and quality of exercise for developing and maintaining cardiorespiratory, musculoskeletal, and neuromotor fitness in apparently healthy adults: guidance for prescribing exercise. *Med Sci Sports Exerc* 43:1334–1359

Gaster M, Staehr P, Beck-Nielsen H, Schrøder HD, Handberg A (2001). GLUT4 is reduced in slow muscle fibers of type 2 diabetic patients: is insulin resistance in type 2 diabetes a slow, type 1 fiber disease? *Diabetes* 50:1324–1329

LaBotz M, Griesemer BA, AAP Council on Sports Medicine and Fitness (2016) Use of performance-enhancing substances. *Pediatrics* 138:e20161300

Lewis GD, Farrell L, Wood MJ, Martinovic M, Arany Z, Rowe GC, ... Gerszten RE (2010). Metabolic signatures of exercise in human plasma. *Sci Transl Med* 2:1–13

Moon HY, Becke A, Berron D, Becker B, Sah N, Benoni G, Janke E, Lubejko ST, Greig NH, Mattison JA, Duzel E, van Praag H (2016) Running-induced systemic cathepsin b secretion is associated with memory function. *Cell Metab* 24:332–340

National Collegiate Athletic Association. (n.d.) Drug Testing. www.NCAA.org/health-and-safety/policy/drug-testing

Nes BM, Janszky I, Wisloff U, Stoylen A, Karlsen T (2013). Age-predicted maximal heart rate in healthy subjects: the HUNT fitness study. *Scand J Med Sci Sports* 23:697–704

Nystoriak MA, Bhatnagar A (2018) Cardiovascular effects and benefits of exercise. *Front Cardiovasc Med* 5:135

Safdar A, Tarnopolsky MA (2018) Exosomes as mediators of the systemic adaptations to endurance exercise. *Cold Spring Harb Perspect Med* 8:a029827

Song Z, Ghochani M, McCaffery JM, Frey TG, Chan DC (2009) Mitofusins and OPA1 mediate sequential steps in mitochondrial membrane fusion. *Mol Biol Cell* 20:3525–3532

Tanner CJ, Barakat HA, Dohm GL, Pories WJ, MacDonald KG, Cunningham PRG, ... Houmard JA (2002). Muscle fiber type is associated with obesity and weight loss. *Am J Physiol Endocrinol Metab* 282:E1191–E1196

Trewin AJ, Berry BJ, Wojtovich AP (2018) Exercise and mitochondrial dynamics: Keeping in shape with ROS and AMPK. *Antioxidants (Basel)* 7:7–28

Thomou T, Mori MA, Dreyfuss JM, Konishi M, Sakaguchi M, Wolfrum C, Rao TN, Winnay JN, Garcia-Martin R, Grinspoon SK, et al. (2017) Adipose-derived circulating miRNAs regulate gene expression in other tissues. *Nature* 542: 450–455

Van Loon LJC, Greenhaff PL, Constantin-Teodosiu D, Saris WHM, Wagenmakers AJM (2001). The effects of increasing exercise intensity on muscle fuel utilization in humans. *J Phys* 536:295–304

Werner CM, Hecksteden A, Morsch A, Zundler J, Wegmann M, Kratzsch J, Thiery J, Hohl M, Bittenbring JT, Neumann F, Böhm M, Meyer T, Laufs U (2019) Differential effects of endurance, interval, and resistance training on telomerase activity and telomere length in a randomized, controlled study. *Eur Heart J.* 40:34–46

Whitham M, Parker BL, Friedrichsen M, Hingst JR, Hjorth M, Hughes WE, Egan CL, Cron L, Watt KI, Kuchel RP, Jayasooriah N, Estevez E, Petzold T, Suter CM, Gregorevic P, Kiens B, Richter EA, James DE, Wojtaszewski JFP, Febbraio MA (2018) Extracellular vesicles provide a means for tissue crosstalk during exercise. *Cell Metab* 27:237–251

Wilson JM, Loenneke JP, Jo E, Wilson GJ, Zourdos MC, Kim JS (2012). The effects of endurance, strength, and power training on muscle fiber type shifting. *J Strength Cond Res* 26:1724–1729

World Anti-Doping Agency. (2014). "What We Do." http://www.wada-ama.org/en/World-Anti-Doping-Program/

Yan Z, Okutsu M, Akhtar YN, Lira VA (2011). Regulation of exercise-induced fiber type transformation, mitochondrial biogenesis, and angiogenesis in skeletal muscle. *J Appl Physiol* 110:264–274

3 Autonomic Pharmacology and Stress

Abstract

The autonomic nervous system maintains many of our life-supporting functions. The synapse, whether it is between nerve, muscle, or gland cells, is a central target for drug design. The parasympathetic fibers use acetylcholine as the neurotransmitter and are called cholinergic. The sympathetic fibers use norepinephrine at their terminal synapses and are called adrenergic. Sympathetic fibers also innervate the adrenal medulla, causing the release of adrenaline (mostly epinephrine). Different adrenergic receptor subtypes show tissue-specific distribution and responses. Stimulation of the adrenergic system is part of the fight or flight response and is related to how we respond to stressful situations. The HPA axis is also important in this response, as the potent corticosteroid released from the adrenal cortex also primes many tissues for the survival response. Regular exercise may replace the normal physical activity of our ancestors, which allowed them to cope with challenges to their survival. Sleep is an essential component of good health, as time is needed for the body to repair from the previous day and prepare for the next.

CASE EXAMPLE

Megan keeps running and running, except she no longer actually *runs*. Now that her first child is in first grade, it is a little easier. Megan just turned 29 and thought she was ready for a career, marriage, and kids, but these days she just can't seem to keep up with everything. Every day is filled, tax season is coming, and her job as a CPA always goes crazy this time of year. And now her Dad, Bob, had this 'heart event' and has a couple of stents. She rarely gets a good night's sleep—she can't seem to relax with everything that is happening. The good news is that she and the kids eat pretty healthy. But she has gained some weight and just doesn't feel good about her appearance— which may be affecting her relationship with her husband Brad. She knows what she has to do to combat all the stress in her life—she has made a decision! She will get up an hour earlier than everyone and go for a run. Running always helped in the past. When she was a collegiate soccer player, sleeping was never an issue—though life sure seemed a lot simpler back in college.

Learning Objectives

1 Become familiar with the organization of the nervous system.
2 Distinguish the roles of the parasympathetic and sympathetic nervous systems.
3 Learn the essential features of a synapse.
4 Distinguish the different adrenergic receptor subtypes.
5 Understand the importance of the fight or flight response.
6 Learn the difference between acute and chronic stress.
7 Consider how exercise improves health and combats stress.

Introduction

This chapter will cover basic aspects of the nervous system, with emphasis on exercise and pharmacological applications. We will also look at the stress response and what happens when it does not resolve and becomes chronic. Finally, we will briefly examine the basics of sleep as it relates to maintaining good health.

The Nervous System

Distinctions can be made between the two parts of the nervous system. The **central nervous system (CNS)** generally involves the brain and spinal cord. Since the brain and spinal cord are tightly interconnected, they are often grouped together and referred to as the **cerebrospinal axis**. The **peripheral nervous system (PNS)** generally involves nerves leading to and from the spinal cord. Nerves that transmit output from the cerebrospinal axis are called **efferent fibers**. Nerves that transmit information from the body back to the cerebrospinal axis are called **afferent fibers**. We will concentrate most of our discussion on the efferent pathways, as they are the more relevant pharmacologically and in regard to exercise. They also tend to be better understood than the afferent pathways. The efferent fibers are distinguished as being either voluntary or involuntary.

The Voluntary versus the Involuntary Nervous System

The **voluntary nervous system**, also known as the somatic nervous system, is responsible for voluntary body movement and sensory information processing. The voluntary nervous system includes the **somatic nerves** that synapse in the cerebrospinal axis (the spinal cord) and extend myelinated fibers to skeletal muscles. A **synapse** is where two nerve cells (neurons) form a connection. A grouping of synapses is called a **ganglion**. The myelinated fibers are characterized by **myelin**, an electrically insulating layer that can dramatically speed the transmission of the nerve signals from the brain, which then can get a very quick response by our skeletal muscles. Myelinated somatic fibers, when severed, result in atrophy of the target muscle cells.

The **involuntary nervous system** is also called the **autonomic nervous system (ANS)**. It works without our conscious control of its activities. It is distinguished from the somatic (voluntary) nervous system in many important ways. It innervates smooth muscle, cardiac tissue, and secretory glands—just about everything except skeletal muscle. It controls breathing, digestion, body temperature, sweating, blood pressure, and secretions from glands. The autonomic nervous system forms ganglions outside the spinal cord. The post-ganglionic fibers are not myelinated, so the signaling from the cerebrospinal axis is not as fast as that of the somatic nerves. Curiously, when severed, target organs and glands often maintain some type of spontaneous activity—the central control is lost, however.

Parasympathetic and Sympathetic Nervous Systems

The efferent component of the ANS is divided into two distinct systems, the **parasympathetic nervous system (PSNS)** and the **sympathetic nervous system (SNS)** (see Figure 3.1). The PSNS is relatively limited in its range, extending pre-ganglionic fibers from the cerebrospinal axis to ganglions relatively close to or even within their target tissues; therefore, the post-ganglionic fibers can be very short (see Figure 3.2). The ratio of post-ganglionic fiber number to pre-ganglionic fiber number is close to 1:1 for many targets. The SNS has relatively short pre-ganglionic fibers. The fibers form ganglions close to the spinal cord, and there can be communication between ganglions. Moreover, the post-ganglionic fibers in the SNS are relatively long and can fork and form multiple connections with target tissues (a process called ramification). The ratio of the number of pre-ganglionic fibers to that of post-ganglionic fibers can exceed 1:20. The result of this arrangement is that the sympathetic nervous system has a more diffuse discharge, with possible overlapping transmission of its signals.

Generally, sympathetic innervation dominates cardiovascular function, and parasympathetic innervation dominates urinary and GI functions. The sympathetic innervations of the autonomic nervous system produce ideal effects during the fight or flight response (discussed in detail below). In those organs receiving dual innervation (from both systems), the parasympathetic innervations in some cases produce opposing effects to the sympathetic innervations. For example, in the case of the heart and the iris of the eye, the innervations from the two systems are antagonistic. In other cases, such as the sexual response, they work together.

Figure 3.1 Schematic overview of the nervous system.

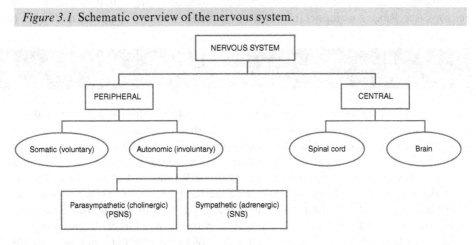

Legend: The relationship between voluntary and involuntary effector nervous systems is shown in schematic form.

Figure 3.2 Comparison of the autonomic and somatic nervous systems.

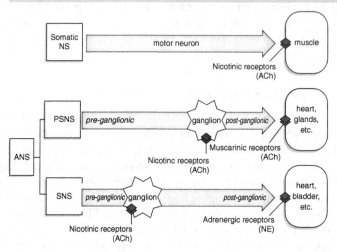

Legend: The autonomic nervous system contains the sympathetic nervous system (SNS) and the parasympathetic nervous system (PSNS). The SNS has short pre-ganglionic fibers and long post-ganglionic fibers. The PSNS has long pre-ganglionic and short post-ganglionic fibers. The somatic nervous system is included for comparison—note the nicotinic receptors at the neuromuscular junction. NE, norepinephrine; Ach, acetylcholine.

Neurotransmitters are chemicals that transmit a signal from one neuron to another neuron or a target cell (discussed in the next section). Acetylcholine is the transmitter at the synapses in the ganglions in both the SNS and PSNS systems; however, different neurotransmitters are released in the two systems at the synapses for the target organs (see Figure 3.2). The chemical nature of the transmitter provides the name for its receptor. Post-ganglionic parasympathetic neurons release acetylcholine and are called **cholinergic** neurons. Post-ganglionic sympathetic neurons release norepinephrine (formerly called noradrenaline) and are called **adrenergic** neurons, for historical reasons (see Box). An important point to be made in terms of pharmacology is that

Adrenaline versus Epinephrine

Adrenergic neurons are so named because they innervate the adrenal medulla and cause the release of adrenaline. Adrenaline's name was changed to epinephrine years ago, but the older nomenclature persists. It is made more confusing with the closely related neurotransmitter called norepinephrine, which was previously called noradrenaline. Many still refer to the hormonal output of the adrenal medulla as **adrenaline** (it is actually about 80:20 epinephrine:norepinephrine) and use the term **epinephrine** (and **norepinephrine**) to distinguish its role at nerve terminals. The term noradrenaline has largely been forgotten. Many of the responses caused by activation of the sympathetic nervous system are similar to the actions of adrenaline on the body (the fight or flight response).

neurotransmitters and their receptors are all potential drug targets. We will discuss this later in the chapter.

The role of the sympathetic nervous system and the adrenal medulla (sympatho-adrenal system) becomes apparent under circumstances of stress. When the body responds to a wide variety of possible stressors, the sympatho-adrenal system plays a critical role in a wide number of responses: the regulation of body temperature, mobilization of glucose, vascular responses under a wide variety of conditions (including exercise), enhanced resistance to fatigue, and other protective responses. The sympatho-adrenal system can discharge as a unit, preparing the body for the fight or flight response. In contrast, the parasympathetic system is more concerned with energy conservation and maintenance of organ function during times of minimal activity. It is organized mainly for discrete and localized discharge. It slows the heart rate and lowers blood pressure. It stimulates secretions and activity in the GI tract to help absorb nutrients. It empties the bladder and rectum and helps protect the retina from excessive light.

Neurotransmission

Nerve cells (neurons) receive and transmit signals. The signals can be transmitted to other nerve cells, muscle cells (neuromuscular junctions), or glands (neuroendocrine junctions). As mentioned earlier, the point where two cells come in close contact is called a synapse. The action potential (i.e., the signal) travels along the axon (the fine extension from the cell body to the target cell) until it reaches the synapse (see Figure 3.3). Here, in order to reach the next cell in the pathway, the signal must cross the synaptic cleft—the space between the two cells. To cross this space, the action potential triggers a membrane depolarization in the pre-synaptic cell (the cell transmitting the signal). The membrane depolarization causes an influx of calcium ions (Ca^{2+}) that trigger the fusion of synaptic vesicles with the pre-synaptic cell's plasma membrane. The contents of the vesicles (neurotransmitters) are released and travel across the cleft to bind and stimulate receptors on the post-synaptic cell (the cell receiving the signal) membrane, triggering an event in the cell and the perpetuation of the signal. If the post-synaptic cell is a neuron, then the signal will continue to the next synapse. If the post-synaptic cell is muscle, it will probably contract; if it is a gland, then the target cells will probably secrete an endocrine factor or hormone. It should be noted that some neurotransmitters have an inhibitory activity that makes the post-synaptic membrane refractory (resistant) to incoming signals for some period of time. The predominant inhibitory neurotransmitter in the mammalian brain is gamma-aminobutyric acid (GABA), a derivative of the amino acid glutamate. Interestingly, glutamate, besides being an amino acid found in proteins, is an important excitatory neurotransmitter in the brain.

The synapse is where most of the action, pharmacologically speaking, takes place. In most cases, the different neurons synthesize and store their particular neurotransmitter; many different transmitters have been identified. Once the transmitter is released, it is subjected to metabolism, or it is taken back up and stored by the pre-synaptic cell. The post-synaptic cell can express different versions of the neurotransmitter receptor, giving rise to a variety of possible biological responses. Pharmacologists take advantage of this fundamental form of communication between cells when they develop drugs. Drugs are designed to:

Figure 3.3 Architecture of a synapse.

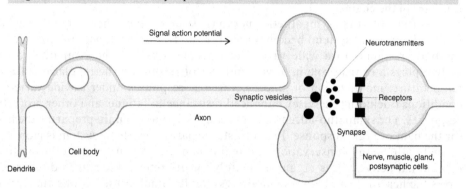

Legend: A highly schematic drawing of a dendrite synapsing at an effector cell, such as another neuron, a muscle cell, or a gland cell. When the action potential arrives at the synapse, the resulting fusion of the synaptic vesicles at the pre-synaptic membrane causes the release of neurotransmitters that diffuse across the synaptic cleft to stimulate receptors in the post-synaptic membrane, thereby perpetuating the signal.

- Affect neurotransmitter synthesis, storage, release, and metabolism.
- Bind the different versions of receptors; they can either block (antagonists) or enhance (agonists) signaling.
- Target downstream events that occur in response to activation of the receptor by the neurotransmitter.

Cholinergic Pharmacology

As discussed previously, acetylcholine is released by post-ganglionic parasympathetic neurons. It is made in the pre-synaptic terminal and released into the synaptic cleft upon signal. Upon release, it rapidly diffuses and activates acetylcholine receptors on the post-synaptic membrane. Termination of acetylcholine involves rapid degradation by the enzyme acetylcholinesterase. There are two major cholinergic receptor subtypes, and their names reflect their selective binding of two different agonists found in nature (refer back to Figure 3.2). Naturally occurring chemical compounds are produced by a large variety of organisms, including plants, fungi, animals, and bacteria. Though chemically complex, many of these natural products are grouped together and called **alkaloids**. Many alkaloids have potent biological activity. Important examples of alkaloids with cholinergic activity include nicotine (from plants) and muscarine (from fungi). Pharmacologists distinguish two major types of cholinergic receptors:

1   *Nicotinic receptors* are located in skeletal muscle endplates (where somatic nerves synapse) and autonomic ganglia (both sympathetic and parasympathetic). The receptors are components of ion channels that respond to acetylcholine or nicotine, causing membrane depolarization and perpetuation of the signal. They do not respond to muscarine. Agonists acting at these sites are "ganglionic" or "neuromuscular" agents.
2   *Muscarinic receptors* are located at synapses innervated by parasympathetic fibers. They respond to acetylcholine and the alkaloid muscarine. There are several

different receptor subtypes, and each is a G-protein–coupled receptor. They are located on autonomic effector cells. Agonists acting at these sites are cholinergic agents, producing a parasympatho*mimetic* effect (mimicking stimulation of the PSNS). Antagonists are anti-cholinergic agents, producing parasympatho*lytic* effects (blocking the effects of the PSNS). Acetylcholine has equivalent affinity for both types of receptors, but certain agonists and antagonists show selectivity.

3   The most commonly used cholinergic drugs are pilocarpine and bethanechol, both of which are muscarinic agonists. Pilocarpine, for example, is often used in patients suffering from glaucoma, because it produces **miosis**—the constriction of the pupil. Bethanechol is used to help manage urinary retention; it stimulates contraction of the bladder muscles to aid expulsion of urine. Pilocarpine and bethanechol have a longer duration of action than acetylcholine because they are poor substrates (substances on which enzymes act) for the enzyme acetylcholinesterase.

Adrenergic Pharmacology

Epinephrine (adrenaline) is released as a hormone from the adrenal medulla. Postganglionic sympathetic neurons release the related compound norepinephrine (once called noradrenaline) as a neurotransmitter. The term *adrenergic* comes from adrenaline. Remember that adrenaline was renamed epinephrine, but the root word has remained.

Adrenergic neurotransmitters are made in nerve terminals. The starting point is the amino acid tyrosine, which in two steps is converted into dopamine (see Figure 3.4). Dopamine is a neurotransmitter, found primarily in the brain. Dopamine can be converted into norepinephrine. Norepinephrine is the predominant neurotransmitter in the ANS and is also used in certain parts of the brain. Norepinephrine is converted into epinephrine in a limited number of neurons and in the adrenal medulla. Epinephrine is released predominantly from the adrenal gland. These compounds are members of a group of related chemicals called **catecholamines**. Whether a cell or nerve ending produces dopamine, norepinephrine, or epinephrine depends on which enzymes in the pathway are expressed. For example, the genes that code for the enzymes dopamine-β-hydroxylase and N-methyltransferase are active in adrenal cells but not in dopaminergic nerves. The result is that adrenal cells make norepinephrine and epinephrine, but dopaminergic cells can only produce dopamine.

Termination of adrenergic transmitters is more complex than termination of the neurotransmitter acetylcholine, which is rapidly degraded by acetylcholinesterase. In the case of adrenergic transmitters, termination of signaling involves re-uptake and metabolism. The re-uptake occurs mostly at the nerve ending or, to a lesser extent, the post-synaptic cell. Diffusion out of the synapse and into the circulation can also occur, with metabolism eventually occurring in liver cells. The diffusion of norepinephrine away from the synapse into the surrounding circulation depends on the level of sympathetic nerve activity. High levels of sympathetic activity increase the amount of norepinephrine that diffuses away from the synapse and can reach additional targets. This effect, called **spillover,** can be observed following intense exercise or high levels of stress—situations when sympathetic activity is elevated. Monoamine oxidase (MAO) and/or catechol-O-methyltransferase (COMT) inactivate the transmitters (Figure 3.4), with MAO playing a more critical role at the synapse.

Adrenergic receptors exist in two major types: α and β. There are two α and three β subtypes. α-1 receptors are localized in arteries and veins and cause constriction. Their

Figure 3.4 Catecholamine biosynthetic pathway.

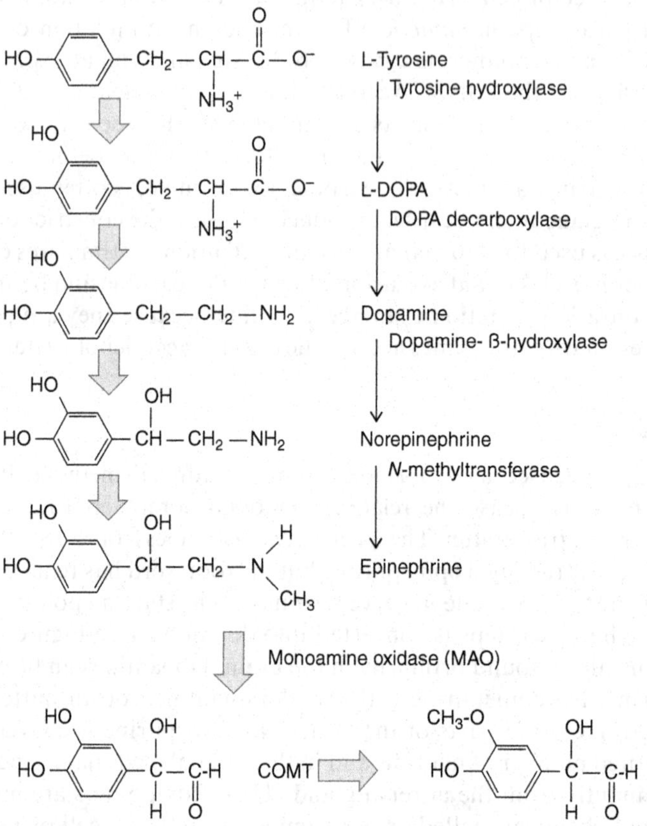

Legend: The pathway for the production of biologically active neurotransmitters is shown. Neurons differ in the terminal enzyme that they express, creating either dopaminergic or norepinergic synapses. Epinephrine is mostly found in the adrenal medulla and a few limited number of nerve endings.

activation increases blood pressure. Vasoconstriction caused by α-1 agonists improves hemostasis at surgical sites. α-1 agonists are also used as decongestants. Norepinephrine and epinephrine have similar affinities on α-receptors. α-2 receptors have been described on pre-synaptic fibers and are considered less pharmacologically important.

β-1 receptors are localized in the heart and other sites (see Table 3.1). Norepinephrine and epinephrine similarly increase heart rate and contractility through β-1 receptors. β-2 receptors are located primarily in the airways and vasculature; they mediate bronchodilation and vasodilation. Epinephrine has a much stronger effect than norepinephrine on β-2 receptors. β-3 receptors have been described more recently with the development of selective agonists (Coman, Păunescu, Ghiţă, et al. 2009). Progress has been slow in describing these "atypical beta receptors" due to limited availability of selective agonists and antagonists, as well as differences in β-3 activity in humans compared to experimental rodents. Based on molecular evidence, β-3 receptors are widely distributed throughout the body, but their functional importance is unclear. They seem to exert influence on metabolic activity. For instance, their presence in brown fat (adipose tissue abundant in hibernating mammals) may involve control of thermogenesis and body temperature (Coman et al.).

Table 3.1 Responses to beta-adrenergic stimulation

Tissue	Effect	Receptor Subtype
Heart	Positive chronotropic effect (increase heart rate)	β-1
	Positive inotropic effect (increase contraction force)	β-1
	Increased automaticity and conduction velocity	β-1
Kidney	Increased renin secretion	β-1
Skeletal muscle	Increased contractility	β-2
	Stimulation of glycogenolysis	β-2
	Stimulation of triglyceride hydrolysis	β-2
	Potassium uptake	β-2
Liver	Stimulation of glycogenolysis	β-2
Lung	Bronchial smooth muscle relaxation	β-2
Vascular smooth muscle	Relaxation	β-2
Bronchiolar smooth muscle	Relaxation	β-2
GI and uterine smooth muscle	Relaxation	β-2
Adipose tissue	Stimulation of lipolysis, thermogenesis	β-3 (β-1, β-2)

Because the response of various effector organs to the differing autonomic innervations is known (see Table 3.2), we can predict the action of drugs that mimic or antagonize the actions of these nerves. Commonly prescribed direct-acting adrenergic agonist drugs, for example, can be specific for the different receptor subtypes (α-1, β-1, and β-2). In contrast, indirectly acting drugs can (1) displace neurotransmitters from storage granules (amphetamine), (2) block re-uptake (cocaine), or (3) block inactivating enzymes (MAO inhibitors). Adrenergic antagonists are available for each receptor subtype (α-1, β-1 or β-2 -blockers). Propranolol (Inderal) is the prototype beta-blocker that is non-selective for β-1 and β-2 receptors and was widely used for hypertension and cardiac arrhythmias; better, more specific drugs are prescribed today. Receptor agonists (i.e., sympathomimetics) and antagonists (i.e., β-blockers) are discussed in more detail in later chapters.

Fight or Flight Response and Stress

Everyone has experienced the adrenaline rush that comes with being frightened (think of the car running off the road, hearing a loud noise in the middle of the night, or coming to bat in the bottom of the ninth with the winning run on third and two outs). Remarkable changes occur to one's physiology. This response, sometimes referred to as the fight or flight response, has been studied extensively. It is an adaptive response

Table 3.2 Responses of various effector organs to innervation from sympathetic and parasympathetic nervous systems

Organ System/Target	Sympathetic Effect (Receptor)	Parasympathetic Effect

Heart
  Sino-atrial node
  Atria
  Atrio-ventricular node
	Accelerates (β1 > β2)
	Increase contractility (β1 > β2)
	Increases conduction (β1 > β2)
		Decelerates
		Decrease contractility
		Decreases conduction

Blood vessels	Constrict (α-1, α-2) Dilate (β-2)	Minimal
Bronchial smooth muscle Bronchial glands	Relaxes (β-2) Decrease secretion (α-1) Increase secretion (β-2)	Contracts Stimulate secretion
GI motility and tone GI secretions	Decrease (α-1, α-2, β-1, β-2) Are inhibited (α-2)	Increase Increase

Skin
  Pilomotor muscle
  Sweat glands
	Contracts (α-1)
	Localized secretion (α-1)
		No effect
		Generalized secretion

Bladder	Relaxes (β-2)	Contracts

Metabolic functions
  Liver
  Liver
  Fat cells
  Kidney
	Gluconeogenesis (β-2, α-1)
	Glycogenolysis (β-2, α-1)
	Lipolysis (β-1, β-2, β-3)
	Renin release (β-1)
		No effect

Eye
  Radial muscle of iris
 	
  Circular muscle of iris
	Contracts (α-1) (mydriasis: pupil dilation)
	No effect
		No effect
		
		Contracts (miosis: pupil contraction)

Legend: Sites of the major innervations of the autonomic nervous system, with the adrenergic receptors indicated; the receptor subtypes are detailed further in Table 3.1. The parasympathetic effects are largely mediated by muscarinic receptors.

that aids in our survival. Whether we are trying to chase down something for dinner or avoiding becoming the dinner of another creature, the physiological and psychological changes that occur help us respond to a wide variety of stressors. The fight or flight response also illustrates the many connections between mind and body.

Fight or Flight Response and the Brain

The fight or flight response involves different regions of the brain. Part of the very rapid response is the brain's telling the adrenal medulla to release adrenaline (epinephrine and norepinephrine). The sympathetic nervous system also prepares the organism to react quickly. An adrenaline surge causes a rapid change in various organ systems, similar to the adrenergic responses mentioned previously. Heart rate and blood pressure increase, blood flow redirects to the muscles, fuel is mobilized

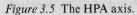
Figure 3.5 The HPA axis.

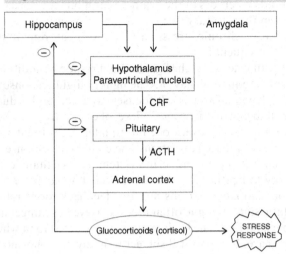

Legend: The major players in the HPA axis are shown. Various regions of the brain affect the release of corticotropin-releasing factor (CRF). CRF stimulates the pituitary gland at the base of the brain to release adrenocorticotropic hormone (ACTH). ACTH travels through the bloodstream to stimulate the adrenal cortex to release compounds called glucocorticoids or corticosteroids. They vary structurally in different species, but they are all very potent hormones with a variety of targets. Some of the negative feedback loops are shown.

(primarily fat and glucose), respiration improves, and even perspiration increases. Blood flow is decreased to the GI-tract, liver, kidneys, and sexual organs.

A slower, maintenance response is also initiated in the brain during a stress event. This response involves the **HPA axis**, so named because it involves the hypothalamus, the pituitary gland, and the adrenal cortex (see Figure 3.5). In this response, the hypothalamus signals the pituitary with corticotropin-releasing factor (CRF) to release adrenocorticotropic hormone (ACTH). ACTH stimulates the adrenal cortex to release glucocorticoids. In humans, the predominant glucocorticoid is cortisol. After a period of time, which can vary depending on the type of stress event, the body returns to its original state. Cortisol binds to sites in the brain and inhibits the release of CRF, leading to a decrease in the release of ACTH. Cortisol also inhibits the release of ACTH, ultimately resulting in a decrease in cortisol levels. Therefore, as cortisol levels rise, new cortisol release eventually becomes inhibited by this negative feedback control mechanism.

Cortisol is a very potent steroid hormone with many diverse functions. It prepares the body for the stressful event, such as by mobilizing fuel. Cortisol causes an increase in levels of blood glucose, as well as fats and amino acids. In pathological conditions, such as Cushing's disease, where cortisol levels remain elevated, the pancreas becomes overworked as it tries to provide enough insulin to compensate for the chronically high level of blood glucose. The result can be diabetes as the pancreas loses its ability to regulate blood sugar levels. Prolonged elevated levels of cortisol also stimulate muscle protein breakdown as a source of fuel. Cortisol can suppress parts of the immune system and decrease inflammation. It is such a strong immunosuppressant that it is often given as a drug (prednisone) for the treatment of inflammation (Chapter 11), diseases of the immune system, or organ transplantation. Similar drugs with glucocorticoid activity are useful for treating asthma (see Chapter 7). Normally, the negative feedback loop works when cortisol binds receptors in the brain and inhibits the release of CRF and the release of ACTH from the pituitary (see Figure 3.5). However, in certain diseases or situations of prolonged or chronic stress, cortisol levels can remain elevated, producing many negative consequences.

During the response to a stressor that activates the fight or flight response, additional neural circuits come into play, which redirect behavior. The fight or flight response increases alertness and causes heightened awareness. It focuses attention and reduces perception of pain. Athletes refer to being in "the zone," a level of concentration where time seems to slow down and injuries can be overlooked until later. Life-threatening situations also trigger this high level of focused attention. The combined responses of the brain, the sympathetic nervous system, the endocrine system, and virtually every organ in the body optimize energy utilization and ready the body for the immediate task—survival. Once the stressor dissipates, various negative feedback loops return the body to its normal, homeostatic state. Fatigue often follows, as well as hunger and thirst, as basic functions come back on line. The brain may remain excited for a while; after all, it just survived a major scare. It is also still subject to many neurohormonal agents, including pain suppressors (e.g., endogenous opioid and cannabinoid molecules, discussed in more detail in Chapter 11) and mood elevators, responsible for a state of mind sometimes described as "runner's high."

Consequences of Chronic Stress

Problems occur when the fight or flight response is prolonged or persistent. Persistent stress is sometime referred to as **allostatic load**, to distinguish the consequences of persistent and possibly pathological levels of stress from the effects of minor stressful events. Our ability to deal with stress is part of normal adaptive behavior. Most of the time, we just cope with whatever has caused the event. However, if we become overstressed, these same physiological changes can extend for prolonged periods of time and become unhealthy. Constant worries about money, jobs, relationships, and so forth can create a pathological condition resulting from prolonged overactivation of many of the same physiological systems involved in the fight or flight response.

Extensive study of the effect of stress on health dates back to Hans Selye's work in the 1930s. For example, overstressed rats have larger adrenal glands, GI ulcers, muscle atrophy, and a suppressed immune system. The effect of allostatic load has also been extensively studied in humans (McEwen 1998). Most of the problems associated with chronic stress can be traced to an overactive adrenal cortex and medulla, and the consequences of elevated levels of cortisol and adrenaline. Additional endocrine systems are affected by chronic stress, including growth hormone, thyroid hormone, and gonadal hormones (Tsatsoulis & Fountoulakis 2006).

Humans who are overstressed complain of sleep disorders, muscle aches, headaches, and fatigue. They may have high blood pressure and an elevated heart rate. The response to stress is in itself stressful and can perpetuate the unhealthy condition. Overstressed individuals also often complain of depression, anxiety, nervousness, or irritability. Many of these people self-medicate with alcohol, smoke cigarettes, or experience binges of overeating. They may overuse prescription medications or illegal street drugs. Physicians and researchers have argued for decades that many of the diseases plaguing modern-day humans can be explained by overactivity of the adrenal gland brought on by prolonged stress (Tsatsoulis & Fountoulakis). Continued, elevated levels of potent cortisol and adrenaline can disrupt biorhythms and create havoc with neurohormonal feedback loops, disrupting homeostatic mechanisms. For instance, stress may contribute to migraine headaches, asthma, difficulty in regulating blood glucose in diabetics, hypertension, anxiety, depression, and drug abuse. Prolonged elevated cortisol can be toxic to nerves in the hippocampus, causing memory disorders and cognitive impairment (Sapolsky 2000). Stress-induced elevation of CRF in parts of the brain can contribute to the detrimental effects of an unresolved stress response (Stern 2011).

Stress can modulate the gut microbiome (discussed in Chapter 1), which, in turn, can modify the host stress response and affect host health. A wide variety of stressors (psychological stress, circadian disruption, sleep deprivation, noise, physical activity, and diet) alter the composition, function and metabolic activity of the gut microbiota, including beneficial or detrimental effects on host health (Karl, Hatch, Arcidiacono, et al. 2018). Hopefully in the near future, the gut microbiome can be manipulated to mitigate adverse stress responses by using a nutritional approach.

Although the influence stress plays in many human disorders is open to debate, its influence is important to keep in mind when we consider drug therapy for some of the previously mentioned physical conditions. Finding and dealing with sources of stress can have therapeutic benefit, and any drug therapy should take this into account.

Exercise and Stress

Stressors, those things that cause stress, can range widely and differ for different people. Different stressors can be distinguished. **Threat stress** causes fearfulness, distress, and feelings of being overwhelmed and not in control. There is increased HPA activity and often an increased appetite, especially in children. In contrast, **challenge stress** results from an event like an oral presentation, an exam, or a race. Challenge stress can be a good stress, because it is something we can tackle and overcome. When faced with a challenge, the brain finds a solution to meet it. A challenge stressor increases SNS activity and can decrease appetite.

Exercise causes changes in the body similar to those caused by a challenge stress, not the types of changes observed with allostatic load. These physiological changes primarily involve the adrenergic response; they are similar in many ways to the effects of the fight or flight response. The increase in adrenergic activity causes activation of α and β receptors and the responses listed in Table 3.2. The heart increases its rate and force of contraction, while the vasculature redirects blood flow to muscle and limits flow to less critical organs. Epinephrine and norepinephrine increase in the blood markedly during exercise, ranging from 1.5 to 20 times basal concentrations, depending on duration and intensity (Zouhal, Jacob, Delamarche, Gratas-Delamarche 2008). Besides the cardiovascular and respiratory adjustments, they mobilize energy substrate utilization. Besides making up about 20% of the catecholamines released from the adrenal medulla, norepinephrine can 'spillover' as exercise intensity increases. Since norepinephrine is the predominant adrenergic neurotransmitter, as ANS activity increases, norepinephrine can diffuse from synaptic sites and enter the bloodstream. Norepinephrine is also very active in certain brain regions involved in the stress response, where it modulates the action of other prevalent neurotransmitters that play a more direct role (Zouhal et al.).

The HPA response is complex due to inputs from different regions of the brain. Threat stressors can be uncontrolled and involuntary, and associated with levels of fear. Exercise is generally controlled and voluntary, but it also involves a demand for energy. As exercise intensity or duration increases, this energy demand creates a challenge to homeostasis, triggering the HPA axis to respond. For many individuals, the threshold for response occurs over about 60% VO_2max or after about 90 minutes at lower intensities. Level of fitness is important, as physically fit individuals have a reduced HPA output at similar exercise intensities (Luger, Deuster, Kyle, et al. 1987; Duclos, Corcuff, Rashedi, et al. 1997).

The HPA response has neuronal, hormonal, and inflammatory components following release of glucocorticoids (cortisol in humans) from the adrenal cortex (Sapolsky, Romero, & Munck 2000). During intense exercise, cortisol works to help the body meet the energy demands and prepare muscle cells for more work if needed. It stimulates the liver to make glucose (a process called gluconeogenesis), helps muscle cells consolidate glycogen reserves, and helps to maintain normal vascular integrity and responsiveness. It also helps keep muscle cell inflammation in check and protects against an overreaction of the immune system to exercise-induced muscle damage. When challenged, whether by exercise or a stressful situation, individuals who are physically fit release less cortisol (Figure 3.6), show less cardiovascular activation, and recover from cardiovascular activity faster than their less fit counterparts (Rimmele, Seiler, Marti, et al. 2009; see Box for details). Cortisol levels return to normal after about two hours in both trained and untrained individuals following exercise or situations causing acute stress (Duclos et al.).

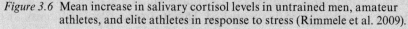

Figure 3.6 Mean increase in salivary cortisol levels in untrained men, amateur athletes, and elite athletes in response to stress (Rimmele et al. 2009).

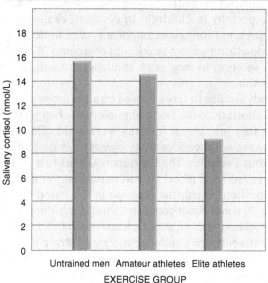

Legend: Subjects were asked to perform five minutes of public speaking and five minutes of solving math problems out loud in front of observers and cameras. The subjects were grouped based on their levels of regular physical activity: Untrained men (n = 24), Regular joggers (Amateur athletes, n = 50), and Marathon runners (Elite athletes, n = 18). Values are the mean absolute increase in salivary cortisol. P = 0.01 for comparison of elite to untrained men; the difference between untrained and amateur men is not significant.

Does Level of Fitness Help in Dealing with Stress?

Are regular exercisers better equipped to deal with stress? Do professional athletes show the same stress response as untrained individuals? If the stressor is competition related, similar to an athlete's specialty, then his or her HPA response may be tempered, but the cardiovascular response may be heightened. What about the response of regular exercisers and elite athletes to a psychosocial stressor? A study by Rimmele and colleagues (2009) examined this problem. They compared elite athletes (marathon-level runners), amateur athletes (regular joggers), and untrained men. The stressor included public speaking in front of strangers and cameras (a simulated job interview) and solving math problems out loud. The researchers monitored cortisol levels in saliva to determine the HPA response and heart rate for the sympathetic response. All participants showed worsened mood with an increased state of anxiety. Interestingly, the elite athletes had a significantly blunted cortisol response, whereas the amateur and untrained men were indistinguishable in their responses (see Figure 3.6). Moreover, the elite and amateur athletes both had reduced heart rates relative to the untrained men.

Psychological stress has been proposed as a major contributor to the progression of cardiovascular disease. Combined stress (psychological and physical) can exacerbate these cardiovascular responses, which may contribute to mortality risks experienced by some occupations (e.g., firefighting and law enforcement) (Huang, Webb, Zourdos, & Acevedo 2013). Physical activity provides benefit for the cardiovascular response to acute stress. It has immediate psychological benefits relative to other therapeutic treatments and is an effective adjuvant therapy for depression and anxiety (more details in Chapter 9). Aerobically trained individuals exhibit lower sympathetic nervous system activity (e.g., heart rate and blood pressure) and improved recovery time in response to physical and/or psychological stress. Resistance training also attenuates cardiovascular responses and improves mental health. This enhanced functionality may facilitate a reduction in the incidence of stroke and myocardial infarction (Huang et al.).

Aerobic exercise training helps protect against ROS-induced lipid peroxidation and decreases the occurrence of ROS-associated diseases such as Alzheimer's disease. Regular exercise is beneficial in up-regulating the protection against oxidative stress. The immune system adapts positively to physical activity. Physical fitness elicits a more resilient immune defense and greater protection from stress. In response to acute psychological stress, improved physical fitness is associated with diminished pro-inflammatory responses. The diminished pro-inflammatory response occurs following aerobic exercise or resistance exercise. In particular, this response to resistance training is a component of the repeated bout effect—when the same resistance exercise is performed subsequently, the damage response in muscle is attenuated. Release of immunoregulators (e.g., cytokines) during recovery lessens during chronic training, providing an explanation for the reduction in the stress response following resistance training. However, over-training increases cortisol, produces signs of the stress response, and can decrease performance. Over-training results when insufficient time is allowed for recovery between intense bouts of exercise.

Repeated exposure to a stressor, such as exercise, will produce an adaptive response to stressors in general. Regular exercise helps buffer acute and chronic responses to stress. This property supports the cross-stressor hypothesis. Because the body is regularly exposed to this 'good' stressor, it has a lower stress response in general and is more efficient at dealing with stress. Higher levels of other stressors or threat are needed to release similar amounts of stress hormones. Exercise seems to give the body a chance to practice dealing with stress. The more sedentary we get, the less efficient our bodies become in responding to stress.

The body's response to stress and exercise is obviously very complex and involves many physiological, biochemical, and psychological processes. Since exercise is one of the best-established ways of coping with stress and preventing stress-related diseases, many theories attempt to explain how this may work:

- Exercise is known to improve a person's quality of sleep and relaxation (more details below). Quality sleep is essential for many aspects of good health, and regular exercise can help combat stress-induced sleep disorders. Relaxation following exercise can counter the muscle tension that is associated with stress.
- Parasympathetic nerve activity increases during recovery after exercise and helps decrease heart rate and blood pressure.
- Regular exercisers are more fit and release lower levels of the stress hormones.
- Resistance training can lead to lower resting levels of cortisol.
- Exercise can provide an outlet for anger or anxiety.
- Exercise can provide quiet time for inner solitude and introspection.
- Exercise that extends for 20 minutes or more can release significant amounts of endorphins, cannabinoids, and other neurochemicals. These substances produce analgesia and a sense of euphoria—"runner's high."
- Regular exercise contributes to improved self-esteem and feelings of self-worth.

The fight or flight response is an important adaptive survival response, deeply rooted in our biology. However, modern-day stress often does not result in physical activity, either fight or flight. Today, most of the stress is psychosocial. Our bodies still undergo these massive biochemical shifts and still contain all of these circulating factors in response to stress, but our activity level often is minimal. The body prepares for physical challenges that never occur. It mobilizes glucose and other nutrients that it doesn't burn. The byproducts of the response build up and have deleterious effects, especially with prolonged stress and high allostatic load. Regular exercise simulates the physical component of the fight or flight response. The byproducts of stress are metabolized and the body returns to homeostatic balance faster, reducing the negative consequences of psychosocial stress (Huang et al.; Tsatsoulis & Fountoulakis). Physically fit individuals withstand the effects of stress better than unfit individuals. They have lower levels of the stress hormones (norepinephrine, epinephrine, and cortisol) than unfit individuals at comparable exercise intensities, resulting in lower heart rate and blood pressure. Regular exercise can reduce the allostatic load. An exerciser who says something like "Got to go sweat out the toxins" might not be far from the truth.

Sleep and the Role of Exercise

Sleep is a highly conserved behavior across animal evolution. It is characterized by relatively suppressed sensory activity (a higher threshold needed to gain attention), inhibition of most voluntary muscles, and altered consciousness. The internal circadian clock promotes sleep each night. Prolactin is secreted during sleep, and during deep sleep, growth hormone is released in bursts. Sleep alternates between two distinct modes: non-REM sleep and REM sleep. REM stands for "rapid eye movement," and REM sleep is a distinct behavioral state from non-REM sleep (discussed below). During sleep, the body is essentially in an anabolic state, restoring the immune system and most tissues. Sleep is vital to maintain mood, memory, and cognitive function. It is also important in maintaining body weight. Humans suffer from a diverse collection of sleep disorders. Some disorders may involve artificial light (not an issue with our ancestors) or blue light from computer and phone screens.

Sleep has its most profound effect on the brain. Non-REM sleep occurs first, transitioning through three phases—N1, N2, and N3. N1 is the transitional period, sometimes called Relaxed Wakefulness. It is relatively brief. N2 is light sleep and can make up almost half of the total sleep period. N3 is characterized as slow-wave or deep sleep, also called delta sleep. During this phase, body temperature and heart rate fall, and the brain uses less energy. The cycle of alternate non-REM and REM sleep takes an average of 90 minutes, occurring four to six times in a good night's sleep of about eight hours. The cycle usually proceeds in the order: N1 → N2 → N3 → N2 → REM. REM sleep consists of a smaller portion of total sleep time, and is characterized by desynchronized and fast brain waves besides the rapid eye movement. Dreams occur during REM sleep. There is a greater amount of deep sleep earlier in the night, while the proportion of REM sleep increases in the two cycles just before natural awakening.

Sleep loss negatively affects exercise performance and the physiological response to exercise (Fullagar, Skorski, Duffield, et al. 2015). Certain tests of maximal physical effort or gross motor performance can be maintained following sleep loss. However, sleep loss can cause slower cognitive function and less accurate cognitive performance in sport-specific functions. Poorer sleep quality and quantity can produce an autonomic nervous system imbalance, mimicking over-training syndrome. Moreover, increases in pro-inflammatory cytokines following sleep loss could promote immune system dysfunction and negatively impact the recovery process to exercise (Fullagar et al.).

How might exercise improve sleep? As discussed in Chapter 2, mitochondria use a lot of oxygen to make ATP, and generate many free radicals (Reactive Oxygen Species—ROS) as a result. The byproducts of mitochondrial activity create 'oxidative stress,' and oxidative stress affects lifespan, aging, and degenerative disease. With physical activity and training, this oxidative stress triggers repair and adaptive responses (discussed in Chapter 2). However, a key feature in this process is the need for sufficient quality sleep. Disruption in sleep can increase oxidative stress, as can a poor-quality diet and environmental chemicals. Antibiotic treatment or drugs for acid reflux can alter the gut microbiome and contribute to oxidative stress, as does prolonged high blood sugar levels and excess weight. Oxidative stress takes a toll on nerves, blood vessels, eyes, skin, muscle, and causes us to age.

Oxidative stress helps regulate sleep and provides a link between chronic lack of sleep and shorter lifespans. Sleep provides a recovery process for stress and oxidative stress. Without it, stress and oxidative stress add up, damaging mitochondria, nerves, and blood vessels. During deep sleep, repair mechanisms such as autophagy activate; growth hormone and other hormones are released that stimulate tissue repair. Repair takes time. Not enough time leads to accumulated cell damage, potential cancer cells not being eliminated by monitoring systems, and signs of aging. Not only is fatigue likely from too little sleep, but there is also potential for memory loss, weight gain, and increased sensitivity to pain.

Studies in fruit flies have linked oxidative stress and sleep (Kempf, Song, Talbot, et al. 2019). Oxidative stress influences sleep-control neurons which act as on/off switches in flies and probably other animals including humans. If the neurons are electrically active, the fly is asleep; when they are silent, the fly is awake. This activity is regulated via two antagonistic potassium channels named Sandman and Shaker. Increased current through Shaker supports sleep and increased current though Sandman produces wakefulness. The oxidized status of the coenzyme NADP/NADPH regulates Shaker current. As oxidative stress increases over the course of the day, the oxidative state (NADP) increases relative to the reduced state (NADPH), the Shaker potassium current increases, and sleep is promoted (Kempf et al.). After sleeping, NADPH levels are re-established, Sandman activity increases relative to Shaker, and wakefulness is promoted. The result is that sleep occurs when energy metabolism and mitochondrial function need time to recover; exercise or physical activity contributes to reaching the point to initiate sleep.

Elder Concerns

Older adults can be more susceptible to stress and its harmful effects. Some individuals define themselves by their career and do not handle retirement well. The elderly may feel like a burden to their family or that they do not feel needed. They fear the loss of independence, such as not being able to live independently or continue driving. With increasing age and decreasing health, they can lose control over their daily routines. Healthcare costs and managed care can cause considerable stress over money. Older people outlive their spouse, other family members, friends, and pets, increasing their sense of isolation. They usually have heart issues, digestive problems, hearing and vision loss, and dental issues—all contributing factors to a decrease in physical activity. The immune system also loses its responsiveness, making them more susceptible to viruses (i.e., COVID-19) and other infectious agents.

Aging weakens the body's ability to respond to stress, possibly due to the inability to terminate the production of glucocorticoid in response to stress. The elderly are less responsive in regions of the brain responsible for shutting off glucocorticoid production following a stressful event. The elevated cortisol levels can contribute to the suppressed immune system found in the elderly population. The effect of aging on the immune system is an area of active investigation and outside the scope of this chapter. Briefly, aging can decrease the number and function of T cells, contributing to a poorer immune response. There is reduction in the production of cytokines, the molecular communicators of the immune response. Neutrophils from elderly donors have poorer phagocytic function and diminished ability to fight off infections, such as pneumonia. Age-related changes and stress can affect many hormonal systems, including sex steroid production. Some sex steroids provide immune protection, but their effect can be overcome with elevated glucocorticoid levels (Vitlic et al. 2014).

To combat stress, the elderly need to maintain a regular exercise program that suits their current state of health. They need to eat a well-balanced diet and maintain their social connections. Learning and practicing relaxation techniques and meditation can help reduce stress and help them focus on things they can control and still enjoy doing.

Conclusion

The autonomic nervous system maintains many of our life-supporting functions. The synapse, whether it is between nerve, muscle, or gland cells, is a central target for drug design. Sympathetic fibers also innervate the adrenal medulla, causing the release of adrenaline, part of the fight or flight response. Corticosteroid released from the adrenal cortex also primes many tissues for the survival response. Regular exercise helps us cope with stress. Sleep is an essential component of good health, as time is needed for the body to repair from the previous day and prepare for the next.

Key Concepts Review

adrenaline
adrenergic
afferent fiber
alkaloid
autonomic nervous system (ANS)
catecholaminecentral nervous system (CNS)
cerebrospinal axis
cholinergic
efferent fiber
epinephrine
ganglion

HPA axis
involuntary nervous system
myelin
neurotransmitterparasympathetic nervous system (PSNS)
peripheral nervous system (PNS)
somatic nerve
spillover
sympathetic nervous system (SNS)
synapse
voluntary nervous system
threat stress and challenge stress

Review Questions

1   Compare and contrast the sympathetic and parasympathetic nervous systems.
2   What is meant by allostatic load, and how does it differ from stressing over a single test?
3   Explain three ways drugs can affect the signals transmitted by nerve cells.
4   How might exercise lessen the effects of stress?
5   Describe some of the theories that attempt to explain the body's paradoxical response to exercise.
6   What are the key physiological changes that occur during the fight or flight response? How do they help in survival?

References

Coman OA, Păunescu H, Ghiţă I, Coman L, Bădărăru A, Fulga I (2009) Beta 3 adrenergic receptors: molecular, histological, functional and pharmacological approaches. *Romanian J Morph Embryol* 50:169–179

Duclos, M, Corcuff J-B, Rashedi M, Fougere V, Manter G (1997) Trained versus untrained men: different immediate post-exercise responses of the pituitary adrenal axis: A preliminary study. *Eur J Appl Physiol* 75:343–350

Fullagar HH, Skorski S, Duffield R, Hammes D, Coutts AJ, Meyer T (2015) Sleep and athletic performance: the effects of sleep loss on exercise performance, and physiological and cognitive responses to exercise. *Sports Med* 45:161–186

Huang C-J, Webb HE, Zourdos MC, Acevedo EO (2013) Cardiovascular reactivity, stress, and physical activity. *Frontiers Physiol* 4:1–13

Karl JP, Hatch AM, Arcidiacono SM, Pearce SC, Pantoja-Feliciano IG, Doherty LA, Soares JW (2018) Effects of psychological, environmental and physical stressors on the gut microbiota. *World J Diabetes* 9:138–140

Kempf A, Song SM, Talbot CB, Miesenböck G (2019) A potassium channel β-subunit couples mitochondrial electron transport to sleep. *Nature* doi: 10.1038/s41586-019-1034-5. [Epub ahead of print]

Luger A, Deuster PA, Kyle SB, Gallucci WT, Montgomery LC, Gold PW, Loriaux DL, Chrousos GP (1987) Acute hypothalamic-pituitary-adrenal responses to the stress of treadmill exercise. *New Engl J Med* 316:1309–1315

McEwen BS (1998) Stress, adaptation, and disease: allostasis and allostatic load. *Annal NY Acad Sci* 840:33–44

Rimmele U, Seiler R, Marti B, Wirtz PH, Ehlert U, Heinrichs M (2009) The level of physical activity affects adrenal and cardiovascular reactivity to psychosocial stress. *Psychoneuroendocrinology* 34:190–198

Sapolsky RM (2000) Glucocorticoids and hippocampal atrophy in neuropsychiatric disorders. *Arch Psychiatry* 57:925–935

Sapolsky RM, Romero L, Munck AU (2000) How do glucocorticoids influence stress responses? Integrating permissive, suppressive, stimulatory, and preparative actions. *Endo Rev* 21:55–89

Stern CM (2011) Corticotropin-releasing factor in the hippocampus: eustress or distress? *J Neurosci* 31:1935–1936

Tsatsoulis A, Fountoulakis S (2006) The protective role of exercise on stress system dysregulation and comorbidities. *Ann NY Acad Sci* 1083:196–213

Vitlic A, Lord JM, Phillips AC (2014) Stress, ageing and their influence on functional, cellular and molecular aspects of the immune system. *Age (Dordr)* 36: 9631.

Zouhal H, Jacob C, Delamarche P, Gratas-Delamarche A (2008) Catecholamines and the effects of exercise, training and gender. *Sports Med* 38:401–423

Section II

Cardiovascular and Respiratory Drugs

4 Beta-Blockers and Cardiovascular Disease

Abstract

There is continued debate over whether monotherapy with beta-blockers is recommended for hypertension and other forms of cardiovascular disease. Several large clinical trials suggest that beta-blockers may not be as effective as other drugs (or drug combinations) in preventing severe cardiovascular events. However, beta-blockers remain widely prescribed for many types of cardiovascular disease, including congestive heart failure, coronary artery disease, angina, arrhythmia, and hypertension. They are often prescribed in combination with other drugs for hypertension and cardiovascular disease, particularly diuretics.

The hemodynamic, metabolic, and ion balance effects of beta-blockers on exercise have been studied extensively. Less information is available on the newer, third-generation drugs, as these drugs have been widely available in the United States only since the early 2000s. The third-generation drugs may have improved profiles of exercise-related effects, but most beta-blockers decrease exercise heart rate, blood pressure, and cardiac output. Beta-blockers make it difficult to use target heart rate effectively as a measure of exercise intensity. In highly fit individuals, beta-blockers may cause bradycardia. Beta-blockers, especially the non-cardioselective beta-blockers, have ergolytic effects on aerobic exercise. They affect lipid utilization and blood sugar regulation, making their use in diabetics restricted. Exercise should still be encouraged for people with cardiovascular disease, even those who are taking beta-blockers, as exercise-dependent improvements in cardiovascular health are still observed.

CASE EXAMPLE

Megan's 64-year-old mom, Wilma, needs to have her right knee replaced. Wilma was a good athlete in her own right, back in the 70s, when Title IX started to change the landscape for girl's and woman's athletics. She was a good volleyball player and kept playing on beaches and rec centers until tearing her ACL. Now everything she does causes her knee to ache—so she has agreed to have it replaced. The orthopedic surgeon requires a pre-op medical evaluation a month in advance of her procedure. An EKG is part of this evaluation. Electrocardiography (EKG or ECG) is a painless, non-invasive procedure that records the heart's electrical activity and can help diagnose arrhythmias. An arrhythmia is a condition in which the heart beats too quickly, too slowly, or irregularly. Wilma is diagnosed with atrial fibrillation, an arrhythmia distinguished by a fast and irregular heart rhythm. In her case, the two chambers in the upper part of the heart (atria) are beating a little too fast and out of sync with the lower chambers (ventricles). The result is a fast and very irregular heartbeat. A-fib is fairly common and the odds of having it increase with age. It helps explain why she sometimes felt dizzy or out of breath just going up some stairs. Her doctor prescribes a beta-blocker. Beta-blockers are prescribed when the heart rate needs to be slowed and for irregular heartbeats (palpitations), angina (chest pain), and high blood pressure. Wilma's A-fib is not too serious, but must be managed before her operation. She will need a follow up EKG and other heart testing before getting her new knee.

Learning Objectives

1   Consider the importance of cardiovascular disease worldwide.
2   Understand the basics of heart function.
3   Understand the causes and progression of cardiovascular disease.
4   Learn how beta-blockers exert their effect.
5   Distinguish how the various classifications of beta-blockers work.
6   Understand how exercise can lower the risk of heart disease.
7   Learn how beta-blockers affect exercise performance.
8   Learn why beta-blockers are banned for certain types of competition.

Introduction

Diseases of the cardiovascular system are a major cause of death worldwide. The next three chapters will deal with drugs that treat different aspects of cardiovascular disease. In this chapter, we will focus on the class of drugs called beta-blockers and how they affect the function of the heart and why they are used to treat cardiovascular disease. Beta-blockers are widely prescribed, though they are no longer considered a 'first line' drug for high blood pressure. Many people continue to take beta-blockers for high blood pressure, though often in combination with other drugs or because they have additional symptoms amenable to beta-blocker treatment. In Chapter 5, we will look more closely at high blood pressure (hypertension) and its treatment. We will explore drugs that modulate the renin-angiotensin regulatory loop and a class of drugs called calcium channel blockers. In Chapter 6 we will examine diuretics, drugs that work in the kidney to control water and electrolyte balance. Diuretics continue to be one of the first-line agents for the treatment of hypertension.

In Chapter 3, we discussed the sympathetic nervous system, the fight-or-flight response, and how chronic stress can increase heart rate and blood pressure. Adrenergic signaling is a central component of these complex responses. Drugs were discovered that had beta-receptor antagonist activity, and these drugs were effective at modulating or treating problems associated with adrenergic-dependent responses. These beta-receptor antagonists became commonly known as **beta-blockers**. Beta-blockers were routinely prescribed for hypertension, although the results from several large clinical studies have questioned their widespread use (Che, Schreiber, & Rafey 2009). Evidence-based guidelines from the Eighth Joint National Committee have also de-emphasized the use of beta-blockers as a first-line agent for hypertension (JNC 8 2014). Unfortunately, 75% of the large-scale trials that questioned whether beta-blockers provide an effective treatment used the beta-blocker atenolol (Ripley & Saseen 2014), which was introduced in 1976. The use of beta-blockers for hypertension in other countries such as Canada continues to be discussed (Poirier & Tobe 2014). Many newer beta-blockers are available with properties that differ from atenolol.

Clinically, beta-blockers are generally well tolerated. Newer beta-blockers with vasodilatory properties may have even fewer unwanted effects and improve endothelial cell function—the cells that form the lining of blood vessels and regulate vessel activity. Beta-blockers are widely prescribed, and millions of people take them for hypertension, especially individuals with co-morbidities such as angina or arrhythmias. We will briefly cover heart function and coronary artery disease, arrhythmias, and heart failure. Patients suffering from cardiovascular disease are often treated with a drug or combination of drugs that works best for their condition. Beta-blockers and the other major classes of drugs in this section are used to help control blood pressure, heart function, and fluid volume, all critical in the management of cardiovascular disease.

Exercise physiologists and pharmacologists have studied beta-blockers extensively over the last 50 years, and much is known about their effect on exercise performance. There are antagonists specific for each receptor subtype, making these drugs of great utility for researchers to tease out how different tissues respond to epinephrine and norepinephrine—or the adrenaline rush of the fight-or-flight response. The beta-blockers have been wonderful tools to understand the role of the sympathetic nervous system during exercise.

The Basics of Heart Function

As you may remember from anatomy or physiology classes, the heart is a complex pump divided into the right and the left side, essentially to keep oxygen-rich blood from mixing with oxygen-poor blood (Figure 4.1). Each side has an **atrium** to collect the blood and a **ventricle** to pump the blood to its destination. The right atrium collects oxygen-poor blood that has circulated through the body, and the right ventricle pumps that blood to the lungs through the pulmonary arteries. The lungs oxygenate the blood and return it to the left atrium. The left ventricle pumps this blood throughout the body to supply tissues with oxygen and nutrients. Four valves within the heart keep the blood moving in the correct direction, from chamber to chamber. Each valve opens and closes once per heartbeat.

During a heartbeat, muscle cells relax to fill and contract to pump. Relaxation is called **diastole** and contraction is called **systole**. During diastole, the left and right ventricles relax and fill with blood coming from the upper chambers, the matching left and right atria. During systole, the ventricles contract and pump blood to the lungs or body, with the right ventricle contracting a little bit before the left ventricle. The ventricles then relax and fill with blood coming from the atria, and the cycle repeats. Electrical impulses keep the heart beating in a rhythmic fashion. A signal conduction system begins high in the right atrium and travels through specialized pathways to the ventricles, so the heart beats with a coordinated rhythm (Figure 4.1). The **pacemaker** high in the right atrium is called the **sinoatrial (SA) node**. The pacemaker creates the rhythmic impulses necessary for heartbeats. Modified cardiac cells in the SA node trigger cardiac contraction following input from the parasympathetic and sympathetic nervous systems, although the pacemaker activity can independently generate 60 to 100 beats per minute. The **atrioventricular (AV) node** electrically connects the atria to the ventricles. The wave of contraction started in the SA node activates the AV node to cause contraction of the ventricles after the atria have emptied. A properly

Figure 4.1 Blood flow through the heart.

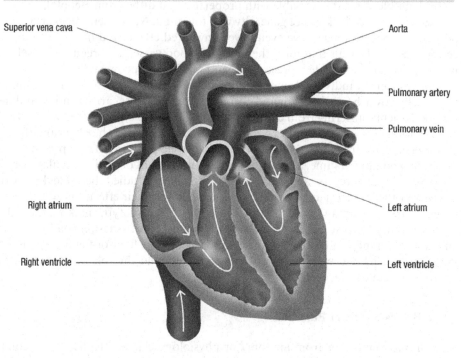

Superior vena cava

Aorta

Pulmonary artery

Pulmonary vein

Right atrium

Left atrium

Right ventricle

Left ventricle

Legend: The direction of blood flow is indicated by the arrows.

functioning heart provides the exchange of oxygen-poor blood for oxygen-rich blood and distributes it throughout the body.

Causes of Cardiovascular Disease

The term *cardiovascular disease* can refer to many different types of heart or blood vessel problems, often resulting from damage to the heart or blood vessels.

Arteriosclerosis

Healthy arteries are flexible and strong. As we age, our artery walls can become thick and stiff. This process is called **arteriosclerosis**, or hardening of the arteries. During arteriosclerosis, as artery walls thicken, become stiff, and lose their elasticity, blood flow becomes restricted to tissues and organs. Arteriosclerosis may occur in any artery of the body, but the disease is most serious when it attacks the coronary arteries, which feed the heart with oxygen and nutrients. Decreased blood flow through the coronary arteries can cause a heart attack.

The most common type of arteriosclerosis is called **atherosclerosis**, which is caused by plaque buildup in a blood vessel. Plaques result from the accumulation of fats, cholesterol, and other substances in and on artery walls. When this buildup occurs, atherosclerotic vessels lose their flexibility and flow capacity. Plaques are a source of inflammation, which can also decrease vessel function, and they can become unstable and trigger a blood clot. Clot formation and inflammation can severely restrict blood flow and cause a cardiac event. Atherosclerosis is preventable in many cases (e.g., a better diet and exercise) and is treatable with drugs (discussed more in Chapter 10). However, acute cases can require insertion of stents or by-pass surgery.

The major risk factors for cardiovascular disease are conditions and behaviors that contribute to atherosclerosis, including untreated hypertension, an unhealthy diet, a lack of exercise, and cigarette smoking. Figure 4.2 shows a simplified flow diagram of events leading up to heart failure.

Angina

If blood flow to the heart is compromised, so that heart tissue lacks a sufficient source of oxygenated blood, chest pains (**angina**) result. To determine whether blood flow to the heart is compromised, a doctor will administer a stress test, which places the patient's heart under an exercise load. Unfortunately, sometimes the "stress test" is unplanned and occurs outside of a doctor's office (such as when a person shovels snow in the driveway), and a heart attack with a trip to the emergency room results. Cardiologists also have a variety of imaging techniques that allow them to determine if blood flow to the heart is compromised.

Figure 4.2 Events leading to heart failure.

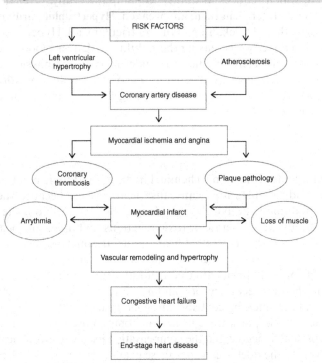

Legend: A simplified flow chart of the major events in the pathophysiology leading to end-stage heart disease is shown. Risk factors include hypertension, hyperlipidemia, diabetes, smoking, diet, and lack of physical activity (adapted from Dzau 1989).

Arrhythmias

A normal heart has rhythm: an orchestrated opening and closing of the valves and conduction of the contraction mechanism across the heart. Abnormal heart rhythms are called **arrhythmias**. Arrhythmias can result from congenital heart defects, coronary artery disease, or valvular heart disease. Other conditions that can lead to arrhythmias include smoking, drug abuse, excessive use of alcohol or caffeine, and stress. Individuals with diabetes or untreated hypertension can also develop arrhythmias. They can also result from prescription medications, over-the-counter medications, or dietary supplements. Arrhythmias are more likely to develop if an area of the heart contains scarred tissue or other defects resulting from diseased or deformed tissue. These damaged areas can interfere with the electrical impulses that must properly start and travel through the heart. A fatal arrhythmia is unlikely in most people without some sort of trigger, such as an electrical shock or a drug overdose.

Cardiomyopathy

Cardiomyopathy is a cardiovascular disease that involves the thickening or enlarging of heart muscle, the causes of which are complex and only partly understood. Possible causes of cardiomyopathy include genetics, drug and alcohol abuse, exposure to toxins or infections, and birth defects. There are three types of cardiomyopathy: dilated, hypertrophic, and restrictive. In the most common type, **dilated cardiomyopathy**, the left ventricle becomes enlarged, which reduces its ability to pump forcefully. Over time, the muscles of the left ventricle stretch, lengthen, and weaken. **Hypertrophic cardiomyopathy** involves abnormal growth and thickening of the ventricular wall. Hypertrophic left ventricles stiffen and lose capacity, decreasing their ability to deliver blood to the body. Failure can occur when a hypertrophic heart is under load during physical activity, and the heart tries to meet the increased demand. **Restrictive cardiomyopathy** is rare, and its cause is unknown. It results from the heart losing elasticity and becoming unable to fill or eject properly.

Other Causes

The heart can also be the target for infections, chemical irritants, and toxic reactions. Drug abuse with cocaine and amphetamine can cause heart issues, because these drugs have strong sympathomimetic activity. Other drugs, such as antibiotics (e.g., penicillin or sulfonamides), can cause allergic or toxic reactions that affect the heart. Certain viruses, bacteria, and parasites can infect heart tissue. In some of these cases, the heart valves suffer. Valves can be damaged by rheumatic fever, infections, and certain medications. Some people are born with a congenital form of valvular disease.

A healthy, well-functioning heart is necessary for maintaining a high quality of life. Regular exercise, a good diet, and not smoking contribute to good heart health. Sometimes, however, genetics, infectious diseases, or a toxic insult can compromise heart function. The body can often compensate to a degree, but the compensation itself can create health issues over time. Annual trips to the doctor can spot these changes before they progress into serious disease. Lifestyle changes may help cardiovascular function, but sometimes drug intervention is needed. In the next section we will discuss one of the most widely prescribed class of medication for cardiovascular disease and hypertension.

Drug Treatment for Arrhythmia and Other Heart-Related Issues

First-line drugs used to treat heart disease work by a variety of mechanisms with recommendations for their use updated every couple of years, based on evidence from large trials. For example, many of the drugs used to treat arrhythmia have multiple modes of action, making any classification imprecise. The Vaughan Williams classification was introduced in 1970 and is generally accepted with its known limitations. The five main classes of antiarrhythmic agents are classified:

Class I agents block sodium (Na^+) channels and Na^+ influx.
> Examples: propafenone (Rhythmol), flecainide (Tambocor), lidocaine, procainamide, quinidine

Class II agents are anti-adrenergic agents, primarily beta blockers.
> Examples: propranolol, metoprolol, cavedilol

Class III block potassium (K^+) channels and K^+ efflux.
> Examples: dronedarone (Multaq), sotalol (Betapace), amiodarone (Cordarone), dofetilide (Tikosyn)

Class IV agents affect calcium channels and the AV node.
> Examples: verapamil, diltiazem

Class V agents work by other or unknown mechanisms.
> Examples: adenosine, digoxin

Class I antiarrhythmic agents interfere with different (Na^+) channels and are separated into subgroups by their effect on cardiac action potentials. They are often used in conjunction with other agents. Sodium channel blockers are also used as local anesthetics and anticonvulsants. Class II agents include beta-blockers, detailed in this chapter. Class III agents predominantly block potassium channels, thereby prolonging repolarization. They are prescribed in special circumstances or in hospital settings. Others are only prescribed when other treatments are ineffective or not well tolerated. Class IV agents include calcium channel blockers, which are covered in Chapter 5. Class V agents include digoxin, a cardiac glycoside that is used in congestive heart failure and for irregular heartbeats, though its use is limited due to its narrow therapeutic window. It is considered a third-line treatment with others drugs more effective and safer.

How Do Beta-Blockers Work?

Beta-blockers relieve stress on the heart by slowing the heartbeat and decreasing the force with which the heart muscle contracts. The resulting decrease in cardiac output should cause a decrease in blood pressure. Beta-blockers are prescribed to prevent abnormally fast heart rates (tachycardia) and irregular rhythms (arrhythmias), such as atrial fibrillation. Beta-blockers are a mainstay treatment of congestive heart failure. Since beta-blockers slow the heart's rate, the heart's demand for oxygen decreases. Hence, these drugs may be useful in treating chest pain (angina) that occurs when the oxygen demand of the heart exceeds the supply. Long-term use of beta-blockers helps manage chronic heart failure. Beta-blockers improve survival after a heart attack, and they also rduce blood vessel contraction throughout the body. In addition, beta-blockers can be prescribed for glaucoma, migraine headaches, anxiety, certain types of tremors, and hyperthyroidism.

Beta-blockers are antagonists of beta-adrenergic receptors. There are two pharmacologically relevant types of beta-receptors, and they differ in their distribution throughout the body (see Chapter 3). A third type, the β-3 receptors, are found in adipose tissue and have a poorly described role in fat metabolism and will not be considered further. The heart and kidney have higher densities of β-1 receptors than β-2. The lungs, arterioles, and GI-tract are richer in β-2 receptors than β-1. Some beta-blockers are **nonselective**, with similar activity toward type 1 and type 2 receptors. Propranolol, for example, is a nonselective beta-blocker that is still prescribed. Other beta-blockers have been developed that have selectivity for either the β-1 or β-2 subtype. Atenolol is an example of a beta-blocker with greater affinity for β-1 receptors, and it is prescribed at the rate of about 25 million prescriptions per year in the United States, down from over 40 million several years ago. Since the heart has a high percentage of the β-1 subtype, atenolol and similar drugs are called **cardioselective beta-blockers.**

Most receptor antagonists bind the receptor at a similar site as the endogenous agonist, but without triggering the usual receptor response. However, some beta-blockers have low-level agonist activity at the receptor. These beta-blockers are much less potent agonists than endogenous epinephrine or norepinephrine, so they ultimately block the endogenous response to stress or exercise. Although they have weak agonist activity, their blocking activity is generally greater than their agonist activity, so they are called **beta-blockers with intrinsic sympathomimetic activity (ISA).**

Nitric Oxide and Vasodilation

Nitric oxide (NO) was discovered as a major vasodilator in the 1980s and was the Molecule of the Year (*Science* magazine) in 1992. NO plays an important role in the protection against the onset and progression of cardiovascular disease. It helps regulate blood pressure and inhibits platelet aggregation and leukocyte adhesion (important in plaque formation). A loss of sensitivity to the vasodilative effects of NO or low NO production results in increased vascular tone and elevated blood pressure. Some of the newer drugs used for hypertension (e.g., the beta-blocker nebivolol, discussed below) can improve vasodilation by increasing the NO response.

NO has a wide variety of biological activities. NO is synthesized from the amino acid arginine in a two-step reaction by the enzyme nitric oxide synthase. Three isoforms of this enzyme activity have been described, with the endothelial isoform the most important for vasodilation. Acetylcholine, cytokines, or platelet-derived factors can stimulate endothelial nitric oxide synthase through a calcium- and calmodulin-dependent pathway, increasing NO synthesis. The NO diffuses rapidly through membranes into smooth muscle cells and binds and activates a cyclic GMP synthase, causing an increase in cyclic GMP. The elevated cyclic GMP levels cause relaxation in the smooth muscle cells by several different mechanisms, including decreasing calcium entry, hyperpolarization, and activation of myosin light chain phosphatase. NO, in addition to causing vasodilation in smooth muscle cells, plays an important role in kidney function. Diabetics can have decreased NO activity, which can lead to blood flow problems in their extremities.

Table 4.1 Classifications of beta-blockers

Nonselective beta-blockers. These beta-blockers have similar affinity for β-1 and β-2 receptors.
EXAMPLES: Propranolol and nadolol

Cardioselective beta-blockers. These beta-blockers are more selective toward the β-1 subtype of receptor than β-2. They were developed to have less of an effect in the lungs and peripheral tissues where β-2 receptors are located. In the heart, β-1 receptor blockers decrease the rate and the force of contraction, thereby decreasing cardiac output and reducing blood pressure. Even though they are called cardioselective, they also block β-1 receptors in the kidney and in the periphery. The cardioselective drugs represented the "second generation" of beta-blocker development.
EXAMPLES: Metoprolol and atenolol

Beta-blockers with ISA. These beta-blockers have low-level agonist activity at the receptor, while blocking activity of endogenous epinephrine or norepinephrine to bind the receptor. Although pharmacologically interesting because of this property, they are not prescribed much anymore.
EXAMPLE: Pindolol

Third-generation beta-blockers. These drugs are distinguished by the fact that they cause vasodilation, by increasing NO activity or blocking α-1 receptors.
EXAMPLES: Nebivolol and carvedilol

Third-generation beta-blockers are relatively new to the U.S. market and are distinguished by the fact that they cause vasodilation. Nebivolol is highly selective for β-1 receptors, and can cause vasodilation by triggering nitric oxide formation in the endothelium (Fongemie & Felix-Getzik 2015). Carvedilol blocks both types of beta receptors and α-1 receptors in the vasculature. The activation of α-1 receptors causes constriction of blood vessels, so blocking these receptors contributes to the vasodilatory effects (DiNicolantonio, Lavie, Fares, et al. 2013). These newer beta-blockers may confer beneficial effects on cardiovascular mortality and morbidity, compared to atenolol. See Table 4.1 for additional information about the classifications of beta-blockers.

Beta-blockers' primary mechanism involves their direct effect on the heart, decreasing the rate and force of contraction. The resulting decrease in cardiac output lessens arterial pressure, producing a decrease in blood pressure. However, beta-receptors are distributed throughout the body, and other responses to these drugs can occur. For example, renin release from kidney cells is mediated by β-1 receptors via input from the sympathetic nervous system. Renin activates the angiotensin pathway, which causes an increase in blood pressure, so beta-blockers could lower blood pressure through this mechanism. The extent of this effect is hard to quantify, but it has been observed under certain conditions (Holmer, Hengstenberg, Mayer, et al. 2001). Some beta-blockers, such as propranolol, can pass the blood–brain barrier and have central effects, such as reduced release of epinephrine and norepinephrine. Third-generation beta-blockers, for example, nebivolol, can increase nitric oxide, with the resulting vasodilation. Carvedilol is a beta-blocker that can also antagonize peripheral α-1 receptors, causing vasodilation. Beta-blockers clearly decrease the pressor (blood pressure) response to norepinephrine and epinephrine during exercise. They also reduce the pressor response to the catecholamines associated with stress and allostatic load.

To summarize, the many different beta-blockers on the market share the property of being antagonists to β-1, β-2, or both receptor subtypes. These receptors are distributed throughout the body as part of the sympathetic nervous system, creating a wide spectrum of possible physiological responses. Additionally, beta-blockers differ in that some have additional targets, such as nitric oxide production or alpha-receptors. This wide spectrum of potential activities allows beta-blockers to be prescribed for a wide variety of conditions, as mentioned earlier.

Exercise Pharmacology and Beta-Blockers

Patients with cardiovascular disease are still encouraged to be physically active and engage in some type of exercise program. Beta-blockers, though widely prescribed for cardiovascular disease and hypertension over the last several decades, can affect exercise performance. In some special cases, these effects may be helpful, but, for the most part, drugs other than beta-blockers are now preferred for individuals who are competitive athletes. There is considerable literature on the positive effects of physical activity on heart health. We will briefly cover some newer findings and then examine some of the issues with the prescription of beta-blockers.

Exercise and Cardiovascular Disease

Physical activity helps modulate systemic inflammation, including the gut microbiome, and may be beneficial to controlling atherosclerosis and overall cardiovascular health. Atherosclerosis, the main driver of cardiovascular disease, is now recognized as an inflammatory disorder. Physical activity has an important role in cardiovascular health, the inflammatory role of atherosclerosis, and supporting the microbiome as a positive regulator of inflammation (Fernandez, Clemente, & Giannarelli, 2018).

The heart has a high energy requirement that is satisfied largely by its preferred oxidation of fatty acids. During exercise, acute metabolic changes occur with an increase in whole-body glucose metabolism increasing proportionately to intensity. Fatty acid metabolism also gradually increases during exercise, particularly during moderate intensity. However, a stressed heart with pathological hypertrophy relies heavily on glucose metabolism through an acceleration of glycolysis. Regular exercise in these individuals promotes metabolic remodeling in the heart, which is associated with physiological cardiac growth. Regular exercise enhances fatty oxidation and normalization of glycolysis, a therapeutic strategy to correct the metabolic phenotype of the hypertrophied heart. Exercise-induced decreases in glycolytic activity stimulate physiological cardiac remodeling, and metabolic flexibility is important for maintaining mitochondrial health in the heart (Fulghum & Hill 2018).

Resistance exercise improves many cardiovascular disease risk factors, and is associated with reduced all-cause mortality. In a study of 12,591 participants (mean age 47 years) over 10 years, resistance exercise was assessed by a self-reported medical history questionnaire. The analysis showed that one session of resistance exercise per week, independent of aerobic exercise, was associated with reduced risks of CVD and all-cause mortality. Those meeting the resistance exercise criteria also had decreased BMI over this time frame (Liu, Lee, Li, et al. 2019).

The potential cardioprotective effects of regular exercise are many and diverse. They overlap with many of the health-related concerns discussed elsewhere in this text. Here is a list of some of them (Quindry & Franklin 2018):

Anti-atherosclerotic—improved blood lipid profile (Chapter 10); lower blood pressure (Chapter 5); reduced adiposity (Chapter 12); decreased inflammation (Chapter 11); increased insulin sensitivity (Chapter 12)

Antiarrhythmic—increased vagal (parasympathetic) tone; decreased adrenergic activity

Anti-ischemic—increase nitric oxide; increase coronary blood flow; decrease myocardial oxygen demand

Anti-thrombotic—decrease platelet adhesiveness; decrease blood viscosity

Cardiac Remodeling—anatomical and biochemical

Psychologic—decrease stress; decrease depression and anxiety (Chapter 9)

Pharmacokinetic Concerns

The numerous beta-blockers on the market differ in their water and lipid solubility. The more water-soluble ones, such as atenolol and nadolol, do not effectively cross the blood–brain barrier and, therefore, have less centrally mediated effects. They are eliminated primarily by the kidneys. The more lipid-soluble drugs, such as propranolol and metoprolol, can cross the blood–brain barrier and exert central effects. They are excreted primarily by liver-dependent mechanisms. Beta-blockers have elimination half-lives that range from three to four hours for propranolol to 14 to 24 hours for nadolol (Wallin & Shah 1987; Che et al.).

During exercise, the blood flow to the liver and kidneys decreases as the intensity level increases. Therefore, drugs that are highly dependent on the liver and kidneys for their elimination, such as the beta-blockers described above, are said to be flow-limited, and they may have altered pharmacokinetic properties with exercise at moderate to high levels of intensity. Generally, research is limited on the effect of exercise on the pharmacokinetics of these drugs. The limited number of studies on the effect of exercise on clearance of beta-blockers suggest that this effect is variable. The more water-soluble drugs (e.g., atenolol and nadolol) will be affected by decreased blood flow to the kidneys, since that is the primary site of their elimination. The more lipid-soluble drugs (e.g., propranolol and metoprolol) will be affected by decreased blood flow to the liver, since they are excreted by liver-dependent mechanisms. In an older study on beta-blockers, exercise at 70% VO_2max showed a decreased volume of distribution for propranolol and an increase in its plasma concentration. However, under the same conditions, no difference was observed with atenolol (van Baak, Mooij, & Schiffers 1992). As stated above, beta-blockers have elimination half-lives that range from 3 to 24 hours, and these times could be affected by prolonged or high intensity of exercise, depending on the particular drug. For the average patient exercising at low to moderate intensities, the changes in elimination rates are expected to be minor and transient. An altered dosing strategy is probably not needed. However, beta-blockers are on the WADA Prohibited List for certain sports (discussed below under PES Watch), and extended elimination times that result from exercise could lead to positive drug tests.

Pharmacodynamic Concerns

As exercise intensity increases, sympathetic activity also increases, and the adrenal gland releases circulating adrenaline (epinephrine and norepinephrine). Beta-blockers, however, antagonize the sympathetic nervous system and circulating epinephrine and norepinephrine. What, therefore, is the result of exercise on the effectiveness of beta-blockers? The drugs' effect on the physiological response to exercise has been studied extensively since the 1970s and summarized in review articles (e.g., van Baak 1988). In general, exercise does not override the effects of beta-blockers on the heart in elite athletes, hypertensive patients, or patients with arrhythmias. The good news for hypertensive patients is that they can exercise, and the drugs will still reduce their blood pressure. The bad news is that taking beta-blockers might reduce exercise-induced changes in their physiology, as discussed below. Use of a target heart rate to measure exercise intensity is problematic when beta-blockers are suppressing the heart rate. Are the beneficial effects of exercise similarly blunted? The answer is not clear-cut, as discussed below, and depends on the type of beta-blockers used. Beta-blockers that are more cardioselective may have advantages over older, nonselective drugs.

Cardiovascular Effects

The sympathetic nervous system mediates the fight-or-flight response and plays a major role in the physiological changes that occur during exercise. Therefore, we expect beta-blockers to antagonize many of the actions of epinephrine and norepinephrine and suppress the physiological response to exertion. Recall from Chapter 2 that VO_2max (oxygen utilization at maximal exercise) is a measurement of physical effort. Because improved VO_2max indicates improved physical fitness, we can use VO_2max to assess the effects of these drugs. VO_2max depends on cardiac output and the difference in O_2 concentration between arterial and venous circulation. As discussed in Chapter 2, cardiac output (Q) is the result of heart rate (HR) times the stroke volume (SV): $Q = HR \times SV$. Therefore, heart rate, stroke volume, cardiac output, and VO_2max are parameters that describe O_2 utilization during exercise. Since VO_2max is directly related to heart rate, heart rate can be used as a measure of exercise intensity and a measurable target during exercise. Exercise increases stroke volume over time as the individual becomes fit, causing the increase observed in VO_2max. A decrease in heart rate, including resting heart rate, is expected in trained individuals with increased stroke volume.

When the heart rate starts to increase to meet an increase in demand, such as physical activity, the parasympathetic input decreases proportionally. Less inhibitory input on the heart allows the heart rate to increase to about 100 beats per minute (bpm). As demand continues to increase and the heart rate needs to exceed 100 bpm, sympathetic input increases, and norepinephrine stimulates the rate and force of contraction. Beta-blockers decrease both resting and exercise heart rate. During rest, inhibition of beta-receptors allows parasympathetic input to become more pronounced, and heart rate decreases. During exercise, beta-blockers reduce the sympathetic input, and the increase in heart rate will be lessened. Therefore, taking beta-blockers results in an impact on an exercise regimen that is based on target heart rate. Exercisers on beta-blockers need to rely on other measures of exercise intensity (e.g., resistance level on an elliptical machine or breathing rate while jogging) or adjust their target heart rate downward.

During mild exercise, beta-blockers with ISA decrease heart rate less than beta-blockers without ISA (reviewed in van Baak 1988). The weak agonist activity with beta-blockers with ISA is observed when epinephrine and norepinephrine levels are low. At a high intensity of exercise, the elevated levels of epinephrine and norepinephrine minimize the difference between beta-blockers with or without ISA, resulting in similar decreases in heart rate. For well-trained athletes, who already have a relatively low resting heart rate, a beta-blocker with ISA would be better—it may reduce the possibility of **bradycardia**. Bradycardia is the condition where the resting heart rate becomes too low (less than 60 bpm) to pump sufficient oxygenated blood to the body.

A limitation of many of these drug studies is that they are done after subjects have taken the drug for a week or two to stabilize their blood pressure response. The treatment of cardiovascular disease or hypertension is expected to be a long-term proposition for most patients. They will probably be taking antihypertensive drugs the remainder of their lives. Only limited studies have compared different types of beta-blockers following months of treatment. Studies where the subjects have been on these drugs for months often show little difference between the first and second generations of beta-blockers (van Baak, Bohm, Arends, et al. 1987). In one study, for example, cardioselective beta-blockers, following long-term use, show little difference from non-specific beta-blockers in terms of decreased heart rate during exercise (Lund-Johansen 1983). Initially, patients may benefit from cardioselective drugs with ISA, but the limited long-term studies suggest that differences in heart rate become minimal after several months of treatment, especially at higher exercise intensities (van Baak 1988). Drugs with strong ISA may have slightly less effect on heart rate than other beta-blockers at low to moderate exercise intensities (Lund-Johansen), but these drugs are rarely prescribed anymore.

The effect of beta-blockers on blood pressure during exercise has also been studied. Blood pressure (BP) depends on cardiac output (Q) times the systemic vascular resistance (SVR): $BP = Q \times SVR$. Since cardiac output depends on heart rate, and heart rate is decreased by beta-blockers, blood pressure should similarly be decreased. Each class of beta-blockers suppresses the increase in blood pressure during exercise. With chronic treatment (i.e., six months), differences in blood pressure are minimal between the different types of beta-blockers (van Baak et al. 1987).

Pulmonary Effects

Sympathetic input improves ventilation during exercise, in part by smooth muscle relaxation and dilation of bronchioles. Beta-blockers antagonize this response and decrease expiratory flow rate and tidal volume (Joyner, Jilka, Taylor, et al. 1987). The decrease in volume of air movement is compensated partially by an increase in respiratory rate, causing faster and shallower breathing. Because of these effects on breathing, beta-blockers can exacerbate asthma. Beta-blockers are not for athletes who suffer from asthma or exercise-induced bronchoconstriction (see Chapter 7).

Metabolic Effects

Humans store considerably more energy in the form of fat compared to carbohydrates, which are stored primarily in the form of glycogen. Fat is stored primarily as triglycerides in cells called fat cells or **adipocytes**. Lipolysis, the cleavage of triglycerides into one part glycerol and three parts fatty acid (see Chapter 2), is stimulated by epinephrine. The "free" fatty acids, also referred to as non-esterified fatty acids, enter the bloodstream, where moderately working skeletal muscle transports and oxidizes them for ATP production. Adipose (fat) tissue receives direct sympathetic input to stimulate lipolysis and mobilize fat reserves, and this process may have all three beta-receptor subtypes involved. During exercise, circulating epinephrine is a major stimulus for lipolysis. During high-intensity exercise (generally over 75% VO_2max), however, rates of fat oxidation cannot keep up with the demand for energy, and rates of muscle glycogenolysis increase as carbohydrates contribute a higher percentage of the energy needed for ATP production. Beta-blockers impair the sympathetic stimulation of adipocytes to increase lipolysis (Wijnen, van Baak, de Haan, et al. 1993). The nonselective and cardioselective drugs have a similar inhibitory effect on adipose tissue (Cleroux, Nguyen, Taylor, & Leenen 1989).

In muscle cells, β-2 receptors stimulate glycogenolysis, lipolysis, and K^+ reuptake. Therefore, as exercise intensity increases, the response to epinephrine is blunted more by non-specific beta-blockers than by the cardiospecific drugs. Figure 4.3 illustrates the magnitude of the effect caused by propranolol, a non-specific beta-blocker (Wijnen et al.). Eleven normotensive volunteers rode a cycle ergometer at 70% of their maximum workload for two trials, after taking either propranolol or placebo. The drug caused a pronounced decrease in glycerol or glucose mobilization, resulting in a higher blood lactate, implying greater reliance on anaerobic metabolism in the muscle cells. The beta-blocker also inhibited the epinephrine-stimulated uptake of K^+ by the muscle cells.

In another study, the cardioselective drug atenolol had a smaller effect on muscle cell lipolysis than that of the nonselective drug nadolol. In the fat cells, there was no difference (Cleroux et al.). In this study, the exercise was submaximal to exhaustion, and no difference was observed for the two different beta-blockers for muscle cell glycogenolysis, probably due to epinephrine's lack of effect at this low level of exercise intensity.

Nebivolol, a third-generation drug with high affinity for β-1 receptors, also causes vasodilation, because it increases nitric oxide levels in the endothelium. When compared to atenolol, it had a similar effect on blood pressure but had a smaller inhibitory effect on glycerol and free fatty acid production (Van Bortel & van Baak 1992). In a pilot study with 18 hypertensive subjects, nebivolol significantly reduced heart rate and blood pressure but did not significantly affect VO_2 or RPE (Table 4.2; Predel, Mainka, Schillings, et al. 2001). The study also showed that nebivolol did not significantly change lipid or lactate levels (Predel et al.). In another study with a total of 60 hypertensive subjects, atenolol caused an elevation of blood sugar and lipid profile after 24 weeks of treatment, whereas nebivolol did not (Badar, Hiware, Shrivastava, et al. 2011).

Endurance and Training Effects

Beta-blockers diminish submaximal exercise capacity in active hypertensive individuals. Most classes of beta-blockers similarly depress exercise heart rate, blood pressure, and cardiac output. At submaximal exercise, beta-blockers impede lipolysis in adipose tissue. The nonselective beta-blockers also decrease lipolysis in skeletal muscle, resulting in less available free fatty acids for muscles to use for fuel. Glycogenolysis is mostly unchanged by beta-blockers at submaximal exercise intensities; at maximal

Figure 4.3 Effect of beta-blockade during endurance exercise.

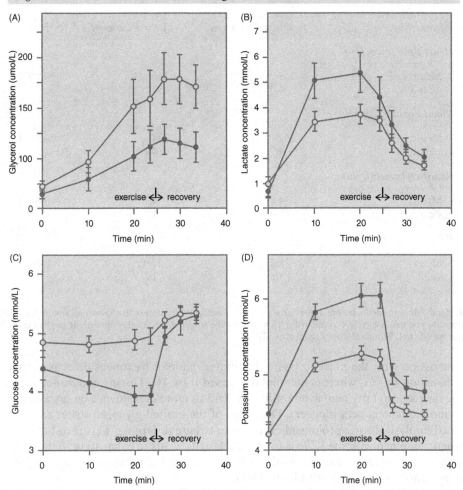

Legend: Eleven normotensive volunteers rode a cycle ergometer at 70% of their maximum workload for two trials, after taking propranolol (closed circles) or placebo (open circles). A: Plasma glycerol levels are shown during exercise and ten minutes of recovery cycling at 75 watts. Mean response with standard error of the mean shown. B: Plasma lactate concentrations. C: Plasma glucose concentrations. D: Plasma potassium concentrations.

output, however, it is reduced as epinephrine levels rise. Plasma levels of K^+ increase, as these drugs block beta-adrenergic stimulation of K^+ reuptake in skeletal muscle. Loss of K^+ from working muscle is a contributor to fatigue and normally, epinephrine stimulates K^+ reuptake. The negative effects at submaximal exercise occur with each class of beta-blockers but are more pronounced with nonselective beta-blockers than with cardioselective beta-blockers.

In one study, eight sedentary, healthy male subjects performed exercise tests using cycle ergometers (Cleroux et al.). After one week of treatment with atenolol, nadolol, or placebo, the subjects exercised at a workload that led to exhaustion in one hour during the pretest phase. The study showed endurance decreased significantly more with nadolol (nonselective) than with atenolol (cardioselective). The mean time to

Table 4.2 Effect of nebivolol during exercise

Parameter	Before Treatment	After Treatment	P
Heart Rate (min–1)			
Mean	168	146	0.0001
s.e.m.	4.3	4.6	
Blood Pressure (mmHg)			
Mean	232	204	0.0001
s.e.m.	4.3	4.1	
Relative Oxygen Uptake			
Mean	34.8	34.1	0.64 NS
s.e.m.	2.0	1.9	
RPE			
Mean	18.2	17.9	0.53 NS
s.e.m.	1.5	1.8	

Legend: Measurements before and after six weeks of nebivolol treatment are shown following a maximal exercise test using a cycle ergometer for 18 hypertensive subjects. s.e.m.: standard error of the mean, NS: not significant. Modified from Predel et al. (2001).

exhaustion with the placebo was ±71 minutes; nadolol treatment decreased time to exhaustion by 6%, whereas atenolol decreased it by 4%. During endurance exercise, the decrease in fatty acid availability can lead to more dependence on glycogenolysis in individuals on beta-blockers. Depletion of the limited glycogen stores and diminished lipolysis during prolonged exercise contribute to fatigue. This metabolic effect, when combined with the K^+ loss from muscle cells, leads to exhaustion. Beta-blockers significantly decrease submaximal performance and endurance in normotensive and hypertensive individuals (van Baak 1988).

In addition, training can be compromised when beta-blockers are used chronically, as subjects do not see the same degree of improvement in their VO_2max with training as individuals who are not taking the drug. However, chronic users of beta-blockers who exercise regularly can still see improvement in their fitness level (Westhoff, Franke, Schmidt, et al. 2007). Although exercising patients who are taking beta-blockers may become somewhat discouraged because of the slow improvement in their fitness and weight loss, the exercise is still causing beneficial physiological changes, if not to the same level as for individuals who are not taking beta-blockers. The newer generation of beta-blockers, such as nebivolol, apparently is less likely to cause these negative effects (Van Bortel & van Baak; Predel et al.; Badar et al.).

Elder Concerns

Several issues continue to spark debate concerning cardiovascular disease and hypertension in the elderly. Examples include what the target should be for blood pressure, the choice of first-line antihypertensive therapy, and the role of drug combination therapy. Concerns include managing dose and side effects as people age and deal with different levels of severity of cardiovascular disease. The concern is that drug-treatment should not create more issues while keeping the elderly's risk of a cardiac event low. Contemporary guidelines advocate a diagnostic threshold of 140/90 mmHg in adults. In high-risk patients with diabetes and renal failure, there may be a lower blood pressure target, as 'the lower the better' practice is generally accepted for most patients. However, the current JNC8 recommendation defined a higher blood pressure target of 150/90-mmHg for people above the age of 60 years, based on randomized controlled trials that showed little difference in morbidity statistics with the slightly higher blood pressure target. This JNC8 recommendation continues to be debated (Currie & Delles 2018) after it generated a 'minority report' that outlined the argument for lower target blood pressure of 140/90 or less (Wright, Fine, Lackland, et al. 2014). One of the minority arguments is that age substantially increases risk for cardiovascular events. They argue there is no justification for different target blood pressures for those older or younger than 60, similar to recommendations by groups in Europe and Canada. Persons aged 60 to 79 years are at higher risk than those who are younger and therefore should have similarly aggressive treatment and target blood pressure. However, the minority report did agree that a systolic blood pressure goal of less than 150 mm Hg for frail persons aged 80 years or older was a reasonable alternate approach to addressing the concern that elderly patients are at higher risk for treatment-related serious events.

Beta-blockers were a mainstay of hypertension treatment for many decades and continue to be widely used though other drugs are now recommended as first-line treatment (more in Chapter 5). Since the JNC7 recommendation came out in 2003, beta-blockers are no longer recommended to treat hypertension in patients older than age 60 unless they have another indication, such as heart failure or ischemic heart disease. Diuretics (Chapter 6) are superior to beta-blockers in reducing cardiovascular and all-cause mortality and are the first-line drug of choice for hypertension (JNC 7 2003; JNC 8). Patients over 60 with ischemic heart disease or heart failure are still prescribed beta-blockers, as well as older patients with hypertension who need multiple agents to control their blood pressure. Metoprolol is inexpensive and proven to reduce mortality in patients with a history of myocardial infarct or heart failure and is considered superior to atenolol (Schumann & Hickner 2008).

Health Risks

Most people who take beta-blockers experience few or only minor side effects. For example, beta-blockers can constrict blood vessels and reduce circulation to the hands and feet, and some people complain of cold hands and feet. Others, however, may experience lethargy, depression, confusion, and impotence. Beta-blockers are contraindicated under conditions of bradycardia (pulse less than 60 bpm) or **symptomatic hypotension** (blood pressure of less than 90/60 mmHg), when dizziness, vertigo, or fainting can occur.

In recent years, there has been debate over whether to use beta-blockers in elderly patients (Che et al.; JNC 8). Beta-blockers are not as effective as other choices in this population, in terms of cardiovascular disease outcomes (Brouwers, Courteau, Cohen, et al. 2014). In addition, the side effects are not as well tolerated in older patients. The kidneys excrete atenolol, and kidney function declines with age, so the drug will not be eliminated as quickly from the body. Dosage should be adjusted for the elderly and for patients with renal impairment, starting at the low end of the dosing range. The elderly also have a greater likelihood of decreased hepatic or cardiac function, and they are often taking other drug therapies or have concomitant diseases.

Beta-blockers should also be avoided for asthmatics, as they can cause bronchoconstriction. The cardioselective (β-1) blockers are not as potentially harmful for asthmatics as the non-specific drugs, but even the cardioselective drugs have some activity toward β-2 receptors in the lungs and peripheral tissues. Asthmatics often take β-2 agonists for their condition, as we will discuss in Chapter 7.

In addition, beta-blockers are not recommended for diabetics (JNC 8). In insulin-dependent diabetics, beta-blockers may block signs of low blood sugar (hypoglycemia), such as rapid heartbeat or tremors, which occur if blood sugar falls too low. It is important for diabetics who are taking beta-blockers to monitor their blood sugar closely. Whether beta-blockers can contribute to Type 2 diabetes and metabolic syndrome is still under debate (Che et al.; Carella, Antonucci, Conte, et al. 2010). The sympathetic nervous system plays a critical role in regulating blood sugar during times of stress or physical activity, so beta-blockers potentially will disrupt these normal processes. However, the newer beta-blockers, such as carvedilol, have more favorable effects on metabolic parameters than atenolol (Leonetti & Egan 2012), and along with other beta-blockers like labetalol are sometimes considered diabetes-friendly (as opposed to the 'un-friendly' atenolol and metoprolol). Future large-scale studies may support re-evaluation of third-generation beta-blockers as a useful therapy for diabetics with hypertension and cardiovascular disease.

The beta-blockers carvedilol and nebivolol have vasodilatory properties and have been evaluated in the treatment of patients with heart failure. They lower heart rate and blood pressure similarly in patients with chronic heart failure, and improve left ventricular function (Karabacak, Doğan, Tayyar, et al. 2015). Resting heart rate plus 20 to 30 bpm is a simplified substitute for calculating heart rate at the anaerobic threshold during exercise, a useful tool for exercise prescription. For patients undergoing beta-blocker therapy, resting heart rate plus 20 bpm is recommended. In patients with subacute myocardial infarction, carvedilol treatment did not significantly change the heart rate at the anaerobic threshold. Therefore, exercise prescription based on heart rate plus 30 bpm is feasible in this patient population (Nemoto, Kasahara, Izawa, et al. 2019).

PES Watch

Beta-blockers have ergolytic properties, including suppression of exercise heart rate and decreased mobilization of energy reserves, such as glucose and free fatty acids. However, both the NCAA and USOC test for and ban beta-blockers in several competitions. The competitions that ban these drugs generally require a steady hand and calm nerves, such as shooting competitions, archery, gymnastics, and synchronized swimming. Since beta-blockers slow heart rate and suppress the fight-or-flight response, they presumably could give an unfair advantage in these types of competition. Actors and politicians have been known to use beta-blockers to reduce symptoms of stage fright.

Drugs and supplements that increase nitric oxide production (e.g., the third-generation beta-blocker nebivolol) could potentially improve oxygen and nutrient delivery to exercising muscles, thus improving exercise performance and recovery mechanisms. However, the results of studies have been mixed, with untrained individuals showing some improvement not observed in highly trained subjects (Bescós, Sureda, Tur, & Pons 2012). WADA has commissioned studies on some drugs (e.g., Viagra) and supplements that increase nitric oxide, but has not put these substances on the list of banned substances.

Conclusion

There is continued debate over whether monotherapy with beta-blockers is recommended for hypertension and other forms of cardiovascular disease (Che et al.). However, beta-blockers remain widely prescribed for many types of cardiovascular disease, including congestive heart failure, coronary artery disease, angina, arrhythmia, and hypertension. Beta-blockers make it difficult to use target heart rate effectively as a measure of exercise intensity. Beta-blockers, especially the non-cardioselective beta-blockers, have ergolytic effects on aerobic exercise.

Key Concepts Review

adipocyte
angina
arrhythmia
arteriosclerosis
atherosclerosis
atrioventricular (AV) node
atrium
β-1 receptor
β-2 receptor
beta-blocker
beta-blocker with ISA
bradycardia
cardiomyopathy
cardioselective beta-blocker

chronotropic
diastole
dilated cardiomyopathy
dromotropic
hypertrophic cardiomyopathy
inotropic
left ventricular hypertrophy (LVH)
nonselective beta-blocker
pacemaker
restrictive cardiomyopathy
sinoatrial (SA) node
systole
third-generation beta-blocker
ventricle

Review Questions

1 What is meant by "beta-blockers with ISA"? What advantages might these drugs have? Disadvantages?
2 What property makes some beta-blockers cardioselective?
3 What are the effects of beta-blockers on exercise physiology?
4 A serious walker (5 miles/day) notices that she has stopped losing weight since starting her new prescription of propranolol (non-cardioselective, without ISA). She also fatigues more quickly than she used to. What can you offer her as an explanation?
5 The NCAA and USOC have banned beta-blockers from many types of competition. Why?

References

Badar VA, Hiware SK, Shrivastava MP, Thawani VR, Hardas MM (2011) Comparison of nebivolol and atenolol on blood pressure, blood sugar, and lipid profile in patients of essential hypertension. *Indian J Pharmacol* 43:437–440

Bescós R, Sureda A, Tur JA, Pons A (2012) The effect of nitric-oxide-related supplements on human performance. *Sports Med* 42:99–117

Brouwers FM, Courteau J, Cohen AA, Farand P, Cloutier L, Asghari S, Vanasse A (2014) Beta-blockers are associated with increased risk of first cardiovascular events in non-diabetic hypertensive elderly patients. *Pharmacoepidem Drug Safety* DOI: 10.1002/pds.3675

Carella AM, Antonucci G, Conte M, Di Pumpo M, Giancola A, Antonucci E (2010) Antihypertensive treatment with beta-blockers in the metabolic syndrome: a review. *Curr Diabetes Rev* 6:215–221

Che Q, Schreiber MJ, Rafey MA (2009) Beta-blockers for hypertension: Are they going out of style? *Cleve Clin J Med* 76:533–542

Cleroux J, Nguyen PV, Taylor AW, Leenen FHH (1989) Effects of beta1- versus beta1 plus beta 2-blockade on exercise endurance and muscle metabolism in humans. *J Appl Physiol* 66:584–554

Currie G, Delles, C (2018) Blood pressure targets in the elderly. *J Hyper* 36:234–236

DiNicolantonio JJ, Lavie CJ, Fares H, Menezes AR, O'Keefe JH (2013) Meta-analysis of carvedilol versus beta 1 selective beta-blockers (atenolol, bisoprolol, metoprolol, and nebivolol). *Am J Cardiol* 111:765–769

Dzau VJ (1989) Clinical implications for therapy: possible cardioprotective effects of ACE inhibition. Br J Clin Pharmac 28: 183S–187S

Fernandez DM, Clemente JC, Giannarelli C (2018) Physical activity, immune system, and the microbiome in cardiovascular disease. *Front Physiol* 9:763

Fongemie J, Felix-Getzik E (2015) a review of nebivolol pharmacology and clinical evidence. *Drugs* 75:1349–1371

Fulghum K, Hill BG (2018) Metabolic mechanisms of exercise-induced cardiac remodeling. *Front Cardiovasc Med* 5:127

Holmer SR, Hengstenberg C, Mayer B, Engel S, Löwel H, Riegger GA, Schunkert H (2001) Marked suppression of renin levels by beta-receptor blocker in patients treated with standard heart failure therapy: a potential mechanism of benefit from beta-blockade. *J Intern Med* 249:167–172

JNC 7: Chobanian AV, Bakris GL, Black HR, Cushman WC, Green LA, Izzo JL, Jones DW, Materson BJ, Oparil S, Wright JT, Roccella EJ (2003) Seventh report of the joint national committee on prevention, detection, evaluation, and treatment of high blood pressure. *Hypertension* 42:1206–1252

JNC 8: James PA, Oparil S, Carter BL, Cushman WC, Dennison-Himmelfarb C, Handler J, Lackland DT, LeFevre ML, MacKenzie TD, Ogedegbe O, Smith SC, Svetkey LP, Taler SJ, Raymond R. Townsend RR, Wright JT, Andrew S, Narva AS, Ortiz E (2014) 2014 Evidence-based guideline for the management of high blood pressure in adults report from the panel members appointed to the Eighth Joint National Committee (JNC 8) *JAMA* 311:507–520

Joyner MJ, Jilka SM, Taylor JA, Kalis JK, Nittolo J, Hicks RW, Lohman TG, Wilmore JH (1987) Beta-blockade reduces tidal volume during heavy exercise in trained and untrained men. *J Appl Physiol* 62:1819–1825

Karabacak M, Doğan A, Tayyar Ş, Özaydın M, Erdoğan D (2015) Carvedilol and nebivolol improve left ventricular systolic functions in patients with non-ischemic heart failure. *Anatol J Cardiol* 15:271–276

Leonetti G, Egan CG (2012) Use of carvedilol in hypertension: an update. *Vasc Health Risk Manag* 8:307–322

Liu Y, Lee DC, Li Y, Zhu W, Zhang 1, Sui 5, Lavie CJ, Blair S (2019) Associations of resistance exercise with cardiovascular disease morbidity and mortality. *Med Sci Sports Exerc* 51:499–508

Lund-Johansen P (1983) Central haemodynamic effects of beta-blockers in hypertension. A comparison between atenolol, metoprolol, timolol, penbutolol, alprenolol, pindolol and bunitrolol. *Eur Heart J* 4(suppl D):1–12

Nemoto S, Kasahara Y, Izawa KP, Watanabe S, Yoshizawa K, Takeichi N, Kamiya K, Suzuki N, Omiya K, Matsunaga A, Akashi YJ (2019) Effect of carvedilol on heart rate response to cardiopulmonary exercise up to the anaerobic threshold in patients with subacute myocardial infarction. *Heart Vessels.* doi:10.1007/s00380-018-01326-5

Poirier L, Tobe SW (2014) Contemporary use of beta-blockers: clinical relevance of sub-classification. *Can J Cardiol* 30:S9–S15

Predel HG, Mainka W, Schillings W, Knigge H, Montiel J, Fallois J, Agrawal R, Schramm T, Graf C, Giannetti BM, Bjarnason-Wehrens B, Prinz U, Rost RE (2001) Integrated effects of the vasodilating beta-blocker nebivolol on exercise performance, energy metabolism, cardiovascular and neurohormonal parameters in physically active patients with arterial hypertension. *J Human Hypertension* 15:715–721

Quindry JC, Franklin BA (2018) Cardioprotective Exercise and Pharmacologic Interventions as Complementary Antidotes to Cardiovascular Disease. *Exerc Sport Sci Rev* 46:5-17

Ripley TL, Saseen JJ (2014) Beta-blockers: a review of their pharmacological and physiological diversity in hypertension. *Ann Pharmacother* 48:723–733

Schumann S-A, Hickner J (2008) When not to use beta-blockers in seniors with hypertension. *J Fam Pract* 57:18–21

van Baak MA, Bohm RO, Arends BG, van Hoof ME, Rahn, KH (1987) Long-term antihypertensive therapy with beta-blockers: submaximal exercise capacity and metabolic effects during exercise. *Int J Sports Med* 5:342–347

van Baak MA (1988) Beta-adrenoreceptor blockade and exercise. An update. *Sports Med* 4:209–225

van Baak MA, Mooij JM, Schiffers PM (1992) Exercise and the pharmacokinetics of propranolol, verapamil and atenolol. *Eur J Clin Pharmacol* 43:547–550

Van Bortel LM, van Baak MA (1992) Exercise tolerance with nebivolol and atenolol. *Cardiovasc Drugs Ther* 6:239–247

Wallin JD, Shah SV (1987) Beta-adrenergic blocking agents in the treatment of hypertension. Choices based on pharmacological properties and patient characteristics. *Arch Intern Med* 147:654–659

Westhoff TH, Franke N, Schmidt S, Vallbracht-Israng K, Zidek W, Dimeo F, van der Giet M (2007) Beta-blockers do not impair the cardiovascular benefits of endurance training in hypertensives. *J Hum Hypertens* 21:486–493

Wijnen JAG, van Baak MA, de Haan C, Stuijker Boudier HAJ, Tan FS, Van Bortel LMAB (1993) Beta-blockade and lipolysis during endurance exercise. *Eur J Clin Pharmacol* 45:101–105

Wright JT Jr, Fine LJ, Lackland DT, Ogedegbe G, Dennison Himmelfarb CR (2014) Evidence supporting a systolic blood pressure goal of less than 150 mm Hg in patients aged 60 years or older: the minority view. *Ann Intern Med* 160:499–503

5   Cardiovascular Drugs and Hypertension

Abstract

For the treatment of hypertension and other mild forms of cardiovascular disease in physically active individuals, better choices than beta-blockers are available. The calcium channel blockers provide control of blood pressure during exercise without negative impact on heart rate, exercise capacity, or metabolism. Drugs that interact with the angiotensin regulatory system provide good control of blood pressure with few documented negative effects on the heart or exercise metabolism. ACE inhibitors reduce angiotensin II–mediated events and enhance the vasodilatory effects of bradykinin. Angiotensin receptor blockers significantly decrease angiotensin II activity mediated by type 1 receptors, but they lack the effects mediated by bradykinin that are enhanced by the ACE inhibitors. Inhibitors of angiotensin activity do not negatively impact heart rate, oxygen utilization, or metabolism during exercise.

CASE EXAMPLE

Bob, Megan's Dad, is close to retirement. He actually isn't that ready to retire, but the sports agency he started is applying some not-to-subtle pressure for him to give up the reins. It probably is a good idea anyway—he has been burned out for a while now. His health has taken a beating. He had bad chest pains last year and ended up getting a stent put into his left anterior descending artery. He is off the blood thinners except for a daily baby aspirin. Years ago, when he was first diagnosed with hypertension, he took the beta-blocker atenolol and did not like it. He had been working out a lot back then, and felt like he was perpetually stuck at 80% effort. Now his doctor is telling him he is pre-diabetic and has signs of metabolic syndrome. She has him on enalapril (an ACE inhibitor, defined below), a common prescription for hypertension, particularly in people with diabetes mellitus. He needs to make some lifestyle changes before things get that bad and he becomes diabetic. Take the dog for a long walk every morning and evening. Cut back on the coffee. Cut back on the IPAs. Eat healthier. And stop smoking.

Learning Objectives

1   Learn the importance of hypertension worldwide.
2   Understand how hypertension is defined and what causes it.
3   Understand the role of angiotensin II in control of blood pressure.
4   Distinguish how ACE inhibitors and angiotensin receptor blockers work.
5   Learn how calcium channel blockers exert their effect.

6   Learn what distinguishes the different calcium channel blockers.
7   Appreciate why ACE inhibitors and calcium channel blockers are considered first-line treatments for hypertension in competitive athletes.

Introduction

In Chapter 4, we saw that beta-blockers are widely prescribed for cardiovascular disease. Although they usually are well tolerated and can be low in cost, beta-blockers can have a negative effect on the heart and suppress energy substrate utilization, especially during exercise. Many other drug choices are currently available. We will look at several classes of drugs in some detail: angiotensin-converting enzyme (ACE) inhibitors, angiotensin receptor blockers (antagonists), calcium channel blockers, and the α-receptor antagonists. The ACE inhibitors and angiotensin receptor blockers (often called ARBs) have overlapping mechanisms and are grouped together as angiotensin inhibitors. The ACE inhibitors block the formation of angiotensin II, and the ARBs antagonize angiotensin II receptors; both types of treatments decrease angiotensin II activity. Each of these drugs is used to treat hypertension and other types of cardiovascular disease, such as angina, arrhythmias, and cardiac myopathies. First, let's review the basics of hypertension and the effect of exercise before covering the pharmacology of these drugs.

Hypertension

About 50 million Americans have **hypertension**, or high blood pressure. There may be as many as one billion sufferers worldwide, leading to approximately seven million deaths per year due to hypertension (JNC 7 2003). Awareness of hypertension is improving, and about 60% of the American population with hypertension is receiving treatment. This improvement in treatment correlates with favorable trends in morbidity and mortality attributed to hypertension (JNC 7). Hypertension is graded from the systolic and diastolic blood pressure (Table 5.1, JNC 7). Blood pressure is normal if both systolic and diastolic pressure criteria are met. High blood pressure is diagnosed if either the indicated systolic or diastolic condition is met. The JNC 8 recommendation is to commence treatment if blood pressure exceeds either 140 (systolic) or 90 (diastolic) for ages 30 to 59. For individuals 60 and older, the recommendation is 150/90 (JNC 8 2014). The recommendation for those over 60 has triggered discussion and was mentioned under Elder Concerns in Chapter 4.

Hypertension can result from increased blood volume, increased cardiac output, or increased total vascular resistance (the sum of resistance in peripheral vasculature).

Table 5.1 Classification of stage of hypertension based on blood pressure

Classification	Systolic Blood Pressure (mm Hg)	Diastolic Blood Pressure (mm Hg)
Normal	<120	<80
Prehypertension	120–139	80–89
Stage 1 Hypertension	140–159	90–99
Stage 2 Hypertension	≥160	≥100

Aging, sympathetic overactivity, exposure to toxins, and genetic defects can damage critical cells in the kidney or vasculature, also causing high blood pressure. Metabolic syndrome, with insulin resistance and elevation in insulin levels, leads to increased sympathetic activity and hypertension, and the number of patients with metabolic syndrome, prediabetes, or diabetes continues to increase. Approximately 5% of patients with hypertension have a secondary etiology that leads to an elevation in blood pressure; this is termed **secondary hypertension**. For these individuals, the hypertension is potentially curable when the underlying cause is treated. Chronic kidney disease is the most common cause of secondary hypertension. Impaired renal function can worsen blood pressure control by reducing sodium and water excretion, leading to volume retention and hypertension. Another cause is when blockage of the renal artery leads to less perfusion of the kidney and activation of the renin-angiotensin-aldosterone system. Activation of this hormonal circuit leads to retention of sodium and water and worsening blood pressure control. Pheochromocytoma, a type of tumor in the adrenal gland, results when chromaffin cells become cancerous in the adrenal medulla or sympathetic ganglia. These cancer cells produce and secrete excess catecholamines, causing fluctuations in blood pressure or sustained hypertension. With treatment of these diseases, the associated hypertension may resolve.

The other 95% of high blood pressure cases are referred to as **primary** (also commonly referred to as "essential") **hypertension**, where the primary cause is unclear. The risk of becoming hypertensive increases with age in almost all contemporary societies. Hypertension results from a complex interaction of genes and environmental factors. However, its genetic basis is poorly understood, even though potential genes have been identified. Environmental factors that may contribute to hypertension include chronic stress, obesity, cigarette smoking, caffeine intake, and vitamin D deficiency. Insulin resistance, which is common in obesity and a component of metabolic syndrome, is also thought to contribute to hypertension. Lifestyle factors that lower blood pressure include exercise, weight loss, reduced alcohol intake, and diets low in salt and high in fruits and vegetables (e.g., Dietary Approaches to Stop Hypertension [DASH diet]).

Many different theories have been proposed to attempt to explain primary hypertension. An increase in total peripheral resistance while cardiac output functions normally could account for many cases of primary hypertension. The rise in peripheral resistance has many different causes. Problems with salt and water handling in the kidneys cause an increase in blood volume, which increases peripheral resistance and blood pressure. Abnormalities in the sympathetic nervous system can increase peripheral resistance with or without an increase in cardiac output. In many patients, both the kidney and the sympathetic nervous system are probably involved to differing degrees. Additional mechanisms that could increase peripheral resistance include vascular inflammation and endothelial cell dysfunction. As we age, increased peripheral resistance is mainly attributable to the narrowing of small arteries and arterioles. A decrease in peripheral venous compliance may also contribute to hypertension. Decreased peripheral compliance can increase venous return and the amount of blood entering the heart, ultimately causing heart issues and problems maintaining blood pressure.

Undiagnosed hypertension and the resulting long-term elevation of blood pressure cause a decline in cardiovascular health. Problems associated with untreated hypertension include coronary and peripheral artery diseases, myocardial infarcts, chronic renal failure, strokes, aneurysms, and heart failure. Individuals with untreated hypertension can develop **left ventricular hypertrophy (LVH)**, a major contributor to heart disease. This pathological condition occurs when muscle cells in the left ventricle grow in size due to the increased load caused by prolonged elevated blood pressure. The left ventricle loses its ability to respond to short-term loads placed on it during stress or exercise. Therefore, patients with LVH display diminished exercise capacity, and those with serious LVH should do low-intensity exercise to minimize the chance of impaired vasodilation, myocardial ischemia, or fatal arrhythmias. Endurance athletes usually have some LVH, but it is not associated with a similar disease etiology.

Treating Hypertension

Patients with hypertension may have a combination of increased sympathetic activity, increased peripheral resistance, elevated angiotensin II, and/or increased blood volume. Therefore, the major approaches to treating hypertension focus on drugs that:

* antagonize the sympathetic nervous system (beta-blockers),
* inhibit angiotensin II activation (ACE inhibitors),
* block angiotensin II receptors (ARBs),
* cause relaxation of smooth muscle cells in the vasculature (calcium channel blockers), or
* decrease blood volume (diuretics; see Chapter 6).

Control of blood pressure is a complex physiological process, involving the central nervous system, heart, vasculature, and kidneys. When lifestyle changes and regular exercise are insufficient in management of blood pressure, drugs are needed. More than 100 drugs are available to treat hypertension. Diuretics and beta-blockers have been prescribed for years and are relatively inexpensive, safe, and effective. However, other classes of drugs have been released in recent years and have gained a large portion of the market. Large-scale studies have attempted to determine whether the new drugs are sufficiently better to warrant their higher cost (ALLHAT 2002). They concluded that diuretics are a superior treatment for hypertension and this finding was further validated with studies on patients with diabetes, renal disease, and metabolic syndrome (Einhorn, Davis, Wright, et al. 2010). Diuretics, particularly when combined with the drug classes listed above, are a significant part of the JNC 8 guidelines for the treatment of hypertension in adults (JNC 8). Newer beta-blockers have not been a component of large randomized control trials and are not included in the JNC 8 recommendations. The other classes of drugs—calcium channel blockers, ACE inhibitors, and ARBs—are recommended under particular circumstances. Drugs such as the ARBs, however, can be considerably more expensive, and their long-term potentials for adverse effects are either not known or have caused some to re-evaluate their use, especially in comparison to diuretics (ALLHAT; Einhorn et al.; JNC 8).

Though the determination of which drugs to prescribe may be somewhat controversial, there is no controversy concerning the need for individuals to regulate their blood pressure properly. Combinations of drugs are needed for many hypertensives. The dire consequences of untreated high blood pressure, including LVH and other cardiovascular diseases, are a major burden on health care in throughout the world. It is estimated that 40% of the USA's population with hypertension is not being adequately treated (JNC 7). It is easy to see that this is a major concern of the medical community and a significant area of research and development for the drug industry, due to the potential return on their investment. Exercise, diet, and lifestyle play important roles in the management of hypertension. As we will see, there is extensive overlap in the physiological response to exercise and the mechanism of action for many of these drugs.

Exercise and Hypertension

Physical activity improves cardiovascular health and decreases morbidity (JNC 7). Exercise stimulates catecholamine secretion, increases cardiac output, and redistributes blood flow. Improvements in cardiopulmonary function correlate with improved metabolic and hormonal function in regular exercisers. Long-term, regular exercise leads to a relative decrease in catecholamine output at comparable exercise levels. Although increasing exercise intensity causes an increase in blood pressure, the increase in blood pressure lessens as fitness level improves. Well-trained individuals have a larger stroke volume and a lower resting blood pressure than untrained individuals.

For individuals with hypertension, regular exercise can help lower blood pressure, but the magnitude is limited (reported decreases range from 2 mmHg to 12 mmHg), and the effect levels off over time (Cardoso, Gomides, Queiroz, et al. 2010). A single episode of aerobic exercise decreases blood pressure during the post-exercise period in normotensive and hypertensive subjects, with hypertensives often having a greater decrease (Cardoso et al.; Fagard & Cornelissen 2007). This phenomenon has been referred to as post-exercise hypotension. The effect lasts for several hours, making it of clinical relevance for these patients.

Many factors may influence the magnitude and duration of post-exercise hypotension. For example, the time of day when the exercise occurs can have an effect, since blood pressure normally has a diurnal rhythm (higher during the day, lower at night). Also, women tend to have a lower-magnitude response. The intensity and duration of the physical activity also show variation in the many published studies (Cardoso et al.). Chronic aerobic training can reduce blood pressure in hypertensive subjects. Meta-analysis of randomized controlled studies involving endurance training in hypertensives showed a significant decrease in blood pressure (Fagard & Cornelissen). Data from this study also showed that the 30 hypertensive study groups analyzed had significantly lowered systemic vascular resistance (7.1%), plasma norepinephrine (29%), and plasma renin activity (20%). In another study of 88 patients with hypertension, including 39 women, a moderate-intensity continuous training protocol (60% VO_2max) was compared to an aerobic interval training protocol (85% to 90% VO_2max; Molmen-Hansen, Stolen, Tjonna, et al. 2012). Compared to a no-exercise control group, both exercise protocols lowered blood pressure, with the interval training protocol showing a greater decrease than the moderate-intensity protocol. Total peripheral resistance was significantly reduced only in the interval-training group, suggesting that the blood pressure–reducing effect of exercise in hypertensives is intensity dependent (Molmen-Hansen et al.). High-intensity intermittent training, as observed during training for soccer (football), also improved the cardiovascular health profile in sedentary, pre-menopausal women (Mohr, Lindenskov, Holm, et al. 2014). This 15-week recreational soccer training treatment resulted in a marked reduction in blood pressure and caused a series of changes in body composition, lipid profile, and cardiovascular fitness, contributing to a large overall reduction in risk factors for cardiovascular disease.

The effect of resistance training on blood pressure has been less clear, due to the limited number of studies (Fagard & Cornelissen). A more recent meta-analysis involved 33 study groups and 1,012 participants (Cornelissen, Fagard, Coeckelberghs, & Vanhees 2011). This analysis supports dynamic resistance training as a way to decrease blood pressure, increase peak VO_2, and decrease body fat and plasma triglycerides. This study also provides support for isometric handgrip training in the management of high blood pressure. However, the lack of published studies using large, randomized controlled trials limits the conclusions that can be drawn and an understanding of the mechanisms involved (Cornelissen et al.). Resistance training also provides musculoskeletal benefits and is an important complement to aerobic training. However, weight training can cause a spike in blood pressure (called exercise hypertension), with extremely high blood pressures recorded during maximal lifts; this type of weight lifting is not recommended for hypertensives. Following stabilization of treatment and evaluation from a physician, dynamic or isometric resistance training is a valuable addition to an exercise prescription.

On the basis of this research, patients who are taking drugs to control their hypertension are encouraged to exercise regularly. Competitive athletes and sport and exercise enthusiasts interested in training and improving their fitness level need to understand how antihypertensive drugs work. Exercisers with high blood pressure prefer antihypertensive drugs that:

- have little or no myocardial depressive effect during exercise.
- are not arrhythmogenic (capable of inducing cardiac arrhythmias).
- do not inhibit blood flow to muscles.
- do not affect energy substrate (lipid, carbohydrates) utilization.

Angiotensin Inhibitors

As discussed previously, control of blood pressure is a complex physiological process, involving the central nervous system, heart, vasculature, and kidneys. The **renin-angiotensin system** helps regulate blood pressure, aldosterone levels, and electrolytes. Genetic analysis of hypertension in humans has found a large number of genes involved in the renin-angiotensin system, suggesting that defects in this pathway contribute to the genetic disposition to high blood pressure. The causative role of the genetic variation in the pathophysiology of humans is debated, but the renin-angiotensin system clearly plays a part in renal failure, vascular disease, and heart failure, in addition to hypertension. The complex pathway involves many tissues and feedback loops, providing many possible gene candidates for altered or improper activity causing disease. Angiotensin II is the most important molecule in this regulatory loop, and drugs have been developed that slow its production or act as antagonists at its receptors. After examining the renin-angiotensin system in some detail, we will discuss both classes of drugs: the angiotensin-converting enzyme inhibitors and the angiotensin receptor blockers. See Table 5.2 for the properties of these drugs.

Figure 5.1 illustrates some of the components of the renin-angiotensin system. The renal cortex (outer region of the kidneys) senses decreases in blood pressure and responds by releasing **renin** into the circulation. Renin release is also caused by sympathetic stimulation and circulating epinephrine. Sodium depletion can also stimulate renin release. Renin is a protease that cleaves the circulating protein **angiotensinogen**

Table 5.2 Summary of angiotensin inhibitor properties

	ACE inhibitors	ARBs
Examples	Captopril, enalapril, benazepril, and many others	Losartan, valsartan, and many others
Indications	Hypertension, heart failure, diabetes	Hypertension, heart failure
Effects	Reduce angiotensin II levels, reduce vasoconstriction, reduce aldosterone secretion	Antagonize angiotensin II receptors, reduce vasoconstriction, reduce aldosterone secretion
Half-life	Two to ten hours	Four to six hours, 12 hours for newer drugs
Bradykinin effect	Increase	No change
Angiotensin receptor AT_1R	No effect	Inhibition
Angiotensin receptor AT_2R	No effect	Stimulation
Side effects	Dry cough, angioedema, hyperkalemia, teratogenic	Similar but with less dry cough

Source: This table contains content derived from Burnton et al. and Katzung, Masters, & Trevor (2012).

to form **angiotensin I**, a peptide that is 10 amino acids in length and has little activity. Angiotensin I is further cleaved to a peptide of only eight amino acids, called **angiotensin II**. A number of different proteases in the body can do this, but the predominant one is called the **angiotensin-converting enzyme (ACE)**.

Angiotensin II is a very potent vasoconstrictor. Its actions can be separated into fast and slow responses. **Fast angiotensin II responses** include direct vasoconstrictor activity, causing an increase in total peripheral resistance. The vasoconstriction is caused by activation angiotensin II receptors (AT_1 receptors) in blood vessels. Angiotensin II also increases sympathetic activity by increasing norepinephrine release and blocking its re-uptake. It can also cause the release of catecholamines (i.e., epinephrine and norepinephrine) from the adrenal medulla. **Slow angiotensin II responses** include increasing sodium reabsorption in the kidney and stimulating the release of **aldosterone** from the adrenal cortex. Aldosterone is a potent hormone that stimulates the kidney to reabsorb sodium. As a result of greater sodium reabsorption during urine formation, the body retains water. These responses contribute to decreased urine output and an increase in blood volume, which raises blood pressure. Additionally, angiotensin II stimulates several areas of the brain involved in thirst and sodium appetite to increase thirst (Fitzsimons 1998). Thirst stimulates the drinking of fluids, resulting in an increase in blood volume, which, in turn, contributes to an increase in blood pressure. Angiotensin II also plays an important role in tissue remodeling and cardiac hypertrophy. It can stimulate certain cells to grow, such as in the ventricles, and thereby can have long-lasting effects on cardiovascular physiology.

Figure 5.1 The renin-angiotensin-aldosterone pathway.

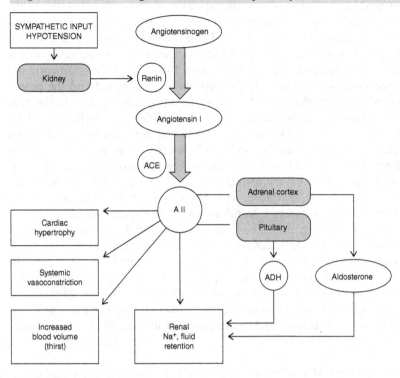

Legend: Major components in the renin-angiotensin system are shown, with the many physiological roles for angiotensin II (A II) indicated.

How Do ACE Inhibitors Work?

Individuals who possess genetic changes that disrupt the normal control mechanism associated with the renin-angiotensin system can have elevated blood pressure. Some hypertensive patients have elevated renin activity or express a highly active version of ACE. ACE inhibitors can be very effective in treating these individuals. Since ACE inhibitors are effective in decreasing ACE activity, the formation of angiotensin II is slowed. Lower angiotensin II levels reduce its contributions to raising blood pressure in patients with the genetic predispositions mentioned above. ACE inhibition also decreases the body's ability to raise blood pressure when the renin-angiotensin system is activated. Therefore, ACE inhibitors suppress vasoconstriction and limit excessive retention of salt and water.

ACE as a Target for Rational Drug Design

Years ago, when the details of the renin-angiotensin system were being worked out, pharmacologists realized that if an inhibitor of ACE could be found, it could possibly serve as a drug to decrease blood pressure. The drug captopril was developed as an **ACE inhibitor**, in an early example of rational drug design: the targeting of a known enzyme (here, ACE) for drug development.

ACE is found in the lining of endothelial walls, particularly in the lung. The enzyme can be considered an **ectoenzyme**, because it is attached to the cell's exterior, so that its activity is extracellular. The enzyme has two similar catalytic sites, each of which contains zinc (Zn^{2+}). ACE cleaves two amino acids off the C-terminal end of peptides; hence, it is referred to as a peptidyl dipeptidase. Known substrates for ACE include the peptides angiotensin I and the potent vasodilator bradykinin. Whereas the predominant role for ACE is in the production of angiotensin II, the activity toward bradykinin is also important for blood pressure control. Bradykinin stimulates the release of prostacyclin (a type of prostaglandin) and nitric oxide, both of which cause a decrease in peripheral resistance and a lowering of blood pressure. ACE was discovered to be the same enzyme as kininase, the enzyme responsible for the inactivation of the bradykinin. Inhibition of ACE, therefore, will slow the inactivation of bradykinin, causing an indirect vasodilatory effect due to higher bradykinin levels.

The genetics of ACE are also interesting and are possibly involved in diseases such as hypertension. The ACE gene shows polymorphisms, meaning there is allelic variation—different versions of the gene. The gene either has an insertion (the I-allele) or a deletion (the D-allele). The frequency of the D- or I-allele varies in the human population as individuals will have either a D/D, an I/D, or an I/I genotype. The D-allele results in higher activity, suggesting that individuals expressing it may have higher angiotensin II levels and a corresponding increase in blood pressure.

Captopril was the first ACE inhibitor, developed through structure-based design in the late 1960s and early 1970s. Its success in controlling blood pressure led to the development of many other derivatives that have longer half-lives and fewer side effects. Enalapril (Vasotec) is a widely prescribed example. It reaches a peak blood level in three to four hours and has a plasma half-life of about 11 hours. Other common ACE inhibitors are benazepril (Lotensin) and lisinopril (Zestril). They all work primarily by decreasing total peripheral resistance and have little or no effect on cardiac output or heart rate. ACE inhibitors are also useful in treating chronic kidney disease and nephropathies, especially in diabetics. These drugs are thought to decrease capillary pressure and improve renal hemodynamics, particularly in the glomeruli (clusters of blood vessels that filter blood from the urine; see Chapter 6). ACE inhibitors are effective for the treatment of chronic heart failure and post-myocardial infarct, probably because they decrease peripheral resistance and fluid retention. They are useful in treating left ventricular hypertrophy, possibly because they impair angiotensin II's effect on hypertrophic growth and myocardial remodeling.

How Do Angiotensin Receptor Blockers Work?

Whereas ACE inhibitors decrease ACE activity, angiotensin receptors mediate the diverse physiological responses to angiotensin II. **Angiotensin receptor blockers (ARBs)**, such as valsartan and losartan, block angiotensin II AT_1 receptors. The AT_1 receptors mediate most of the fast and slow responses caused by angiotensin II, detailed above. These drugs are now widely prescribed for hypertension and congestive heart failure. These receptor antagonists are very specific for AT_1 receptors and are very potent blockers. They are referred to as "insurmountable antagonists," because even at high concentrations of angiotensin II, their antagonism cannot be completely reversed. Use of angiotensin receptor blockers causes an increase in blood levels of angiotensin II, possibly in compensation for the reduced angiotensin II receptor activity. Other angiotensin receptor subtypes are insensitive to this group of angiotensin receptor blockers and may become inappropriately stimulated by the elevated levels of angiotensin II. The possible negative consequences and possible side effects of elevated angiotensin II have generated controversy, particularly in terms of whether they increase the likelihood of myocardial infarct (Strauss & Hall 2006). Numerous additional studies do not support a significant increase in the risk of myocardial infarct, but they also do not support a lower risk, even though angiotensin receptor blockers effectively lower blood pressure. Angiotensin receptor blockers are approved for the treatment of hypertension. Their efficacy is similar to the ACE inhibitors and other antihypertensive drugs. Some of the angiotensin receptor blockers have been approved for diabetic nephropathy, stroke prophylaxis, and certain conditions of myocardial infarction. They help protect kidney function in diabetics. ACE inhibitors are generally considered the first-line choice, with angiotensin receptor blockers prescribed if ACE inhibitors are ineffective or not well tolerated (i.e., dry cough; 2013 ACCF/AHA Guideline).

Angiotensin receptor blockers provide a more complete inhibition of angiotensin II activity than ACE inhibitors. Because the body contains other enzymes besides ACE that can produce angiotensin II, some level of angiotensin II can still be generated after administration of ACE inhibitors. In contrast to ACE inhibitors, angiotensin receptor blockers have no effect on bradykinin activity (discussed more in Box).

Exercise Pharmacology of ACE Inhibitors and Angiotensin Receptor Blockers

Pharmacokinetic Concerns

Of the ACE inhibitors, captopril has a very short half-life and contains a sulfhydryl component that can leave a bad taste in the mouth. Enalaprilat is a second-generation ACE inhibitor that can be given IV, but it cannot be absorbed orally. It was chemically modified into a pro-drug, called enalapril, that can be taken orally but requires metabolism for activation. Most of the other widely prescribed ACE inhibitors are given orally as a pro-drug requiring metabolism and activation in the liver. Elimination of ACE inhibitors is primarily by the kidneys.

Several ACE inhibitors are given at reduced dosage in patients with renal insufficiency. Moderate to intense exercise might be expected to alter the active drug's activation and elimination, extending the time to peak levels and its moderate half-life (about 11 hours). Several of the angiotensin receptor blockers, such as losartan and valsartan, also have liver metabolites with significant activity and depend on the liver for clearance. Their dosage is adjusted in individuals with hepatic insufficiency. One could expect intense exercise and decreased flow to the liver to extend their bioavailability.

Pharmacodynamic Concerns

ACE inhibitors and angiotensin receptor blockers provide cardio protection and cardio reparative activity (Dzau 1989; Motz & Strauer 1996). These beneficial effects on the cardiovascular system are enhanced with an exercise program. Regular exercise reduces resting blood pressure and helps control risk factors for hypertension and cardiovascular disease (excessive weight, elevated blood lipids, elevated insulin and blood sugar, and so forth).

These drugs decrease resting blood pressure and generally temper the increase in blood pressure during exercise. In an early study, nine patients with hypertension took captopril for seven days and performed a graded submaximal exercise test (Manhem, Bramnert, Hulthén, & Hökfelt 1981). Blood levels of norepinephrine and epinephrine increased to the same level with or without captopril, suggesting that the drug did not affect the sympathetic nervous system. Blood pressure was lower with the drug at rest and during exercise, with no difference in heart rate (Manhem et al.). In a study with 17 hypertensive patients, the ACE inhibitor cilazapril reduced total peripheral resistance at rest and during handgrip isometric exercise (see Table 5.3). Maximal exercise level and lactate concentrations were largely unaffected by cilazapril (Kleinbloesem, Erb, Essig, et al. 1989).

In another study with 16 patients with mild to moderate essential hypertension, six weeks of captopril decreased blood pressure with no effect on heart rate (van Baak, Koene, Verstappen, & Tan 1991). During a maximal exercise test, captopril had little effect on blood pressure and heart rate, unlike the beta-blocker atenolol, which significantly decreased both. Maximum workload and VO₂max were close to placebo levels with captopril, whereas atenolol caused significant decreases (see Table 5.4). In a submaximal endurance test, both drugs reduced exercise duration, but the decrease in duration was greater with atenolol.

Table 5.3 The effect of cilazapril on hypertensive patients during isometric exercise

	At Rest		Isometric Exercise	
Parameter	Placebo	Cilazapril	Placebo	Cilazapril
Systolic BP (mm Hg)	144 ± 13	131 ± 15**	168 ± 17	152 ± 16**
Diastolic BP (mm Hg)	103 ± 8	93 ± 12**	116 ± 10	109 ± 11*
Heart Rate (bpm)	76 ± 12	73 ± 0	81 ± 12	79 ± 12
TPR (dyn s cm⁻³)	2416 ± 749	2005 ± 569*	2760 ± 927	2448 ± 855*

Legend: Hypertensive patients ($n = 17$) were tested with a handgrip isometric exercise protocol after three weeks of treatment with either cilazapril or placebo in a double-blind crossover study. BP: blood pressure; TPR: total peripheral resistance. $*p < 0.05$; $**p < 0.01$ (compared to placebo). Data modified from Kleinbloesem et al.

Table 5.4 Effect of captopril on work rate and oxygen uptake at maximal aerobic exercise

Condition	Wmax (W)	VO₂max (liter/min)	Heart Rate max (bpm)
Placebo 1	237 ± 11	3.38 ± 0.13	174.8 ± 3.0
Placebo 2	238 ± 11	3.30 ± 0.13	171.7 ± 3.4
Atenolol	221 ± 11	3.08 ± 0.16	128.9 ± 3.7
Captopril	234 ± 14*	3.33 ± 0.13*	171.9 ± 3.0**

Legend: Hypertensive patients ($n = 16$) were treated with a randomized double-blind crossover design. After treatment with placebo for six weeks, atenolol or captopril was given for a six-week period, followed by another six weeks with a placebo (wash-out period), and then a final six weeks with the other drug. For the maximal exercise test, at the end of each six-week period, subjects were subjected to incremental increases of work rate using cycle ergometers until exhaustion. $*p < 0.05$; $**p < 0.01$ (atenolol vs. captopril). Data modified from van Baak et al.

A newer ACE inhibitor (trandolapril) was used in a study with 20 young, healthy males to test the effect of the drug on maximum workload using cycle ergometry (Predel, Rohden, Heine, et al. 1994). Drug treatment did not significantly alter maximum power, RPE, VO_2, free fatty acids, glucose, insulin, cortisol, or growth hormone (Predel et al.). Monotherapy with trandolapril was more effective than captopril in regulating blood pressure during exercise on a treadmill until exhaustion (Carreira, Tavares, Leite, et al. 2003). The trandolapril group had lower peak diastolic blood pressure and a greater increase in exercise capacity than the captopril group.

Very little research is available on the effect of angiotensin receptor blockers on exercise. One prospective study compared an angiotensin receptor blocker to a calcium channel blocker on the inflammatory and thrombotic response during exercise in 60 hypertensive patients (Liakos, Vyssoulis, Michaelides, et al. 2012). Six months after normalization of blood pressure from taking the drug, the patients underwent maximal treadmill exercise testing, with blood samples taken at rest and during peak exercise. The angiotensin receptor blocker group had less exercise-induced markers of inflammation than the calcium channel blocker group, suggesting that angiotensin receptor blockers may have a protective effect in exercising hypertensive patients (Liakos et al.).

Available research is consistent with the expectation that inhibitors of angiotensin activity have nominal direct effect on the heart during exercise and have little or no negative effects on mobilization of energy reserves. These drugs have minimal effect on oxygen utilization and capacity. There is some evidence that exercise duration may be decreased somewhat, but not to the extent observed with beta-blockers (van Baak et al.). The positive outcomes associated with training and exercise are expected to occur when these drugs are being used. The beneficial effect on heart and vasculature remodeling with these drugs probably improves with regular aerobic exercise (Dzau; Omvik & Lund-Johansen 1993; Carreira et al.).

Health Risks of ACE Inhibitors and Angiotensin Receptor Blockers

ACE inhibitors and angiotensin receptor blockers should be discontinued during pregnancy, as they have teratogenic potential. ACE inhibitors can cause a dry cough and angioedema. **Angioedema** is similar to urticaria (hives), but there is rapid swelling deeper in the dermis below the skin, often around the eyes and lips. It possibly involves bradykinin. These side effects are less pronounced with angiotensin receptor blockers. There has been some controversy as to health-related problems associated with angiotensin receptor blockers, with conflicting reports indicating a risk of cancer with their use. A comprehensive meta-analysis concluded that angiotensin receptor blockers did not increase the risk of cancer overall (Azoulay, Assimes, Yin, et al. 2012).

Calcium Channel Blockers

Cardiac and smooth muscle depend on extracellular calcium for excitation-contraction. Extracellular calcium moves into cells through calcium channels following membrane depolarization, along the membrane's electrochemical gradient. The first voltage-activated calcium channel (i.e., those channels that open due to membrane depolarization) was described in heart cells, and other calcium channels have been characterized in neurons and smooth muscle cells (Reuter 1983). The concentration gradient for calcium is steep, as free

The L-type Calcium Channel

The **L-type calcium channel** is the prevalent voltage-activated calcium channel in vascular smooth muscle, cardiac muscle, and the SA and AV nodes. Other voltage-activated calcium channels, such as the T, N, and P channels, are found in a variety of different neurons and tissues.

L-type and other channels are considered voltage-activated (or gated) channels because they open in response to membrane depolarization. The voltage change across the membrane causes a transition of the channel from a first closed, resting state to a second open, calcium-conducting state. The open state can transition to a third non-conducting, inactivated state before the channel returns to the original closed state. When the channel opens, calcium enters the cells along its steep concentration gradient; the resulting rise in intracellular calcium is coupled to many cellular responses, ranging from neurosecretion and muscle contraction to gene expression. These channels can, therefore, transduce electrical signals at the cell membrane into physiologically important signal transduction pathways, often involving the calcium-binding protein calmodulin.

The L-type calcium channel acts as a drug receptor for the calcium channel blockers. A complex of different proteins forms these channels. The complex contains the pore-forming $\alpha 1$ subunit, the intracellular β subunit, and the chemically linked $\alpha 2$ and δ subunits (see Figure 5.2). In some cases, there is a transmembrane γ subunit (not shown in Figure 5.2). Verapamil probably binds the channel from the inside of the cell, and diltiazem and the dihydropyridines probably access their binding sites from the extracellular side (Hockerman, Peterson, Johnson, & Catterall 1997). However, the binding sites for these drug classes are very close to each other and may share common molecular interactions. All three classes of calcium channel blockers bind individually distinct sites on the sixth helical segments of domains III and IV (see Figure 5.2). Binding of the drugs to these sites possibly alters protein–protein interactions at the interface between the two domains.

Each drug class of the calcium channel blockers prefers binding the channel in the open or inactivated state versus the closed state. The protein conformation of the closed state presumably interferes with access of the drug to its binding state. Once bound, the different classes of drugs act similarly to allosteric inhibitors, probably by distorting flexible portions of the protein at structural interfaces between domains within the protein subunits. The result is a decrease in calcium current, which causes relaxation of muscle cells. The relaxation in vascular smooth muscle causes a decrease in vascular resistance and a lowering of blood pressure. In the heart, a decrease in calcium conduction depresses contractility and suppresses automaticity and conduction. The different classes of channel blockers differ in their effect on the heart, as detailed later in this chapter.

calcium is maintained at very low levels inside cells. The resulting spike in intracellular calcium concentration can trigger a variety of responses, depending on the cell type; examples include contraction in muscle cells and secretion in nerve and glandular cells. The increase in intracellular calcium can also stimulate calcium-induced calcium release from intracellular stores, which helps amplify the calcium signal. The brief increase in intracellular

Figure 5.2 Schematic representation of the subunit composition of the L-type calcium channel.

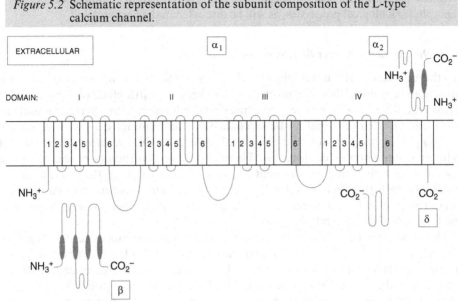

Legend: The α_1 subunit forms the pore with the four helical bundles shown. The long C-terminal tail is the site for regulation by cellular factors. Accessory subunits are shown. The composition of the subunits varies depending on tissue localization. The shaded sixth helical segments of domains III and IV contain amino acid residues important in binding to the different calcium channel blockers (Hockerman et al.).

calcium can also trigger signal transduction pathways dependent on the calcium-binding protein calmodulin. The calcium–calmodulin complex can mediate calcium signals long after the spike in intracellular calcium.

Drugs effective in blocking calcium entry are useful therapeutic agents. When the entry of calcium in the cells is slowed, there is less muscle fiber contraction, vascular smooth muscle is relaxed, vasodilation occurs, and peripheral vascular resistance is decreased. A similar effect is observed in cardiac tissue, where a decrease in calcium entry results in less force of contraction and a lower workload on the heart. The overall result is lower blood pressure (see the Box on the L-type calcium channel).

Drugs that slow calcium entry into cells are called **calcium channel blockers**, **calcium antagonists**, or similar terms. We will use the relatively common term calcium channel blockers. The **phenylalkylamine** class includes verapamil, the first calcium channel blocker that became clinically useful. It is a chemical derivative of papaverine, an alkaloid with weak vasodilator activity originally isolated from the opium poppy plant. Many of the commonly prescribed calcium channel blockers are related to another compound called **dihydropyridine**, and these drugs form a fairly large group. Nifedipine is the most studied member of the dihydropyridine class of drugs, and it is thought that the other members of this class have similar activity to nifedipine. However, the different dihydropyridines can vary in their effect on smooth muscle cells in different vascular beds throughout the body and in their rate of clearance. For example, the commonly prescribed amlodipine (Norvasc) is a member of the dihydropyridine class, but it has a much longer plasma half-life than nifedipine (about 40 vs. 4 hours). Amlodipine is widely prescribed, in part, because once its effective blood level is reached, its effect on blood pressure is relatively smooth and stable. A third chemically distinct type of calcium channel blocker is **diltiazem**. All three chemical variants are relatively specific for the L-type calcium channel, but they vary in their pharmacological properties, as will be discussed in the next section.

How Do Calcium Channel Blockers Work?

All three classes of calcium channel blockers are relatively specific for vascular smooth muscle and cardiac cells. Calcium channel blockers have little effect on skeletal muscle, because, unlike smooth muscle, which uses extracellular calcium, skeletal muscle uses intracellular calcium stored in the sarcoplasmic reticulum for excitation-contraction coupling. Following stimulation of skeletal muscle, calcium release from these intra-cellular stores initiates contraction. Therefore, since contraction of skeletal muscle does not have the same requirement for extracellular calcium, the calcium channel blockers have little effect on skeletal muscle. Cardiac muscle contraction has a mixture of control mechanisms with regard to calcium; calcium channels are also important to the function of the SA and AV nodes.

The different types of calcium channel blockers have varying effects on heart mus-cle, the AV and SA nodes, and vascular smooth muscle (Table 5.5). Verapamil, a drug in the phenylalkylamine class, depresses heart function to a greater degree than the dihydropyridine drugs. Verapamil can cause a mild decrease in heart rate and can reduce cardiac output, due to its depressive effects on cardiac muscle cells and the AV and SA nodes. The dihydropyridine drugs are more potent for vascular muscle cell relaxation than verapamil or diltiazem. Smooth muscle cells respond at relatively low plasma concentrations of the dihydropyridine drugs, and therefore, there is a greater effect on smooth muscle than cardiac muscle at the recommended dose. Diltiazem has somewhat intermediate activity between verapamil and nifedipine (see Table 5.5). Blocking calcium influx causes relaxation of the smooth muscle cells in the arterial wall. The result is a decrease in peripheral resistance and a drop in blood pressure. Nifedipine and verapamil can also inhibit smooth muscle contraction in the GI-tract, resulting in constipation. Newer drugs, such as amlodipine, have less of a GI-effect.

The various pharmacological properties of the calcium channel blockers (see Table 5.5) allow them to be prescribed for different indications. Verapamil and others are also prescribed because of their anti-angina or anti-arrhythmic activity. As stated earlier, angina occurs when blood supply to the heart is insufficient to meet the oxygen demand. This is particularly true during exertion, giving rise to exertional angina. The depression of cardiac activity caused by verapamil is thought to decrease the oxygen demand on the heart, thereby reducing angina. Suppressed activity at the SA and AV nodes, also an effect of the drug, can help with certain types of arrhythmias.

Exercise Pharmacology of Calcium Channel Blockers

Pharmacokinetic Concerns

Very little data are available on how exercise affects the pharmacokinetic properties of calcium channel blockers. The calcium channel blockers are highly lipophilic and subject to considerable and variable first-pass metabolism by the liver. The result is a wide range of drug levels in the plasma among individuals. These drugs are mainly cleared by metab-olism and depend on intact liver blood flow and function for normal rates of elimination (McAllister, Hamann, & Blouin 1985). Metabolism of diltiazem and verapamil gives rise to active metabolites. Absorption, distribution, and elimination are affected by age and

Table 5.5 Relative specificity of the three major classes of calcium channel blockers

Property	Verapamil	Diltiazem	Nifedipine	Amlodipine
Drug Class	Phenylalkylamine	Benzothiazepine	Dihydropyridine	Dihydropyridine
Indications	Angina, hypertension, arrhythmias	Angina, hypertension	Angina	Angina, hypertension
Plasma half-life (hours)	6	3–4	4	30–50
Vasodilation*	4×	3×	5×	5×
Depression of cardiac contractility*	4×	2×	1×	1×
Suppression of SA node (automaticity)*	5×	5×	1×	1×
Suppression of AV node (conduction)*	5×	4×	None	None
Toxic effects	Hypotension, myocardial depression, constipation, edema	Hypotension, dizziness, flushing, bradycardia	Hypotension, dizziness, flushing, nausea, constipation, edema	Headache, edema

Legend: Properties of the three major classes of calcium channel blockers are shown. Verapamil and diltiazem are the main representatives of their respective classes. Nifedipine was the first heavily studied dihydropyridine, and several drugs of this class are now on the market. They are thought to have similar cardiovascular effects. Amlodipine (Norvasc) is widely prescribed and is included for comparison. Rows marked * indicate the relative cardiovascular effects for the different drugs, with rankings between "None" and "5×" (prominent).
Source: This table contains content derived from Burnton, Chabner, Chabner, and Knollman (2011).

pathological conditions, suggesting that intense exercise could also have an effect on liver function and increase blood levels of these drugs. However, these drugs have a relatively high therapeutic index, and usually there is no need for monitoring of treatment.

Pharmacodynamic Concerns

When considering the interaction of calcium channel blockers and exercise, keep in mind the differences in specificity shown in Table 5.5. Verapamil has greater effects on the heart, while amlodipine has greater effect on the vasculature. Studies have examined calcium channel blockers' effect on exercise and the effect of exercise on these drugs' ability to manage the patient's symptoms. Generally, these drugs exert an immediate and sustained lowering of blood pressure.

In the case of nifedipine, a single dose causes rapid vasodilation, which could decrease exercise performance. However, nifedipine is not usually given for long-term control of hypertension. It is used for acute cases of angina, not for maintenance therapy, because of its short plasma half-life.

Amlodipine is much more widely prescribed for hypertension because its long plasma half-life produces a much more stable response in patients. Amlodipine is a strong vasodilator and has little or no negative **chronotropic** (heart rate), **inotropic** (force of contraction), or **dromotropic** (conduction velocity) effects in the heart. Normal individuals who took amlodipine for two weeks showed no change in resting heart rate, blood pressure, or catecholamine response during exercise. There was also no significant change in oxygen uptake at the anaerobic threshold or at maximum exercise with amlodipine (Stankovic, Panz, Klug, et al. 1999; Lay, Bjorksten, Stainsby, & Blake 2001). However, other studies with hypertensive patients have found a decrease in blood pressure at rest and during exercise. When amlodipine was administered for 11 months to 18 hypertensive patients, resting blood pressure was decreased, largely due to a decrease in total peripheral resistance (Lund-Johansen, Omvik, White, et al. 1990). In this study, exercise at three levels of intensity showed a similar suppression in blood pressure at all three levels, with no change in heart rate. Studies that used a similar protocol with diltiazem found essentially the same results (Lund-Johansen & Omvik 1990).

In a placebo-controlled crossover study with ten hypertensive subjects, amlodipine treatment for two weeks decreased resting blood pressure but did not affect heart rate, VO_2, stroke volume, RPE, free fatty acids, blood lactate, or blood glucose during prolonged submaximal exercise (Gillies, Derman, & Noakes 1996). In a study that used lacidipine, which is closely related to amlodipine, oxygen uptake and heart rate were unchanged at peak exercise, while blood pressure was reduced (Fariello, Boni, Corda, et al. 1991).

We can conclude from these studies that calcium channel blockers do not alter the normal hemodynamic response to exercise or maximal exercise performance. They may suppress exercise blood pressure to a similar degree as resting blood pressure, but that effect appears to vary among the studies. During sustained exercise, energy substrate metabolism is modulated via the sympathetic nervous system. Amlodipine for two weeks did not cause a change in heart rate or catecholamine response (Lay et al.). Calcium channel blockers also have little documented effect on fat or carbohydrate metabolism. Taken together, these responses to calcium channel blockers suggest that individuals should be able to maintain a regular exercise program, manage their disease symptoms, and still see the positive results of a training regimen.

Most drugs in these classes reduce left ventricular hypertrophy, a common form of cardiomyopathy that can result from prolonged hypertension. Left ventricular hypertrophy can transition into heart failure and left ventricular systolic dysfunction. Exercise plus antihypertensive drugs, however, reduce left ventricular hypertrophy more than drug treatment alone (Kokkinos, Narayan, Colleran, et al. 1995). In another study, patients with left ventricular systolic dysfunction and moderate levels of heart failure were tested for the effects of amlodipine on exercise tolerance, quality of life, and left ventricular function. In a double-blind, placebo-controlled study, 437 subjects were treated for 12 weeks with amlodipine in addition to their existing therapy. No significant difference was found with amlodipine treatment in the patients' exercise tolerance and quality of life measures. Left ventricle function did improve marginally in the patients on amlodipine, suggesting that amlodipine may offer only a marginal improvement for patients with heart failure, with no documented negative effects (Udelson, DeAbate, Berk, et al. 2000).

Amlodipine does have a marked effect on patients with angina. One study showed a lower frequency of angina events and lower consumption of nitroglycerin (glycerol trinitrate; Kinnard, Harris, & Hossack 1988). Patients in this study also saw an increase in peak oxygen consumption. Another study found that angina patients taking amlodipine showed less myocardial ischemia (Taylor 1994), consistent with the drug's ability to reduce systemic resistance and improve blood flow to the heart, which allows the heart to receive sufficient oxygen to meet its workload demands. Compared to those who took a placebo, patients who took 10 mg of amlodipine showed a 48% increase in exercise time to the onset of angina and a 31% increase in total exercise time (Taylor). They also had fewer angina attacks per week and took less glycerol trinitrate.

In summary, these drugs help individuals with a range of cardiovascular issues to maintain and benefit from an exercise program. These drugs generally have little suppression of cardiac activity, especially when compared to beta-blockers. Moreover, they have negligible effect on energy mobilization and respiratory activity. Patients with cardiomyopathy, such as left ventricular hypertrophy, also benefit from these drugs, in conjunction with an exercise program.

Health Risks of Calcium Channel Blockers

The toxicity of these drugs is often related to extensions of their calcium channel blocking activity. Excessive inhibition of calcium influx can cause serious issues with the heart, including bradycardia, cardiac arrest, or congestive heart failure. Other, less toxic side effects, which usually do not require discontinuance of therapy, include nausea, dizziness, edema, and constipation (see Table 5.4).

Alpha-Blockers

Norepinephrine stimulates α-1 receptors on vascular smooth muscle, causing vasoconstriction and raising blood pressure. **Alpha-blockers,** such as prazosin (Minipress) and doxazosin, are antagonists for the α-1 receptor, and, thus, can lower blood pressure. Though currently considered second-line agents for hypertension, they are prescribed in certain cases, such as hypertension related to pheochromocytoma (a tumor of the adrenal gland, causing unregulated production of catecholamines) and other diseases involving poor circulation. Side effects following the first dose ("first dose phenomenon") are usually overcome after several doses. The most prevalent side effect is a rapid drop in blood pressure, and so it is recommended to take this drug at bedtime. This type of hypotension, which can cause dizziness or fainting, is called **orthostatic** or **postural hypotension** and can occur when the person stands up after sitting for a while. Alpha-blockers can decrease exercise diastolic blood pressure, and they have little effect on cardiac output. With alpha-blockers, most studies report little or no effect on lactate, VO_2, duration, or performance with moderate exercise (Fahrenbach, Yurgalevitch, Zmuda, & Thompson 1995). Their usefulness as a treatment for hypertension has been overshadowed in recent years with the introduction of newer drugs, such as the angiotensin receptor blockers, but their neutral or possible beneficial effects during exercise have been known since the 1990s (Lund-Johansen, Hjermann, Iversen, & Thaulow 1993).

Elder Concerns

Sarcopenia represents a major health problem, affecting almost 50 million people worldwide with an expectation of continued increase as the world population ages. As we discussed in Chapter 2, questions remain as to whether sarcopenia in the elderly is an inevitable consequence of aging or is the result of a combination of different aging-related causative factors (i.e., chronic obstructive pulmonary disease (COPD), diabetes, hypertension, cardiovascular disease, etc.). Also contributing are years of chronic drug treatment in many of the elderly and the altered pharmacokinetics of drugs that occurs with aging. The elderly often have altered sensitivities to the many possible side effects of the drugs they take.

Sarcopenia involves the progressive impairment in skeletal muscle strength caused by loss of type II skeletal muscle fibers and overall muscle quality. Alterations in calcium cycling during excitation-contraction, mitochondrial dysfunction, metabolic disorders, and insulin resistance are implicated as possible contributors to loss of muscle power and increased fatigability. There is also age-related decline of the sex hormones, growth hormone, and vitamin D, with an increase in pro-inflammatory agents. The pool of satellite cells is depleted in the elderly, leading to sarcopenia and susceptibility to injuries due to the loss of capacity for muscle regeneration. As we saw in Chapter 2, poor diet and lack of physical activity contribute to loss of muscle mass and strength, regardless of age.

Therapeutic approaches to impede or reverse sarcopenia are limited. Manipulation of the population of satellite or stem cells may be an approach in the future, but is not available currently. Exercise and diet are essential components of therapy for sarcopenia. Few pharmacological interventions have been effective in relieving the degradative process. More recently, investigation of the role of the renin-angiotensin system in skeletal muscle suggests a potential benefit of angiotensin-converting enzyme (ACE) inhibitors and angiotensin receptor blockers in sarcopenia (Sartiani, Spinelli, Laurino, et al. 2015).

The renin-angiotensin system regulates perfusion and regeneration capacity of skeletal muscle. Angiotensin II infusion in rodents leads to skeletal muscle wasting, increased apoptosis, enhanced muscle protein breakdown, and decreased appetite. Furthermore, angiotensin II infusion inhibits skeletal muscle stem cell (satellite) proliferation, leading to lowered muscle regenerative capacity (Delafontaine & Yoshida 2016). In humans, elevated stress hormones increase angiotensin II. Many individuals suffering from hypertension have defects in the renin-angiotensin system. Elevated levels of angiotensin II, working through the AT_1 receptors, initiate similar responses found in the animal studies, including muscle wasting diseases and sarcopenia. Humans with the insertion allele in the ACE gene (see Box concerning ACE inhibitors) have reduced ACE activity and have lower angiotensin II. They respond better to training with increased muscle mass—perhaps by having less angiotensin II and less AT_1 receptor activation. In summary, elevated angiotensin II levels have negative effects on muscle and lower angiotensin II levels have a positive effect, suggesting drugs that interfere with angiotensin production or function may have potential in treating muscle wasting conditions like cachexia and sarcopenia.

A possible role for angiotensin receptor blockers and ACE inhibitors in supporting muscle health is being investigated. Blockade of the AT_1 receptor with angiotensin receptor blocker treatment improved muscle remodeling and protected against disuse atrophy (Burks, Andres-Mateos, Marx, et al. 2011). When ACE is inhibited after drug treatment, a second enzyme (ACE2) produces a shorter angiotensin fragment called angiotensin (1-7); it binds and stimulates the AT_2 receptor and the Mas receptor but not the AT_1 receptor. Activation of AT_2 receptors can be considered the 'good arm' of the renin-angiotensin system and is thought to counter-balance AT_1 receptor activity. AT_2 receptor activation (and possibly the Mas receptor) stimulates satellite cell activity and muscle cell growth. Additionally, AT_1 receptor blockade by angiotensin receptor blockers causes an increase in angiotensin II (the body compensates for the blocked receptor by making more angiotensin II) and may spillover to increase activity at the AT_2 receptor. Therefore, ACE inhibitors and angiotensin receptor blockers have therapeutic potential in sarcopenia as they slow or block AT_1 receptor function and encourage AT_2 receptor activity. Blockade of the renin-angiotensin system with these drugs can protect satellite cells and promote muscle regeneration with functional improvement (Sartiani et al.). In an experiment to try and confirm this idea, losartan was used in a trial of elderly men that performed a single bout of heavy resistance training. Losartan did not affect the number of satellite cells per muscle fiber in the days following a single bout of heavy resistance exercise, but it did decrease myostatin expression—a muscle-specific hormone (myokine) that suppresses muscle growth (Heisterberg, Andersen, Schjerling, et al. 2018). Therefore, losartan may contribute to muscle cell growth by lowering myostatin activity, in addition to its possible indirect activation of AT_2 receptors—and by efficiently blocking AT_1 receptors. Research on ACE inhibitors and angiotensin receptor blockers continues as they may provide a therapeutic approach to muscle wasting diseases and sarcopenia.

PES Watch

Management of hypertension and other cardiovascular issues in competitive athletes raises some concerns (Bruno, Cartoni, & Taddei 2011). We learned in the previous chapter that the NCAA and USOC test for beta-blockers in certain competitions. Diuretics, a first-line choice for hypertension (discussed in the next chapter), are also on the banned list. The NCAA and USOC do not ban calcium channel blockers, ACE inhibitors, angiotensin receptor blockers, or alpha-blockers. These drugs, however, are sometimes formulated in combination with beta-blockers or diuretics, which are banned. An alpha-blocker could be a good choice for an athlete who has hypertension if the individual tolerates the side effects (primarily the postural hypotension), but these drugs are not used very often as a monotherapy. For competitive athletes, therefore, the drugs of first choice are the calcium channel blockers and ACE inhibitors (Bruno et al.).

Conclusion

The calcium channel blockers provide control of blood pressure during exercise without negative impact on heart rate, exercise capacity, or metabolism. ACE inhibitors reduce angiotensin II–mediated events and enhance the vasodilatory effects of bradykinin. Inhibitors of angiotensin activity do not negatively impact heart rate, oxygen utilization, or metabolism during exercise. ACE inhibitors and angiotensin receptor blockers may have a use in treating sarcopenia or muscle-wasting diseases.

Key Concepts Review

ACE inhibitor

aldosterone

alpha-blocker

angioedema

angiotensin I

angiotensin II

angiotensin-converting enzyme (ACE)

angiotensin receptor blocker (ARB)

angiotensinogen

calcium antagonist

calcium channel blocker

dihydropyridine

diltiazem

ectoenzyme

fast angiotensin II responses

hypertension

L-type calcium channel

orthostatic hypotension

papaverine

phenylalkylamine

postural hypotension

prehypertension

primary hypertension

renin

renin-angiotensin system

secondary hypertension

slow angiotensin II responses

stage 1 hypertension

stage 2 hypertension

symptomatic hypotension

Review Questions

1   Bill, our deconditioned, recently divorced 50-something exec driving that new BMW, wants to drop some weight and look good. He has high blood pressure. What kind of exercise regime would you recommend?

2   Mary enjoys running and likes to compete in 10K races and half marathons. She also is diagnosed with high blood pressure. What are her options for regulating her blood pressure while maintaining a training schedule and remaining competitive?

3   How do ACE inhibitors affect blood pressure?

4   Why do calcium channel blockers mostly affect smooth muscle, with little effect on skeletal muscle?

5   How do calcium channel blockers reduce blood pressure?

References

2013 ACCF/AHA Guideline for the Management of ST-Elevation Myocardial Infarction: A Report of the American College of Cardiology Foundation/American Heart Association Task Force on Practice Guidelines. *J Am Coll Cardiol* 61:e78–e140

ALLHAT: Officers and Coordinators for the ALLHAT Collaborative Research Group. The Antihypertensive and Lipid-Lowering Treatment to Prevent Heart Attack Trial (2002) Major outcomes in high-risk hypertensive patients randomized to angiotensin-converting enzyme inhibitor or calcium channel blocker vs. diuretic: The Antihypertensive and Lipid-Lowering Treatment to Prevent Heart Attack Trial (ALLHAT). *JAMA* 288:2981–2997

Azoulay L, Assimes TL, Yin H, Bartels DB, Schiffrin EL, Suissa S (2012) Long-term use of angiotensin receptor blockers and the risk of cancer. *PLoS One* 7:e50893. doi:10.1371/journal.pone.0050893

Bruno RM, Cartoni G, Taddei S (2011) Hypertension in special populations: Athletes. *Future Cardiol* 7:571–584

Burks TN, Andres-Mateos E, Marx R, Mejias R, Van Erp C, Simmers JL, Walston JD, Ward CW, Cohn RD (2011) Losartan restores skeletal muscle remodeling and protects against disuse atrophy in sarcopenia. *Sci Transl Med* 3:82ra37

Burnton L, Chabner BA, Chabner B, Knollman, B (2011) *Goodman and Gilman's The Pharmacological Basis of Therapeutics,* 12th ed. New York: McGraw Hill, p. 756

Cardoso CG, Gomides RS, Queiroz ACC, Pinto LG, Lobo FS, T Tinucci, Mion Jr D, Forjaz CLM (2010) Acute and chronic effects of aerobic and resistance exercise on ambulatory blood pressure. *Clinics* 65:317–325

Carreira MA, Tavares LR, Leite RF, Ribeiro JC, Santos AC, Pereira KG, Velarde GC, Nóbrega AC (2003) Exercise testing in hypertensive patients taking different angiotensin-converting enzyme inhibitors. *Arq Bras Cardiol* 80:133–137

Cornelissen VA, Fagard RH, Coeckelberghs E, Vanhees L (2011) Impact of resistance training on blood pressure and other cardiovascular risk factors: a meta-analysis of randomized, controlled trials. *Hypertension* 58:950–958

Delafontaine P, Yoshida T (2016) The renin-angiotensin system and the biology of skeletal muscle: mechanisms of muscle wasting in chronic disease states. *Trans Am Clin Climatol Assoc* 127:245–258

Dzau VJ (1989) Clinical implications for therapy: possible cardioprotective effects of ACE inhibition. *Br J Clin Pharmac* 28:183S–187S

Einhorn PT, Davis BR, Wright JT, Rahman M, Whelton PK, Pressel SL, ALLHAT Cooperative Research Group (2010) ALLHAT: still providing correct answers after 7 years. *Curr Opin Cardiol* 25:355–365

Fagard RH, Cornelissen VA (2007) Effect of exercise on blood pressure control in hypertensive patients. *Eur J Cardiovasc Prev Rehabil* 14:12–17

Fahrenbach MC, Yurgalevitch SM, Zmuda JM, Thompson PD (1995) Effect of doxazosin or atenolol on exercise performance in physically active, hypertensive men. *Am J Cardiol* 75:258–263

Fariello R, Boni E, Corda L, Muiesan ML, Agabiti-Rosei E (1991) Exercise-induced modifications in cardiorespiratory parameters of hypertensive patients treated with calcium antagonists. *J Hypertens Suppl* 3: S67–S72

Fitzsimons JT (1998) Angiotensin, thirst, and sodium appetite. *Physiol Rev* 78:583–686

Gillies HC, Derman EW, Noakes TD (1996) Effects of amlodipine on exercise performance and cardiovascular and skeletal muscle function in physically active hypertensive patients. *Clin Drug Invest* 12:135–145

Heisterberg MF, Andersen JL, Schjerling P, Bülow J, Lauersen JB, Roeber HL, Kjaer M, Mackey AL (2018) Effect of Losartan on the acute response of human elderly skeletal muscle to exercise. *Med Sci Sports Exerc* 50:225–235

Hockerman GH, Peterson BZ, Johnson BD, Catterall WA (1997) Molecular determinants of drug binding and action on L-type calcium channels. *Annu Rev Pharmacol Toxicol* 37:361–396

JNC 7: Chobanian AV, Bakris GL, Black HR, Cushman WC, Green LA, Izzo JL, Jones DW, Materson BJ, Oparil S, Wright JT, Roccella EJ (2003) Seventh report of the joint national committee on prevention, detection, evaluation, and treatment of high blood pressure. *Hypertension* 42:1206–1252

JNC 8: James PA, Oparil S, Carter BL, Cushman WC, Dennison-Himmelfarb C, Handler J, Lackland DT, LeFevre ML, MacKenzie TD, Ogedegbe O, Smith SC, Svetkey LP, Taler SJ, Raymond R. Townsend RR, Wright JT, Andrew S, Narva AS, Ortiz E (2014) 2014 Evidence-based guideline for the management of high blood pressure in adults report from the panel members appointed to the Eighth Joint National Committee (JNC 8) *JAMA* 311:507–520

Katzung BG, Masters SB, Trevor AJ (2012) *Basic & Clinical Pharmacology*, 12th ed. New York: McGraw Hill

Kinnard DR, Harris M, Hossack KF (1988) Amlodipine in angina pectoris: effect on maximal and submaximal exercise performance. *J Cardiovasc Pharmacol* 12(Suppl 7): S110–S113

Kleinbloesem CH, Erb K, Essig J, Breithaupt K, Belz GG (1989) Haemodynamic and hormonal effects of cilazapril in comparison with propranolol in healthy subjects and in hypertensive patients. *Br J Clin Pharmac* 27:309S–315S

Kokkinos PF, Narayan P, Colleran JA, Pittaras A, Notargiacomo A, Reda D, Papademetriou
V (1995) Effects of regular exercise on blood pressure and left ventricular hypertrophy in
African-American men with severe hypertension. *N Engl J Med* 333:1462–1467

Lay L, Bjorksten AR, Stainsby GV, Blake DW (2001) Effect of amlodipine on cardiopulmonary
performance in volunteers. *Clin Exp Pharmacol Physiol* 28:25–27

Liakos CI, Vyssoulis GP, Michaelides AP, Chatzistamatiou EI, Theodosiades G, Toutouza
MG, Markou MI, Synetos AG, Kallikazaros IE, Stefanadis CI (2012) The effects of angiotensin receptor blockers vs. calcium channel blockers on the acute exercise-induced inflammatory and thrombotic response. *Hypertens Res* 35:1193–1200

Lund-Johansen P, Omvik P (1990) Effect of long-term diltiazem treatment on central haemody-
namics and exercise endurance in essential hypertension. *Eur Heart J* 11:543–551

Lund-Johansen P, Omvik P, White W, Digranes O, Helland B, Jordal O, Stray T (1990) Long-
term haemodynamic effects of amlodipine at rest and during exercise in essential hypertension. *Hypertension* 8:1129–1136

Lund-Johansen P, Hjermann I, Iversen BM, Thaulow E (1993) Selective alpha-1 inhibitors: first-
or second-line antihypertensive agents? *Cardiology* 83:150–159

Manhem P, Bramnert M, Hulthén UL, Hökfelt B (1981) The effect of captopril on catecholamines, renin activity, angiotensin II and aldosterone in plasma during physical exercise in
hypertensive patients. *Eur J Clin Invest* 11:389–395

McAllister RG Jr, Hamann SR, Blouin RA (1985) Pharmacokinetics of calcium-entry blockers.
Am J Cardiol 55:30B–40B

Mohr M, Lindenskov A, Holm PM, Nielsen HP, Mortensen J, Weihe P, Krustrup P (2014) Football training improves cardiovascular health profile in sedentary, premenopausal hypertensive women. *Scand J Med Sci Sports* 24:36–42

Molmen-Hansen HE, Stolen T, Tjonna AE, Aamot IL, Ekeberg IS, Tyldum GA, Wisloff U,
Ingul CB, Stoylen A (2012) Aerobic interval training reduces blood pressure and improves
myocardial function in hypertensive patients. *Eur J Prev Cardiol* 19:151–160

Motz W, Strauer BE (1996) Improvement of coronary flow reserve after long-term therapy with
enalapril. *Hypertension* 27:1031–1038

Omvik P, Lund-Johansen P (1993) Long-term hemodynamic effects at rest and during exercise of newer antihypertensive agents and salt restriction in essential hypertension: review of
epanolol, doxazosin, amlodipine, felodipine, diltiazem, lisinopril, dilevalol, carvedilol, and
ketanserin. *Cardiovasc Drugs Ther* 7:193–206

Predel HG, Rohden C, Heine O, Prinz U, Rost E (1994) ACE inhibition and physical exercise:
studies on physical work capacity, energy metabolism, and maximum oxygen uptake in well-
trained, healthy subjects. *J Cardiovasc Pharmacol* 23(suppl 1):S25–S8

Reuter H (1983) Calcium channel modulation by neurotransmitters, enzymes and drugs. *Nature* 301:569–574

Sartiani L, Spinelli V, Laurino A, Blescia S, Raimondi L, Cerbai E, Mugelli A (2015) Pharmacological perspectives in sarcopenia: a potential role for renin-angiotensin system blockers?
Clin Cases Miner Bone Metab 12:135–138

Stankovic S, Panz V, Klug E, Di Nicola G, Joffe BI (1999) Amlodipine and physiological responses to brisk exercise in healthy subjects. *Cardiovasc Drugs Ther* 13:513–517

Strauss MH, Hall AS (2006) Angiotensin receptor blockers may increase risk of myocardial
infarction: unraveling the ARB-MI paradox. *Circulation* 114:838–854

Taylor SH (1994) Usefulness of amlodipine for angina pectoris. *Am J Cardiol* 73:28A–33A

Udelson JE, DeAbate A, Berk M, Neuberg G, Packer M, Vijay NK, Gorwitt J, Smith WB,
Kukin ML, LeJemtel T, Levine TB, Konstam MA (2000) Effects of amlodipine on exercise
tolerance, quality of life, and left ventricular function in patients with heart failure from left
ventricular systolic dysfunction. *Am Heart J* 139:503–510

van Baak MA, Koene FMM, Verstappen FTJ, Tan ES (1991) Exercise performance during captopril and atenolol treatment in hypertensive patients. *Br J Clin Pharmac* 32:723–728

6 Diuretics

Abstract

Diuretics are widely prescribed for hypertension and other cardiovascular diseases. They generally work by blocking Na^+ reuptake from the filtrate back into the blood. As a result, water follows the loss of Na^+, and diuresis results. Loop diuretics block the $Na^+/K^+/2Cl^-$ symporter in the thick ascending limb. Thiazide diuretics block a Na^+/Cl^- symporter in the distal convoluted tubule. The potassium-sparing diuretics either block a Na^+ channel or antagonize aldosterone in the collecting tubule system. Other diuretics, such as carbonic anhydrase inhibitors and osmotic agents, have limited indications. Diuretics are taken by athletes to drop weight or to mask other illegal substances in their urine. Their use can decrease plasma volume and impair normal vasodilatory response to exercise. Hypovolemia initiates cardiovascular adjustments to preserve blood pressure (i.e., maintain venous return and cardiac output), at the expense of regulation of body temperature. Hypovolemia causes changes in circulation, decreasing the ability to thermoregulate, by both evaporative cooling (i.e., sweat) and cooling by radiation. Although hypovolemic exercisers still sweat, creating an even more negative water balance, their sweat rate and the related cooling effect can be reduced. This problem can be exacerbated in warm, humid weather, leading to heat exhaustion.

Exercise causes shifts in electrolyte distribution, and diuretics can exacerbate their loss. K^+ loss with diuretics leads to earlier muscle fatigue and may affect the heart during intense exercise. Salt loss can result in an increased chance of muscle cramps and/or cardiac arrhythmias. Performance can be suppressed after rapid dehydration and rehydration, and decreased duration/stamina would be expected. Athletes and exercise enthusiasts who are taking diuretics other than potassium-sparing drugs should eat fruit such as bananas or drink sport drinks with electrolytes to help alleviate salt and water imbalance and prevent hypokalemia. Thiazide diuretics (and related sulfonamides) can cause photosensitivity, so individuals taking these drugs should use sunscreen and avoid the sun during midday hours.

CASE EXAMPLE

Back in her college days, Megan made a bad mistake. Her roommate was taking a weight-loss supplement called StarCaps. It was also supposedly good for bloating and digestion issues, which is why Megan tried it. Between her training schedule, soccer practice, classwork, and trying to find an internship, she was constantly dealing with stomach issues. Her less than healthy diet probably also contributed. The pills seemed to help—maybe at least a little. The problem occurred when she got the notice that her name had been selected for random drug testing. She didn't even consider the StarCaps. After all, they were organic and all-natural—a blend of papaya, garlic, and a bunch of other herbs from Peru. The shock came when the coach called her in and said she had flunked the drug test. For Megan, the news could have been worse. This drug test was out of season and school-administered—not the NCAA-sanctioned test from last season's trip to the NCAA tournament. She was still in trouble—but a positive test at the NCAAs could have had a one-year suspension. Her coach told her she had tested positive for bumetanide—a diuretic. The coach asked her "Why are you taking a diuretic?" Megan said "I did not take a diuretic." Coach asks "Have you started taking any new medicines or supplements?" That's when it hit her—the stupid pills from her roommate. But a diuretic in a weight-loss pill? Luckily, she only got a stern lecture about not trusting supplements and was put on 'probation' for essentially the rest of her time as a collegiate athlete.

About this time, several NFL players and other professional athletes were not so lucky and got up to one-year penalties for testing positive for bumetanide after taking this supplement. The maker of the supplement was fined. Why are diuretics banned? As we will see, they generally are ergolytic with negative effects on salt and water balance. However, they can cause rapid weight-loss following excessive urination and act as a masking agent to make detection of PES more difficult.

Learning Objectives

1   Understand the basics of kidney function and urine formation.
2   Appreciate the usefulness of diuretics.
3   Learn how diuretics exert their effect.
4   Understand the effect of diuretics on water and electrolyte balance.
5   Learn why diuretics are ergolytic.
6   Understand why athletes abuse them.
7   Appreciate the seriousness of misused diuretics.

Introduction

Diuretic drugs have been a mainstay in the treatment of hypertension and heart failure for decades. Their effectiveness was re-established in the ALLHAT report (2002) and the report of the Eighth Joint National Committee (JNC-8 2014). **Diuretics** induce loss of water and solutes, through a process called diuresis. They effectively treat those patients who are geriatric, obese, and/or African American. These groups of individuals respond well and often tolerate diuretics better than other drugs prescribed for hypertension. These drugs are also used for correcting water and sodium retention observed in congestive heart failure. They have the additional benefit of decreasing stroke rate. Once widely used for hypertension, they have been largely displaced in the market by newer classes of drugs, such as the calcium channel blockers, ACE inhibitors, and angiotensin receptor blockers (discussed in Chapter 5). However, large-scale clinical studies have suggested that diuretics provide a safe and inexpensive alternative to many of these new drugs, especially those that are not yet available as generics (ALLHAT; JNC-8).

Renal Physiology

The kidneys play a critical role in whole-body homeostasis by precisely maintaining overall water and salt balance. They do this by filtering the body's extracellular volume the equivalent of 16 times a day. Most of the filtrate is reabsorbed, and the rest is eliminated during urine formation. The **nephron** is the fundamental unit of the kidney involved in this process. Figure 6.1 illustrates the basic features of a nephron. The nephron contains the glomerulus and its associated capillary bed, where filtration takes place. It also has an extended system of tubules where regulated reabsorption occurs, taking up to 99% of the original filtrate. The remaining filtrate accumulates in the collecting ducts on its way to the bladder. Each of the tubule segments is subdivided into many substructures, due to variation in function and the cells that are present. For our purposes, the major anatomical features are labeled in Figure 6.1. The reabsorption process comes with a significant energy cost in that much of the transport is active and requires the input of energy in the form of ATP. Therefore, the kidneys are very active in terms of oxygen consumption and ATP production. Diuretic drugs target functions in different segments of the nephron with their primary site of activity indicated in Figure 6.1. These targets will be expanded upon and discussed below.

Figure 6.1 Schematic view of the nephron.

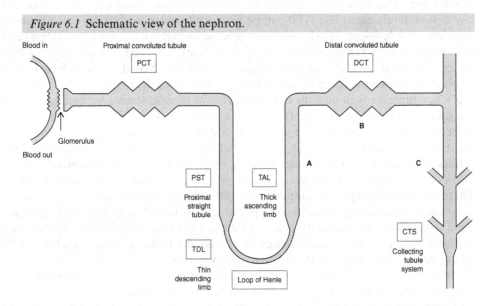

Legend: Major anatomical features of a simplified nephron are identified. Letters identify locations where major classes of diuretics exert their primary effects:

A = loop diuretics

B = thiazide diuretics

C = potassium-sparing diuretics

These primary sites of drug action will be expanded upon in upcoming figures. For clarity, additional possible sites of action are not shown.

PCT: proximal convoluted tubule; PST: proximal straight tubule; TDL: thin descending limb; TAL: thick ascending limb; DCT: distal convoluted tubule; CTS: collecting tubule system.

Renal physiology is complex. It involves many neuronal and hormonal levels of control, which are only partly understood. One of the key indicators of renal function is the **glomerular filtration rate**, the rate of flow of filtered fluid through the kidneys. An increase in glomerular filtration rate will increase urine output. The clearance rate for a drug is similar to the glomerular filtration rate if the kidneys do not reabsorb the drug. The glomerular filtration rate is controlled by arterial blood pressure and arteriole diameter, thereby providing global (blood pressure) and local (vessel diameter) control. Sympathetic activity and the renin-angiotensin-aldosterone system have significant input in the kidneys. We saw in the previous chapter the central role for the kidney in the renin-angiotensin-aldosterone system. Moreover, **autacoids** also act on the kidneys. Autacoids (also called paracrine factors) are locally produced molecules that exert their effect locally. For the kidneys, examples of important autacoids include a number of different prostaglandins. **Prostaglandins** are a family of signaling molecules produced in response to a wide variety of stimuli. They are discussed in more detail in Chapters 7 and 11. One example is PGE_2. It enhances diuretic function by slowing salt and water reabsorption (more details below) and increasing urine production.

The nucleoside adenosine is another autacoid that has a role in kidney function. Different triggers cause the release of adenosine, including hypoxia (low oxygen conditions). The increase in adenosine levels causes stimulation of adenosine receptors that decrease blood flow and the glomerular filtration rate. The decrease in blood being filtered results in less work that needs to be done by the kidney to reabsorb sodium and other ions. This decrease in workload on the kidneys is critical, because low oxygen levels mean less ATP can be produced, which means less is available to the kidneys. Adenosine, besides decreasing urine formation, can increase sodium and possibly potassium reabsorption by related mechanisms. The weak adenosine antagonists, caffeine (from coffee) and theophylline (from tea), have diuretic activity in part by blocking adenosine receptors (see Chapter 14 for more details).

Kidney function is important in many different disease states. As we discussed in the previous two chapters, hypertension can result from several conditions, such as defects in the renin-angiotensin system. Blood pressure depends on blood volume, and the kidneys control salt and water retention; increased salt and water retention results in increased blood volume. Fluid retention and an increase in blood volume also occur during congestive heart failure, which, once again, involves the kidneys. There are also many types of kidney diseases that have a genetic basis or are acquired as we age. Certain drugs can also damage kidney function. The kidneys, therefore, are good targets for drug intervention for a wide variety of common ailments, particularly hypertension and heart failure. Drugs that target the kidneys are also useful to help relieve edema (swelling) resulting from a variety of causes.

The negative water and salt balance that diuretics produce may be useful in people with congestive heart failure or hypertension, but it can have a negative effect on exercise performance. As we will see, diuretics can have ergolytic effects. Moreover, their use is banned by most sport governing agencies. Some athletes use diuretics to drop weight quickly (wrestlers, boxers, bodybuilders, gymnasts, etc.). Some athletes have also used diuretics as masking agents for performance-enhancing substances, such as anabolic steroids.

How Do Diuretics Work?

Most diuretics are **natriuretic**: they inhibit sodium (Na^+) reabsorption in the kidney. Because of osmosis, water accompanies the loss of sodium during urine formation, and urine output increases following diuretic administration. Other electrolytes can be lost, including potassium (K$^+$), causing **hypokalemia** (low blood K$^+$ level) by the process **kaliuresis (K$^+$ loss)**. Table 6.1 lists the three major classes of diuretics and their relative activity. As you can see, **loop diuretics** have the greatest efficacy (the highest rate of urine production); furosemide (Lasix) is the prototype drug. The **thiazide diuretic** class is the most prescribed class of diuretics, with hydrochlorothiazide (HCTZ) the most common drug. The **potassium-sparing drugs**, such as spironolactone or dyrenium, are usually prescribed in combination with thiazide or loop diuretics to minimize loss of potassium.

Other less frequently prescribed diuretics include **carbonic anhydrase inhibitors** (e.g., acetazolamide) and **osmotic agents.** The carbonic anhydrase inhibitors are used for high-altitude mountain sickness and glaucoma (as eye drops). They are relatively weak diuretics and are not usually prescribed as a single agent. Osmotic agents are not absorbed into cells and help pull water from various compartments of the body, increasing the urinary excretion of all electrolytes. They can be given orally (isosorbide) or intravenously (mannitol) to increase the osmolality (as their concentration increases) in plasma and the tubular fluid. They are freely filtered and have limited reabsorption. They have limited applications, such as pre-surgery to reduce edema, or for kidney dialysis issues. We will concentrate our discussion on the three main classes of diuretics listed in Table 6.1, as these are the drugs widely prescribed and banned by most governing bodies associated with sports. Drugs that are agonists and antagonists of vasopressin receptors are also becoming available, and we will discuss them briefly.

Loop Diuretics

Loop diuretics are sometimes called "high ceiling" diuretics, because they have the greatest efficacy (Table 6.1). Most of their activity occurs in the thick ascending limb of the loop of Henle in the kidney, where they target the Na$^+$/K$^+$/2Cl$^-$ (sodium/potassium/chloride) symporter (see Figure 6.1). A symporter couples the transport of ions along their concentration gradient with the movement of other ions against their concentration gradient. This symporter is localized along the apical membrane of the epithelial cells that separate the lumen from the blood supply in the interstitial space (see Figure 6.2). The lumen contains the filtrate destined to become urine. The symporter uses the thermodynamic drive of Na$^+$ moving into the cell along its concentration gradient. This thermodynamic drive is coupled to the movement of K$^+$ and Cl$^-$ into the cell against their concentration gradients. The symporter is electrically neutral, so for each Na$^+$ and K$^+$ that enter the cell, two Cl$^-$ also enter. The low concentration of

Table 6.1 Efficacy and duration of major classes of diuretics

Drug	Volume (mL/min)	pH	K$^+$ loss (mM/L)	Half-life (hours)
Control	1	6.0	15	
Loop diuretics Furosemide (Lasix)	8	6.0	10	2–3
Thiazides Hydrochlorothiazide (HCTZ)	3	7.4	25	3–6
Potassium-sparing Triamterene (Dyrenium)	2	7.2	5	4–6

Legend: Relative values are given to allow comparison of features of the three major classes of diuretics.

Figure 6.2 Site of action of loop diuretics in the thick ascending limb.

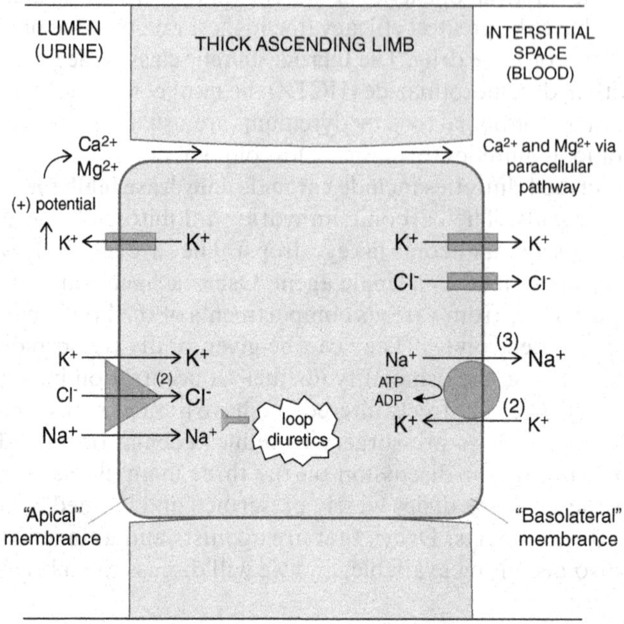

Legend: The lumen where the filtrate is processed to become urine is indicated on the left, and the interstitial compartment that enters into the bloodstream is indicated on the right. The epithelial cells indicated orient with their apical membranes toward the lumen and their basolateral membranes toward the blood flow. The Na^+/K^+ pump, which uses ATP to maintain the ion gradients, is indicated in the basolateral membrane. The $Na^+/K^+/2Cl^-$ symporter is indicated in the apical membrane. The other transport processes mentioned in the text are indicated. The font size of the ion suggests relative concentration levels.

Na^+ and relatively high concentration of K^+ inside cells are maintained by the Na^+/K^+ pump localized along the basolateral membrane oriented toward the interstitial space. The Na^+/K^+ pump uses ATP to transport Na^+ and K^+ against their concentration gradients. For each ATP used, three Na^+ are pumped out and two K^+ are pumped into cells. Cl^- exits the cell along its concentration gradient through Cl^- channels in the basolateral membrane.

The increase in intracellular K^+ that results from the $Na^+/K^+/2Cl^-$ symporter and the Na^+/K^+ pump is dissipated by diffusion through K^+ channels located in both apical and basolateral membranes. The passive movement of K^+ back into the lumen builds up the positive charge potential in the luminal space. To compensate for the positive charge buildup, paracellular (transport *between* neighboring cells) movement of Mg^{2+} and Ca^{2+} occurs from the lumen to the interstitial space. This transport of Mg^{2+} and Ca^{2+} is essential to minimize their loss during urine formation (Figure 6.2).

Loop diuretics bind the Cl^- binding site on the $Na^+/K^+/2Cl^-$ symporter and slow activity. The decrease in Na^+ uptake from the lumen results in more Na^+ and water being excreted during urine formation. By blocking $Na^+/K^+/2Cl^-$ symporter activity, loop diuretics also cause loss of K^+, Mg^{2+}, Ca^{2+}, and Cl^-. Normally, about 25% of the Na^+ load is handled in the thick ascending limb, with the other major sites of Na^+ reabsorption occurring earlier, such as in the proximal convoluted tubule (see Figure 6.1). Considerably less Na^+ reabsorption occurs downstream of the thick ascending limb.

As a result of loop diuretics, Na^+ not reabsorbed in the thick ascending limb is generally excreted in urine, as the rest of the nephron does not have the capacity to "undo" what has been done in the thick ascending limb.

Thiazide Diuretics

In the distal convoluted tubule, only about 10% of the filtered Na^+ and Cl^- remains to be reabsorbed (Figure 6.1). The primary transporter in cells lining the distal convoluted tubule is an electrically neutral Na^+ and Cl^- symporter. This symporter is the target for thiazide diuretics (see Figure 6.3). Thiazide diuretics interfere with Na^+ or Cl^- binding, so the thiazide-binding site may overlap or alter both ion-binding sites. The Na^+/K^+ pump in the basolateral membrane is again the key activity, as it uses ATP to set up the Na^+ and K^+ concentration gradients, keeping Na^+ concentration low inside cells. In the apical membrane, the Na^+/Cl^- symporter couples the energy associated with Na^+ entering cells along its gradient to the movement of Cl^- against its concentration gradient. As levels of Cl^- level increase in these cells, it exits the cell passively through a Cl^- channel in the basolateral membrane. Thiazide diuretics effectively inhibit the Na^+/Cl^- symporter, decreasing Na^+ reabsorption. Decreasing Na^+ reabsorption results in Na^+ and water excretion and an increase in urine volume.

Ca^{2+} transport is also important in the distal convoluted tubule. Ca^{2+} enters cells from the filtrate through apical calcium channels, along its concentration gradient. Utilizing the energy of Na^+ entering the cell along its gradient, a Na^+/Ca^{2+} antiporter

Figure 6.3 Site of action of thiazide diuretics in the distal convoluted tubule.

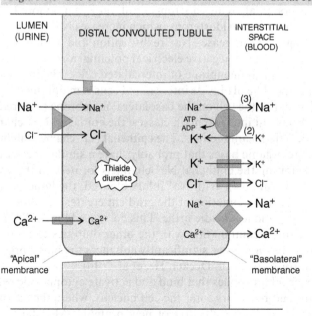

Legend: The orientation is the same as in Figure 6.2. The Na^+/K^+ pump is indicated in the basolateral membrane. The Na^+/Cl^- symporter is shown in the apical membrane. The other transport processes mentioned in the text are indicated.

in the basolateral membrane moves Ca^{2+} in the opposite direction and out of the cell. Parathyroid hormone works in these cells to increase Ca^{2+} reabsorption. It stimulates the calcium channel activity, thereby reducing Ca^{2+} loss in the urine.

Potassium-Sparing Diuretics

The collecting tubule system is a group of tubular structures that link the distal convoluted tubule to the ureter. The cells lining the collecting tubule system are critical in determining the final composition of urine, though they are responsible for only 2% to 5% of the total NaCl reabsorption. These cells contain mineral corticoid receptors, making them responsive to hormones such as aldosterone. Aldosterone is a mineral corticoid (steroid hormone) released by the adrenal cortex as part of the renin-angiotensin-aldosterone system (discussed in Chapter 5). This site is also important in K^+ secretion, especially following diuretic treatment. Multiple cell types exist in the collecting tubule system, including **principal cells** and **intercalated cells**. Principal cells regulate Na^+, K^+, and water transport, while intercalated cells deal more with acid/base balance and H^+ and bicarbonate transport (see Figure 6.4).

Principal cells have the Na^+/K^+ pump in the basolateral membrane using ATP to maintain the Na^+ and K^+ gradients. There are separate Na^+ and K^+ channels in the apical membrane. Na^+ enters and K^+ exits cells along their gradients. However, Na^+ entry exceeds K^+ exit, so the lumen develops a negative charge potential. The negative potential in the lumen drives Cl^- transport from the lumen to the blood by both Cl^- channels and a paracellular Cl^- pathway (Figure 6.4). The negative potential also helps draw K^+ out of the cells. This K^+ effect is more pronounced following loop or thiazide diuretic therapy. The higher level of Na^+ in the lumen that results from diuretic treatment means more Na^+ entering the principal cell and a stronger negative charge potential. The larger potential creates a stronger pull on K^+, and more K^+ can be lost as a result of diuretic treatment. Aldosterone, which increases Na^+ channel and Na^+/K^+ pump activity, dramatically increases Na^+ reabsorption and K^+ loss by this mechanism. The increase in the lumen's negative electrical potential also increases the activity of the H^+ pump in the apical membrane of intercalated cells. The increase in pump activity acidifies the urine. The pH inside intercalated cells is maintained by coincident transport of HCO_3^- out of the cell on the basolateral membrane (Figure 6.4).

The potassium-sparing drugs fall into two main classes: the epithelial Na^+ channel inhibitors and the mineralocorticoid antagonists. The **epithelial Na^+ channel inhibitors** amiloride and triamterene are organic bases that probably share a similar mechanism of action. They work by inhibiting the epithelial Na^+ channels located on the apical membrane of principal cells (Figure 6.4). With Na^+ influx blocked, the lumen's negative electrical gradient is reduced. Attenuation of the gradient creates less pull on K^+ and H^+, resulting in less K^+ loss and less acidic urine. This decreased loss of K^+ in the urine makes these drugs useful in combination with the other diuretics to minimize loss of potassium. For example, triamterene significantly enhances the blood pressure lowering effect of hydrochlorothiazide (Tu, Decker, He, et al. 2016).

Mineralocorticoids are steroid hormones that bind and activate cytoplasmic receptors. Activated, hormone-bound receptors enter the cell nucleus, where they activate genes. Gene activation results in the production of new proteins. Aldosterone increases the activity of the apical Na^+ channel and the Na^+/K^+ pump, increasing Na^+ reabsorption significantly. Available **aldosterone antagonists** include spironolactone and

Figure 6.4 Site of action of potassium-sparing diuretics in the collecting tubule system.

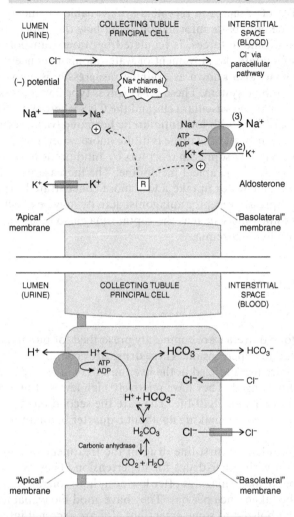

Legend: A. Principal cells: the orientation is the same as in Figure 6.2. The Na^+/K^+ pump is indicated in the basolateral membrane. The Na^+ channel is indicated in the apical membrane. The aldosterone receptor is indicated by R. The other transport processes mentioned in the text are indicated. B. Intercalated cells: the role of carbonic anhydrase is shown, along with a proton (H^+) pump in the apical membrane and the HCO_3^- Cl^- antiporter in the basolateral membrane.

eplerenone. Their antagonist activity depends on the levels of endogenous aldosterone and other mineralocorticoids. Stimulation of the renin-angiotensin system increases aldosterone, but these drugs antagonize the ability of aldosterone to increase the Na^+ reabsorption machinery. The result is less Na^+ uptake and weak diuresis, along with less secretion of K^+. By two rather different mechanisms, these two different classes of potassium-sparing diuretics act as relatively weak diuretics, but they spare K^+ loss. The potassium-sparing diuretics are useful as adjunct therapy with other diuretics or other drugs for hypertension, such as calcium channel blockers or beta-blockers.

Agonists and Antagonists of Vasopressin Receptors

Limited **agonists** and **antagonists of vasopressin receptors** are available or under development, and so we will provide only basic information about how they work. Water movement, besides following osmotic forces, is regulated by water transporters called **aquaporins**. Aquaporins facilitate the movement of water along its concentration gradient. **Antidiuretic hormone**, also known as **arginine vasopressin**, is active in cells further down the collecting tubule system. These cells express type 2 vasopressin receptors, which distinguishes them from vascular cells and the CNS where type 1 receptors are expressed. Under conditions with low antidiuretic hormone (vasopressin) activity, there is low water permeability and the urine is dilute (more water, lower salt concentration). Activation of the type 2 vasopressin receptors by antidiuretic hormone leads to recruitment of aquaporin-2 to the apical membrane. The increase in water transporter activity results in greater water uptake and a more concentrated urine. Therefore, future drugs with vasopressin receptor antagonist activity may be effective diuretics. Vasopressin receptor antagonists such as the vaptans may also be useful in treating critically ill patients with hyponatremia.

Exercise Pharmacology of Diuretics

Pharmacokinetic Concerns

Furosemide and several other loop diuretics are commonly prescribed for pulmonary edema, congestive heart failure, and hypertension. These drugs are generally well absorbed when taken orally. They are metabolized in the liver and the kidneys to some extent. They are also excreted unchanged. They have relatively high levels of binding to serum proteins and overall have a short half-life. They are the second most common diuretics detected during PES testing, making up about a quarter of all diuretics detected in positive drug tests.

The thiazide diuretics are considered a first-line drug in the treatment of hypertension, alone or in combination with other drugs for hypertension. They are also prescribed for different types of edema. Thiazides offer low cost, high tolerance, and good compliance, as they can be taken once per day. They have good bioavailability when taken orally. They are metabolized to some extent but also are excreted intact. The half-life of available thiazides ranges from short (minutes) to long (days). This class of compounds also shows a range of non-specific binding to plasma proteins. The thiazide diuretics are the most frequently detected diuretics during drug testing, with HCTZ regularly coming in at number one.

Among the potassium-sparing diuretics, channel-blocking drugs such as amiloride and triamterene have low efficacy and are usually used in combination with one of the other diuretics. They have relatively low availability when taken orally. Amiloride has a 20-hour half-life, and triamterene's is about five hours. They are not detected very often during drug testing.

Mineral corticoid antagonists (e.g., spironolactone) have good availability when taken orally, but they are metabolized extensively. Some of the metabolites do retain antagonist activity, however. These drugs have relatively high binding to serum proteins and overall have a short half-life. They are usually prescribed in combination with other diuretics. They make up a small percentage of positive doping samples.

Sustained exercise decreases blood flow to liver and kidneys due to shunting of blood to working musculature. Flow-limited diuretics, with short half-lives, could have enhanced effect, with slower clearance from the system. Exercise also causes acute, negative water balance. Consistent exercise training can decrease resting and exercise blood pressure and is a great adjuvant treatment for hypertension in many patients. Negative water balance and lower blood pressure following exercise could be augmented by the actions of diuretics. Water loss during exercise still occurs even when an individual is **hypovolemic** (i.e., has a decrease in the volume of plasma) following diuretic treatment. Renal perfusion decreases with increasing levels of exercise. When an individual exercises at 60% VO$_2$max, significant decreases are observed in glomerular filtration rate, urine flow, and water or osmolyte clearance. The decrease in urine formation with increasing intensity of exercise correlates with increased blood levels of aldosterone, antidiuretic hormone (vasopressin), and plasma renin activity (Freund, Shizuru, Hashiro, & Claybaugh 1991).

Exercise causes a decrease in intracellular K$^+$ as K$^+$ moves out of muscle cells into intravascular spaces. Epinephrine (which rises during exercise) stimulates K$^+$ reuptake through β-2 receptors, but diuretics can increase K$^+$ loss (kaliuresis) during or following exercise. The increased K$^+$ load arriving at the kidneys during exercise is not reabsorbed as efficiently in the presence of loop or thiazide diuretics. Potassium is necessary for nerves and muscles to repolarize and fire again. When potassium levels are low, cells do not repolarize as efficiently and are unable to fire repeatedly, causing fatigue and weakness. It is very important to follow K$^+$ balance during diuretic treatment.

Pharmacodynamic Concerns

A common therapeutic use of diuretics is to treat hypertension or to treat congestive heart failure. These patients will probably take these drugs every day for the rest of their lives. Exercise in these patients, even when it is limited or moderate in intensity, contributes to improved exercise capacity, helps improve (or maintain) cardiovascular function, and reduces cardiovascular morbidity and mortality (Faris, Flather, Purcell, et al. 2002). Most of the studies on the effect of diuretics on exercise performance were done in the 1980s and 1990s following acute treatment. We will review studies that show how use of these drugs can be detrimental to performance and health, as well as cause disqualification from competition.

There are two major issues with the use of diuretics: volume depletion and electrolyte loss. Both of these issues come into play during exercise. When the body is hypohydrated but continuing to work, normal cardiovascular responses are altered and the body's ability to dissipate heat is compromised. As we will see below, performance also suffers, even following rehydration.

Thermoregulation

There are two major mechanisms for staying cool while exercising: **radiant cooling** and **evaporative cooling.** Exercise causes muscle tissue to warm up. To dissipate heat, radiant cooling occurs as circulation shunts blood from the viscera (internal organs) via vasoconstriction to muscle, where vessels are vasodilating. The increased blood flow to the working muscles absorbs some of the heat, in addition to providing oxygen and nutrients. Blood is also redirected to the skin. Peripheral vasodilation near the surface of the body allows heat to dissipate, producing radiant cooling. As exercise continues, cardiac output increases to meet the needs of the working musculature. The result is that the heat picked up in the muscle tissue radiates and dissipates at the skin's surface. Exercisers often look flushed because of the large amount of blood circulating near the body's surface. However, this type of surface heat dissipation depends on the external temperature and is less effective when the environment is warm. Moreover, the increased blood flow to the surface also increases the rate of perspiration. Sweat evaporating from the skin results in a significant cooling effect. With heavy exercise, especially in warm temperatures, the exerciser sweats profusely. This evaporative cooling is the main mechanism by which heat is dissipated during exercise.

Hypohydration causes detrimental effects on thermoregulatory mechanisms. Diuretics decrease plasma volume acutely, particularly in athletes who are taking them for illegal purposes. Long-term hypertensives taking diuretics see stabilization of plasma volume over time. Subjects with decreased plasma volume from diuretics continue to sweat during exercise; however, a decrease in plasma volume will reduce blood flow to the skin, needed for heat loss, because central venous return is favored over blood flow to skin. As venous return worsens with water loss from exercise combined with diuretics, stress on the cardiovascular system increases. A decrease of about 10% in plasma volume reduces stroke volume, cardiac output, and VO_2max (Nadel, Fortney, & Wenger 1980; Caldwell, Ahonen, & Nousiainen 1984). To maintain cardiac output and blood pressure, the heart rate increases and arteries constrict, further compromising blood flow to the skin. The result is less radiant and evaporative cooling, an increase in body temperature, and an increased likelihood of heat exhaustion or even death.

Performance

Few studies have been conducted concerning athletic performance with individuals who chronically use diuretics. We do know that plasma volume stabilizes in individuals using diuretics long term. However, diuretics are widely abused by athletes who want to drop weight quickly or mask other illegal drugs (Cadwallader, de la Torre, Tieri, & Botre 2010). Problems arise when athletes take a single dose for rapid weight loss, such as for a competition with weight classes. Athletes may also take several doses to increase urine production with the hope of increasing the clearance rate of other illegal performance-enhancing substances they have taken. Diuretics decrease VO_2max (Caldwell et al.), making them ergolytic when taken acutely; dehydrated individuals are at a disadvantage even at the start of a competition. In addition, K^+ loss (common with use of diuretics) contributes to muscle fatigue. Regular exercise training causes influx of water into the intravascular space, known as plasma volume expansion, generating exercise-induced hypervolemia. Plasma volume expansion is a beneficial adaptation of chronic exercise that improves cardiovascular performance and thermoregulatory capability. Diuretics can interfere with this normal adaptation to regular exercise (Convertino 1991). Therefore, some of the benefits associated with training are negated with even short-term use of diuretics.

Sport Drinks

Back in the mid-1960s, researchers at the University of Florida wanted to help their football team, the Gators, deal with heat and heat-related illnesses. The researchers reasoned that the excessive sweating during intense exercise was causing a significant loss of water and electrolytes. Moreover, the heavy workload on these athletes was probably drawing down their carbohydrate (i.e., glycogen) stores. The researchers formulated a new carbohydrate-electrolyte beverage that replaced the key components lost through sweating and exercise. They called their concoction Gatorade. An 8-ounce serving contains 110 mg Na^+, 30 mg K^+, and 14 grams of sugar. The players responded well. Use of Gatorade spread from college football to professional football and eventually became widespread in all sports at all levels. Even professional race car drivers have a Gatorade In-Car Drinking System, which is now considered an essential piece of racing equipment. Newer formulations of Gatorade target endurance athletes with higher levels of Na^+ and the inclusion of additional electrolytes (200 mg Na^+, 90 mg K^+, 6 mg Ca^{2+}, and 3 mg Mg^{2+}). Other companies have produced a series of alternative products that compete in the sport drink market. Additional beverages, such as so-called energy drinks, often include high levels of caffeine, B vitamins, and herbal products. Their use for electrolyte replacement is not recommended, and the high levels of caffeine may cause a positive drug test in some cases (see Chapter 14).

Consumption of beverages that contain electrolytes and carbohydrates is recommended when there is greater than a 2% body weight reduction after prolonged exercise (American College of Sports Medicine 2007). Drinking too much water when dehydrated under these conditions can result in **hyponatremia**, the condition of insufficient sodium in the body fluids outside cells (Rosner & Kirven, 2007). The low concentration of sodium in the blood that can result (water intoxication) is rare, but it can be a serious medical emergency. The need for electrolyte replacement depends on exercise intensity, duration, weather, and individual differences in sweat rate. Sodium and potassium help replace electrolyte losses from sweat, and sodium also helps stimulate thirst.

Carbohydrates can be obtained from energy bars and foods such as bananas or other fruits, as well as from sport drinks. Athletes should remember that performance depends on hydration state, so they should hydrate before and during exercise. After exercise, athletes should drink 20 to 24 ounces for every pound lost and consume a 3:1 to 4:1 ratio of carbohydrate to protein to help replenish glycogen stores, depending on the length and type of training (American Dietetic Association; Dietitians of Canada; American College of Sports Medicine, et al. 2009). A beverage hydration index has been developed (Maughan, Watson, Cordery, et al. 2016). Many different beverages were tested in a randomized trial—essentially the volume of urine produced after drinking the test beverage expressed relative to the standard treatment of the same volume of water. Most beverages tested in this study were not significantly different than water, except for an oral rehydration formula and milk. Milk should not be too surprising, as it has more sodium than sports drinks (Maughan et al.).

As mentioned earlier, both exercise and diuretics decrease plasma volume. Exercise causes a reduction in plasma volume as fluid shifts from vascular to extravascular spaces, prior to when sweating occurs. Considerable literature shows decreases in performance following heat stress–induced dehydration during exercise. In an older study, sweat loss of 4% body weight caused a 12% decrease in plasma volume and a significant decrease in muscle performance. Following rehydration, muscle performance was still depressed compared to that of the control subjects (Torranin, Smith, & Byrd 1979). In another study, seven collegiate wrestlers who lost close to 5% of their body weight while exercising in rubber suits during a 36-hour weight-loss period had reduced upper body but not lower body strength (Webster, Rutt, Weltman 1990). Anaerobic power and anaerobic capacity were significantly reduced in the dehydrated state. When these athletes were tested on a treadmill, peak velocity was decreased by 6.5%, VO_2peak was reduced by 6.7%, and treadmill time to exhaustion was significantly reduced by 12.4% (all measures were $p < 0.05$, Webster et al.). Clearly, heat-induced fluid and electrolyte loss can affect performance and require supplementation for endurance exercise (Sawka & Montain 2000) and muscle strength and power (Judelson, Maresh, Anderson, et al. 2007).

Few studies have examined the short-term effects of dehydration following diuretic use. One study looked at the use of furosemide in a group of eight runners (Armstrong, Costill, & Fink 1985). The diuretic treatment decreased plasma volume around 10%. The times for a 1500-meter run were not significantly altered, but times for the 5,000- and 10,000-meter runs were significantly increased. When these participants were tested indoors on a treadmill, there was no significant difference in VO_2 at submaximal or maximal levels of work. However, the mean time to exhaustion was significantly decreased in the diuretic-treated group. Therefore, dehydration due to the diuretic treatment caused a more pronounced effect in the trials of longer duration.

In a widely quoted study, 62 non-endurance athletes (weight lifters, wrestlers, boxers, and judoka) were separated into three experimental groups and a control group (Caldwell et al.). The experimental groups decreased their body weight by about 4% in one of three ways. One group used furosemide, another group spent excessive time in a sauna, and the third exercised over a period of 48 hours with limited fluid intake to decrease their body weight. The groups that became hypohydrated from diuretics or the sauna had a significantly decreased VO_2max compared to the exercise-treated group. The authors of this study concluded that not only the degree of water loss but also the method itself could affect physical performance (Caldwell et al.). During exercise, the body normally responds to conserve electrolytes and regulate temperature, using sympathetic and renin-angiotensin regulatory mechanisms. Diuretic hypohydration can affect performance more than exercise-induced, because of greater K^+ loss and problems with thermoregulation following use of diuretics.

Elder Concerns

Inadequate hydration in the elderly is associated with increased morbidity and mortality. In a survey of community-dwelling elderly ($n = 170$), roughly 1/3 were not aware that fluid overload occurs in heart failure or kidney failure (Picetti, Foster, Pangle, et al. 2017). A majority of respondents were not aware that improper hydration or changes in hydration status can result in confusion, seizures, or death. About 60% of respondents overestimated the amount of fluid loss at which moderately severe dehydration symptoms occur, and 60% did not know fever can cause dehydration. Promoting health literacy should improve outcomes related to hydration-associated illnesses in the elderly.

Age-related changes in the kidney include a decreased number of functional glomeruli with some compensatory hypertrophy of remaining nephrons (Weinstein & Anderson 2010). Total kidney volume remains stable through about age 50, with declining cortical volume compensated with an increase in medullary volume. After about age 50, the compensation lessens and total kidney volume starts to decrease, with an associated decrease in glomerular filtration rate. Nephrosclerosis increases from 2.7% in healthy young individuals (under 29) to 73% for healthy individuals over age 70. Aging also results in larger and more numerous renal cysts. The decline in glomerular filtration rate can be misdiagnosed as chronic kidney disease. Mortality data supports the use of a lower range of glomerular filtration rate to define normal in the elderly (Weinstein & Anderson). Since the elderly retain less reserve capacity of renal function, they are at higher risk for chronic kidney disease and acute kidney injury as they continue to age.

Normal aging of kidney function is of clinical relevance to managing elderly patients. Lower doses of water-soluble medications that are cleared through kidneys may be warranted. Non-steroidal anti-inflammatory drugs (NSAIDs) can have negative effects on the kidneys, so their use should be monitored closely. Age-related kidney functional decline has very little effect on life expectancy, and alone, should not exclude motivated older individuals from kidney donation (Weinstein & Anderson).

Health Risks

Common side effects with diuretics include problems that result from volume depletion and low blood sodium. Because of the critical importance of sodium, potassium, and calcium in most of the body's normal functions, regular monitoring of electrolytes is recommended, especially in the geriatric population. Elderly patients, who often have poorer eating habits, are less active, and can have compromised kidney or other organ function, can be particularly sensitive to some of these side effects. These side effects include:

- Frequent urination, which may last for several hours after a dose or disrupt sleep.
- Dizziness or lightheadedness, especially when getting up from a lying or sitting position.
- Dehydration, resulting in dizziness, extreme thirst, and excessive dryness of the mouth.
- Nausea, vomiting, blurred vision, confusion, headache, increased perspiration (sweating), and restlessness.
- Electrolyte abnormalities:
  - Hyponatremia (low blood sodium level)
  - Hypokalemia (low blood potassium level)
  - Weakness, tiredness, muscle cramps (consider potassium supplements)
  - Loss of appetite
  - Arrhythmia (abnormal heart rhythm), coma, death.

A number of serious health risks are associated with exercise and the use of diuretics, for both exercising hypertensive patients and athletes who use the drugs improperly:

- Dehydration impairs temperature control, possibly leading to heat exhaustion, especially in warm and humid conditions.
- Electrolyte balance can be disrupted, with possible increased rate of loss, leading to cramps and arrhythmias.
- Thiazide diuretics are associated with photosensitivity.
- Diuretics can decrease exercise duration and capacity.

PES Watch

Diuretics are on the WADA list of banned substances. Detection by the NCAA or USOC can result in disqualification. Although acute use of diuretics is ergolytic, diuretics are used to mask other drugs in urine and so are referred to as a masking agent. The increased rate of urine production makes a more dilute urine and may help speed up clearance of other drugs from the system. Urine is tested for its specific gravity and must have a minimum specific gravity to be considered valid. Athletes are provided with approved fluids to drink while they are waiting for their tests. If the urine is too dilute (the specific gravity is too low), then the test is not valid. Athletes also may use diuretics when they are trying to make weight for sports with weight limits. Some professional athletes may also use them if their contract stipulates a maximum weight. Bodybuilders and others use diuretics to get that "cut" look.

For competitive athletes with hypertension, the drugs of first choice are the calcium channel blockers and ACE inhibitors (Bruno, Cartoni, & Taddei 2011). For competitors who have a bona fide therapeutic purpose for diuretics, usually for hypertension, they (with their doctors) can apply for a therapeutic use exemption. A therapeutic use exemption allows patients to use substances or methods that are on the List of Prohibited Substances or Methods if they have prior approval by the appropriate committee, well in advance of the competition.

During the 2008 NFL season, several players tested positive for a diuretic and were given suspensions. However, they were able to appeal the ruling, saying that the diuretics were in an NFL-approved supplement but not listed in the ingredients on the label. The case went to court, and the players ultimately ended up serving suspensions.

Conclusion

Diuretics are widely prescribed for hypertension and other cardiovascular diseases. They generally work by blocking Na^+ reuptake from the filtrate. Water follows the loss of Na^+, and diuresis results. Diuretics are taken by athletes to drop weight or to mask other illegal substances in their urine. Hypovolemia initiates cardiovascular adjustments to preserve blood pressure at the expense of regulation of body temperature. Exercise causes shifts in electrolyte distribution, and diuretics can exacerbate their loss. K^+ loss with diuretics leads to earlier muscle fatigue, cramps, and may affect the heart during intense exercise. Performance can be suppressed after rapid dehydration and rehydration, with a probable decrease in duration/stamina. Fruit or sport drinks with electrolytes help alleviate salt and water imbalance and prevent hypokalemia.

Key Concepts Review

agonists and antagonists of
  vasopressin receptors
antidiuretic hormone
aquaporin
arginine vasopressin
autacoid
carbonic anhydrase inhibitor
diuretic
epithelial Na+ inhibitor
evaporative cooling
glomerular filtration rate
hypokalemia
hyponatremia

hypovolemic
intercalated cell
kaliuresis (K+ loss)
loop diuretic
mineralocorticoid antagonist
natriuretic
nephron
osmotic agent
potassium-sparing drug
principal cell
prostaglandin
radiant cooling
thiazide diuretic

Review Questions

1   How can diuretics contribute to over-heating in exercisers, particularly in warm weather?

2   Some athletes use diuretics to gain an unfair advantage. What advantage is gained? What is the risk, besides disqualification?

3   Most diuretics are kaliuretic. How does that property affect exercisers?

4   When is it a good idea for athletes and exercisers to drink a sport drink, and when should they just drink water?

References

ALLHAT (2002) Major outcomes in high-risk hypertensive patients randomized to angiotensin-converting enzyme inhibitor or calcium channel blocker versus diuretic. *JAMA* 288:2981–2997

American College of Sports Medicine (2007) American College of Sports Medicine Special Communication position stand. Exercise and fluid replacement. *Med Sci Sports Exerc* 39:377–390

American Dietetic Association; Dietitians of Canada; American College of Sports Medicine, Rodriguez NR, Di Marco NM, Langley S (2009) American College of Sports Medicine position stand. Nutrition and athletic performance. *Med Sci Sports Exerc* 41:709–731

Armstrong LE, Costill DL, Fink WJ (1985) Influence of diuretic-induced dehydration on competitive running performance. *Med Sci Sports Exerc* 17:171–174

Bruno RM, Cartoni G, Taddei S (2011) Hypertension in special populations: Athletes. *Future Cardiol* 7:571–584

Cadwallader AB, de la Torre X, Tieri A, Botre F (2010) The abuse of diuretics as performance-enhancing drugs and masking agents in sport doping: pharmacology, toxicology and analysis. *Br J Pharmacol* 161:1–16

Caldwell JE, Ahonen E, Nousiainen U (1984) Differential effects of sauna-, diuretic-, and exercise-induced hypohydration. *J Appl Physiol* 57:1018–1023

Convertino VA (1991) Blood volume: its adaptation to endurance training. *Med Sci Sports Exerc* 23:1338–1348

Faris R, Flather M, Purcell H, Henein M, Poole-Wilson P, Coats A (2002) Current evidence supporting the role of diuretics in heart failure: a meta analysis of randomized controlled trials. *Int J Cardiol* 82:149–158

Freund BJ, Shizuru EM, Hashiro GM, Claybaugh JR (1991) Hormonal, electrolyte, and renal responses to exercise are intensity dependent. *J Appl Physiol* 70:900–906

JNC 8: James PA, Oparil S, Carter BL, Cushman WC, Dennison-Himmelfarb C, Handler J, Lackland DT, LeFevre ML, MacKenzie TD, Ogedegbe O, Smith SC, Svetkey LP, Taler SJ, Raymond R, Townsend RR, Wright JT, Andrew S, Narva AS, Ortiz E (2014) 2014 Evidence-based guideline for the management of high blood pressure in adults report from the panel members appointed to the Eighth Joint National Committee (JNC 8) *JAMA* 311:507–520

Judelson DA, Maresh CM, Anderson JM, Armstrong LE, Casa DJ, Kraemer WJ, Volek JS (2007) Hydration and muscular performance: does fluid balance affect strength, power and high-intensity endurance? *Sports Med* 37:907–921

Maughan RJ, Watson P, Cordery PA, Walsh NP, Oliver SJ, Dolci A, Rodriguez-Sanchez N, Galloway SD (2016) A randomized trial to assess the potential of different beverages to affect hydration status: development of a beverage hydration index. *Am J Clin Nutr* 103:717–723

Nadel ER, Fortney SM, Wenger CB (1980) Effect of hydration state of circulatory and thermal regulations. *J Appl Physiol Respir Environ Exerc Physiol* 49:715–721

Picetti D, Foster S, Pangle AK, Schrader A, George M, Wei JY, Azhar G (2017) Hydration health literacy in the elderly. *Nutr Healthy Aging* 4:227–237

Rosner MH, Kirven J (2007) Exercise-associated hyponatremia. *Clin J Am Soc Nephrol* 2:151–161

Sawka MN, Montain SJ (2000) Fluid and electrolyte supplementation for exercise heat stress. *Am J Clin Nutr* 72:564S–572S

Torranin C, Smith DP, Byrd RJ (1979) The effect of acute thermal dehydration and rapid rehydration on isometric and isotonic endurance. *J Sports Med Phys Fitness* 19:1–9

Tu W, Decker BS, He Z, Erdel BL, Eckert GJ, Hellman RN, Murray MD, Oates JA, Pratt JH (2016) Triamterene enhances the blood pressure lowering effect of hydrochlorothiazide in patients with hypertension. *J Gen Intern Med* 31:30–36

Webster S, Rutt R, Weltman A (1990) Physiological effects of a weight loss regimen practiced by college wrestlers. *Med Sci Sports Exerc* 22:229–234

Weinstein JR, Anderson S (2010) The aging kidney: physiological changes. *Adv Chronic Kidney Dis* 17:302–307

7   Respiratory Agents

Abstract

Respiratory diseases are common. Environmental factors, such as smoking, particulates, allergens, and so forth, can be causative agents or can trigger episodes of coughing. COPD is a progressive disease, and drugs can relieve only some of the symptoms. Asthma, however, can be managed with drugs and exercise in many cases. During an asthmatic attack, coughing and wheezing can result from bronchiolar constriction and inflammation. Drugs that cause relaxation of the bronchiolar smooth muscle provide short-term relief; these include the β-2 agonists and the anti-muscarinics. Other drugs used for long-term control, such as anti-inflammatory steroids and leukotriene receptor antagonists, target the inflammation component and make the bronchiolar tissue less reactive. Asthmatics can also suffer bouts of shortness of breath and wheezing following exercise, especially in cold, dry air. This exercise-induced bronchoconstriction can be treated with short-acting β-2 agonists or, in some cases, reduced by pretreatment with leukotriene receptor antagonists.

Although inhaled β-2 agonists have not been shown to have ergogenic properties, systemic long-acting β-2 agonists may have doping potential. For example, clenbuterol, though not approved for human use in the United States, is readily available and increases fast-twitch muscle fiber size and activity. Many athletes have failed drug tests by testing positive for clenbuterol. For those athletes that need an inhaled β-2 agonist because of asthma or exercise-induced bronchoconstriction, many sports governing bodies have dropped the requirement of a therapeutic use exemption.

CASE EXAMPLE

Megan played competitive soccer from an early age. Megan is an asthmatic, and she has suffered coughing bouts since she was a young girl. Although this is somewhat counterintuitive, Megan's asthma improved once she started playing soccer and training with the local "elite" team. She rarely used her corticosteroid-containing inhaler after she became fit. Late in the fall season of her first year on the varsity team, she had a coughing fit about five minutes after a strenuous workout—she could hardly breathe from the restricted airflow. It went away after about 90 minutes but her coach told her to see her family doctor. Megan was diagnosed with exercise-induced bronchoconstriction and got a prescription for an inhaler with albuterol. Albuterol, a widely used bronchodilator, is commonly used as a "rescue" or "quick-relief" medication during an asthmatic attack. Moreover, if taken before exercise, albuterol may prevent exercise-induced bronchoconstriction. As a junior in high school, Megan was not subjected to testing, but didn't want to take something banned by the NCAA. Albuterol, because it is a β-2 receptor agonist, has properties similar to epinephrine (and norepinephrine) and has been heavily scrutinized. When inhaled, however, β-2 agonists are not ergogenic and are now permitted by WADA (with urine threshold limits). When she got to college, Megan needed a therapeutic use exemption for her inhaled albuterol.

Learning Objectives

1   Understand the basics of pulmonary exercise physiology.
2   Learn what happens to respiratory function with asthma.
3   Appreciate the issues associated with exercise-induced bronchoconstriction.
4   Learn how bronchodilators work.
5   Learn why anti-inflammatory drugs are useful in treating asthma.
6   Distinguish the effect of inhaled versus systemic β-2 agonists on exercise performance.
7   Understand how the extent of exercise-induced bronchoconstriction can be minimized.

Introduction

The lungs circulate a lot of air in and out of the body over the course of our lifetime. During physical activity, the amount of air that enters our lungs can increase significantly. Our body naturally adjusts the rate and depth of breathing based on the demand. However, in some disease states respiratory responses are impaired, and drug therapy may be needed. How does respiratory activity affect exercise performance? Does exercise improve respiratory performance? These are some of the questions that this chapter attempts to answer. After a brief review of pulmonary exercise physiology, we will examine different classes of drugs used to treat asthma and other diseases associated with respiration. We will also examine evidence for the ergogenic activity of some of these drugs.

The Respiratory System

Air inhaled through the nose or mouth is warmed and humidified as it makes its way to the trachea, where the breathing passage splits into two bronchi, serving the left and right lungs. Some of these passageways are equipped to filter out debris in the incoming air. The lungs contain a system of branching tubes that form smaller bronchi, which, in turn, branch into smaller tubes called **bronchioles**. Each terminal bronchiole divides into two respiratory bronchioles, which branch again, forming alveolar ducts. The alveolar ducts branch into smaller ducts and eventually terminate, creating thin-walled sacs called **alveoli**. The alveoli are highly vascularized with blood and lymph vessels and nerve input. Alveoli are very efficient in the diffusion of gases. The extensive branching, forming smaller and smaller units, creates an enormous number of alveoli and a corresponding amount of surface area for gas exchange. The total cross-sectional area in the lungs for gas exchange has been estimated between 500 and 1,000 square feet! Flow of air through the lungs is partially controlled by the autonomic nervous system. Sympathetic input (adrenergic) causes relaxation of smooth muscle cells controlling the airway's diameter and, hence, increases airflow. Parasympathetic input (cholinergic) causes smooth muscle contraction and decreases airflow (Housh, Housh, & DeVries 2012). Airflow and lung capacity are measured by a common office test called spirometry. **Spirometry** measures how much air is inhaled, how much air is exhaled, and how quickly it is exhaled. Spirometry is used to diagnose asthma, chronic obstructive pulmonary disease (COPD), and other conditions that affect breathing.

The rate of breathing (**frequency**) and depth (**tidal volume**) of respiration require a sophisticated control system to maintain homeostasis under conditions ranging from sleep to maximal exertion. In the lower brain stem resides the **respiratory control center**, below the thalamus and including the pons and medulla. The control center is responsible for the automatic and rhythmic innervation of the muscles that control breathing. The rate and depth of breathing are also controlled by the respiratory control center based on input from the brain, neural input from working muscles and joints, and humoral input (signaling molecules in the blood), to meet the demands for oxygen. Humoral factors include pH and carbon dioxide (CO_2). Breathing rate will increase with an increase in carbon dioxide and an acidification (lower pH, higher H^+ concentration) of blood. Receptors in the control center and throughout the periphery detect the partial pressure of CO_2 and pH. For example, carotid bodies, chemoreceptors located in the carotid artery, are stimulated by low partial pressure of arterial oxygen, high partial pressure of carbon dioxide, and a more acidic pH. Under these conditions, the carotid bodies signal the control center to increase breathing rate. The increased breathing rate increases the partial pressure of oxygen, lowers the partial pressure of carbon dioxide, and increases pH.

Lung ventilation rate (volume of breathing per minute) is the result of two variables: frequency and tidal volume. At maximal exercise, breathing rate can increase from a resting rate of less than 10 breaths per minute to over 30 breaths per minute. Tidal volume similarly can increase, from around 500 ml to 2,500 ml during maximal effort. Total lung ventilation, therefore, increases from about 7 liters per minute to 150 liters per minute or more during intense exercise (Housh et al.). During exercise, it is more efficient to increase tidal volume than breathing frequency because of the volume of space made up by the conducting portion of the airways ("dead space" that is not involved in air exchange). A slower frequency of breathing with larger tidal volume results in more efficient air exchange in the alveoli (Neder, Dal Corso, Malaguti, et al. 2003). Adrenergic input during exercise increases airway diameter, causing an increase in tidal volume. In general, if lung function values are within a normal range, exercise performance will not be limited by the lung's ability to oxygenate blood. In elite athletes with high cardiac output, the lung's capacity may become a factor during maximal exercise, due to the unusually high amount of blood arriving at the lungs from the heart.

Training improves the efficiency in breathing, not by changes in alveoli, but by reducing the metabolic acidosis that occurs during exercise. During exercise, the pH of the blood becomes acidic because of the increase in CO_2 levels and higher metabolic activity (more acid equivalents are produced, including lactic acid). In trained individuals, the more efficient use of oxygen results in less carbon dioxide and lactic acid with less metabolic acidosis. The decrease in metabolic acidosis causes less stimulatory input into the respiratory control center and a lower drive to increase ventilation. Endurance training also increases the oxidative capacity of respiratory muscles, which may be related to increased expression of β-2 receptors (Sato, Shirato,

Tachiyashiki, & Imaizumi 2011). The increased oxidative capacity of the muscles that control breathing makes them more efficient at making ATP at similar exercise intensities, compared to untrained subjects. Endurance training also improves other measures of lung volume and capacity, providing better alveolar ventilation and improved athletic performance. The result is that the **ventilation equivalent for oxygen** (the number of liters of air breathed for every 100 ml of oxygen consumed) decreases as the result of training (Wasserman, Hansen, Sue, et al. 1999). In other words, less air has to move through the lungs to get the same amount of oxygen.

VO_2 max (rate of maximal oxygen consumption) depends on oxygen transport to working muscles and working muscles' use of oxygen to produce ATP, as discussed in Chapter 2. VO_2 max measures an individual's level of cardiorespiratory fitness and regular training can increase VO_2max. Oxygen transport depends on cardiac output and the hemoglobin concentration in the blood, and training improves cardiac output. Muscle ATP production and oxygen utilization are improved with regular training through increased mitochondrial activity (size and number), increased myoglobin level, and increased levels of enzymes involved in oxidative metabolism (see Chapter 2 for details). Therefore, aerobic exercise training improves factors related to both oxygen transport and oxygen utilization.

In normal individuals exercising at moderate to high intensities, lung function does not limit performance, because the respiratory system has sufficient reserve capacity to provide sufficient oxygen. As stated above, in elite endurance athletes working at maximum intensity, gas exchange in the lungs may not keep up fully with the increase in cardiac output, exceeding the reserve capacity. In individuals suffering from respiratory disease, reduced lung capacity can negatively impact exercise performance and require drug therapy, as we will see.

Asthma

The Centers for Disease Control (CDC) estimate that 1 out of 12 Americans suffers from asthma, with an 8.4% incidence rate in children and 7.7% in adults. An **asthma exacerbation** or attack results from the narrowing of bronchial airways. Associated with this constriction of airway smooth muscle is the inflammation of the bronchial mucosa. The inflammation can lead to increased responsiveness (called **hyperresponsiveness**) to inhaled stimuli, which can trigger recurrent bouts of shortness of breath, wheezing, and spasm of the muscle cells in the bronchioles (**bronchospasm**). Stimuli can include a variety of triggers, such as cigarette smoke (Burke, Leonardi-Bee, Hashim, et al. 2012), allergens (mold, dust mites, pollen, animals, etc.), or gastroesophageal reflux disease. Wheezing attacks are associated with a tightness in the chest. Over time, asthmatics develop thickening of the airway passages, a consequence of hyperplasia (increased cell production) and inflammation in the airway tissues, resulting in chronic respiratory impairment (Stewart, 2012).

The underlying causes of asthma are not fully known. Genetics, environment (e.g., exposure to pollutants and/or cigarette smoke), and viral infections may all be factors. Allergies and hypersensitivity reactions may also be a major cause of asthma. One theory to explain asthma focuses on the role of **immunoglobulin E (IgE)**, one of the many types of antibodies (also called immunoglobulins, abbreviated Ig). The IgE hypothesis proposes that allergens (an allergen is any substance that can cause an allergic reaction) stimulate the release of this specific IgE class of antibodies. The IgE antibodies bind and stimulate **mast cells**. Mast cells are found in association with blood vessels and nerves and in proximity to surfaces that interface with the external environment. Stimulated mast cells release a wide range of factors that we will be discussing, including histamine and lipid mediators called **eicosanoids** (e.g., prostaglandins, thromboxanes, and leukotrienes) that are important in many aspects of the inflammatory response. Mast cells are a critical component in allergic asthma, but animal models and other evidence suggest that the allergen-stimulation and IgE hypothesis for asthma are not sufficient to explain the complexity of the disease (Mukherjee & Zhang 2011).

In addition, non-allergenic agents can also trigger the constriction of bronchioles (**bronchoconstriction**) and **bronchial hyperreactivity** observed with asthmatic attacks. Hyperreactivity is the condition observed in asthmatics where bronchospasm is easily triggered. Non-allergic triggers can include smoke, perfume, household cleaners, and cold, dry air. Though the underlying causes of asthma are not completely known, the prevalence of asthma and its impact on our health-care system are significant. Underutilized treatment probably contributes significantly to the costs associated with emergency care for individuals suffering from severe asthma attacks (National Center for Environmental Health 2014).

Treatment strategies can be thought of as "short-term relievers" or "long-term controllers." For short-term relievers, the drug target is the problematic contraction of smooth muscle in the airways. Long-term controllers are used to manage the inflammation and associated edema in the lungs. Because asthma is a chronic disease, daily medication is often necessary to control symptoms. Mild to moderate asthma can be relieved with β-2 agonists that cause smooth muscle relaxation in the bronchioles. In the case of long-term controllers, a number of different drug classes are used, and we will discuss their relative merits below. Individuals who have frequent attacks requiring long-term control may need inhaled anti-inflammatory steroids. A common treatment, Advair, contains an inhaled mixture of both a "reliever" (the β-2 agonist salmeterol) and a "controller" (the anti-inflammatory steroid fluticasone).

Exercise-Induced Bronchoconstriction

Exercise-induced bronchoconstriction results from loss of heat and water from the respiratory track. Endurance athletes exchange a lot of air. This large amount of ventilation can lead to drying of airways and greater intake of pollutants and allergens. Exercise can precipitate *bronchospasm* (fits of coughing) and, rarely, **anaphylaxis** (a severe allergic reaction).

Exercise-induced bronchoconstriction can occur frequently in asthmatics, especially when they are exercising in cold, dry air. Exercise-induced bronchoconstriction has also been called exercise-induced asthma, but the condition is distinct from asthma, even if common in asthmatics. Although the terms are often used interchangeably, some prefer the term exercise-induced bronchoconstriction because asthma is not a prerequisite to having exercise-induced bronchoconstriction. The recommendation is to avoid the term exercise-induced asthma and instead use the term **exercise-induced bronchoconstriction with asthma** for asthmatics. The term exercise-induced bronchoconstriction is used for non-asthmatics (Randolph 2009). Factors that may increase the prevalence of exercise-induced bronchoconstriction with asthma include the severity of asthma, respiratory infections, and urbanization.

Many successful athletes have asthma. At least 8% of Olympic athletes have documented asthma and airway hyperresponsiveness (Fitch 2012). An estimated 70% to 90% of asthmatics can suffer exercise-induced bronchoconstriction. In the general population, 7% to 20% of the population may suffer some form of exercise-induced bronchoconstriction (Randolph). Therefore, in addition to asthmatics, otherwise healthy athletes may need bronchodilators or anti-inflammatory drugs to treat exercise-induced bronchoconstriction.

Endurance training and dryness in the airways are probably major factors for individuals who suffer exercise-induced bronchoconstriction (Kemp 2009). During exercise, airways usually function normally, but after exercise stops, a 50% decline in pulmonary airflow can occur within five to ten minutes. The **forced expiratory volume in one second** (**FEV_1**) is a useful measurement for respiratory function. Significant decreases in FEV_1 are observed in asthmatics and those suffering exercise-induced bronchoconstriction. Recovery from exercise-induced bronchoconstriction usually occurs within 90 minutes following cessation of exercise.

The use of inhaled β-2 agonists can decrease the severity of the bronchoconstriction. Drugs such as albuterol, a β-2 agonist, have the potential to be ergogenic when taken orally and have been on the list of banned substances. However, when these drugs are inhaled, their effect is limited mostly to the lungs, and the competitor before 2013 had to obtain a therapeutic use exemption (Pluim, de Hon, Staal, et al. 2011). Even the newer, long-acting β-2 agonist formoterol does not improve endurance performance compared to placebo when inhaled (Carlsen, Hem, Stensrud, et al. 2001). This situation raises an interesting philosophical point: should these drugs be construed as ergogenic in people with respiratory limitations, because they reverse the detrimental effects on lung function? Or are the limitations in lung function observed in asthmatics similar to other diseases (fever, hypertension, allergies, etc.) that require drug therapy? Current thinking supports the latter, as inhalation of these drugs more likely returns these individuals to a more normal respiratory activity and, thus, is permissible. In 2013, WADA removed its requirement for a therapeutic use exemption and added urinary thresholds for the three most commonly inhaled β-2 agonists, listed in Table 7.1. However, the NCAA still requires a physician's support for a therapeutic use exemption.

Chronic Obstructive Pulmonary Disease

As discussed, asthma and exercise-induced bronchoconstriction are conditions that are reversible with drug treatment. In contrast, **chronic obstructive pulmonary disease (COPD)**, which is also characterized by narrowing of airways and low airflow, is poorly reversible and generally becomes progressively worse over time. It is characterized by persistent airflow limitation, progressive breathlessness on exertion, cough, and sputum production. The incidence of COPD increases with age, with most cases occurring in people over 50 years old (Decramer, Janssens, & Miravitlles 2012). Cigarette smoking is the leading cause of COPD, and inhalation of other potentially hazardous chemicals or particles can contribute to the disease. COPD and related emphysema require more serious intervention (e.g., oxygen supplementation, surgery, or even lung transplantation), though long-acting β-2 agonist and muscarinic antagonist (also called anticholinergics) inhalers are used as treatment. Exercise capacity is greatly diminished in COPD patients. However, a mild exercise program, along with cessation of smoking, is part of the pulmonary rehabilitation plan that can improve the quality of life in these patients. Our discussion will focus mainly on asthma and exercise-induced bronchoconstriction.

How Do Respiratory Drugs Work?

The drugs used to treat asthma and exercise-induced bronchoconstriction are diverse in mechanism, as we will see. They can mimic sympathetic input or antagonize parasympathetic input in the lungs. They can dampen the allergic response by slowing the release of histamine from mast cells or antagonizing histamine receptors. They can also mimic the immunosuppressive activity of the adrenal corticosteroids, such as cortisol. Other weak beta-agonists (sympathomimetics) are not as good at bronchodilation and not used for asthma or exercise-induced bronchoconstriction, though they can be used as over-the-counter decongestants (see Chapter 8). Emphasis will be placed on those drugs most commonly prescribed for asthma and exercise-induced bronchoconstriction. We will first cover drugs that cause bronchodilation, then drugs that are anti-inflammatory, and then the methylxanthines (see Table 7.1).

Table 7.1 Examples of medications discussed in this chapter

Drug Class	Example	Function	Dosing
β-2 Agonists	Albuterol (salbutamol)	Reliever/bronchodilator	As needed or up to 4 puffs per day
	Salmeterol	Reliever/bronchodilator	12 hours
	Formoterol	Reliever/bronchodilator	
	Clenbuterol	Not approved in the United States for humans	12 hours
Anticholinergics or Muscarinic antagonists	Ipratropium	Reliever/bronchodilator	3–4 times per day
	Tiotropium	Reliever/bronchodilator	24 hours
Corticosteroids	Fluticasone *combined with salmeterol* (Advair)	Controller/ anti-inflammatory	2 puffs twice a day
	Budesonide *combined with formoterol* (Symbicort)	Controller/ anti-inflammatory	2 puffs twice a day
Leukotriene Modifiers	Montelukast	Controller/ anti-inflammatory	24 hours
Mast-Cell Stabilizers	Cromolyn, nedocromil	Controller/ anti-inflammatory	2 puffs 4 times per day
Antihistamines	Diphenhydramine (Benadryl)	Controller/ anti-inflammatory	4–6 hours
	Loratadine (Claritin)	Controller/ anti-inflammatory	12–24 hours
	Fexofenadine (Allegra)	Controller/ anti-inflammatory	24 hours
Methylxanthines	Theophylline	Controller	Variable

Bronchodilators

Bronchodilators are usually administered in **nebulizers** or **metered-dose inhalers**. A nebulizer is a device that turns a liquid solution into a fine mist and delivers the drug through a face mask or mouthpiece over the course of about ten minutes. The alternative to nebulizers is the metered-dose inhaler. The metered-dose inhaler has several advantages, including quicker delivery (two puffs in 30 seconds), lower cost, and fewer systemic side effects.

β-2 Agonists

The inhaled **β-2 agonists** stimulate β-2 receptors in the bronchial tree, causing relaxation of smooth muscle cells and bronchodilation. Although isoproterenol is the prototype β-agonist, newer drugs have been developed that are more β-2 receptor specific and have longer duration. Albuterol is a β-2 agonist that is widely used for asthma and exercise-induced bronchoconstriction. It is relatively short acting and used for acute asthmatic attacks or given prior to exercise. Albuterol has almost pure β-2 activity, with little direct effect in the CNS or heart. When inhaled, it has less systemic effects; however, repeated heavy use causes desensitization and tolerance to its effects.

Longer-acting β-2-agonists, such as salmeterol and formoterol, have become more popular for treatment of asthmatics. Controversy over their use arose when a report linked salmeterol with asthma-related hospitalizations, implying that prolonged bronchodilation increased the chance of inflammation (Lang 2006). In 2005, the FDA released a health advisory concerning the possible deleterious effects of long-acting β-2 agonists. Though strongly debated for a time, changes were made in delivery of long-acting β-2 agonists: an anti-inflammatory steroid is combined with long-acting β-2 agonists in inhalers. For example, fluticasone is often included with salmeterol (Advair), and budesonide is included with formoterol (Symbicort).

The β-2-agonists can be taken orally as a maintenance therapy, but their side-effect profile and the possibility of tolerance limit their usefulness. The inhaled β-2 agonists provide fast and effective relief during asthmatic attacks in most sufferers. The systemic effects of oral β-2 agonists do have ergogenic potential, and their use is banned by most sports governing bodies. The ergogenic effects of long-acting β-2 agonists on skeletal muscle will be discussed later in the chapter.

Muscarinic Antagonists/Anticholinergics

Parasympathetic input causes constriction of airway smooth muscle cells; anticholinergics antagonize cholinergic receptors and cause relaxation with bronchodilation. Ipratropium is the primary anticholinergic used for pulmonary disease. It is relatively fast acting and can help protect against bronchospasm and decrease mucus secretion. It is given for acute attacks or prior to exercise for exercise-induced bronchoconstriction. However, ipratropium is considered inferior to β-2 agonists in terms of potency and is usually combined with a short-acting β-2 agonist, such as albuterol. It is administered in metered-dose inhalers or nebulizers. Newer, long-acting muscarinic antagonists, such as tiotropium, are useful in COPD but not currently approved for asthma treatment in children. The long-acting muscarinic antagonists may prove useful as add-on treatments in asthma patients who do not respond well to β-2 agonists and corticosteroid therapy (Rogers & Hanania 2015). Other long-acting muscarinic antagonists are coming to market and may be considered first-line agents in some types of COPD (D'Urzo, Peter Kardos, & Wiseman 2018).

Anti-Inflammatory Drugs

Inflammation is a complex process and is discussed in more detail in Chapter 11. Inflamed tissue has increased blood flow and capillary permeability that allows plasma fluids and leukocytes (white blood cells) access to the area. To combat inflammation, synthetic corticosteroids are used as potent suppressors of the immune system. Other drugs decrease the production of chemical mediators of inflammation such as the leukotriene modifiers. Additional drugs target the triggers of the inflammation by stabilizing mast cells or antagonizing histamine.

Inhaled Synthetic Corticosteroids

Corticosteroids (cortisol) suppress aspects of the immune system, as shown in Figure 7.1. They are effective at inhibiting the infiltration of asthmatic airways by immune cells (e.g., mast cells and leukocytes). At the molecular level, corticosteroids inhibit the production of inflammatory **cytokines**. Cytokines are molecules released by immune cells to communicate with other cells in the immune system. This complex communication network between different lineages of leukocytes is essential for the

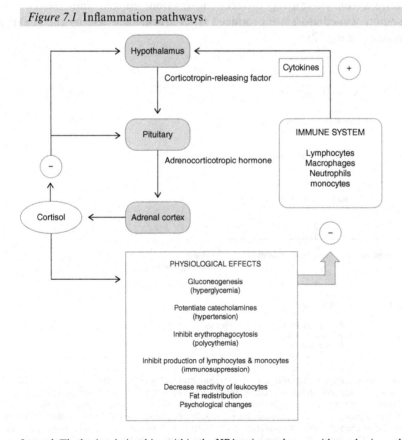

Figure 7.1 Inflammation pathways.

Legend: The basic relationships within the HPA axis are shown, with emphasis on the inflammatory response. Several of the biological effects of cortisol, the corticosteroid, are listed, as well as how they feedback on cells in the immune system. CRF: corticotropin-releasing factor; ACTH: adrenocorticotropic hormone.

functioning of the immune system. The suppression of cytokine production by corticosteroids helps decrease the level of inflammation and leukocyte infiltration in the airways of patients with asthma.

Synthetic corticosteroids are used for persistent or chronic asthma. They are not used for acute attacks. Inhalation minimizes the adverse effects associated with long-term use of steroids. Regular use of corticosteroids can decrease the frequency of asthma exacerbations. Corticosteroids do not cause relaxation of bronchial smooth muscle cells directly, though they may help potentiate β-2 agonists. Corticosteroids are very potent and have wide-ranging effects (see Figure 7.1). When inhaled in moderate doses, however, systemic effects can be minimized, and the drugs provide effective long-term control for asthma.

Leukotriene Modifiers

Arachidonic acid, a polyunsaturated omega-6 fatty acid (discussed in Chapters 11 and 13), is the source for many eicosanoids, a large group of lipid-like signaling molecules. The eicosanoids (e.g., leukotrienes, prostaglandins, thromboxanes) play a central role in inflammation. Leukotrienes are involved in many inflammatory responses and are released from a variety of inflammatory cells present in the airways. In asthma, leukotrienes have a role in causing bronchoconstriction, edema, and mucus production. These potent mediators are produced from **arachidonic acid** by the enzyme **5-lipoxygenase** (see Figure 7.2).

Figure 7.2 Production of eicosanoids.

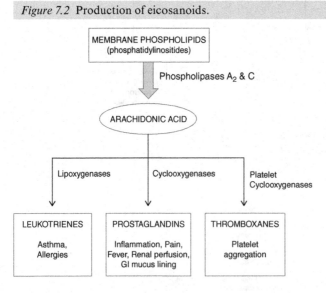

Legend: Eicosanoids, a large group of lipid-like signaling molecules derived from the fatty acid called arachidonic acid, include leukotrienes, prostaglandins, and thromboxane. Arachidonic acid is a component of phospholipids that make up the membranes of cells. When cells respond to stimuli that are part of the inflammatory response, enzymes cleave arachidonic acid from membrane phospholipids. Arachidonic acid is then chemically converted to a variety of different eicosanoids by the enzymes shown in the figure. Cell types differ depending on the pathway in which they are present or the pathway that is activated following stimulation.

Leukotriene modifiers, drugs that target leukotriene signaling, include a newer group of respiratory anti-inflammatory agents. Zileuton is a 5-lipoxygenase inhibitor. Zafirlukast and montelukast are leukotriene receptor antagonists. These drugs are used in maintenance therapy for asthma and decrease the frequency of asthma exacerbations. They are not for acute attacks. Their daily use helps manage exercise-induced bronchoconstriction. They are not as potent as corticosteroids in their anti-inflammatory effect, but they decrease the frequency of asthma attacks to a similar level. They have the advantage of being taken orally, as children sometimes don't like to use inhalers.

Zileuton is the least prescribed because of possible liver toxicity. Zafirlukast and montelukast have relatively low toxicity, with montelukast often being preferred because it can be taken once a day without regard to meals. These drugs are not on the WADA list of banned substances and are probably suitable for use during athletic competition.

Mast-Cell Stabilizers

Recall that mast cells are a critical component of asthma, as they release a wide range of factors that are important in many aspects of the inflammatory response. The class of drug called **mast-cell stabilizers** probably also affects the membranes of other cells, possibly by blocking membrane channels involved in the secretory response. The overall result is that the response to allergens is diminished somewhat in mast cells and other responsive cells.

The mast-cell stabilizers cromolyn and nedocromil are relatively safe but not very potent. Their main attribute is that they can provide a protective effect against asthma attacks, such as occupational asthma (chemical or particulate triggers) and exercise-induced bronchoconstriction. They are found in non-prescription preparations for intranasal administration. Once widely used, these drugs are rarely prescribed anymore because the corticosteroids provide superior control. These drugs do not affect smooth muscles and do not treat bronchospasms. As mentioned, these drugs probably affect the membranes of other cells, as well, possibly by blocking membrane channels involved in the secretory response. The overall result is that the response to allergens is diminished somewhat in mast cells and other responsive cells.

Antihistamines

Histamine is released from mast cells and basophils (a type of white blood cell) in response to allergens. It acts locally in the immune response and can be a trigger for inflammation. Histamine also causes increased permeability in the vasculature. As a result, leukocytes and serum proteins gain access to the affected area, fueling the inflammation response with increased mucus secretion, bronchial hyperresponsiveness, and airway smooth muscle constriction. In the nasal passages, histamine can cause rhinorrhea (running nose). It can make eyes red and itchy. A large number of **antihistamines** are on the market, and all of these antihistamines are H_1-receptor antagonists. The older antihistamines, such as Benadryl, are available over the counter. They tend to cause drowsiness because they cross the blood–brain barrier and antagonize receptors involved in sleep and wakefulness. In fact, some of these older antihistamines have been marketed to promote sleep. Newer antihistamines (e.g., Claritin and Allegra, also available OTC) do not cross the blood–brain barrier and do not cause drowsiness. They generally have a longer half-life and can be taken once per day. Even though they have similar effectiveness to the older drugs, they are more expensive.

The many prescription antihistamines available differ mainly in potency, side-effect profile, and tissue selectivity. The H_1-receptor antagonists are generally not considered an asthma medication or prescribed for exercise-induced bronchoconstriction. They are used to combat allergies and can be used in conjunction with asthma medications to help control and minimize allergy-induced asthma. However, possible drug interactions and side-effect profiles need to be monitored when drug-treated asthmatics use H_1-receptor antagonists. Antihistamines are also useful for other allergic reactions, such as urticaria (hives, associated with hot temperatures or sun exposure) or anaphylaxis (a serious, potentially life-threatening allergic reaction). Though exercise-induced anaphylaxis is rare, antihistamines are an adjunct therapy for this disorder. Curiously, H_2-receptor antagonists, such as cimetidine (Tagamet) or famotidine (Pepcid), are also widely used, but for completely different reasons. H_2-receptors are found in the stomach and are involved in acid secretion, hence, H_2-receptor antagonists have been used to treat heartburn because they inhibit gastric acid secretion in the stomach.

Methylxanthines

Methylxanthines, a class of drugs that includes caffeine (see Chapter 14) and theophylline, have been used for long-term management of asthma and COPD. Although theophylline is inexpensive as a maintenance drug, its use has decreased due to the potency and usefulness of β-2 agonists and corticosteroids available in recent years. Monitoring the plasma level of theophylline is important, because it has a relatively narrow therapeutic window and undesirable side-effect profile (anorexia, nausea, headache, anxiety, and possible seizures and arrhythmias at elevated doses). Newer oral formulations of theophylline, however, are absorbed better, and time-release formulations help better manage blood levels, making theophylline a useful adjunct therapy for asthma and pulmonary disease. Theophylline works well when used in conjunction with corticosteroids in inhalers, and it is also available as a suppository. Although no longer considered a first-line agent as a respiratory drug, theophylline is still useful in many applications, including COPD.

Theophylline's mechanism of action remains largely unknown, with many potential targets identified (discussed in detail in Chapter 14). Although the methylxanthines may act directly on the respiratory control center, they may also affect inflammation in the lungs. Theophylline has antagonist activity toward certain types of adenosine receptors, including those found on human mast cells (i.e., A_{2B}; Fozard 2003). Adenosine is a neuromodulator involved in many diverse processes, including control of blood flow, inflammation, and response to ischemia. It also plays a key role in asthma. Adenosine concentrations in exhaled breath are increased in asthmatics, and increases in plasma adenosine accompany exercise-induced bronchoconstriction. Genetically modified mice with elevated adenosine levels manifest an "asthma" phenotype in lungs, with pulmonary inflammation and airway remodeling. This phenotype includes mast-cell degranulation, increased mucus secretion, and bronchial hyperresponsiveness. The changes in these mice are reversed by an enzyme therapy that reduces adenosine levels. The asthma-related changes in adenosine concentration found in the mice are also attenuated by theophylline. In addition, theophylline blocks the pro-inflammatory effects of adenosine in allergen-challenged mice. Antagonism of adenosine signaling is a potential avenue for drug treatment of asthma (Fozard).

Drug Treatment Options to Prevent Exercise-Induced Bronchoconstriction

As stated earlier, many athletes suffer an acute narrowing of their airways upon completion of a vigorous workout. Their airways are hyperresponsive to allergens or cold, dry air. Several drug options are available to ease the severity of these symptoms. In the case of β-2 agonists, tolerance can occur with chronic use (Haney & Hancox 2005). Montelukast, a leukotriene receptor antagonist, is effective in the treatment of exercise-induced bronchoconstriction and does not show tolerance. In the study shown in Figure 7.3, inhaled salmeterol, a long-acting β-2 agonist, is compared to montelukast in 47 patients with exercise-induced bronchoconstriction (Philip, Pearlman, Villarán, et al. 2007). The exercise challenge consisted of running on a treadmill for six minutes at a workload that increased heart rate to 80% to 90% of each individual's maximum heart rate. While running, patients breathed dry air at room temperature supplied through a mask from a compressed air tank. When administered two hours before exercise, both drugs improved airway function and caused a more rapid recovery. When administered 8.5 hours before exercise, both drugs improved the initial decrease in FEV_1, but only montelukast sped the return to normal. If the drugs are taken 24 hours before the exercise challenge, only montelukast treatment is significantly different from placebo and salmeterol. These results suggest that maintenance therapy with montelukast can be effective in treating exercise-induced bronchoconstriction.

Edelman, Turpin, Bronsky, et al. (2000) examined the change in protection of salmeterol versus montelukast against exercise-induced bronchoconstriction over eight weeks of drug treatment. This double-blind experiment had more than 90 participants per group. The average age of the participants was about 26, and almost half the participants were female. After eight weeks of treatment with montelukast, no loss in protection was observed. However, those treated with salmeterol showed a loss of protection over the time of treatment. After eight weeks on salmeterol, more than half of the participants showed a lack of protection against exercise-induced bronchoconstriction. The results support the conclusion that tolerance can occur with the chronic use of β-2 agonists; however, tolerance was not evident in the montelukast group.

Exercise Pharmacology of Respiratory Agents

Pharmacokinetic Concerns

The clearance of many of these different bronchodilators is flow-limited during exercise. Some drugs, such as theophylline, have half-lives of four to six hours. Most people don't exercise for over an hour, so the effect is not clinically relevant. For endurance athletes, it may have more of an effect. Theophylline, with its potential side effects (anorexia, nausea, headache, anxiety, and possible seizures and arrhythmias at elevated doses), should be monitored in aggressively training patients. Exercise-induced increases in ventilation increase the chance of exposure to allergens, which may stimulate histamine reactions, and histamine levels in blood can increase following exercise. Therefore, individuals taking antihistamines may experience compromised therapeutic effectiveness and may need to increase their dose. Exercise also increases bronchodilation through the release of catecholamines. This effect is additive to the effects of the drug albuterol. Training increases bronchodilation in elite athletes and improves ventilation in older, deconditioned individuals. Therefore, exercise can compromise antihistamines but augment bronchodilators.

Pharmacodynamic Concerns

As discussed earlier, the lungs, in general, do not limit exercise performance. In normal individuals, exercise is limited more by cardiac output and peripheral oxygen utilization than by ventilation. Since O_2 to the lungs is generally not limiting to exercise performance, augmentation with bronchodilators would not affect performance, unless there is pulmonary disease. In people with airflow problems, a lower VO_2max correlates with a lower FEV_1 (forced expiration volume). Lung function may limit exercise capacity for individuals with asthma or the elderly. By definition, patients with COPD have limited capacity for exercise.

Exercise also improves asthma control in adults (Dogra, Kuk, Baker, & Jamnik 2011). Exercise may increase the number or sensitivity of beta-receptors in the airways, similar to the beta-receptor response observed in skeletal muscle (Sato et al.). Exercise and bronchodilators, however, have a complex relationship. Bronchodilation and air exchange improve with training; bronchodilation after maximum effort has been documented in elite athletes with asthma, and a single dose of albuterol augmented

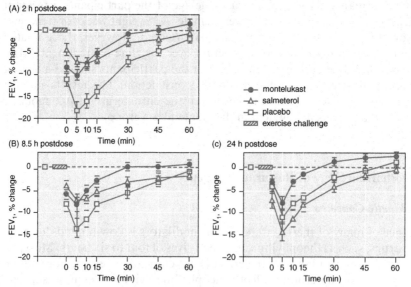

Figure 7.3 Comparison of salmeterol and montelukast for the treatment of exercise-induced bronchoconstriction.

Philip G, Pearlman DS, Villáran C, Legrand C, Loeys T, Langdon RB, Reiss TF (2007). Used with permission

Legend: Salmeterol, montelukast, or a placebo were given at the indicated times before an exercise challenge. The mean (± standard error) percent changes in FEV_1 are shown for 60 minutes following the completion of exercise (Philip, Pearlman, Villarán, et al. 2007).

this response (Todaro 1996). Many studies, however, show significant bronchodilation with no benefit to performance. Despite these findings, many endurance athletes, such as participants in triathlons, will take a couple of "puffs" from a β-2 agonist inhaler to try to improve their performance. These participants may experience a psychological effect, even if there is no measurable gain in performance.

Inhaled β-2 Agonists

Generally, since β-2 agonists are usually inhaled, their systemic bioavailability is relatively low and their effects on heart rate minimal. Moreover, with the heart containing predominantly β-1 receptors, β-2 agonists, such as albuterol, have little direct effect on heart rate. Besides being the prevalent receptors in lung tissue, β-2 receptors are prevalent in skeletal muscle, and their expression can increase with exercise (Sato et al.). In adipocytes, breakdown of triglycerides to release free fatty acids is mostly under β-1 control. The breakdown of skeletal muscle triglycerides is mostly under β-2 control. As discussed in Chapter 3, epinephrine works at both receptors, so during exercise both sources of fat are utilized.

Systemic β-2 agonists should preferentially activate muscle lipid breakdown. At maximum levels of exercise, when endogenous catecholamines are at high levels systemically, an additional effect of acutely inhaled β-2 agonists is not expected. Chronic exposure to systemic β-2 agonists could produce an ergogenic effect on skeletal muscle, and limited studies, primarily with clenbuterol, are discussed below. A compounding factor, however, is that tolerance develops with regular use of inhaled β-2 agonists over the course of several weeks (Edelman et al.), so ergogenic effects from inhaled β-2 agonists could be limited.

Inhaled β-2 agonists have been studied extensively to determine if they have an ergogenic effect. Since many athletes require treatment for asthma or exercise-induced bronchoconstriction, the question is whether they gain a performance benefit by inhaling these drugs. Most of the evidence compiled in a large meta-analysis suggests that β-2 agonists do not provide an ergogenic benefit when inhaled at recommended doses (Pluim et al.). In a subsequent study, high-dose inhaled albuterol had no acute effect on oxygen uptake or aerobic capacity in healthy athletic men (Elers, Mørkeberg, Jansen, et al. 2012). Dickinson, Hu, Chester, and colleagues (2014) found that daily doses of albuterol at the upper limit allowed by WADA did not improve running performance in 5-kilometer time trials. However, terbutaline, a β-2 agonist no longer available in the United States, was found to increase muscle strength and sprint performance in trained men (Hostrup, Kalsen, Bangsbo, et al. 2014). In this study, peak power and mean power increased subjects' performance on the Wingate test, with an associated increase in plasma lactate, suggesting that high-dose terbutaline use should be restricted during competition. In a follow-up study, a high dose of inhaled terbutaline was evaluated during maximal sprint cycling (Kalsen, Hostrup, Söderlund, et al. 2016). In a randomized double-blind cross-over design, nine moderately trained men conducted a ten-second cycle sprint after inhalation of either 15 mg of terbutaline or placebo. A muscle biopsy sample was collected before and within ten seconds after the sprint; they were analyzed for metabolites and muscle fiber types. Terbutaline treatment increased power output, associated with increased rates of glycogenolysis and glycolysis. Terbutaline also counteracted the reduction in ATP in Type II fibers, suggesting that terbutaline may postpone fatigue development in these fibers (Kalsen et al., 2016). However, in another study, oral terbutaline at supraphysiological dose did not change oxygen uptake in non-asthmatic athletes (Sanchez, Borrani, Le Fur, et al. 2013).

When the three approved β-2 agonists (Table 7.1) were inhaled combined at permitted doses, swim ergometer sprint performance and maximal voluntary contraction were improved (Kalsen, Hostrup, Bangsbo, & Backer 2014). In these elite swimmers, however, no improvement in an exhaustive swim performance test was observed. To date, the majority of the evidence supports the WADA decision to allow inhaled β-2 agonists below a specified dose. The performance potential of these drugs is such that monitoring their levels in urine is necessary to eliminate abuse.

Systemic β-2 Agonists

Systemic β-2 agonists may have ergogenic effects, but the data are limited (Pluim et al.). Most studies have used the relatively short-acting albuterol. In a more recent study, Sanchez, Collomp, Carra, and colleagues (2012) found that orally administered albuterol was ergogenic for a sprint exercise, with significantly higher blood lactate concentrations in the drug-treated group. They also found that an acute treatment was more effective than three weeks of treatment (Sanchez et al., 2012). Oral albuterol also increased performance on the Wingate test in elite male athletes after acute or two weeks of treatment (Hostrup et al.). Formoterol was more potent than salmeterol in causing skeletal muscle hypertrophy with minimal cardiac hypertrophy, when injected intraperitoneally daily for four weeks in rats (Ryall, Sillence, & Lynch 2006). Formoterol also caused skeletal muscle hypertrophy in mice, associated with an increase in muscle protein synthesis and a decrease in muscle protein degradation (Koopman, Gehrig, Léger, et al. 2010). Formoterol is more specific toward β-2 receptors than clenbuterol, a β-2 agonist that has been studied extensively since the 1990s.

Available in Europe, clenbuterol is a potent, long-acting β-2 agonist that is not approved for humans in the United States. Called a "repartitioning agent," it may enhance fat burning while promoting lean muscle mass. In Europe and the United States, clenbuterol was used in livestock to improve muscle mass, but has since been banned. Clenbuterol is also used as a bronchodilator in racehorses, and there are post-race blood and urine limits for racehorses in most states. Quarter horse racing now bans clenbuterol entirely. Interestingly, after prolonged use (21 days), airway function decreases in horses. A widely cited article on clenbuterol (Prather, Brown, North, & Wilson, 1995) reviewed the use of clenbuterol in animals, and, even then, the authors were alarmed by the notion of its unsupervised use in humans. Some consider the drug to be an anabolic steroid substitute, and it can be obtained over the Internet. Prominent baseball players and other professional athletes have tested positive for using clenbuterol. Swimmers have been disqualified from the Olympics for taking the drug. The 2010 Tour de France winner, Alberto Contador, tested positive, blaming tainted meat as the source of the small amount of clenbuterol found in his urine sample. His defense was not accepted, however, and he was stripped of his title.

Studies on clenbuterol may help illustrate the possible ergogenic effects of long-acting β-2 agonists taken systemically. For example, clenbuterol treatment for 14 days in sedentary rats increased lean muscle mass, but the rats showed faster fatigue (Dodd, Powers, Vrabas, et al. 1996). Other cellular changes suggested drug treatment caused a shift toward a fast-twitch phenotype. Clenbuterol-treated rats were compared to rats on an eight-week progressive isometric force program (Mounier, Cavalié, Lac, & Clottes 2007). Each treatment resulted in an increase in muscle mass and induced a consistent slow-to-fast phenotype change without increasing activities of glycolytic enzymes.

The results of clenbuterol treatment in rodents suggested a possible use for clenbuterol in muscle-wasting diseases in humans (dystrophy, AIDS, cancer, etc.), and there has been considerable interest in studying the use of β-2 agonists and muscle-wasting diseases. However, long-term use has serious negative effects. Clenbuterol or other β-2 agonists cause hypertrophy of fast skeletal muscle fibers with toxic effects on slow fibers, probably due to effects on calcium homeostasis (Sirvent, Douillard, Galbes, et al. 2014). Long-acting β-2 agonists cause excessive stimulation of β-2 receptors. Moreover, the β-2 agonists cause down-regulation of β-2 receptors in slow-twitch muscle, minimizing their usefulness in muscle-wasting diseases (Sato et al.). These drugs can also cause hypertrophy and dysfunction of the heart (Ryall, Schertzer, Murphy, et al. 2008).

Clenbuterol was also tested on patients' recovery of muscle area and strength after knee surgery. In this randomized, double-blind, placebo-controlled study, 20 male patients were treated for four weeks postoperatively, followed by a two-week washout period. In the operated leg, clenbuterol treatment caused a more rapid rehabilitation of strength in knee extensor muscles. The strength in the unoperated leg improved after six weeks of training. However, at the end of the six weeks, absolute strength was not significantly different between the placebo and treated groups (Maltin, Delday, Watson, et al. 1993).

What can be concluded from the limited data? Chronic use of β-2 agonists taken systemically may have anabolic properties and be ergogenic. They can cause muscle development and improve strength performance. However, their side-effect profile and possible negative physiological effects in the long term suggest they should be used only limitedly and with caution.

β-2 Agonists, Muscle Hypertrophy, and Muscle Fiber Type

Exercise can increase the size of muscle cells, a process called hypertrophy. Inactivity, unloading ("taking the weight off," such as by using crutches or a sling), or disease can cause a decrease in muscle size, a process called atrophy. At the cellular level, hypertrophy results from an increase in protein content, and atrophy results from a decrease in protein content. We will focus here on the hypertrophic response. The increase in protein content in cells is due to an increase in the rate of protein synthesis and a decrease in the rate of protein degradation. Muscle cell proteins have a relatively high rate of turnover, with the balance between synthesis and degradation very tightly regulated. The response of muscle cells to exercise is mediated largely by adrenergic input from epinephrine and norepinephrine. Skeletal muscle expresses considerably more β-2 receptors than β-1 receptors. Therefore, β-2 agonists can significantly influence muscle protein levels. This property gives β-2 agonists, particularly long-acting ones such as clenbuterol, doping potential when taken systemically, and, as discussed, this anabolic property also suggests a possible role for these drugs in the treatment of muscle-wasting diseases (Sato et al.).

When activated, β-2 receptors increase cyclic AMP (adenosine monophosphate) levels and can activate additional signal transduction pathways. Genes coding for muscle proteins are activated, and the rate of new protein synthesis increases. The rate of protein degradation also decreases after β-2 receptor activation, by both of the principal mechanisms for protein degradation in muscle (ubiquitin-mediated protein degradation and calcium-dependent protein degradation). Interestingly, fast-twitch fibers are more responsive than slow-twitch fibers to β-2 receptor stimulation, and they show a greater hypertrophic response. This greater response of the fast-twitch muscle cells may be due to less desensitization of the adrenergic receptors. With prolonged agonist treatment, β-2 receptors in slow-twitch muscle become less responsive, but that does not occur in fast-twitch muscle.

Another mechanism involves the way muscle cells are programmed to respond (Sato et al.). Fast- and slow-twitch muscle cells differ in expression of gene control proteins, so when signals enter the nucleus following stimulation of β-2 receptors, different genes are expressed in the different types of muscle cells. One result of this differential gene expression is that long-acting β-2 agonists cause switching of slow-twitch (type I fibers) to the physiology of fast-twitch (type II) fibers. Although based largely on animal experiments, considerable evidence shows that β-2 agonists cause hypertrophy and increased responsiveness of fast-twitch muscle cells (Sato et al.).

The type of exercise can also differentially affect muscle fiber types, as discussed in Chapter 2. Strength training ultimately improves force generation. The improved ability to generate force is related to increases in muscle mass, fiber cross-sectional area, and protein content. When clenbuterol was given orally to rats in conjunction with an eight-week strength-training program (progressive isometric force), no additive effect on muscle mass and force generation was observed (Mournier et al.; Sato et al.). One explanation is that during weight training, the high levels of epinephrine sufficiently occupy fast-twitch receptors, and no additional gain is seen with the agonist treatment.

A different response is observed with endurance training. Endurance training causes an increase in mitochondrial mass, increased levels of enzymes for oxidative metabolism, increased expression of slow contractile proteins, and improved insulin-dependent glucose uptake. Endurance training also causes fast muscle fibers to switch to a slow-fiber phenotype. Clenbuterol's ability to switch slow fibers to fast fibers is suppressed with endurance training (Lynch, Hayes, Campbell, & Williams 1996). These results suggest that endurance training's effect on the metabolic capabilities of muscle cells occurs at moderate levels of β-2 receptor occupation, enhancing slow-twitch muscle function. High levels of β-2 agonist activity, such as observed with clenbuterol, enhance fast-twitch muscle function. When clenbuterol is combined with endurance training, the drug-dependent switch of slow-twitch fibers to fast-twitch is not observed, and the exercise-dependent switch of fast to slow is also lessened. The normal responses of muscle tissue to different types of exercise (and corresponding receptor occupation) are altered when long-acting β-2 agonists are present.

Other Respiratory Agents

Ipratropium (anti-muscarinic) had no effect on cardiac, pulmonary, and other parameters of exercise in both asthmatics and non-asthmatics. Leukotriene antagonists are effective in treating exercise-induced bronchoconstriction, and they do not affect heart rate or VO_2

and do not have ergogenic properties. Nedocromil (a mast-cell stabilizer) has no effect on VO_2max in master athletes. Inhaled corticosteroids also do not have a documented effect on cardiovascular, metabolic, or pulmonary measures of exercise. However, they may exert systemic effects on the HPA axis. One study examined whether inhaled corticosteroids affected the HPA response to exercise. Eleven healthy males were placed on two weeks of inhaled corticosteroids (fluticasone twice daily). They performed a 30-minute bout of exercise on a cycle ergometer at approximately 70% of peak work rate before and after the start of treatment. After inhaled corticosteroid treatment, a blunted exercise response was observed for cortisol, adrenocorticotropin, and growth hormone (Schwindt, Zaldivar, Eliakim, et al. 2010). Although use of corticosteroids in children is considered safe (Pedersen 2006), results such as these and others suggest that chronic use of inhaled corticosteroids in children and athletes should be monitored.

Theophylline inhibits bronchoconstriction, increases circulating epinephrine, enhances free fatty acid mobilization, increases cardiac output, and causes CNS stimulation, so it has some ergogenic properties. However, it also has a diuretic effect, antagonizes adenosine, and decreases production of erythropoietin (a hormone that acts on stem cells of the bone marrow to stimulate red blood cell production), so it has ergolytic properties, as well. The complex response to theophylline during exercise is the sum of all these effects. Theophylline can increase resting heart rate, but it has little effect on exercise heart rate. Theophylline also has a CNS effect, stimulating respiration at the medulla by increasing sensitivity to CO_2. The drug, however, has no effect on VO_2 in non-asthmatics. Theophylline inhibits exercise-induced bronchoconstriction in a dose-dependent manner (Magnussen, Reuss, & Jörres 1988).

Elder Concerns

Lung function deteriorates progressively with age and the elderly can suffer from shortness of breath and other pulmonary diseases (MacNee, Rabinovich, & Choudhury 2014). Is the decreased lung function due to 'normal' aging or the result of underlying disease? Aged lungs are characterized by a progressive reduction in FEV1 of about 20 ml per year. As we age, there is a decrease in chest wall compliance and elastic recoil with a decrease in respiratory muscle strength. Deterioration in alveolar structure results in a decrease in the surface area for gas exchange. These age-related changes can result in lower oxygen levels in the blood and decreased ability to eliminate carbon dioxide.

Many chronic inflammatory diseases accelerate the aging process. COPD has been considered a disease of accelerated lung aging and can provide a mechanistic link for associated symptoms and comorbidities. Animal models of premature aging show structural changes in the lungs and skeletal muscle that resemble those in COPD. Residual volume in the lung is increased and respiratory muscle strength is decreased in patients with COPD, similar to aging. Wrinkle formation and elastin degradation in the skin is related to emphysema and arterial stiffness in patients with COPD, providing a link between skin aging, COPD, and cardiovascular risk (MacNee et al.).

Aging may result from accumulated damage from exposure to noxious agents over time (e.g., cigarette smoke) that potentially accelerate the process of aging. Oxidative stress is also involved in aging and is prevalent in the lungs, blood cells, and muscle in COPD patients, especially smokers. Oxidative stress causes mitochondrial dysfunction and damage to mitochondrial DNA. It can lead to shortening of telomeres (discussed in Chapter 2) and smokers (current and former) have shortened telomeres in white blood cells and lung tissue, the extent of which depends on pack-years smoked. Cell death in lung tissue is enhanced and the capacity for cell replacement decreases in COPD and is far more accelerated than normal aging. Chronic inflammation becomes a major problem in these patients.

Exercise has a positive outcome in the elderly and those with COPD. One study used over 4,000 participants of the Canadian Longitudinal Study on Aging (Dogra, Good, Buman, et al. 2018). Among participants with asthma, those engaged in strengthening activities were less likely to report poor perceived health, poor mental health, or unhealthy aging. Among those with COPD, the most sedentary group more frequently reported poor perceived health, poor mental health, and unhealthy aging. These authors concluded that higher physical activity levels and lower sedentary time provided lower healthcare use and better quality of life in older patients with respiratory disease (Dogra et al. 2018).

Health Risks

β-2 agonists can induce skeletal muscle tremor, such as shaky hands. Headache, anxiety, nausea, and cardiac arrhythmias are additional side effects. Systemic β-2 agonists can affect skeletal muscle function and have negative effects on the heart. Anticholinergics can increase heart rate and cause blurred vision. Drowsiness from some antihistamines can affect performance and worsen when combined with alcohol. Long-term use of corticosteroids at high doses may affect bone mineral density. However, exercise is good for bone mineral density, so with inhaled low doses for maintenance therapy, fewer complications are expected. Other side effects of inhaled corticosteroids include nasal irritation and possible nosebleeds (epistaxis). Theophylline has the greatest potential for adverse effects, because it has a relatively narrow therapeutic window. As stated earlier, theophylline can cause anorexia, nausea, headache, anxiety, arrhythmias, and possible seizures at elevated doses.

Non-Drug Prevention of Exercise-Induced Bronchoconstriction

Although drug treatment may be required to prevent the development of exercise-induced bronchoconstriction, there are some things that can be done to prevent flare-ups (Ali, Norsk, & Ulrik 2012). Warming up prior to exercising and cooling down after exercise can help prevent exercise-induced bronchoconstriction. For individuals with allergies that act as a trigger, exercise should be limited when the pollen count is high. Similarly, they should exercise indoors, if possible, when outdoor temperatures are extremely low or air pollution levels are high. When fighting a cold or other respiratory infection, individuals with asthma should restrict exercise, especially cardiovascular exercise. They should breathe through the nose to warm air before it goes into the lungs and should keep the mouth and nose covered during exercise in cold weather, for example, by wearing a heat mask specially designed for outdoor winter athletes. Diets rich in antioxidants (e.g., fresh fruits and vegetables) may help reduce airway inflammation in some people. It is important that people not avoid exercise because of asthma or exercise-induced bronchoconstriction. Staying fit can ease asthma symptoms over time (Bruurs, van der Giessen, & Moed 2013; Wanrooij, Willeboordse, Dompeling, & van de Kant 2014).

PES Watch

In 2013, WADA started permitting specific inhaled β-2 agonists without a therapeutic use exemption. Albuterol (urine threshold 1000 ng/ml) and formoterol (urine threshold 40 ng/ml) may be used as long as they are under the stated threshold. The inhaled β-2 agonists generally clear the system in two to three days. Illegal, high-dose inhalation of β-2-agonists may enhance performance and create a challenging anti-doping issue. Oral use of β-2 agonists is not permitted. Clenbuterol is not licensed for human use in the United States. The NCAA bans all types of β-2 agonists; athletes with a physician's prescription for an inhaled β-2 agonist must complete a therapeutic use exemption. The NCAA has no ban on inhaled corticosteroids. WADA and the U.S. Anti-Doping Agency (USADA) will allow a therapeutic use exemption for inhaled corticosteroids. Ipratropium, theophylline, the leukotriene receptor antagonists, and mast-cell stabilizers are not banned.

Conclusion

Environmental factors, such as smoking, particulates, allergens, and so forth can be causative agents or can trigger episodes of coughing. During an asthmatic attack, coughing and wheezing can result from bronchiolar constriction and inflammation. The β-2 agonists cause relaxation of the bronchiolar smooth muscle and provide short-term relief. Long-term control is managed with anti-inflammatory steroids or leukotriene receptor antagonists. Exercise-induced bronchoconstriction can be treated with short-acting β-2 agonists or, in some cases, reduced by pretreatment with leukotriene receptor antagonists.

Systemic long-acting β-2 agonists may have doping potential and many athletes have failed drug tests by testing positive for clenbuterol. For those athletes that need an inhaled β-2 agonist because of asthma or exercise-induced bronchoconstriction, many sports governing bodies have dropped the requirement of a therapeutic use exemption.

Key Concepts Review

alveoli
anaphylaxis
antihistamine
arachidonic acid
asthma exacerbation
β-2 agonist
bronchial hyperreactivity
bronchiole
bronchoconstriction
bronchodilator
bronchospasm
chronic obstructive pulmonary disease (COPD)
cytokine
eicosanoid
exercise-induced bronchoconstriction

exercise-induced bronchoconstriction with asthma
forced expiratory volume in one second (FEV1)
frequency
histamine (H1)
hyperresponsiveness
immunoglobulin E (IgE)
leukotriene modifier
5-lipoxygenase
lung ventilation rate
mast cell
mast-cell stabilizer
metered-dose inhaler
methylxanthine
nebulizer

respiratory control center
spirometry
synthetic corticosteroid

tidal volume
ventilation equivalent for oxygen

Review Questions

1 Years ago, children with asthma were restricted in their activity to minimize their "spells." Nowadays, asthmatics are encouraged to exercise. Why?
2 Many competitors in Nordic skiing events suffer from exercise-induced bronchoconstriction. What are the signs, why is it happening, and can they do anything about it? Is the treatment that you suggest legal according to the IOC?
3 Jogging in the spring seems to make Jan's allergies worse. Why? What would you recommend she do?
4 Many bronchodilators are powerful β-agonists, but they do not have strong effects on the heart. Why?
5 Should bronchodilators be banned from competitions? What benefits of using these drugs may give a competitor an unfair advantage?

References

Ali Z, Norsk P, Ulrik CS (2012) Mechanisms and management of exercise-induced asthma in elite athletes. *J Asthma* 49:480–486

Bruurs ML, van der Giessen LJ, Moed H (2013) The effectiveness of physiotherapy in patients with asthma: a systematic review of the literature. *Respir Med* 107:483–494

Burke H, Leonardi-Bee J, Hashim A, Pine-Abata H, Chem Y, Cook DG, Britton JR, McKeever TM (2012) Prenatal and passive smoke exposure and incidence of asthma and wheeze: systemic review and meta-analysis. *Pediatrics* 129:735–744

Carlsen K-H, Hem E, Stensrud T, Held T, Herland K, Mowinckel P (2001) Can asthma treatment in sports be doping? The effect of the rapid onset, long-acting inhaled β-2 agonist formoterol upon endurance performance in healthy well-trained athletes. *Respir Med* 95:571–576

Decramer M, Janssens W, Miravitlles M (2012) Chronic obstructive pulmonary disease. *Lancet* 379:7–13

Dickinson J, Hu J, Chester N, Loosemore M, Whyte G (2014) Acute impact of inhaled short acting b2-agonists on 5 km running performance. *J Sports Sci Med* 13:271–279

Dodd SL, Powers SK, Vrabas IS, Criswell D, Stetson S, Hussain R (1996) Effects of clenbuterol on contractile and biochemical properties of skeletal muscle. *Med Sci Sports Exerc* 28:669–676

Dogra S, Kuk JL, Baker J, Jamnik V (2011) Exercise is associated with improved asthma control in adults. *Eur Respir J* 37:318–323

Dogra S, Good J, Buman MP, Gardiner PA, Copeland JL, Stickland MK (2018) Physical activity and sedentary time are related to clinically relevant health outcomes among adults with obstructive lung disease. *BMC Pulm Med* 8:98

D'Urzo AD, Peter Kardos P, Wiseman R (2018) Practical considerations when prescribing a long-acting muscarinic antagonist for patients with COPD. *Int J COPD* 13:1089–1104

Edelman JM, Turpin JA, Bronsky EA, Grossman J, Kemp JP, Ghannam AF, DeLuca PT, Gormley GJ, Pearlman DS (2000) Oral montelukast compared with inhaled salmeterol to prevent exercise-induced bronchoconstriction. *Ann Intern Med* 132:97–104

Elers J, Mørkeberg J, Jansen T, Belhage B, Backer V (2012) High-dose inhaled salbutamol has no acute effects on aerobic capacity or oxygen uptake kinetics in healthy trained men. *Scand J Med Sci Sports* 22:232–239

Fitch KD (2012) An overview of asthma and airway hyper-responsiveness in Olympic athletes. *Br J Sports Med* 46:413–416

Fozard JR (2003) The case for a role for adenosine in asthma: almost convincing? *Cur Opin Pharmacol* 3:264–269

Haney S, Hancox RJ (2005) Tolerance to bronchodilation during treatment with long-acting beta-agonists, a randomised controlled trial. *Respir Res* 61:107

Hostrup M, Kalsen A, Bangsbo J, Hemmersbach P, Karlsson S, Backer V (2014) High-dose inhaled terbutaline increases muscle strength and enhances maximal sprint performance in trained men. *Eur J Appl Physiol* 114:2499–2508

Housh TJ, Housh DJ, DeVries HA (2012) *Applied Exercise and Sport Physiology, 3e*. Scottsdale: Holcomb Hathaway

Kalsen A, Hostrup M, Bangsbo J, Backer V (2014) Combined inhalation of beta2-agonists improves swim ergometer sprint performance but not high-intensity swim performance. *Scand J Med Sci Sports* 24:814–822

Kalsen A, Hostrup M, Söderlund K, Karlsson S, Backer V, Bangsbo J. (2016) Inhaled beta2-agonist increases power output and glycolysis during sprinting in men. *Med Sci Sports Exerc* 48:39–48

Kemp JP (2009) Exercise-induced bronchoconstriction: the effects of montelukast, a leukotriene receptor antagonist. *Ther Clin Risk Manag* 5:923–934

Koopman R, Gehrig SM, Léger B, Trieu J, Walrand S, Murphy KT, Lynch GS (2010) Cellular mechanisms underlying temporal changes in skeletal muscle protein synthesis and breakdown during chronic {beta}-adrenoceptor stimulation in mice. *J Physiol* 588:4811–4823

Lang DM (2006) The controversy over long-acting beta agonists: examining the evidence. *Cleveland Clinic J Med* 73:973–992

Lynch GS, Hayes A, Campbell SP, Williams DA (1996) Effects of β2-agonist administration and exercise on contractile activation of skeletal muscle fibers. *J Appl Physiol* 81:1610–1618

MacNee W, Rabinovich RA, Choudhury G (2014) Ageing and the border between health and disease. *Eur Respir J* 44:1332–1352

Magnussen H, Reuss G, Jörres R (1988) Methylxanthines inhibit exercise-induced bronchoconstriction at low serum theophylline concentration and in a dose-dependent fashion. *J Allergy Clin Immunol* 81:531–537

Maltin CA, Delday MI, Watson JS, Heys SD, Nevison IM, Ritchie IK, Gibson PH (1993) Clenbuterol, a beta-adrenoceptor agonist, increases relative muscle strength in orthopaedic patients. *Clin Sci (Lond)* 84:651–654

Mounier R, Cavalié H, Lac G, Clottes E (2007) Molecular impact of clenbuterol and isometric strength training on rat EDL muscles. *Pflugers Arch* 453:497–507

Mukherjee AB, Zhang Z (2011) Allergic asthma: influence of genetic and environmental factors. *J Biol Chem* 286:2883–2889

National Center for Environmental Health (September 22, 2014) Asthma surveillance data. Centers for Disease Control and Prevention. www.cdc.gov/asthma/asthmadata.htm

Neder JA, Dal Corso S, Malaguti C, Reis S, De Fuccio MB, Schmidt H, Fuld JP, Nery LE (2003) The pattern and timing of breathing during incremental exercise: a normative study. *Eur Respir J* 21:530–538

Pedersen S (2006) Clinical safety of inhaled corticosteroids for asthma in children: an update of long-term trials. *Drug Saf* 29:599–612

Philip G, Pearlman DS, Villarán C, Legrand C, Loeys T, Langdon RB, Reiss TF (2007) Single-dose montelukast or salmeterol as protection against exercise-induced bronchoconstriction. *Chest* 132:875–883

Pluim BM, de Hon O, Staal JB, Limpens J, Kuipers H, Overbeek SE, Zwinderman AH, Scholten RJ (2011) β-2 agonists and physical performance: a systematic review and meta-analysis of randomized controlled trials. *Sports Med* 41:39–57

Prather ID, Brown DE, North P, Wilson JR (1995) Clenbuterol: a substitute for anabolic steroids? *Med Sci Sports Exerc* 27:118–121

Randolph C (2009) An update on exercise-induced bronchoconstriction with and without asthma. *Cur Allergy Asthma Rep* 9:433–438

Rogers L, Hanania NA (2015) Role of anticholinergics in asthma management: recent evidence and future needs. *Curr Opin Pulm Med* 21:103–108

Ryall JG, Sillence MN, Lynch GS (2006) Systemic administration of beta2-adrenoceptor agonists, formoterol and salmeterol, elicit skeletal muscle hypertrophy in rats at micromolar doses. *Br J Pharmacol* 147:587–595

Ryall JG, Schertzer JD, Murphy KT, Allen AM, Lynch GS (2008) Chronic β2-adrenoceptor stimulation impairs cardiac relaxation via reduced SR Ca2+-ATPase protein and activity. *Am J Physiol-Heart Circ Physiol* 294:H2587–H2595

Sanchez AM, Collomp K, Carra J, Borrani F, Coste O, Préfaut C, Candau R (2012) Effect of acute and short-term oral salbutamol treatments on maximal power output in non-asthmatic athletes. *Eur J Appl Physiol* 112:3251–3258

Sanchez AM, Borrani F, Le Fur MA, Le Mieux A, Lecoultre V, Py G, Gernigon C, Collomp K, Candau R (2013) Acute supra-therapeutic oral terbutaline administration has no ergogenic effect in non-asthmatic athletes. *Eur J Appl Physiol* 113:411–418

Sato S, Shirato K, Tachiyashiki K, Imaizumi K (2011) Muscle plasticity and β-2 adrenergic receptors: adaptive responses of β-2adrenergic receptor expression to muscle hypertrophy and atrophy. *J Biomed Biotech* article ID 729598, pages 1–10

Schwindt CD, Zaldivar F, Eliakim A, Shin HW, Leu SY, Cooper DM (2010) Inhaled fluticasone and the hormonal and inflammatory response to brief exercise. *Med Sci Sports Exerc* 42:1802–1808

Sirvent P, Douillard A, Galbes O, Ramonatxo C, Py G, Candau R, Lacampagne A (2014) Effects of chronic administration of clenbuterol on contractile properties and calcium homeostasis in rat extensor digitorum longus muscle. *PLoS One* 9(6):e100281

Stewart A (2012) More muscle in asthma, but where did it come from? *Am J Resp Crit Care Med* 185:1035–1037

Todaro A (1996) Exercise-induced bronchodilation in asthmatic athletes. *J Sports Med Phys Fitness* 36:60–66

Wanrooij VH, Willeboordse M, Dompeling E, van de Kant KD (2014) Exercise training in children with asthma: a systematic review. *Br J Sports Med* 48:1024–1031

Wasserman K, Hansen JE, Sue DY, Casaburi R, Whipp BJ (1999) *Principles of Exercise Testing and Interpretation.* Philadelphia: Lippincott Williams & Wilkins

8 Sympathomimetics

Abstract

Sympathomimetics are a diverse group of drugs that have adrenergic properties. This chapter focused on two main classes of drugs: (1) derivatives of the natural product ephedrine that work primarily in the periphery and (2) the centrally acting stimulants. The ephedrine derivatives are used to alleviate cold symptoms. Their adrenergic activity can be pronounced, but they do not clearly show ergogenic properties. Their approved use during competition continues to generate debate. The centrally acting stimulants are powerful drugs that have abuse potential. They are illegal without a prescription and can cause significant and dangerous side effects when an individual is exercising. However, some of these drugs are useful in treating Attention Deficit/Hyperactivity Disorder. This somewhat paradoxical use of these drugs has helped provide researchers with additional tools for studying how the brain works. Exercise exerts effects in areas of the brain that are also targets for these stimulants. Regular exercise is encouraged as a helpful supplement to drug therapy for Attention Deficit/Hyperactivity Disorder.

CASE EXAMPLE

Megan's first child, Robbie, has been a struggle. It started in pre-school, when he could never settle down. At home, he just seemed like a very active kid—she thought this is just how little boys are. First grade was not much better, and the family doctor tested him to see if he had any auditory or visual causes for his behavior. Robbie was very impulsive, and the other kids tended to keep their distance from him. Robbie's doctor noted that Robbie had many of the symptoms of Attention Deficit/Hyperactivity Disorder (ADHD) and administered a non-invasive brain scan. There is no single test to diagnose ADHD, but Robbie checked enough boxes to try drug treatment. Part of the diagnosis for ADHD is whether the child (or adult) responds characteristically to central acting stimulants. The drug Ritalin does seem to help Robbie as he is 'more normal'. He is able to complete tasks and not be so impulsive (and impolite). It is quite remarkable that a stimulant containing an amphetamine-like drug can cause children and adults with ADHD to 'calm down' and cope with their surroundings. Megan was so surprised by the change, she did a little experiment. She remembered her one roommate using speed (amphetamines) around final exams, as this roommate always waited to the last minute to get anything done. Megan never did speed in college—she knew it was on the banned list, and she already had a strike against her from the diuretic fiasco when she took the stupid supplement. One afternoon, when she was dragging around trying to get the laundry done and the house clean, she took one of Robbie's pills. Yes, Robbie's pills contain a stimulant—she has no doubt. Megan begins to worry about Robbie's long-term health because these are strong drugs. She starts reading about ADHD, and how exercise and sports can help, so this summer it will be T-ball with soccer in the fall—and less screen-time!

Learning Objectives

1   Learn how sympathomimetics work.
2   Distinguish between peripheral and centrally acting sympathomimetics.
3   Learn the medical conditions for which sympathomimetics are used.
4   Appreciate the issues associated with attention deficit and hyperactivity disorder.
5   Understand why centrally acting stimulants are prescribed for ADHD.
6   Understand how ephedrine and related drugs affect athletic performance.
7   Appreciate how exercise may be a useful adjuvant therapy for ADHD.
8   Contemplate the ongoing debate over whether drugs like pseudoephedrine should be banned from competition.

Introduction

Amphetamines are commonly referred to as stimulants. Because they work by stimulating the sympathetic nervous system, they belong to a group of drugs called sympathomimetics. Drugs related to the natural product ephedra are also sympathomimetics. Sympathomimetics have diverse mechanisms, with some drugs having agonist activity and others indirectly increasing the activity of norepinephrine and epinephrine. They also vary in their access to the central nervous system, so some drugs largely affect peripheral responses, whereas others can profoundly change behavior. Since the drugs mimic adrenergic activity, and exercise and stress also involve adrenergic responses, the exercise pharmacology of these drugs explores whether they provide competitive advantage and the negative effects they may exert on the cardiovascular system.

Types of Sympathomimetics and Their Uses

Sympathomimetics are drugs that mimic the actions of norepinephrine (through adrenergic receptors at post-synaptic sites), epinephrine (released from the adrenal gland following stress or intense exercise), and possibly dopamine (active mostly in the central nervous system). See Figure 8.1 for a comparison of the structures of the naturally occurring catecholamines and some of the sympathomimetics discussed in this chapter. Responses to these drugs can be similar to portions of the stress response covered in Chapter 3. Drugs with sympathomimetic activity can be characterized as **specific** (as with β-2 agonists) or **general** (having epinephrine-like effects). Sympathomimetics are distinguished by their mechanism of action. Some of these drugs have agonist activity, and some have indirect mechanisms for increasing levels of endogenous catecholamines. Examples of indirectly acting drugs include those that block reuptake of neurotransmitters at the pre-synaptic membrane, drugs that displace neurotransmitters from their storage sites, and drugs that inhibit metabolic inactivation of the

Figure 8.1 Structures of sympathomimetics compared to naturally occurring catecholamines.

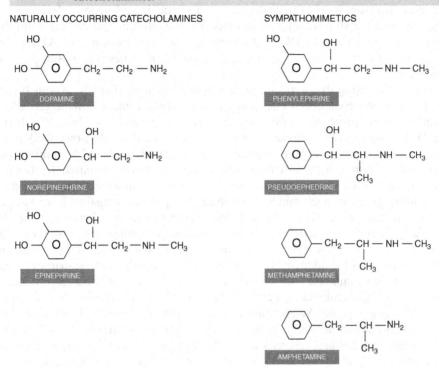

NATURALLY OCCURRING CATECHOLAMINES

DOPAMINE

NOREPINEPHRINE

EPINEPHRINE

SYMPATHOMIMETICS

PHENYLEPHRINE

PSEUDOEPHEDRINE

METHAMPHETAMINE

AMPHETAMINE

neurotransmitters. Sympathomimetic drugs also differ in their access to the central nervous system, with some acting mostly in the periphery and others causing a significant CNS response.

Sympathomimetics are indicated for a variety of conditions. Epinephrine itself is the drug of choice during emergencies involving anaphylactic shock (a severe allergic reaction involving swelling, respiratory distress, and circulation collapse), when it is injected intramuscularly or subcutaneously. People with extreme reactions to things like bee stings or peanuts sometimes carry EpiPens in case of severe allergic reaction. Drugs with largely peripheral effects are used as pressor agents (agents that cause the constriction of blood vessels), usually in a clinical setting. One of the most common uses for sympathomimetics is in formulations for decongestion. They are also used in eye drops. Other sympathomimetics suppress appetite and have been used for weight control. Sympathomimetics used for asthma, including β-2 agonists, were discussed in the previous chapter.

Sympathomimetics with a strong effect on the CNS are prescribed for **narcolepsy, attention deficit / hyperactivity disorder (ADHD),** and some types of sleep disorders. Narcolepsy is a neurological disorder characterized by overwhelming daytime drowsiness. ADHD is a neurobehavioral disorder characterized by the inability to concentrate or maintain attention span. ADHD is estimated to affect 5% to 7% of children aged 4 through 17. About two-thirds of these children are being treated, which means that 3% to 4% of all children are on medication for ADHD. Children with ADHD will often carry some form of the disorder into adulthood. Methylphenidate (Ritalin) is related to the amphetamine family of drugs and has efficacy in treating ADHD. In addition to being prescribed for narcolepsy and ADHD, some of the centrally acting drugs have also been used to treat depression and cocaine addiction. Modafinil is a sympathomimetic with CNS effects marketed as a wakefulness-promoting agent, but has not been approved for ADHD. It has been prescribed off-label for ADHD and there is limited data on its effectiveness; insurance companies may not approve its off-label use.

The centrally acting drugs are frequently abused or used illegally. Amphetamine abuse has reached epidemic proportions, and law enforcement now targets illegal methamphetamine production labs. Amphetamines were widely used by troops during World War II, and methamphetamine was one of the first diet pills prescribed, in the 1950s, due to its ability to suppress appetite. Stimulants are still used by military personnel under certain conditions to overcome fatigue when sleep is limited. In athletics, former Major League Baseball players such as Tony Gwynn have acknowledged the long-standing use of amphetamines in baseball and spoken out against it. In January 2007, the baseball player Barry Bonds failed a drug test for amphetamines; he also became a key figure in a scandal involving performance-enhancing substances. Endurance athletes, such as competitive cyclists, have abused amphetamines for decades.

What are the possible additive effects of powerful sympathomimetic drugs like amphetamine to the stimulation of the sympathetic nervous system associated with intense physical activity? Does mimicking norepinephrine and epinephrine mean that all sympathomimetics are ergogenic? Amphetamines and cocaine can significantly increase blood pressure, which adds to the effect of exercise. They also make it harder for the body to cool, increasing the chance of heat exhaustion. Clearly, the powerful centrally acting stimulants have properties that go beyond the normal physiological response to intense exercise.

How Sympathomimetics Work

As stated earlier, some sympathomimetics have agonist activity, and some have indirect mechanisms for increasing levels of endogenous catecholamines; the latter category includes drugs that block reuptake of neurotransmitters at the pre-synaptic membrane, drugs that displace neurotransmitters from their storage sites, and drugs that inhibit metabolic inactivation of the neurotransmitters. The major catecholamine neurotransmitters in the CNS play many important roles in a wide variety of behaviors and pathological conditions.

The primary mechanism for termination of synaptic transmission by these neurotransmitters is reuptake, the process by which the neurotransmitter is taken back up and stored by the pre-synaptic cell (see Figure 8.2). Different protein transporters in the plasma membrane of the pre-synaptic and post-synaptic cells mediate reuptake. In the post-synaptic membrane, a poorly defined transporter takes up a small percentage of the neurotransmitters. The enzyme catechol-O-methyltransferase (COMT) inactivates the monoamine neurotransmitters in the post-synaptic cell. Transporters in the pre-synaptic membrane take up the vast majority of the synaptic neurotransmitters (see Figure 8.2). After reuptake, monoamine neurotransmitters are transported back into secretory vesicles or metabolized in mitochondria by the enzyme **monoamine oxidase (MAO)**.

There are distinct transporters for dopamine (DA), serotonin (SER), and norepinephrine (NE): DAT, SERT, and NET. These transporters vary in their selectivity toward the monoamine neurotransmitters, and they also differ in their interaction

Figure 8.2 Overview of monoamine neurotransmitter flow.

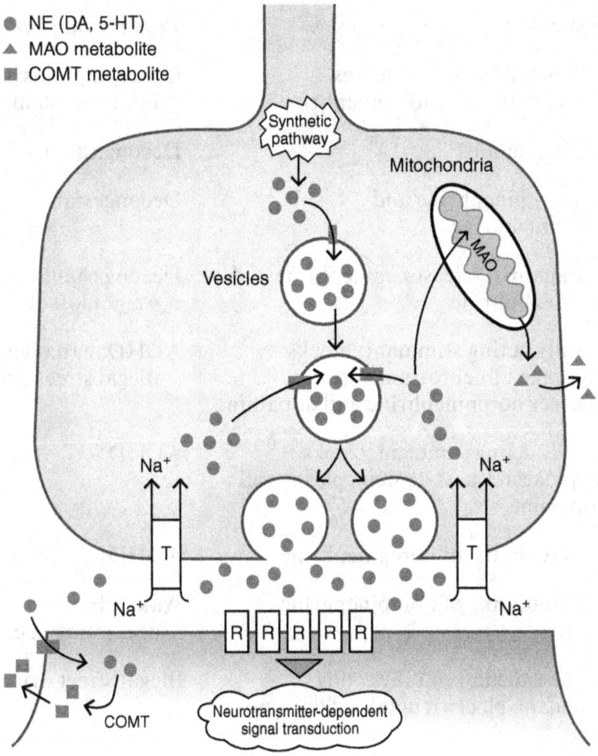

- NE (DA, 5-HT)
- MAO metabolite
- COMT metabolite

Legend: A generic synapse is shown, with some common features for norepinephrine (NE), dopamine(DA), and serotonin (5-HT). In dopamine terminals, dopamine is produced and transported into the secretory vesicles. In norepinephrine-containing terminals, the enzymatic conversion of dopamine to norepinephrine occurs in the vesicle. When the action potential reaches the synapse, some vesicles fuse with the membrane and release their contents into the cleft, and the transmitters diffuse across to stimulate receptors (R) on the post-synaptic cell. The primary termination of the signal occurs by reuptake by the transporter (T). The Na^+ gradient is used to take up the transmitters actively, though the ratio of Na^+ and Cl^- varies with the class of transporter. Once back in the cytoplasm, the transmitter can be taken up into the vesicles or metabolized in mitochondria by monoamine oxidase. A small fraction (about 20%) is taken up by the post-synaptic cell and metabolized by catechol-O-methyltransferase (COMT) in the cytoplasm.

with drugs that block their function (Zhou 2004). Sympathomimetics, such as amphetamine, are effective inhibitors of NET and DAT. Drugs that block DAT and SERT, as well as NET, will be discussed further in the next chapter, as these drugs are used to treat depression and other types of mental illness. Table 8.1 lists the sympathomimetics discussed in this chapter and summarizes their primary actions and indications.

Ephedrine and Related Drugs

Ephedra is a naturally occurring plant alkaloid. The Chinese have used ephedra-containing plant extracts for 2,000 years, primarily as part of herbal therapy for alleviating cold symptoms. Western cultures have used the herbal remedy for about 80 years. The active ingredient is **ephedrine**, a prescription drug, which is often present in commercially available herbal remedies. Taken orally, ephedrine has high bioavailability and long duration. It has a weak CNS stimulatory effect. Ephedrine releases norepinephrine

Table 8.1 Basic information about drugs discussed in this chapter

Drug Name	Primary Action	Primary Indication
Ephedrine	Weak mixed agonist; releases epinephrine and norepinephrine	Cold symptoms; mild stimulant
Phenylephrine	Weak α-1 agonist	Decongestant
Pseudoephedrine	Releases epinephrine and norepinephrine	Decongestant
Phenylpropanolamine	Weak agonist; releases epinephrine and norepinephrine	Decongestant; weight loss
Amphetamine, methamphetamine (Adderall)	Centrally acting stimulant; blocks reuptake of neurotransmitters; releases norepinephrine and dopamine	ADHD; narcolepsy; illegal street drug
Methylphenidate (Ritalin)	Centrally acting stimulant; blocks reuptake; releases norepinephrine and dopamine	ADHD
Atomoxetine	Blocks reuptake of norepinephrine	ADHD
Modafinil	Blocks reuptake of norepinephrine	Wakefulness-promoting agent
Cocaine	Local anesthetic; centrally acting stimulant; blocks reuptake of dopamine	Illegal street drug

from storage sites in sympathetic neurons. It also has weak, non-selective agonist activity for α- and β-receptors. Ephedrine can cause adverse effects, including increased blood pressure, arrhythmias, psychosis, seizure, and death. Pseudoephedrine, one of several compounds related to ephedrine, is less potent, requiring about three times the dose to be equipotent (depending on the response being measured). Other common drugs related to ephedra include phenylephrine and phenylpropanolamine.

Common OTC decongestants, such as Sudafed, contain pseudoephedrine. Pseudoephedrine has limited or very weak agonist activity. It probably works more by displacing norepinephrine from pre-synaptic terminals, resulting in a contraction of vascular smooth muscle in the nasal passages. Vasoconstriction decreases blood flow in nasal passages, thereby decreasing inflammation, swelling, and mucus production. Newer formulations replace pseudoephedrine with phenylephrine. The primary reason for the change is that pseudoephedrine can be converted into methamphetamine illegally, and new laws require that products with pseudoephedrine be sold in limited amounts and require an identification check. Note the similarity between pseudoephedrine and methamphetamine (refer back to Figure 8.1). Unlike pseudoephedrine, phenylephrine cannot be easily converted to methamphetamine. It is rapidly metabolized, however, reducing its bioavailability and making it less effective than pseudoephedrine. The action of phenylephrine is largely due to α-1 agonist activity in the periphery. Recall that α-1 agonist activity causes vasoconstriction by its action on smooth muscle cells. The vasoconstriction can increase blood pressure.

In hospitals, ephedrine-related sympathomimetics are given intravenously to increase blood pressure and heart rate, but they also work orally. Phenylephrine and pseudoephedrine can be taken for decongestion orally or as a nasal spray. Repeated use of these drugs in nasal sprays causes a loss of effectiveness and possible rebound congestion. A related drug called oxymetazoline, a sympathomimetic that is chemically unrelated to ephedrine, is more common in nasal sprays, as it seems to be tolerated better. These sympathomimetics are mydriatic (they cause dilation of the pupil) and are formulated in eye drops. Additional adrenergic agonists (e.g., Propine) are also used in eye drops to treat glaucoma, where they reduce pressure in the eyes by decreasing the amount of fluid in the aqueous humor. Phenylpropanolamine was used in decongestants and to suppress appetite in over the counter products such as Acutrim/Dexatrim. However, phenylpropanolamine can cause strokes and was taken off the shelf in the United States in 2005. Phenylpropanolamine can also be used as a precursor for methamphetamine synthesis, so it is subject to the laws that combat the methamphetamine epidemic.

Sympathomimetics with a Strong CNS Effect

This section discusses sympathomimetics with a strong CNS effect, including amphetamine, related drugs, and cocaine. Figure 8.3 presents a schematic for the drug action of amphetamine and cocaine.

Figure 8.3 Schematic for the action of amphetamine and cocaine.

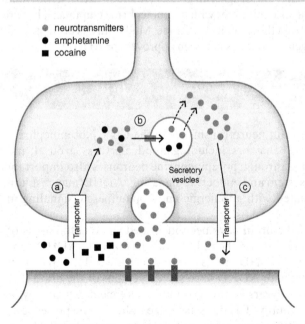

Legend: Cocaine (solid squares) is non-selective toward the three transporters (DAT, NET, and SERT). It acts as a competitive inhibitor, blocking reuptake of neurotransmitters (grey circles) from the synaptic cleft. Amphetamine (black circles) and related drugs are substrates for the transporter and use the transporter to enter the cytoplasm (a). They enter the secretory vesicles and disturb the vesicle's capacity to store transmitters (b). Transmitters leak back into the cytoplasm, causing an increase in their cytoplasmic concentration. If their concentration becomes sufficiently high, the membrane transporter will change directions and move transmitters into the synaptic cleft, significantly increasing transmitter activity and signaling post-synaptically (c) (Torres, Gainetdinov, & Caron 2003).

Amphetamine and Related Sympathomimetics

Amphetamine causes release of neurotransmitters from nerve terminals similar to that caused by ephedrine. Unlike ephedrine, amphetamine readily enters the CNS, causing a stimulant effect on mood and alertness. Amphetamine also interferes with reuptake of norepinephrine by the norepinephrine transporter (NET) in the pre-synaptic membrane. Amphetamine is a substrate for the NET and is transported into the cytoplasm of the pre-synaptic cell. From the cytoplasm, it can enter the storage granules and displace norepinephrine from the vesicle into the cytoplasm (see Box on Treatment of ADHD and Figure 8.3). Other aspects of the normal recycling of norepinephrine into secretory vesicles are perturbed when amphetamine is present. The result is elevated and prolonged levels of norepinephrine at the synapse, causing increased norepinephrine-dependent signaling. Amphetamines may similarly affect dopamine synapses, which could contribute to the elevated mood, wakefulness, appetite suppression, and pleasure responses many feel when taking these drugs. The dopamine-dependent effects can be confirmed with the use of dopamine antagonists. Dopamine antagonists can suppress some of amphetamine's effects, suggesting the involvement of both norepinephrine and dopamine pathways.

Methamphetamine has an even greater CNS effect than amphetamine, probably because it can more easily pass through the blood–brain barrier. Methylphenidate (Ritalin), prescribed for ADHD, is related to the amphetamine family. It also interferes with neurotransmitter reuptake and recycling and has similar abuse potential. Atomoxetine, a newer drug used for ADHD, lacks stimulant activity. It is more selective for norepinephrine reuptake and lacks the abuse potential of the drugs with greater stimulant activity. Modafinil is a chemically unrelated drug that also interferes with norepinephrine reuptake; it has properties and side effects different from those of amphetamine. Modafinil has been prescribed as a wakefulness-promoting agent, and it has not been approved for ADHD.

Sympathomimetics in the Treatment of ADHD

Norepinephrine is an important neurotransmitter in the CNS. Norepinephrine signaling is involved in many behaviors, including mood, alertness, arousal, and regulation of sleep. Signaling through norepinephrine neurons is also important in the autonomic nervous system and endocrine signaling. ADHD may result in part from problems associated with adrenergic and dopaminergic signaling in certain parts of the brain.

Three to four regions of the brain have been identified as potential areas of concern, based largely on brain scans of children with and without ADHD. One hypothesis is that the defect in ADHD brains results from slower development of these brain regions. Patients with ADHD have several regions of the brain that appear smaller and one to two years behind normal development, which may or may not catch up developmentally. The decreased size indicates the presence of fewer cells and a lower density of connections. The affected regions of the brain play a role in processing "inside information" (body functions) and integrating it with "outside information" (perceptions of the world outside). Children (and adults) without ADHD can filter the information and respond accordingly in socially acceptable ways, whereas those with ADHD have trouble filtering and responding appropriately. Much of the brain works in inhibitory mode, suppression of nerve activity is a major control mechanism (Nigg 2001). Patients with ADHD appear lacking in this mechanism: they can "go," but they are slow to "stop." They tend to act "without thinking" or can lack the ability to "say no"—a major component of behavior that most of us learn and identify as self-control.

The regions of the brain that are involved in these functions have significant amounts of norepinephrine and dopamine signaling. Therefore, these underdeveloped regions with less dense connections may respond to stimulant drugs that increase norepinephrine and dopamine transmitter levels in ways that compensate for the missing signaling. The prediction from this model is that in people without ADHD, these drugs act as stimulants, increasing activity in these regions of the brain; in ADHD patients, the drugs increase neurotransmitter activity to help compensate for incomplete circuits and feedback loops.

As stated earlier, the stimulants related to amphetamine used for symptom management of ADHD include methylphenidate (Ritalin) and dextro-amphetamine/amphetamine mixed salts (Adderall). Dextro refers to the D-form of methamphetamine, which is more potent than the L-form, though many preparations are roughly a 50/50 mix. D- and L-forms are isomers, meaning they have the same molecular formula but differ in their stereochemistry (they are mirror images, resulting from the way certain bonds are pointed relative to a common feature). Many biological systems respond differently to D- and L-stereoisomers, presumably because binding to specific sites on proteins is stereospecific. For example, proteins are made only from L-amino acids, and metabolism uses D-glucose.

Ritalin and Adderall work in part by inhibiting NET and DAT, thereby increasing the relative levels of norepinephrine and dopamine at synapses. These drugs are effective in a large percentage of ADHD cases, but they have the potential for misuse and are tightly regulated. As stated earlier, newer drugs have been developed that are more selective and primarily inhibit NET, and these drugs lack some of the stimulant properties associated with abuse. Since they have less effect on dopamine, they have less effect on the pleasure centers of the brain, making them less likely to be addictive. The first non-stimulant drug approved for use in adults with ADHD was atomoxetine (Strattera). It was effective in several large clinical trials, with modest side effects and little abuse potential (Garnock-Jones & Keating 2009). The mechanism of how reuptake inhibitors help manage ADHD is still largely unknown, but their effectiveness in inhibiting NET activity implies a critical role for norepinephrine signaling in normal function in certain regions of the brain (Zhou).

Cocaine

Cocaine use dates back to ancient cultures, in which leaves of the coca plant were chewed to obtain their stimulant properties. The Spanish realized the power in coca leaves when they conquered the indigenous populations of South American countries such as Peru. The indigenous people used extracts of coca for many medicinal purposes, such as pain reduction. The early versions of Coca-Cola used coca extracts until the early 1900s.

The use of cocaine as a local anesthetic for a wide variety of applications has been supplanted by the many synthetic derivatives that have been developed which work better; examples include dental (novocaine) and dermal (lidocaine) applications. The local anesthetic action is probably due to cocaine's ability to bind and block Na^+ channels and suppress action potential transmission in neurons. Cocaine readily enters the CNS, where it acts as a non-selective, competitive inhibitor for the monoamine transporters (Torres et al.). When it binds DAT, it blocks the reuptake of dopamine, causing accumulation at the synapse and an increase in dopaminergic signaling (see Figure 8.3). Since it blocks dopamine reuptake in areas of the brain involved in pleasure and can be smoked, snorted, or injected, it is widely abused. Cocaine's effects are more rapid and intense than those of methamphetamine, and it has a relatively short (38 minute) half-life. Because of the short half-life, coupled with the tolerance that occurs with the "rush" feelings, abusers tend to increase their doses and take them more frequently. Cocaine use has grown steadily worldwide, particularly in more affluent populations. However, its use may have peaked among athletes in the early 1990s. Improved testing and the potential life-threatening effects on the cardiovascular system are some of the reasons for the decline in use among competitive athletes who are subjected to regular drug testing.

Exercise Pharmacology

Pharmacokinetic Concerns

During exercise, the blood level of epinephrine increases markedly, as do levels of dopamine, norepinephrine, and serotonin. The sympathetic response includes shifting metabolism to mobilize energy reserves, activating sweat glands, and stimulating K^+ reuptake by skeletal muscle. Sympathomimetics that are largely restricted to the periphery would be expected to have similar systemic effects on metabolism and K^+ retention, albeit to a lesser extent, due to their lower potency compared to endogenous epinephrine/norepinephrine. At higher exercise intensity, the elevated levels of epinephrine may overcome the contribution of systemic sympathomimetics. Under most conditions, the blood–brain barrier excludes systemic catecholamines from entering the CNS. However, under conditions of high stress or intense exercise, the blood levels of catecholamines can become high enough that some will cross the barrier and exert an effect centrally.

Ephedrine-Related Drugs

The pharmacokinetics of ephedra-related compounds have been studied because of their ergogenic potential. Urine concentration of pseudoephedrine peaks about four hours after the final dose (Chester, Mottram, Reilly, & Powell 2004). Most (about 70%) of the ephedra-related compounds are secreted unchanged by the kidneys (Chester et al.). Pseudoephedrine was detectable in urine 24 hours after final dose. The longer half-life for pseudoephedrine compared to phenylephrine probably results from the lack of an (–OH) group on the ring (see Figure 8.1), so it is not a substrate for one of the enzymes that inactivates the endogenous transmitters (COMT: catechol-O-methyltransferase).

Amphetamines

Amphetamines are readily absorbed from the small intestine and reach maximum levels in the blood in one to two hours. Metabolism of amphetamines varies greatly with different animal species, so animal studies have limited value. For testing purposes in humans, the parent compound is quantified in urine samples; amphetamine can be detected up to 48 hours after ingestion. Tolerance develops in individuals who abuse amphetamines, particularly for those responses related to the high or "feel good" feelings. Therefore, addicts become more prone to the adverse effects; as they increase their doses to get the desired effect, the negative effects on the cardiovascular and respiratory systems can become more pronounced. Amphetamines cause vasoconstriction and an increase in peripheral resistance, giving rise to an increase in blood pressure. The prolonged vasoconstriction also adds to the difficulty in maintaining body temperature, especially while the individual is physically active. Heat diffusion from the skin is diminished. The inability to cool down and possible dehydration can contribute to heat exhaustion. Another side effect of amphetamine use during exercise is reduced sensitivity to pain. Athletes taking amphetamines can sustain more damage when continuing to compete after an injury due to the increased pain tolerance.

Cocaine

Although athletes who use cocaine may perceive improved performance during sports, there is little evidence of actual improvement. To the contrary, perceptual misjudgments increase. The adverse effects of cocaine use, with or without physical activity, can be life-threatening. Similar to amphetamine, cardiovascular problems and the possibility for heat exhaustion are significant. The drug-induced vasoconstriction limits blood flow to the skin, decreasing the dissipation of heat. Cocaine misuse is also associated with cerebrovascular events, such as strokes and seizures. When it is mixed with alcohol, cocaine can cause cardiac arrest, seizures, and respiratory failure. Cocaine is mostly metabolized in the liver, and metabolites are detected in the urine within four hours. Most of the metabolites are below levels of detection after 24 hours, though clearance rates depend on the individual and how the drug is consumed. Certain metabolites can be detected in regular users several days later, when more sensitive techniques are used. Because the drug has a very short half-life, low- to mid-level intensity exercise effects on metabolism and clearance by the kidneys may not be pronounced. High-intensity exercise while on cocaine can cause serious health risks, in addition to possible effects on metabolism and clearance (Avois, Robinson, Saudan, et al. 2006).

Pharmacodynamic Concerns

Ephedrine and Related Drugs

Ephedra (the herbal supplement) and ephedrine (the active component) have been studied for weight loss and athletic performance (Chen, Muhamad, & Ooi 2012). As we will discuss in a later chapter on supplements, the distinction between therapeutic drugs and supplements can become blurred from a patient's or athlete's point of view, though the laws governing their use and distribution require that they be handled differently. A large-scale meta-analysis of 52 controlled trials suggested that moderate short-term weight loss was possible with ephedrine but that long-term weight loss or improved athletic performance was not (Shekelle, Hardy, Morton, et al. 2003). Moreover, the safety issues raised in many studies (i.e., cardiovascular health, psychiatric symptoms, seizures, and death) far outweigh any possible gains in performance.

The oral dose of 24 mg ephedrine did not give beneficial effects on strength, endurance, power, reaction time, hand–eye coordination, speed, or RPE during maximal or sub-maximal exercise. Ephedrine did improve performance on the Wingate test, but the effect was not significantly different from placebo in other tests. When ephedrine is combined with caffeine, the combination often produced improved performance compared to either drug alone (Shekelle et al.; Chen et al., 2012). A critical factor when evaluating the effects of sympathomimetics is the intensity of the exercise. The endogenous catecholamine activity increases with intensity level and may negate a contribution attributable to the drug.

As stated earlier, the drugs related to ephedrine are contained in common OTC preparations used for cold symptoms, nasal sprays, and eye drops. Are these preparations ergogenic, and does their use give a competitive advantage? Limited studies show that oral doses of pseudoephedrine or phenylpropanolamine have little effect on strength, energy metabolism, or oxygen consumption (Gillies, Derman, Noakes, et al. 1996; Swain, Harsha, Baenziger, & Saywell 1997). The few that show some performance gain are at higher than recommended doses and at optimal times following ingestion (Hodges, Hancock, Currell, et al. 2006). A slight increase in heart rate may be observed with phenylephrine and pseudoephedrine, but there is usually no difference from placebo during exercise. Metabolic effects of pseudoephedrine are also not pronounced (Hodges et al.). Phenylpropanolamine can increase blood pressure, and the increase can be additive to the handgrip exercise. Cases of hemorrhagic stroke have been reported following its use. In 2000, the FDA issued an advisory against use of this drug and subsequently removed it from OTC sale in 2005. Phenylpropanolamine is still available OTC in Europe and in the United States as a drug used in veterinary practice. There is little evidence of the expected ergogenic effect by these ephedrine-related drugs. At higher than recommended doses, there are limited reports of gains in performance. The general conclusion may be that as exercise intensity increases, it is hard to distinguish the effect of the drug from the effects of exercise alone.

Ephedra and the News

In the early 2000s, several stories linked the death of athletes to the use of supplements containing ephedra. In many cases, the evidence was circumstantial, and it certainly cannot be given the same weight as placebo-controlled double-blind studies. However, the link between these tragedies and ephedra was made in the press. In the summer of 2001, an overweight and out-of-shape Korey Stringer, an offensive lineman for the Minnesota Vikings, died from apparent heat stroke. He had been fasting to lose weight and had a supplement called Ripped Fuel in his locker. This supplement contained ephedra and caffeine. Although it was reported that ephedra was not detected upon autopsy, it is not clear that it was actually tested. Stringer had been ill and vomiting the night before the practice that led to his overheating and death.

A second case occurred in February of 2003, when a pitcher for the Baltimore Orioles died from apparent heat exhaustion early in training camp in Florida. Steve Belcher was 23, out of shape, and at least 10 pounds over his playing weight from the previous year. He died the day after his body temperature reached 108 degrees. He was known to have high blood pressure and some abnormal liver activity. To lose weight, he had been on a liquid diet and was taking an ephedra-containing supplement called Xenadrine RFA-1. The coroner's report suggested that ephedrine could have been a factor in his death. A third incident involved Rashidi Wheeler, a football player at Northwestern University, who collapsed at practice in the summer in 2003. At first, his cause of death was reported as bronchial asthma, but subsequent reports showed he had ephedrine in his system and the supplement Ultimate Orange in his locker. Subsequent lawsuits have alleged he died of ventricular arrhythmia and that the supplement, which contains ephedra, was involved.

Although these high-profile cases have led most leagues and competition governing bodies to ban ephedra and educate against using supplements containing it, there is limited published research with controlled, double-blind studies on the toxic effects of ephedra (Shekelle et al.; Chen et al. 2012). Of course, for any substance that is toxic or potentially fatal, experiments in humans are not possible. Enough circumstantial evidence existed, however, to cause many sports governing bodies to take action. Major League Baseball distributed information on ephedra that listed known side effects including increased blood pressure, rapid heart rate, seizures, heart attacks, and death. The FDA banned ephedra in 2004, and it was removed from many OTC supplements. Internet sale of herbal extracts claiming to contain ephedra for weight loss still exists, but these products are not regulated and the contents are not guaranteed (see Chapter 13).

Amphetamines and Related Drugs

The centrally acting stimulants, such as amphetamine, reduce fatigue and enhance performance. Amphetamines increase time to exhaustion during treadmill running, cycling, and distance running. As expected, amphetamines increase heart rate and blood pressure, redistribute blood to muscle, and mobilize energy substrates (Avois et al.). The increase in time to exhaustion is related to amphetamine's ability to decrease fatigue. Fatigue can result from limitations imposed by metabolic changes occurring in exercising skeletal muscle, giving rise to "peripheral fatigue" (Swart, Lamberts, Lambert, et al. 2009). As exercise time increases, changes occur in muscle cells (energy supplies, oxygen, K^+, pH, lactate, etc.) that conflict with homeostasis (the body's desire to return to "normal" or "at rest"). Fatigue and exercise performance can also be centrally controlled, with the duration of a bout of exercise determined early, in an anticipatory way ("pacing yourself"), which suggests that the body is maintaining some reserve capacity. In a placebo-controlled crossover study, elite cyclists worked at a prescribed RPE (Swart et al.). Subjects receiving methylphenidate cycled 32% longer and, at the point where the placebo trial terminated, had higher power output (see Table 8.2). They also had greater oxygen consumption, heart rate, ventilatory volume, and blood lactate. These results suggest that we exercise with a centrally controlled reserve and that amphetamine-like drugs allow access to this reserve, thereby delaying fatigue (Swart et al.).

Table 8.2 Effect of methylphenidate on eight elite cyclists

Physiological Variable	Placebo	Methylphenidate
Power (W)	210.6 (30.6)	251.0 (33.1)*
Heart rate (bpm)	148.0 (10.3)	165.3 (10.7)*
VO$_2$ (ml/min)	3,428.3 (500.3)	3,864.8 (610.4)*
Ventilatory volume (l/min)	83.3 (22.4)	92.9 (22.8)*
Lactate (arterial; mmol/l)	1.2 (0.7)	1.7 (1.0)*

Legend: Values are means (SD). The physiological variables were measured at the point of fatigue, which was after 68 (18) minutes during the placebo trial and at the equivalent time for the methylphenidate group. *$p < 0.05$ for differences between trials.

ADHD presents an interesting case for drug and exercise interaction. Children with ADHD may exhibit high levels of restlessness and increased motor activity; they often lack the development of their age-matched peers. ADHD negatively impacts performance in school, family life, and social relationships. Many patients with ADHD respond paradoxically to CNS stimulants compared to individuals without ADHD. They can become calmer and better able to manage their attention span when taking methylphenidate or amphetamine. Sports require a level of focus that causes individuals with ADHD to struggle. Studies with basketball and soccer players with ADHD have shown improved ability to remain in proper position during games and to be more receptive to coaching when on medication. However, some players report loss of spontaneity while taking these powerful drugs (Conant-Norville & Tofler, 2005). The use of drugs on the WADA Prohibited List creates obvious problems in terms of enhanced performance. Atomoxetine (Strattera) is a non-CNS stimulant approved for ADHD. It is a specific norepinephrine uptake inhibitor and has proven effective in ADHD (Garnock-Jones & Keating). It may take several weeks for the individual to benefit fully and adjust to initial side effects. It is not a controlled substance, nor is it on the WADA list.

There is emerging support for the notion that regular exercise and participation in sports can improve some symptoms of ADHD (Berwid & Halperin 2012). Such activities may help children with ADHD improve their neural development and cognitive function. In a six-week study by Kang, Choi, Kang, and Han (2011), 13 children with ADHD participated in a 90-minute athletic activity twice a week, while 15 children with ADHD received education on behavior control (see Figure 8.4). A positive correlation was found between athletic activity and improvement in attention symptoms, cognitive symptoms, and social skills (Kang et al.).

Exercise increases noradrenergic and dopaminergic signaling in regions of the brain that have some overlap with the regions affected by ADHD. The centrally acting stimulants and intense exercise probably share overlapping yet distinct mechanisms (Lenz 2012). Aerobic exercise increased the effectiveness of methylphenidate on clinical symptoms of adolescents with ADHD (Choi, Han, Kang, et al. 2014). Aerobic exercise is beneficial for various executive functions, response time, attention, and behavior (Den Heijer, Groen, Tucha, et al. 2017). Functional MRI was used to examine the underlying neural mechanisms following a single

Figure 8.4 Changes in attention symptoms between the physically active group (sports-cADHD) and inactive group (edu-cADHD).

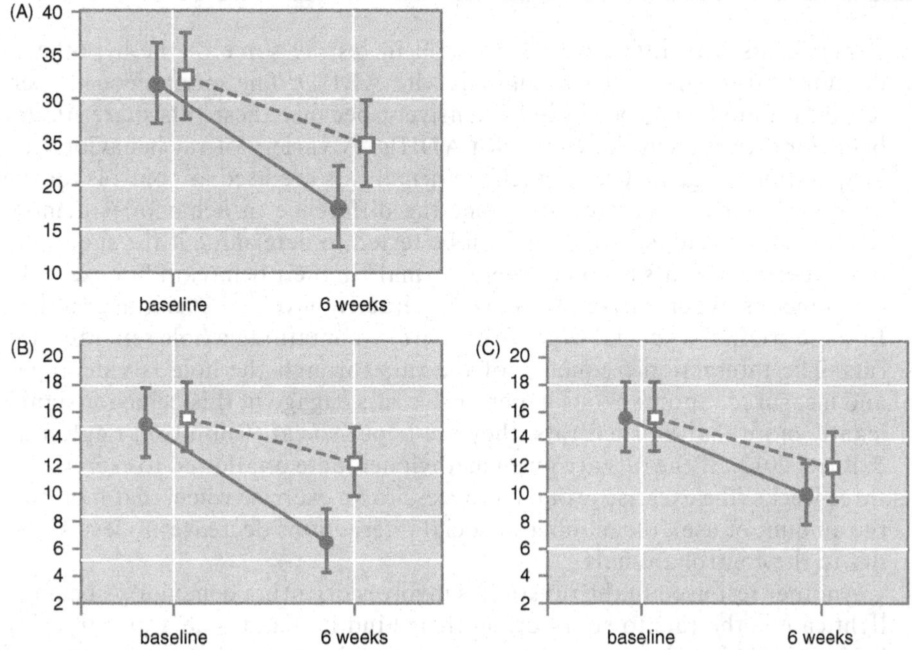

Legend: In a six-week trial, 13 children with ADHD participated in a 90-minute athletic activity (sports-cADHD—filled circle) twice a week, while 15 children with ADHD received education on behavior control (edu-cADHD—square). (a) Total score for K-ARS-PT (ADHD Rating Scale—parent and teacher version), significant difference, $p = 0.04$. (b) Sub-scale score for K-ARS-PT-inattention, significant difference, $p < 0.01$. (c) Sub-scale score for K-ARS-PT-hyperactivity, not significant, $p = 0.17$. See Kang, Choi, Kang, and Han (2011) for additional details.

bout of aerobic exercise in adult patients with ADHD ($n = 23$) (Mehren, Özyurt, Lam, et al. 2019). This study measured attention and executive function compared to age-matched healthy controls ($n = 23$). Continuous stationary cycling (moderate intensity for 30 minutes) significantly improved reaction times in the patients with ADHD but not in healthy controls. ADHD patients with a higher degree of cardiorespiratory fitness showed measurable brain changes with exercise using functional MRI (Mehren et al.).

Exercise produces physical, mental, and emotional benefits without problematic side effects. Timing and dosing strategies that include both drugs and exercise will require optimization, but there is significant support for exercise being an adjunct therapy in controlling ADHD (Lenz; Berwid & Halperin; Mehren et al.). Since different ADHD subtypes have been identified, symptoms of ADHD change with age, and patients vary in their responsiveness to the available drugs, there is a need for alternate or adjunctive therapies. Moreover, the effectiveness of drug therapy in ADHD patients may decrease over time, and the long-term health effects of these powerful and possibly addictive drugs are always a concern. Regular exercise and participation in sports provide potentially helpful alternative therapies.

A Rat Model for Studying ADHD and Exercise

Experiments with rats have been useful in testing some of the hypotheses developed through studies of humans with ADHD. The spontaneous hypertensive rat model has been used extensively, because these rats share similar behavioral traits with humans with ADHD. A variety of rat behaviors can be quantified. Age and sex–matched normal rats are used as controls for the spontaneous hypertensive rats. Once the difference in behavior is demonstrated, then various treatments can be tested to determine if the spontaneous hypertensive rats become "more normal" in their behavior. For example, spontaneous hypertensive rats show hyperactive levels of social interaction. In these studies, a special cage with a barrier containing a hole separates the rats. The interaction frequency of the rats through the hole is videotaped and measured. Spontaneous hypertensive rats engage in this behavior significantly more than normal rats: they are hyper-social (Robinson, Eggleston, & Bucci 2012). If the rats are given methylphenidate or allowed to exercise for three weeks (the exercise group has access to an exercise wheel that monitors the amount of use), the number of social interactions decreases to levels similar to the control animals.

Another test used in the rat studies involves orienting behavior. A beam of light causes the rats to stand up on their hind legs and take notice (rearing behavior). This behavior is not reinforced with a reward. Normal rats will get tired of this trick over time—they habituate to the response—so that they respond less often. Spontaneous hypertensive rats are not able to ignore irrelevant stimuli, so they continue to respond. The exercise group and the drug-treated spontaneous hypertensive rats showed habituation to a level that approached that of normal rats. The authors concluded that exercise was as effective as methylphenidate or atomoxetine in these two behavioral tests (Robinson et al.).

In another study with spontaneous hypertensive rats, the brain levels of dopamine and brain-derived neurotrophic factor were analyzed (Kim, Heo, Kim, et al. 2011). Brain-derived neurotrophic factor is a peptide growth factor involved in healthy brain activity; it will be discussed in greater detail in Chapter 9. Adult male rats were tested for hyperactivity in an "open field test," and spatial learning was tested with an eight-arm maze. Spontaneous hypertensive rats were hyperactive in the field test and made more errors in the maze. However, methylphenidate or exercise for a month caused the spontaneous hypertensive rats to behave more like normal rats (see Figure 8.5). The brains of the rats from the different experimental groups were analyzed for dopamine activity in the striatum and brain-derived neurotrophic factor levels in the hippocampus. Exercise increased levels of dopamine activity and brain-derived neurotrophic factor to levels similar to methylphenidate treatment. These experiments in a rat model for ADHD, in addition to many other studies, strengthen the case for exercise being an effective adjunct therapy for patients with ADHD.

Figure 8.5 Effect of exercise in a rat model for ADHD.

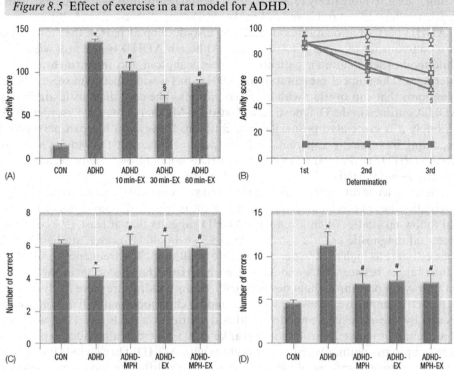

Legend: Groups of 15 rats were randomly assigned to four groups: control, Spontaneous Hypertensive Rats (SHR, ADHD) untreated, SHR (ADHD) with methylphenidate, and SHR (ADHD) with exercise. (A) Treadmill exercise for different lengths of time (10, 30, or 60 minutes) per day for 10 days. $*p < 0.05$ compared to the control group. $\#p < 0.05$ compared to the ADHD group. $\S p < 0.05$ compared to the ADHD 10 min-EX group. (B) Activity in the open field test. Filled square = control group; open circle = ADHD group; filled triangle = ADHD and methylphenidate-treated group; open square = ADHD and 30-minute treadmill exercise group. $*p < 0.05$ compared to the control group. $\#p < 0.05$ compared to the first determination in each group. $\S p < 0.05$ compared to the second determination in each group. (C) Number of correct trials. $*p < 0.05$ compared to the control group. $\#p < 0.05$ compared to the ADHD group. (D) Number of errors in the radial eight-arm maze test. An additional group combining drug and exercise is included. $*p < 0.05$ compared to the control group. $\#p < 0.05$ compared to the ADHD group.

Elder Concerns

ADHD typically starts during childhood or early adolescence and is defined by age-inappropriate levels of inattention and impulsivity interfering with normal functioning. ADHD was initially described in boys, but it was recognized that many girls had been undiagnosed. Typically, in child and adolescent clinics, around 80% of ADHD cases are male, whereas in adult clinics, the proportion of males is closer to 50%. This finding may be due to a couple of reasons. Boys present in clinics with disruptive behaviors and learning problems. Girls display predominantly inattentive symptoms and less overt disruptive behaviors, and may be underrepresented in clinics. The level of hyperactivity in boys declines to the level of the girls with age, suggesting that the expression of core ADHD symptoms is more similar across the sexes in the adult population.

Women are also more likely to seek help for mental health problems than men, increasing their referral rates (reviewed in Franke, Michelini, Asherson, et al. 2018).

ADHD persists into adulthood, and may also develop as part of the aging process or a consequence of damage to the brain. Although ADHD is generally viewed as a childhood-onset condition, patients can meet symptom and impairment criteria at later ages. The clinical presentation of ADHD has a wide spectrum of severity and symptoms that can overlap with other conditions. The core diagnostic attributes of ADHD, outlined in the Diagnostic and Statistical Manual of Mental Disorders (DSM-5), imply it is associated primarily with children. However, a lifespan perspective is becoming increasingly apparent, with the acknowledgement that adults also suffer from ADHD (Franke et al.). For some, ADHD is not outgrown following adolescence and the disorder persists.

The prevalence rate, gender differences, and subtype shifts among the adult ADHD population have been studied (Zalsman & Shilton 2016). Meta-analysis of longitudinal follow-up studies of children with ADHD suggests that at least 15% continue to meet full diagnostic criteria for ADHD at 25 years old. However, studies from Europe estimate as high as 80% persistence into adulthood. The frequency for ADHD in adults ranges between 1.4% and 3.6%. Characteristic changes occur in the profile of ADHD symptoms throughout development. Young children are more likely to display hyperactive-impulsive behavior, while in middle childhood inattentive symptoms increase. By late adolescence and in adulthood, inattention tends to persist, while there is a decline in motor hyperactivity (Franke et al.). There is a broader expression of core symptoms commonly reported by adults with ADHD. They include internal restlessness, ceaseless unfocused mental activity, and a difficulty focusing on conversations. Regulating emotional responses, controlling impulses, maintaining attention, initiating tasks, and problem-solving are problems with self-regulation and executive functions. These symptoms result from deficits across multiple neural networks and cognitive processes and can cause sleep problems, low self-esteem, and subthreshold anxiety and depression (Franke et al.).

Diagnosable ADHD syndrome can arise in adulthood following brain injury. Whether ADHD arises in adulthood without a known cause is controversial and if it occurs, adult-onset ADHD is probably rare. Apparent cases of adult-onset ADHD are mostly due to the existence of undiagnosed or subthreshold childhood ADHD. In subthreshold cases, the onset of symptoms could occur many years later, particularly among those with supportive social environments or high levels of internal strength and intelligence when they were younger (Franke et al.).

Adults with ADHD have similar responses to drugs (methylphenidate, dexamphetamine, and atomoxetine) and psychosocial interventions, to those seen in children and adolescents (Asherson, Buitelaar, Faraone, & Rohde 2016). Despite progress in awareness and diagnosis in adults, treatment of adult ADHD in Europe and many other regions of the world is not yet common practice, and diagnostic services are limited. ADHD is often comorbid with other psychiatric conditions in adults. Multiple Swedish national registers generated 5,551,807 adults aged 18 to 64 years that were assessed for clinical diagnoses of adult ADHD, substance use disorder, depression, bipolar disorder, anxiety, type 2 diabetes mellitus, and hypertension (Chen, Hartman, Haavik, et al. 2018). All comorbid conditions were more prevalent in adults with ADHD (3.9% to 44.7%) than in those without (0.7% to 4.9%), and remained associated in older adults aged 50 to 64. The comorbidity patterns of adult ADHD underscore the severity and clinical complexity of the disorder (Chen et al. 2018).

People living in detention have a much higher incidence of ADHD. A meta-analysis of people living in detention pooled 102 original studies that included 69,997 participants (Baggio, Fructuoso, Guimaraes, et al. 2018). The results are striking; 26.2% of those incarcerated have ADHD—about a 5-fold increase over the general population. The authors call attention to this critical public health issue and suggest that individuals entering detention get screened for ADHD and receive treatment during and after detention. The goal, in addition to improving the health and well-being of people living in detention, is to reduce recidivism and reincarceration, and possibly reduce violence in detention settings (Baggio et al.).

Health Risks

At recommended doses of sympathomimetics for decongestant use, a mild and general adrenergic effect would be noted. During endurance training, endogenous epinephrine probably supersedes the drug effect and its weak agonist activity. Blood pressure can rise to very high levels during weight lifting; use of high levels of these drugs is not recommended, since it could augment the rise in blood pressure. Phenylpropanolamine can cause hemorrhage in normal individuals, especially with a 100 mg dose. These drugs are not recommended for use by hypertensives or diabetics.

Centrally acting stimulants increase blood pressure and can cause left ventricular hypertrophy with prolonged use. Physical and psychological dependence (i.e., addiction) are possible with both amphetamine and cocaine. These drugs also cause issues with the body's cooling ability and can lead to heat exhaustion. Cocaine can significantly increase heart rate and blood pressure, producing a serious health risk (as evident from the deaths of basketball player Len Bias or football player Don Rogers and the many others who have died from cocaine abuse).

PES Watch

Because sympathomimetics have possible ergogenic effects, they have doping potential (Avois et al.). Stimulants like amphetamine and cocaine, usually obtained illegally, are on the WADA Prohibited List. The weaker, mostly systemic acting derivatives of ephedra were moved from the Prohibited List to the Monitored List around 2004. For many years, drugs such as pseudoephedrine have been sold over the counter as decongestants and for weight loss. Their use as performance enhancers has been highly debated. They contributed to 60% of all positive drug tests by the IOC before 2004. In 2004, these drugs were removed from the WADA Prohibited List and placed on the Watch List. The IOC also moved them from their banned substance list to their monitoring program, which means the committee continues to test for them but does not disqualify athletes who test positive.

Are these compounds truly stimulants? Do they not have ergogenic properties? One report published after the changes in 2004 suggested improved times in a 1,500 meter run following pseudoephedrine use at three times the recommended dose (Hodges et al.). Pseudoephedrine was put back on the WADA Prohibited List in 2010, with a urinary threshold of 150 µg/ml. This threshold should allow for the therapeutic use of pseudoephedrine at 60 mg every four to six hours (240 mg per day max; Deventer, Van Eenoo, Baele, et al. 2009). The NCAA and NHL do not ban pseudoephedrine. Ephedrine and methylephedrine have urine thresholds of 10 µg/ml.

To summarize, these drugs are found in a variety of OTC preparations and herbal supplements and have few documented measurable ergogenic effects. Questions concerning an ergogenic effect persist, and pseudoephedrine was put back on the Prohibited List with a new threshold urine concentration to keep competitors from taking excess doses. Additionally, these drugs are often mixed with caffeine, which can obscure or perhaps enhance their effects. These drugs will probably remain a source of debate for years to come.

Most of the CNS stimulants are Schedule II Controlled Substances and require a prescription. They are on the WADA Prohibited List and banned by Olympic committees. The NCAA will offer a drug exemption to qualified individuals with diagnosed ADHD. Cessation of therapy for 24 hours before competition has been suggested to minimize the stimulant contribution during the competition but allow the individual with ADHD to train (and live) effectively.

Conclusion

Sympathomimetics are a diverse group of drugs that have adrenergic properties. The ephedrine derivatives are used to alleviate cold symptoms. The centrally acting stimulants are powerful drugs that have abuse potential. However, some of these drugs are useful in treating ADHD. Exercise affects areas of the brain that are also targets for these stimulants and is encouraged as a helpful supplement to drug therapy for ADHD.

Key Concepts Review

amphetamine
attention deficit and hyperactivity disor-
    der (ADHD)
ephedra
ephedrine

general activity
monoamine oxidase (MAO)
narcolepsy
specific activity
sympathomimetic

Review Questions

1   Why do stimulants (amphetamine and cocaine) and exercise have such a profound effect on blood pressure?
2   Joe is a power lifter. He doesn't want to do anything illegal, but he does take large doses of Sudafed before working out to get pumped up. Why might this be a bad idea?
3   Some people think exercise and physical fitness are important to one's mental state. What do they base this on?
4   ADHD is treated with CNS stimulants, which seems paradoxical. Can exercise play a role in treating children with ADHD?
5   What are the pharmacokinetic and pharmacodynamic effects of ephedrine and related drugs?
6   Rats would seem to be an unlikely experimental model for studying ADHD. How do researchers use spontaneously hypertensive rats to study ADHD?

References

Asherson P, Buitelaar J, Faraone SV, Rohde LA (2016) Adult attention-deficit hyperactivity disorder: key conceptual issues. *Lancet Psychiatry* 3:568–578

Avois L, Robinson N, Saudan C, Baume N, Mangin P, Saugy M (2006) Central nervous system stimulants and sport practice. *Br J Sports Med* 40(suppl 1):i16–i20

Baggio S, Fructuoso A, Guimaraes M, Fois E, Golay D, Heller P, Perroud N, Aubry C, Young S, Delessert D, Gétaz L, Tran NT, Wolff H (2018) Prevalence of attention deficit hyperactivity disorder in detention settings: a systematic review and meta-analysis. *Front Psychiatry* 9:331

Berwid OG, Halperin JM (2012) Emerging support for a role of exercise in attention-deficit/hyperactivity disorder intervention planning. *Curr Psychiatry Rep* 14:543–551

Chen CK, Muhamad AS, Ooi FK (2012) Herbs in exercise and sports. *J Physiol Anthropol* 41:4–10

Chen Q, Hartman CA, Haavik J, Harro J, Klungsøyr K, Hegvik TA, Wanders R, Ottosen C, Dalsgaard S Faraone SV, Larsson H (2018) Common psychiatric and metabolic comorbidity of adult attention-deficit/hyperactivity disorder: a population-based cross-sectional study. *PLoS One* 13:e0204516

Chester N, Mottram DR, Reilly T, Powell M (2004) Elimination of ephedrines in urine following multiple dosing: the consequences for athletes, in relation to doping control. *Brit J Clin Pharm* 57:62–67

Choi JW, Han DH, Kang KD, Jung HY, Renshaw PF (2014) Aerobic exercise and attention deficit hyperactivity disorder: brain research. *Med Sci Sports Exerc* 47:33–39 doi:10.1249/MSS.0000000000000373 [Epub ahead of print]

Conant-Norville DO, Tofler IR (2005) Attention deficit/hyperactivity disorder and psychopharmacologic treatments in the athlete. *Clin. Sports Med* 24:829–843

Den Heijer AE, Groen Y, Tucha L, Fuermaier AB, Koerts J, Lange KW, Thome J, Tucha O (2017) Sweat it out? The effects of physical exercise on cognition and behavior in children and adults with ADHD: a systematic literature review. *J Neural Transm (Vienna)* 124(Suppl 1):3–26

Deventer K, Van Eenoo P, Baele G, Pozo OJ, Van Thuyne W, Delbeke FT (2009) Interpretation of urinary concentrations of pseudoephedrine and its metabolite cathine in relation to doping control. *Drug Test Analysis* 1:209–213

Franke B, Michelini G, Asherson P, Banaschewski T, Bilbow A, Buitelaar JK, Cormand B, Faraone SV, Ginsberg Y, Haavik J, Kuntsi J, Larsson H, Lesch KP, Ramos-Quiroga JA, Réthelyi JM, Ribases M, Reif A (2018) Live fast, die young? A review on the developmental trajectories of ADHD across the lifespan. *Eur Neuropsychopharmacol* 28:1059–1088

Garnock-Jones KP, Keating GM (2009) Atomoxetine: a review of its use in attention-deficit hyperactivity disorder in children and adolescents. *Paediatr Drugs* 11:203–226

Gillies H, Derman WE, Noakes TD, Smith P, Evans A, Gabriels G (1996) Pseudoephedrine is without ergogenic effects during prolonged exercise. *J Appl Physiol* 81:2611–2617

Hodges K, Hancock S, Currell K, Hamilton B, Jeukendrup AE (2006) Pseudoephedrine enhances performance in 1500-m runners. *Med Sci Sports Exer* 38:329–333

Kang KD, Choi JW, Kang SG, Han DH (2011) Sports therapy for attention, cognitions and sociality. *Int J Sports Med* 32:953–959

Kim H, Heo H-I, Kim D-H, Ko I-G, Lee S-S, Kim S-E, Kim B-K, Kim T-W, Ji E-S, Kim J-D, Shin M-S, Choi Y-W, Kim C-J (2011) Treadmill exercise and methylphenidate ameliorate symptoms of attention deficit/hyperactivity disorder through enhancing dopamine synthesis and brain-derived neurotrophic factor expression in spontaneous hypertensive rats. *Neurosci Lett* 504:35–39

Lenz TL (2012) A pharmacological/physiological comparison between ADHD medications and exercise. *Am J Lifestyle Med* 6:306–308

Mehren A, Özyurt J, Lam AP, Brandes M, Müller HHO, Thiel CM, Philipsen A (2019) Acute effects of aerobic exercise on executive function and attention in adult patients with ADHD. *Front Psychiatry* 10:132

Nigg JT (2001) Is ADHD a disinhibitory disorder? *Psychol Bull* 127:571–598

Robinson AM, Eggleston RL, Bucci DJ (2012) Physical exercise and catecholamine reuptake inhibitors affect orienting behavior and social interaction in a rat model of attention-deficit/hyperactivity disorder. *Behav Neurosci* 126:762–771

Shekelle PG, Hardy ML, Morton SC, Maglione M, Mojica WA, Suttorp MJ, Rhodes SL, Jungvig L, Gagne J (2003) Efficacy and safety of ephedra and ephedrine for weight loss and athletic performance, a meta-analysis. *JAMA* 289:1537–1545

Swain RA, Harsha DM, Baenziger J, Saywell RM (1997) Do pseudoephedrine or phenylpropanolamine improve maximum oxygen uptake and time to exhaustion? *Clin J Sport Med* 7:168–17

Swart J, Lamberts RP, Lambert MI, Gibson ASC, Lambert EV, Skowno J, Noakes TD (2009) Exercising with reserve: evidence that the central nervous system regulates prolonged exercise performance. *Br J Sports Med* 43:782–788

Torres GE, Gainetdinov RR, Caron MG (2003) Plasma membrane monoamine transporters: structure, regulation and function. *Nature Rev Neuro* 4:13–25

Zalsman G, Shilton T (2016) Adult ADHD: A new disease? *Int J Psychiatry Clin Pract* 20:70–76

Zhou J (2004) Norepinephrine transporter inhibitors and their therapeutic potential. *Drugs Future* 29:1235–1244

Section III

Frequently Prescribed Medications

Abstract

Mental illness affects a significant portion of the population. Many of these people also suffer from poor cardiovascular health, and some experts feel these different types of illness are more related than they might appear. Many of the common types of mental illness respond to drug therapy. The drugs do not cure the disease, but they help the afflicted individuals cope and function better. Many of these drugs manipulate neurotransmitter levels in the brain. The neurotransmitters are important in how nerve cells communicate with each other. The ability of drugs to change neurotransmitter levels and alter brain function has led to a variety of theories concerning defective neurotransmitter signaling as a contributor to mental illness. Newer theories incorporate neurogenesis, where the production of nerve growth factors such as brain-derived neurotrophic factor (BDNF) can help produce new cells in certain regions of the adult mammalian brain. BDNF also contributes to the plasticity of the brain by increasing synaptic activity and the overall health of neurons. The lack of sufficient neurogenesis and plasticity may contribute to depression, bipolar disease, and age-related decrease in brain function.

Exercise is becoming an important intervention in mental health. Exercise can increase BDNF, neurogenesis, and neuronal plasticity, providing an overlapping model for how drugs and exercise contribute to mental health. Given these benefits combined with our increasing understanding of exercise's ability to combat stress and improve cardiovascular health, it is becoming clear how exercise contributes to a healthy lifestyle.

CASE EXAMPLE

Megan's brother Bo dealt with clinical depression through most of his school years. Bo had bad grades and generally did not "fit in." He was arrested for drugs in ninth grade, and matters seemed to come to a head when Bo spent a couple of nights in the hospital after a suicide attempt. Drug intervention and therapy had some effect, but Bo often fell back into his old behaviors. When Bo was a sophomore in high school, his guidance counselor and his father encouraged him to take part in a school-based program to alter behavior of at-risk adolescents. That was where he discovered running. It took two weeks of supervised, controlled activity with his cohort group, but Bo soon found that running several miles every day in conjunction with taking medication helped him manage his emotions better. He liked the way he felt after running. He also liked the solitary aspect of running. He had hated playing soccer and baseball, because he felt like a failure most of the time and he didn't fit in with the team. But running allowed him to just run. His grades improved, and he eventually was asked to join the cross country team his senior year. He declined, but deep down was pleased that he had been asked. Bo went on to earn his associate's degree at the local community college and is now employed in the hospitality industry. He continues to run every day and to take his medication.

Learning Objectives

1   Appreciate the scope of the problems and the issues associated with mental illness.
2   Learn how the major classes of psychotherapeutic agents work.
3   Appreciate the relationship between a healthy mind and a healthy body, and how exercise can be a powerful adjunct therapy.
4   Understand how exercise can help a person control weight gain associated with antipsychotic drug use.
5   Appreciate how exercise can help a person deal with anxiety.
6   Learn the role of neurogenesis and neuronal plasticity in mental health.
7   Examine the evidence supporting a role for exercise in maintaining good mental health during the aging process.

Introduction

The prevalence of mental illness is hard to estimate for many reasons, including issues with diagnosis, cultural differences in acknowledging mental illness, and lack of health-care coverage. It has been estimated that serious mental illness will affect about 5% of the population with nearly one in five suffering from any mental illness (National Institute of Mental Health, "Statistics"). Treatment with medication and psychotherapy is expensive for individuals suffering from serious mental illness, and the total estimated costs soar when we include those associated with anxiety disorders, mood disorders, and drug or alcohol dependence. If people who experience these disorders at least once in their lifetime are included, the percentage of individuals in the population approaches 40% (National Institute of Mental Health, "Statistics"). Though some have taken issue with the data on the prevalence of mental illness and these other disorders, we can be certain that the overall number of individuals affected is very large. Costs associated with treatment of mental illness are predicted to approach the costs associated with cardiovascular disease. However, many medications are limited in their effectiveness and cause unwanted secondary effects. Unfortunately, they do not cure mental illness; they are just the best drugs available to help manage the disease.

As an adjunct to medication, exercise is becoming an important intervention in mental health. The relationship between mind and body has been studied and expounded upon for ages. Psychosomatic research has shown how changes in mental state can affect the physical state (Vitetta, Anton, Cortizo, & Sali 2005). For example, competitors put on their "game face" and focus to "slow the game down." The physical state also affects the mental state. A healthy body is important for maintenance of a healthy mind, especially as we age. Exercisers are aware of the psychological changes that occur during physical activity and as a result of becoming fit. The fact that improved feelings of well-being and self-esteem follow exercise is well established. Regular exercise can improve clarity of thought, provide better sleep, and lower the risk of dementia later in life (Lövdén, Xu, & Wang 2013; Law, Barnett, Yau, & Gray 2014; Taspinar, Aslan, Agbuga, & Taspinar 2014). Because of its benefits, exercise is being considered as an adjunct therapy for mental illness (Stathopoulou, Powers, Berry, et al. 2006). Compared to the general population, individuals with mental illness are less physically fit, and some of the medications they take may exacerbate the problem (Galper, Trivedi, Barlow, et al. 2006).

This chapter examines the different classifications of psychotherapeutic drugs, including antipsychotics, anxiolytics, antidepressants, and mood stabilizers and how they work to treat different mental disorders: psychosis, anxiety, depression, and bipolar disorder. The chapter also examines whether exercise improves the condition of patients with the different mental disorders and whether exercise alters the action of psychotherapeutic drugs.

Mental Illness

The exact cause of most mental illnesses is not known, and it probably involves a combination of biological, psychological, and environmental factors. Mental illnesses result primarily from abnormal functioning of neuronal circuits or pathways in the brain. Defects or injuries in certain areas of the brain have been linked to some mental conditions. These defects can have a genetic or developmental component. Mental illnesses sometimes run in families, supporting a genetic component to the disease. Susceptibility is passed on to the next generation through inheritance of altered or defective genes. A genome-wide analysis identified specific variants underlying genetic effects shared among five disorders: autism spectrum disorder, attention deficit / hyperactivity disorder (see Chapter 8), schizophrenia, major depressive disorder, and bipolar disorder. Genomic sequence data for the five disorders were obtained from 33,332 cases and 27,888 controls of European ancestry. Four genetic loci were identified and two of them mapped to calcium-channel activity genes with possible effects on psychopathology. These results provide evidence that in the future, genetic analysis will be used for diagnosis of mental illness, replacing the descriptive syndromes in psychiatry (Cross-Disorder Group of the Psychiatric Genomics Consortium 2013). Genetics combined with imaging technology provide even greater possible advances in diagnosis and treatment of complex causes of mental illness (Moore, Sawyers, Adkins, & Docherty 2018).

Mental illness occurs from the interaction of genes and environmental factors (Schmidt 2007). A person who inherits a susceptibility gene for a mental illness does not necessarily develop the illness. How these genes interact with the environment is unique for every person, even identical twins. Environmental influences can occur at any time: in the individual's parents (to be passed along in sperm or eggs), during the individual's time in utero, early in life, or late in life. Environmental factors include drug abuse, trauma, stress, bacterial or viral infection, injury, lack of oxygen to the brain, poor nutrition, toxins, neglect, emotional stress (e.g., loss of a parent or spouse), and so forth. The combination of environmental factors and the expression of genetic variants that increase the susceptibility to mental illness can give rise to a wide variation in symptoms (National Alliance on Mental Illness). Since nerve cells communicate through neurotransmitters, modification of this signaling process by using drugs, psychotherapy, or other adjunct therapies (e.g., programs that increase physical activity) can improve brain function and quality of life, but it cannot cure the disease.

The DSM-V (*Diagnostic and Statistical Manual of Mental Disorders*, 5th ed., published by the American Psychiatric Association in 2013) details mental health disorders for children and adults. Health-care professionals use this manual to diagnose, understand, and treat patients with mental illness. The manual also provides possible causes and statistics on incidence related to age and gender.

Classes of Psychotherapeutic Agents

Psychotherapeutic (sometimes called psychotropic or psychoactive) drugs are those that exert their primary effect on the central nervous system. Classification of these drugs varies in different textbooks, in part because of the complexity of the illnesses they are used to treat. Some of the current classes of drugs were discovered because of their calming or "sedative" side effects when prescribed for other purposes. In the 1950s, tranquilizers of the *phenothiazine* class showed some effectiveness for schizophrenia and other psychotic symptoms and, thus, became known as the "major" tranquilizers. *Benzodiazepine* derivatives such as Librium and Valium effectively reduced anxiety, and these drugs became known as "minor" tranquilizers. Since the mechanisms of action of the major and minor tranquilizers are unrelated, new terminology supplanted the use of the term *tranquilizers*. The major tranquilizers are now called **antipsychotics** or *neuroleptics*, and the minor tranquilizers are called **anxiolytics** (sometimes still grouped with other sedative-hypnotics, such as the barbiturates). A third class of drugs includes **antidepressants**, used for the treatment of major depressive disorder. **Mood-stabilizing drugs**, used for bipolar disorder, are the final class of drugs we will discuss.

Barbiturates (a member of the sedative-hypnotics class of drugs), anti-seizure drugs, psychedelic drugs, and anesthetics will not be covered in detail. Table 9.1 presents an

Table 9.1 Examples of medications discussed in this chapter

Drug Class	Indications	Drug Types	Examples
Antipsychotics	Psychosis, including schizophrenia	Typical (first generation) Atypical (second generation)	phenothiazine risperidone, clozapine, olanzapine
Anxiolytics and sedative-hypnotics	Generalized anxiety disorder (GAD)	Non-benzodiazepines Benzodiazepines	barbiturates, hydroxyzine Librium, Valium, Lorazepam
Antidepressants	Major depressive disorder (MDD)	Monoamine oxidase (MAO) inhibitors Tricyclic antidepressants SSRI SSNRI	Iproniazid Imipramine paroxetine (Paxil), sertraline (Zoloft), escitalopram (Lexapro) duloxetine (Cymbalta)
Mood stabilizing	Bipolar disorder	Lithium salts Antiepileptic Anticonvulsant	lithium carbonate Valproate carbamazepine, lamotrigine

Legend: SSRI: selective serotonin reuptake inhibitor, SSNRI: selective serotonin and norepinephrine reuptake inhibitor.

overview of the different classifications of drugs and sample medications discussed in this chapter.

How Do Psychotherapeutic Drugs Work?

The exact mechanism of action of most psychotherapeutic drugs is not well understood. Moreover, the cause of the diseases they are used to treat is often not well understood. Diagnosis and therapeutic intervention are challenging and complex due to the behavioral and psychological nature of the diseases. In comparison, the pathology associated with cardiovascular disease is known in great detail, with drug targets clearly identified (e.g., cardioselective beta-blockers or ACE inhibitors). However, our overall understanding of how normal processes work in the CNS continues to improve, due in part to the study of mental illness and the effects of psychotherapeutic drugs.

Most drugs acting in the CNS modulate synaptic transmission. They affect neurotransmitter signaling, usually at the synapse. Drugs can alter neurotransmitter release, reuptake, metabolism, or they may act directly on receptors, as we saw in the previous chapter and in Chapter 3. There are many centrally acting neurotransmitters, including dopamine, norepinephrine, GABA (gamma-aminobutyric acid), glycine, glutamate, aspartate, acetylcholine, histamine, NMDA (N-methyl-d-aspartate), and serotonin (5-hydroxytryptamine, 5-HT). Many peptides have been identified that exert effects on the brain and behavior. Agonist and antagonist drugs for specific receptor subtypes have been discovered for many of the neurotransmitter pathways.

Antipsychotic Drugs (Neuroleptics, Major Tranquilizers)

Psychosis is a generic term that includes many types of mental disorders that are manifested by the loss of contact with reality. Psychotic patients often have delusions about who they are and what is happening around them, and they can suffer from auditory or visual hallucinations. Besides these active (or hyperactive) issues, psychotics show negative symptoms, such as social withdrawal, emotional blunting, and lack of motivation. They can suffer from depression, fatigue, and anxiety attacks. The incidence of psychosis is associated with a wide variety of risk factors, including alcohol and drug use, degenerative brain diseases or tumors, dementia (such as Alzheimer's disease), and stroke. As a group, psychotic individuals are less physically fit than the general population, with poor cardiovascular health, and they may have associated hyperglycemia,

Everyday Psychotherapeutics

Three of the most heavily used drugs worldwide affect the central nervous system. These drugs are associated, to a degree, with feelings of well-being. They are potent, and each one causes a level of psychological addiction and physical dependence. Nicotine (smoking, chewing, patch), caffeine (coffee, tea, cola), and ethanol (beer, wine, liquor) all act on the central nervous system. Regular users of any of the three can suffer withdrawal symptoms upon discontinuation. Each of these three drugs will be addressed in later chapters.

obesity, and type 2 diabetes (Saddichha, Manjunatha, Ameen, & Akhtar 2008; Holley, Crone, Tyson, & Lovell 2011).

How Antipsychotic Drugs Work

Psychological intervention requires trained staff and substantial time and expense. Antipsychotic drugs are used to manage psychosis, but their efficacy is often challenged. Several large-scale studies have examined treatment of **schizophrenia** (severe chronic disorder characterized by abnormal perception and behavior) and other conditions with psychotic episodes, raising a variety of issues about the long-term use of antipsychotic drugs (Ballon & Stroup 2013). Typical (first generation) drugs of the **phenothiazine** class have been available since the 1950s. These drugs are thought to work by antagonizing dopamine receptors (D_2) in the brain. They are not very specific in terms of regions of the brain and, therefore, tend to have more secondary effects. Their effectiveness gave rise to the **dopamine hypothesis**, which suggested that hyperactivity of dopaminergic signaling in certain regions of the brain was associated with psychosis. Hyperactivity of subcortical transmission at D_2 receptors is consistent with the antipsychotic action of drugs that cause D_2 receptor blockade. This hyperactivity is episodic in nature and correlates with disease symptomatology. Elevated dopamine synthesis and release in pre-synaptic cells and hyperactivity of receptors in post-synaptic cells have been proposed (Abi-Dargham & Laruelle 2005). The dopamine theory is also supported by the observations that drugs with dopamine agonist activity (e.g., amphetamines and levodopa) increase schizophrenic episodes. Moreover, brain scans show increased dopamine receptor density in certain brain regions of patients with schizophrenia (Knable & Weinberger 1997). However, the dopamine theory is insufficient to describe the complexities observed with schizophrenia. Newer, more effective drugs target additional neurotransmitter receptors (Abi-Dargham & Laruelle). These drugs have demonstrated the limitations of the dopamine hypothesis and have led to a more generalized model for brain dysfunction in psychosis. This new model has led to a multiple-drug approach for treatment (Ballon & Stroup).

The older, first-generation drugs are more effective at treating the active symptoms of the disease (delusions, hallucinations, and hyperactivity) than the negative symptoms (emotional blunting and social withdrawal). These older drugs are still sometimes referred to as the **typical antipsychotics**. They are considerably less expensive than the newer drugs, as they are available as generic drugs, but they also have a higher incidence of side effects, which include muscle rigidity and tremor. These side effects, referred to as extrapyramidal effects, can mimic the symptoms of Parkinson's disease. **Parkinson's disease** is a progressive disorder of the nervous system that causes muscle stiffness or slowing of movement due to loss of neurons in the brain that produce dopamine. The decrease in dopaminergic signaling leads to Parkinson's disease, or, in the case of these drugs that block dopamine action, symptoms resembling Parkinson's disease.

The second-generation drugs, called **atypical antipsychotics**, block dopamine receptors, and some (e.g., risperidone, clozapine, olanzapine) also block serotonin receptors ($5\text{-}HT_2$). These newer drugs cause fewer Parkinson-like effects than the older drugs, but they can still have serious side effects. For example, clozapine can cause agranulocytosis (low white cell count and immune suppression). Another side effect with the newer drugs is rapid weight gain in the first 10 to 12 weeks of use. For example, olanzapine (Zyprexa), a widely prescribed atypical antipsychotic, can cause hyperglycemia, hyperlipidemia, and excessive weight gain. These metabolic changes increase the risk of diabetes. The weight gain can contribute to psychological problems related to lack of self-control, social stigma, and demoralization. These drugs also increase symptoms associated with metabolic syndrome, diabetes, and dyslipidemia.

Although these drugs do manage mental illness in a large portion of the patients, the metabolic side effects have led to lawsuits. For example, in 2007, Lilly, the maker of Zyprexa, agreed to pay up to $700 million to settle 8,000 lawsuits (Berenson 2007). Despite the lawsuit, in 2009 Zyprexa sales worldwide increased 5% to $4.92 billion, ranking it among the top 20 drugs based on total sales. Sales, however, dipped in 2012 when generic versions came on the market. In 2013, the FDA issued a communication regarding deaths following injection of Zyprexa (FDA 2013).

Exercise Pharmacology

The use of antipsychotic medication in the United States and throughout the world continues to increase, partially due to the second-generation antipsychotic medications with decreased extra pyramidal effects. Once prescribed mostly for severe mental illness, the second-generation antipsychotics are now prescribed as adjuvant treatment of mood disorders (Shulman, Miller, Misher, & Tentler 2014). These drugs can negatively impact cardiovascular health in a population that already has a higher incidence of risk factors such as smoking and a sedentary lifestyle. Cardiac problems are a major contributor to the increased risk of all-cause mortality, along with metabolic syndrome, diabetes, hyperlipidemia, and myocarditis.

Many psychiatric conditions are characterized by an increased risk of metabolic syndrome—the cluster of cardiovascular risk factors that include dyslipidemia, abdominal obesity, hypertension, and hyperglycemia. The severity of psychiatric symptoms has a stronger association with abdominal obesity and dyslipidemia than with hypertension. Contributing mechanisms include an unhealthy lifestyle and a poor adherence to medical regimen, which are prevalent among psychiatric patients (Penninx & Lange 2018). Body mass index is as an independent predictor of psychiatric rehospitalization, suggesting that outpatient treatment programs for overweight and obese psychiatric patients might influence readmission rates. The diagnosis and severity of each patient's psychiatric symptoms must be weighed against the individual's medical risk factor profile to determine a rational pharmacotherapeutic approach.

Lifestyle changes and a multi-disciplinary approach to treatment of these patients are needed. Low levels of physical fitness are associated with more severe negative, depressive, and cognitive symptoms. In an early study of 53 obese patients treated with clozapine, dietary control and regular exercise significantly reduced body weight (Wu, Wang, Bai, et al. 2007). The subjects in the study group, who decreased their calorie intake and walked three times per week, also improved their insulin and triglyceride profiles (see Table 9.2). A systematic review evaluated the effects of education, diet, and physical activity on reduction of metabolic syndrome in schizophrenia. Interventions led to significant weight reduction (eight studies), reduced body mass index (five studies), decreased waist circumference (four studies), and lower blood glucose levels (five studies). These lifestyle interventions decrease and manage antipsychotic-induced weight gain and can be delivered without additional drug use, making them a low-cost and safe way to improve quality of life in these patients (Gurusamy, Gandhi, Damodharan, et al. 2018).

Table 9.2 Anthropometric data for clozapine-treated inpatients with schizophrenia

Variable	Baseline Value				Change at Six Months			
	Control Group		Study Group		Control Group		Study Group	
	Mean	SD	Mean	SD	Mean	SD	Mean	SD
BMI (kg/m^2)	30.27	3.31	30.43	4.20	0.35	1.30	−1.59*	1.66
Weight (kg)	77.8	11.2	78.4	11.6	1.0	3.4	−4.2*	4.4
Waist (cm)	97.8	9.7	98.3	7.3	0.3	2.7	−3.3*	4.2

Legend: Anthropometric data at baseline and changes after six months for clozapine-treated inpatients with schizophrenia assigned to a control group ($n = 25$) or study group ($n = 28$) consisting of reduced calorie intake and regular physical exercise (walking 60 minutes three days per week). *Significant difference between control and study group at six months ($p < 0.001$). Data derived from Wu, Wang, Bai, et al. (2007).

Aerobic exercise improves cognitive deficits, total symptom severity (including positive and negative symptoms), depression, quality of life, and global functioning. For example, one meta-analysis included 29 studies and 1,109 patients. Exercise was superior to control conditions in improving total symptom severity, quality of life, global functioning, and depressive symptoms (Dauwan et al., 2016). In a study with 22 multi-episode schizophrenia patients (with 22 matched controls), bicycle ergometer training (30 minutes three time per week for three months) with computer-assisted cognitive training significantly improved overall functioning and performance on specific psychological tests. There was also less severity of negative symptoms (Malchow, Keller, Hasan, et al. 2015). Another meta-analysis showed that exercise significantly reduced psychiatric symptoms in schizophrenic patients (Firth, Cotter, Elliott, et al. 2015), besides improving physical fitness and other cardiometabolic risk factors. Around 90 minutes of moderate-to-vigorous exercise per week improved functioning, co-morbid disorders, and neurocognition. These results suggest that a sufficient dose of exercise, in supervised or group settings, can be feasible and effective interventions for schizophrenia (Firth et al.). However, in this analysis, this level and duration of exercise had no significant effect on body mass index.

One possible conclusion from many of these studies is that patients with mental illness often have poor diet and exercise habits that cause them to be physically unfit. For those patients who can maintain an exercise program and improve their cardiovascular health, there is improvement in their disease symptoms.

Anxiolytic Drugs and Sedative-hypnotics (Minor Tranquilizers)

Normal anxiety, often experienced under stressful conditions, can lead to enhanced productivity or motivation. Although many people work well under pressure, some suffer from anxiety that is chronic and excessive, a condition referred to as **generalized anxiety disorder (GAD).** In some peoples' brains, there are problems in the GABA network (GABA is a neurotransmitter that usually inhibits nerve signaling), and these people are predisposed to types of mental disorders such as GAD. The problem may be in the GABA circuits that modulate stress responses. Loss of this GABA function decreases the ability to suppress or manage the response to stress. Causes for the loss are not clear but it increases with age and correlates with lack of physical activity. In individuals with deficient GABA signaling, stimuli that create anxiety do not initiate sufficient GABA-induced inhibitory signals. The stress response grows unchecked, eventually causing the individual to present with GAD or other phobias. People with GAD are unable to function in normal daily activities. They can have trouble concentrating, suffer recurring headaches, and have very tense muscles. They often have sleep disorders that can compound the problem.

How Anxiolytic Drugs and Sedative-Hypnotics Work

Anxiolytics and sedative-hypnotics enhance GABA signaling and help overcome GABA-related deficiencies in responses to stress. These drugs help individuals with GAD or other phobias manage their day-to-day activities by keeping their anxiety levels down. Drugs used to combat anxiety are generally divided into two categories: **non-benzodiazepines** and **benzodiazepines.** (In some cases, antidepressants are prescribed; these will be discussed below.) The non-benzodiazepines include older, less effective drugs such as barbiturates and hydroxyzine, an older antihistamine with sedative effects. The benzodiazepines are a fairly large class of drugs with varying degrees of anxiolytic, anticonvulsant, muscle relaxant, and sedative properties. They have been used in medical procedures to reduce tension and induce sedation and amnesia for the procedure (e.g., colonoscopy, wisdom teeth extraction). The first benzodiazepine was Librium, one of the drugs mentioned earlier that was serendipitously found to have tranquilizing activity back in the 1950s. In the early 1960s, the derivative diazepam, known as Valium, was released. These drugs, though relatively safe, cause a physical dependence with continued use. Benzodiazepine addiction manifests itself upon discontinuation of long-term use, and the resulting benzodiazepine withdrawal syndrome can be serious because of possible seizures.

Benzodiazepines have been very useful in neuroscience. The benzodiazepine receptor is the $GABA_A$-receptor, one of the prevalent inhibitory receptors in the brain. Upon binding its receptor on the post-synaptic membrane, GABA causes the post-synaptic cell to become non-responsive to excitatory input, blocking the firing of new action potentials. $GABA_A$-receptors act as a ligand-gated Cl^- channel. Upon binding GABA, they transiently open and allow the entry of Cl^- along its concentration gradient (the concentration of Cl^- is much greater outside the cell than inside), causing hyperpolarization. Hyperpolarized cells do not fire new action potentials until they return to normal resting potential.

A typical $GABA_A$-receptor contains five subunits, usually two alpha, two beta, and one gamma subunit. There are multiple genetic variants of each subunit, generating a wide variety of $GABA_A$-receptor subtypes. These different receptor subtypes are expressed in different regions of the brain. The benzodiazepine derivatives differ in their affinity for the subunit subtypes. Their preferential binding to different subtypes helps the different benzodiazepines generate varied effects—such as sedation, anti-anxiety, or muscle relaxation—by binding variant $GABA_A$-receptors in different parts of the brain (Möhler, Fritschy, & Rudolph 2002). When a $GABA_A$-receptor binds a benzodiazepine, the receptor has increased affinity for GABA. The gated Cl^- channel opens with a higher frequency. The greater influx of Cl^- causes hyperpolarization—that is, the inside of the cell becomes more negative—creating an inhibitory post-synaptic potential (IPSP). The IPSP effectively reinforces GABA's inhibitory effects (i.e., it blocks the generation of new action potentials). Barbiturates also bind the $GABA_A$-receptor and cause a similar effect, but at a different site on the receptor than benzodiazepine.

Barbiturates prolong the time the channel is open, causing a greater influx of Cl^- and hyperpolarization. The other major type of GABA-receptor, the $GABA_B$-receptor, does not respond to these classes of sedative-hypnotics and is structurally distinct. The $GABA_B$-receptor is a G-protein–coupled receptor instead of a ligand-gated channel like the $GABA_A$-receptor.

Exercise Pharmacology

Exercise programs may help individuals manage panic disorders and phobias such as agoraphobia (the fear of being outside, in crowds, or in places difficult to escape). In a meta-analysis of six randomized control trials (262 adults with anxiety or stress-related disorders), exercise significantly decreased anxiety symptoms relative to controls (Stubbs, Vancampfort, Rosenbaum, et al. 2017). What intensity of exercise is required to improve patients with anxiety? A systematic review was accomplished assessing the use of exercise (vs. waiting list control groups) in the treatment of anxiety and compared high intensity versus low intensity exercise. Long-term follow-up scores were also analyzed. Fifteen studies were incorporated with a total of 675 patients. Aerobic exercise was effective in the treatment of raised anxiety, with higher intensity exercise showing greater effects than low-intensity programs (Aylett, Small, & Bower 2018).

Extensive animal studies have been done with the benzodiazepines. Aged rats have fewer benzodiazepine/GABA binding sites in their brains than do young rats. Exercise can reverse the age-related decrease in GABA-receptor number (Tehrani, Tate, & al-Dahan 1995). Voluntary exercise in mice is anxiolytic; following two weeks of exercise, mice show reduced anxiety as measured with a variety of tests, such as a startle response (Salam, Foxa, DeTroya, et al. 2009). These results are consistent with the idea that sufficient GABA activity is necessary for normally regulated brain activity to control the anxiety response.

In humans, benzodiazepine (lorazepam) decreases peak power and blood levels of epinephrine and lactate during maximal exercise. In elite athletes, benzodiazepine (lorazepam) suppressed exercise-induced increases in dopamine, epinephrine, and norepinephrine (see Table 9.3) but did not significantly change time to exhaustion at submaximal (85% VO_2max) exercise (Collomp, Fortier, Cooper, et al. 1994). Considerable evidence suggests that the suppression of epinephrine release caused by benzodiazepines during exercise occurs centrally. How might this central suppression contribute to a decrease in anxiety? As discussed in Chapter 3, exercise activates the sympathetic nervous system and the HPA (hypothalamus–pituitary–adrenal) component of the stress and fight or flight response. This response is kept in check partly through suppression of dopaminergic signaling via GABA inhibitory input. The benzodiazepine-induced increase in GABA activity would suppress sympathetic activity and the HPA response to stress or exercise and cause the observed lower circulating catecholamines noted in Table 9.3. However, a peripheral role for benzodiazepines, such as direct suppression of epinephrine release from the adrenal medulla, cannot be ruled out completely.

A meta-analysis of 16 articles contained 922 participants randomized to a resistance exercise training ($n = 486$) or a nonactive group ($n = 436$). It also contained a validated anxiety outcome (Gordon, McDowell, Lyons, & Herring 2017). Resistance exercise training significantly reduced anxiety symptoms. Improvements were not dependent on gender or resistance exercise training protocol. Resistance exercise has anxiolytic effects after both single-bout sessions and long-term training (Strickland &

Table 9.3 Effect of benzodiazepine on circulating catecholamines

Cycling Time	Dopamine (ng/ml)		Norepinephrine (ng/ml)		Epinephrine (ng/ml)	
	Placebo	*BZ*	*Placebo*	*BZ*	*Placebo*	*BZ*
Rest	51	31	358	278	57	52
5 min	115	69*	1,414	1,121	172	129
10 min	193	131*	3,039	2,583*	415	293*
15 min	246	184*	4,170	3,722*	590	428*
End	337	261*	5,780	4,844*	960	631*

Legend: A double-blind randomized protocol using seven male triathletes cycling at 85% maximum oxygen uptake. BZ = benzodiazepine. Values are means. *$p < 0.05$ for difference between placebo and BZ. Data derived from Collomp, Fortier, Cooper, et al. (1994).

Smith 2014). Resistance training at a low-to-moderate intensity (<70% 1 repetition maximum) produces the most reliable decrease in anxiety in a diverse range of populations (e.g., gender and different age groups). Resistance training combined with aerobic exercise caused robust decreases in anxiety. The mechanisms involved are not clear, but some evidence suggests that stress effects on the HPA axis occur concurrently with anxiety. Resistance exercise may modify the HPA response and thus affect stress and anxiety. Another possible mechanism involves brain-derived neurotrophic factor (BDNF), which increases following aerobic exercise of sufficient intensity. BDNF is discussed in more detail in the following sections.

These studies suggest a tentative model. In some peoples' brains, there are problems in the GABA network; these people are predisposed to types of mental disorders such as generalized anxiety disorder. The problem may be in the GABA circuits that modulate stress responses. Loss of this GABA function due to ageing, lack of physical activity, or other causes decreases our ability to suppress or manage our response to stress. In individuals with deficient GABA signaling, stimuli that create anxiety do not initiate sufficient GABA-induced inhibitory signals. The stress response grows unchecked, eventually causing the individual to present with generalized anxiety disorders or other phobias (Figure 9.1).

Anxiolytics enhance GABA signaling and help overcome the GABA-related deficiencies when responding to stress. These drugs help individuals with GAD or other phobias manage their day-to-day activities by keeping their anxiety levels down. In conjunction with anxiolytics, which enhance GABA signaling and help overcome the GABA-related deficiencies in stress responses, exercise can be a useful adjunct therapy—for its maintenance of the GABA-signaling network and its ability to decrease anxiety, as well as for its obvious cardiovascular benefits (see Figure 9.1). Although more research is needed, exercise is an effective treatment for some of the anxiety disorders (reviewed in Asmundson, Fetzner, Deboer, et al. 2013). Available evidence generally supports an exercise prescription tailored to current fitness and physical health as a promising addition to pharmacologic treatment of clinically significant anxiety (Asmundson et al.). A combination of moderate intensity aerobic exercise and low-to-moderate resistance exercise appears to generate the most robust response.

Figure 9.1 Simplified hypothetical scheme as to how exercise and drugs affect anxiety and GABA signaling.

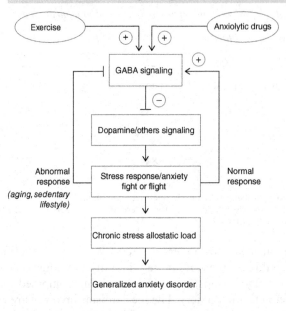

Legend: GABA signaling suppresses regions of the brain involved in fight or flight response/stress/anxiety. Normally, coping mechanisms increase GABA activity, and stress response subsides (arrow labeled Normal Response). As we age, become sedentary, or have defects in the appropriate circuits, this coping mechanism becomes less efficient, and there is less GABA suppression (arrow labeled Abnormal Response). Under the abnormal condition, occasional stress morphs into allostatic load and anxiety, leading to GAD if not dealt with or treated. Exercise and anxiolytic drugs increase GABA activity, increasing the suppression downstream of its signaling, and help strengthen the coping mechanism.

It is important to keep in mind that the sedative-hypnotic drugs can impair physical activity and judgment due to their suppression of adrenal medullary activity (related to the decrease in epinephrine response noted above) and the sedative, muscle relaxing, and hypnotic effects they cause. Whereas some of these effects may be helpful in certain pulmonary or cardiac patients, they may be expected to have negative consequences for certain types of athletic performance. These drugs can also impair driving an automobile, especially in the elderly. Patients taking these drugs can fail field sobriety tests if pulled over while driving, because their driving can be similar to driving under the influence of alcohol.

Antidepressant Drugs

Major depressive disorder (MDD) affects millions of Americans and more than 300 million people worldwide, with estimates approaching 5% of the population (www.who.int/newsroom/fact-sheets/detail/depression). More women are affected than men, and MDD is a major contributor to the overall global burden of disease. People who suffer from MDD have shortened lifetimes (Murri, Ekkekakis, Magagnoli, et al. 2019). Diagnosis can be difficult, and many who suffer may not seek treatment, creating variability in the attempts to quantify the problem. Depression is characterized by significant impairment in social and occupational functioning, and the majority of depressed individuals have recurrent episodes and/or chronic depression. According to the DSM-V, people are diagnosed with MDD if they suffer from the majority of the following symptoms on a daily basis:

- Insomnia
- Depressed mood
- Diminished interest in day-to-day activities
- Significant weight loss (or gain)
- Psychomotor agitation (or retardation)
- Fatigue
- Feelings of worthlessness or guilt
- Diminished ability to concentrate or indecisiveness
- Thoughts of death or suicide.

MDD is being diagnosed increasingly in children, with the annual rate of depression in teenagers and young adults (18- to 25-year-olds) nearly twice that of 26- to 49-year-olds (www.nimh.nih.gov/health/statistics/major-depression.shtml). Depression is closing in on cardiovascular disease as the world's leading cause of death and disability. Depression shows high co-morbidity with cardiovascular disease (Pozuelo, Tesar, Zhang, et al. 2009). Depression in the young can carry into adulthood and contribute to a wide variety of destructive behaviors, including drug and alcohol abuse and suicidal tendencies. Late-life depression may differ in pathophysiology and follow other age-related decline in general health.

Opiates and amphetamines were used in the past to help deal with clinical depression. However, addiction and unwanted side effects limited their usefulness. Isoniazid was developed as an anti-tuberculosis drug and was found to have a general stimulatory effect, possibly due to inhibition of the enzyme diamine oxidase. Iproniazid was developed as a more specific inhibitor of **monoamine oxidase (MAO)**, the enzyme largely responsible for metabolizing and inactivating **catecholamine-derived neurotransmitters**. Other **MAO inhibitors** were developed and widely prescribed for depression in the 1960s and 1970s. These drugs are associated with hepatotoxicity (toxic damage to the liver), and their use is now limited, although an available patch for the drug's delivery apparently has less toxicity.

Imipramine was the first of many **tricyclic antidepressants** that became widely prescribed in the 1970s, replacing the MAO inhibitors. The tricyclic antidepressants block reuptake of several different neurotransmitters, including norepinephrine, serotonin, and dopamine. The tricyclics can also antagonize acetylcholine and histamine receptors. A newer generation of drugs (called SSRI) has become the first line of treatment for depression and certain anxiety or personality disorders. **SSRI** stands for selective serotonin reuptake inhibitor or serotonin-specific reuptake inhibitor. Paxil, Zoloft, and Lexapro are members of this class of drug. Other newer antidepressants on the market include the **SSNRI** class of drugs, such as Cymbalta. These drugs are selective serotonin and norepinephrine reuptake inhibitors. Either by inhibiting the metabolism of neurotransmitters (i.e., MAO inhibitors) or by blocking their reuptake, the drugs cause the effective concentration of the neurotransmitter to increase at its receptor.

The effectiveness of these drugs in treating depression in humans gave rise to the **neurotransmitter hypothesis**, which postulates that depression can result from defective neurotransmitter signaling in the brain. In research with rodents, antidepressant drugs increase the synthesis of new neurons in the brains of adult animals (Malberg, Eisch, Nestler, & Duman 2000), a process called neurogenesis. Similar results were found in primates (Perera, Coplan, Lisanby, et al. 2007). A newer **neurogenesis theory** suggests that depression results from people having low rates of neurogenesis in certain brain regions (Ernst, Olson, Pinel, et al. 2006). Drugs (such as SSRI and SSNRI) stimulate neurogenesis and help maintain "normal" brain function. This theory has been expanded to include neuronal plasticity—these drugs increase neuroplasticity (see Box).

A few specific regions of the adult mammalian brain contain progenitor cells with replication potential. Under proper stimulation, these progenitor cells can divide and differentiate into new neurons and glial cells. It has been postulated that antidepressant drugs promote neurogenesis, thereby providing a therapeutic effect in major depressive disorder. Experiments in rodents support this hypothesis, as antidepressant drugs increase **brain-derived neurotrophic factor (BDNF)** in the hippocampus, and BDNF is an important mediator of neurogenesis (Garza, Ha, Garcia, et al. 2004). Other gene products involved in neurogenesis are also present in these regions of the brain following treatment with antidepressant drugs.

Brain Health, Neurogenesis, and Neuroplasticity

The brain has the capacity to undergo significant change, a quality referred to as **neuroplasticity**. Brain changes have been investigated at the molecular and cellular level. How neuroplasticity contributes to behavior is of great interest in the fields of mental health and aging. What are the important signals that initiate changes in specific regions of the brain? What happens to these processes when we age or suffer from mental illness?

Brain changes and the remodeling of neuronal circuitry result from experiences rich in complexity and novelty. Examples might include learning new processes (a new game or a musical instrument) or experiencing new cultures (traveling to a foreign country). Such sets of complex stimuli involve many areas of the brain. These stimuli help maintain cognitive functions in the brain as we age. In rodents, cognition is related to locomotion, because physical activity increases the chance to experience situations where more brain activity would be a benefit (Fabel & Kempermann 2008). Exercise in humans provides input into similar regions of the brain, primarily the hippocampus, from both centrally acting pathways and signals that come from the periphery and cross the blood–brain barrier (Cotman & Berchtold 2002). In the hippocampus, these stimuli increase the release of neurotrophins (polypeptide growth factors in the brain) such as BDNF and cause the activation of genes involved in plasticity. As a result of these changes in hippocampal activity and the release of neurotrophins, neurogenesis increases, neuronal survival is enhanced, new synapses are made, brain vascularization improves, and learning and maintenance of cognitive function are enhanced.

Plasticity decreases as we age and can be deficient in individuals with certain types of mental illness. With depression and perhaps bipolar disease, lack of neurogenesis and plasticity can be contributing factors to the disease etiology. Problems with generating and receiving the stimuli, or the release of the neurotrophic factors, or how cells respond to these factors—any of these could decrease plasticity. These defects could be manifested by the lack of generation of new neural networks (and lack of maintenance of old ones) that would normally provide adaptation to the environmental stimuli generated by significant life experiences. Drug treatment affects certain signaling pathways that increase neurotrophins such as BDNF, but drugs alone may not provide the rich experience needed to guide neuronal network development (Castren & Rantamaki 2010). Adjunct therapies, such as exercise or other types of rehabilitation, could be necessary for the mentally ill. In terms of aging gracefully, exercise certainly contributes to healthy brain activity, largely by stimulating processes involved in neuroplasticity and helping maintain cognitive function.

Besides the production of new cells, BDNF contributes to neuronal plasticity (see Box) by increasing the branching of axons and dendrites and stabilizing synaptic contacts. BDNF also promotes neuronal survival and growth (Castren & Rantamaki). The increase in BDNF in the rodent brain following antidepressant drug treatment suggests possible ways that antidepressants may work in humans.

Some types of depression may have other causes. For example, late-life depression is hypothesized to result from age-related deficiencies in the cerebrovascular system. Deficient blood flow to regions of the brain impairs cell health and growth. The depression syndrome that results from these changes is often resistant to antidepressant drug therapy.

Exercise Pharmacology

The comparative efficacy of 21 antidepressant drugs for the acute treatment of adults with major depressive disorder was determined from a systematic review and meta-analysis. The analysis included 28,552 citations from 522 trials comprising 116,477 participants. All antidepressants were more effective than placebo. For acceptability, only two drugs were associated with fewer dropouts than placebo, whereas one drug had more dropouts than placebo (Cipriani, Furukawa, Salanti, et al. 2018). Although antidepressants are currently the treatment of choice for major depressive disorder, a significant percentage of patients do not respond to a first-line antidepressant drug and a significant proportion of patients are treatment-resistant. In addition, adherence can be poor, drug combinations increase the risk of side effects, and there is a lag time between starting antidepressants and improvements in mood (Cooney, Dwan, Greig, et al. 2013).

Exercise and physical activity have beneficial effects on the mind as well as the body. The distinction between mind and body is dated, as it is now well recognized that the health of both are intimately related. For example, exercise improves sleep quality and duration, refreshing mental and physical energy for the coming day. Exercise also causes beneficial mental and physical adaptations in the response to stress, including the HPA axis. It dampens inflammatory processes, restores sympathetic balance, and improves cardiorespiratory fitness both in healthy individuals and in individuals with depression (Murri et al.). A Cochrane Review and meta-analysis of 35 randomized controlled trials ($n = 1356$) found that exercise was moderately effective at reducing depressive symptoms relative to a control condition in depressed adults. Subgroup analyses indicated that there was no evidence for a difference in the effectiveness of exercise relative to psychotherapy (seven trials) and pharmacotherapy (four trials) in treating depression (Cooney et al.).

Exercise interventions consisting of three sessions per week for 12 to 24 weeks typically result in a medium to large reduction in the severity of depression, measured by symptom rating scales. The efficacy of exercise seems greater if it is aerobic, delivered in groups, and supervised by an instructor. The efficacy of exercise may be comparable in terms of magnitude to that of psychotherapies or antidepressant medications (Cooney et al.; reviewed in Murri et al.). In depressed individuals, exercise can help ameliorate sleep and appetite issues; it can reduce depressed mood, suicidal ideation, and help depressed patients enjoy life again. The effect of exercise may diminish over time if not continued. However, individuals who regularly engage in moderate physical activity maintain reduced risk of incurring depressive episodes. Exercise in conjunction with the standard medications may provide improved outcomes (Mura, Moro, Patten, & Carta 2014). Moreover, exercise may be effective in individuals with treatment-resistant depression, or those with concerns about drug treatment, such as adolescents or women during or following pregnancy.

Interestingly, exercise stimulates neurogenesis in hippocampal regions of rodent brains similar to that stimulated by antidepressant drugs. Increases in BDNF mRNA expression occur in brains of old and young animals following exercise and antidepressant treatment (see Figure 9.2). Exercise and antidepressant drugs potentiate the

Figure 9.2 BDNF mRNA levels following 14-day treatment of antidepressant and physical activity.

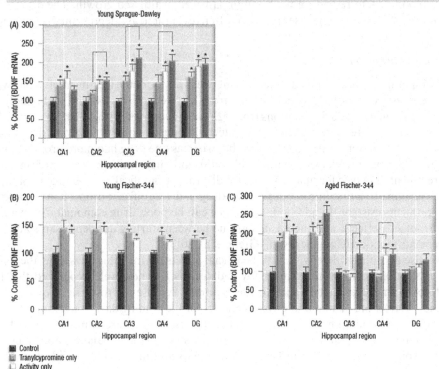

Source: Garza AA, Ha TG, Garcia C, Chen MJ, Russo-Neustadt AA (2004) Exercise, antidepressant treatment, and BDNF mRNA expression in the aging brain. Pharmacol Biochem Behav 77:209–220. Used with permission.

Legend: Hippocampal regional differences in BDNF mRNA levels in response to the four treatment conditions in (A) young (3-month) Sprague-Dawley rats, (B) young (3-month) Fischer rats, and (C) aged (22-month) Fischer rats. Expression of BDNF mRNA was determined in the indicated subregions of the hippocampus of the treated rats. Results are displayed as the percentage of control and represent the mean ±S.E.M. Asterisks denote statistically significant differences from the control group, $p < 0.05$. Bridges between bars denote statistical significance ($p < 0.05$) between the indicated groups (Garza et al.).

expression of BDNF, suggesting the two different treatments may converge at the cellular level (Garza et al.). In addition to increasing BDNF, exercise increases beta-endorphin, vascular endothelial growth factor (VEGF), and serotonin. Serotonin may be a central player in neurogenesis, as indicated by the fact that the SSRI drugs induce BDNF and are effective in the treatment of depression (Ernst et al.). Norepinephrine signaling, part of the response to exercise, may also be involved in increased BDNF expression (Cotman & Berchtold), and this supposition is supported by the effectiveness of drugs like Cymbalta, a SSNRI-class drug. A microarray analysis of 5,000 genes in rat brain following exercise showed changes in gene expression of a large number of genes involved with neuronal growth and plasticity (Tong, Shen, Perreau, et al. 2001).

In humans, aerobic exercise and antidepressant medication also have overlapping regional effects on brain structure. Several brain regions show structural plasticity in response to exercise or in relation to higher levels of fitness, including the hippocampus, anterior cingulate cortex, and the prefrontal cortex. Similar regions show a similar volume increase after antidepressant medications. In depressed adults, these regions have reduced volume. Exercise may also influence white matter connectivity. BDNF may be a key mediator of exercise effects on structural brain markers of depression. BDNF levels are lower in depressed individuals and its level increases with exercise. In an early study, exercise in 35 elderly women with depression caused the normalization of serum levels of BDNF following a single exercise session (Laske, Banschbach, Stransky, et al. 2010). The low initial levels of BDNF in the depressed women increased to levels approaching those of normal women, whose BDNF levels did not change significantly following this protocol. BDNF may mediate the exercise-induced increases in hippocampal volume, similar to animal studies that suggest that exercise relieves depressive symptoms by acting through BDNF pathways (Gujral, Aizenstein, Reynolds, et al. 2017).

A meta-analysis examined the effectiveness of resistance exercise training on depression (Gordon, McDowell, Hallgren, et al. 2018). The total participants in these combined randomized clinical trials included 947 exercisers and 930 as the nonactive control condition. Validated measures of depressive symptoms were assessed at baseline, mid-intervention, and/or post-intervention. Resistance exercise training significantly reduced depressive symptoms among adults regardless of health status, total prescribed volume of resistance exercise training, or significant improvements in strength.

The pathophysiology of late-life depression differs from younger adults. Older patients have higher prevalence of physical illnesses and cognitive impairments. They can also respond less to antidepressant drugs. Exercise is an effective add-on to antidepressant drugs for mild to moderate depression compared to those only receiving antidepressants. Exercisers displayed greater improvements in cognition and autonomic balance (Murri et al.). In depressed older adults, exercise may reduce atrophy, reduce white matter lesion burden, and improve cognitive function. Those with late-life depression tend to be less physically fit and may show greater improvement after starting to exercise, translating to greater neural benefits (Murri et al.). In addition to stimulating neurogenesis, exercise increases vascularization in the brain, helping maintain cognitive function as we age. The adult-neurogenesis hypothesis provides support for exercise antagonizing the effects of aging and helping manage depression and other types of mental illness (Duman, Schlesinger, Russell, & Duman 2008).

The results from these and many other studies suggest that exercise at levels consistent with public health recommendations can be an adjunct treatment option for depression. Exercise is now included in the American Psychiatric Association's treatment recommendations for major depressive disorder (Rethorst & Trivedi 2013). Rethorst and Trivedi provide evidence-based recommendations for prescribing exercise for patients, including aerobic exercise and resistance training.

Mood-stabilizing Drugs

Patients with **bipolar disorder** (referred to as manic-depression in the past) cycle between high (manic) and low (depression) "poles." Though bipolar disorder can be difficult to diagnose, it differs from "unipolar" depression in the mania that occurs, with abnormally elevated mood swings. Patients with bipolar disorder may experience one or more episodes of mania alternating with depressive episodes, or they may have mixed episodes with both mania and depression at the same time. Bipolar disorder is estimated to occur in about 3% of the population, and both genetic and environmental factors are implicated (National Institute of Mental Health, "Bipolar Disorder"). It is often misdiagnosed or underdiagnosed. Treatment can be hindered because patients crave the high-energy, sometimes creative bursts of activity that characterize the manic phase. Onset usually occurs in young adults, and it can be a long-lasting disorder. Episodes of abnormality are associated with distress and increased risk of suicide. The disorder is evaluated with a clinical scale and assigned subtypes.

Triggers for bipolar disorder episodes include stress and loss of daily routines and structure. Individuals with bipolar disorder are prone to binge eating, substance abuse, and depression. Patients with bipolar disorder are often physically unfit, similar to patients with other psychological disorders. They have higher rates of obesity than the general public. The drugs used to treat their illness can contribute to their poor physical state, as weight gain following drug treatment is documented (Keck & McElroy 2003).

Lithium carbonate and other lithium formulations are the "gold standard" mood-stabilizing drugs. **Lithium** was one of the first effective treatments for mania, actually dating back to observations in the late 1800s before its rediscovery in the 1940s. Lithium prevents relapses of manic and depressive episodes, although it may take time to dose the patient effectively. Lithium can be toxic, so it is important to monitor blood levels. For patients who exercise, awareness of lithium's toxicity is very important, because changes in blood volume, such as those caused by dehydration, can drastically alter blood lithium levels.

Lithium's mechanism of action is still unclear, but its effectiveness may be due to its reported inhibition of enzymes such as inositol monophosphatase or GSK-3B (glycogen synthase kinase 3B). Inositol monophosphatase is necessary for the reincorporation of inositol into inositol-containing phospholipids; these phospholipids play a critical role in neurotransmitter signaling. GSK-3B is of interest because it has a role maintaining circadian rhythms. Circadian rhythms regulate many activities, including metabolism and sleep cycles. Lithium may also affect nitric oxide signaling and signaling by the excitatory neurotransmitter glutamate. Although the mechanism of action is still not clear, lithium is effective in managing bipolar episodes.

Other drugs used for bipolar disorder have anticonvulsant activity. Sodium valproate is widely used for this disorder, as well as for epilepsy. Other anticonvulsant drugs used for bipolar disorder include carbamazepine and lamotrigine. These mood stabilizers generally work better at preventing the manic phase. Use of antidepressants (discussed earlier) alone is not recommended, and they are sometimes used in conjunction with a mood stabilizer (National Institute of Mental Health, "Bipolar Disorder"). In individuals with severe manic episodes, the atypical antipsychotic drugs (also discussed earlier) are often prescribed.

For pediatric bipolar disease, an international group of experts completed a selective review of literature regarding differential diagnosis, treatment, and neurobiology (reviewed in Goldstein, Birmaher, Carlson, et al. 2017). For acute mania and/or mixed mania, second-generation antipsychotics are indicated in children and adolescents. Lithium is indicated for the treatment and recurrence prevention of mania in youths aged 12 years and older. Anticonvulsants appear less effective than second-generation antipsychotics or lithium for mania. For depression, the combination of olanzapine (second-generation antipsychotic) and fluoxetine (SSRI antidepressant) is indicated for bipolar disease in youth aged 10 to 17 years old. Some anticonvulsants can improve depression symptoms compared to placebo. Antidepressant monotherapy is not recommended in pediatric bipolar disease. For maintenance therapy, lithium and divalproex (anticonvulsant) slowed recurrence in several studies. A second-generation antipsychotic (aripiprazole) reduced severity of symptoms and improved global functioning compared to placebo. In another study with a different second-generation antipsychotic, bipolar symptoms were reduced, but there was a high occurrence of sedation and significant weight gain. Adjunct treatments (such as exercise or other support programs) target primarily depressive symptoms (Goldstein et al.).

Exercise Pharmacology

Patients who present with bipolar disorder are first stabilized with drug treatment. Alternative, supportive therapies may be added later. Exercise is one of these supportive therapies. It helps stabilize mood in people with bipolar disorder, and it should help suppress the weight gain associated with the disorder and drug therapy. Executive dysfunction, resulting in social and functional impairment, is common during and between mood episodes in bipolar disorder. Adolescents with bipolar disease ($n = 30$) and healthy control subjects ($n = 20$) completed an attention and response inhibition task before and after 20 minutes of cycling at about 70% maximum heart rate. MRI results showed a larger effect in bipolar adolescents than healthy controls after exercise, throughout the ventral prefrontal cortex, amygdala, and hippocampus. Acute aerobic exercise improved executive task function among adolescents with bipolar disorder, and pre-exercise symptoms were absent after exercise (Metcalfe, MacIntosh, Scavone, et al. 2016). A systematic review of physical activity and bipolar disease included 31 studies with 15,587 patients. Sedentary lifestyle varied from 40% to 64.9%. Physical activity was associated with less depressive symptoms, better quality of life, and increased functioning (Melo, Daher Ede, Albuquerque, de Bruin, et al. 2016).

An older review identified several neurobiological targets of physical exercise in bipolar disorder (Alsuwaidan, Kucyl, Law, & McIntyre 2009). Table 9.4 gives a comprehensive list of possible targets of physical activity. In several of these targets, the defective response in bipolar disorder was reversed with exercise. Exercise-induced BDNF and neurogenesis are implicated in the management of bipolar disorder (Phillips 2017b). Figure 9.3 shows a proposed mechanism where exercise causes the release of BDNF,

Table 9.4 Proposed neurobiological targets of physical exercise in bipolar disorder

Neurobiological Mediator	Bipolar Disorder	Effect of Physical Exercise
Norepinephrine (NE)	Lower plasma levels in depression; higher levels in mania	Acutely increases plasma NE; chronically may increase NE in locus coeruleus and dorsal raphe
Serotonin (5-HT)	Altered neurotransmission with decreased $5HT_{1A}$ binding potential	Elevated central 5HT.
Dopamine (DA)	Lower level of DA metabolite detected in depression	Mouse models demonstrate increased DA synthesis
Endocannabinoids	Decreased CB_1 receptor density in anterior cingulate cortex in depression	Increased plasma endogenous cannabinoid (anandamide, see Chapter 15)
Inflammation	Higher levels of proinflammatory cytokines; lower levels of anti-inflammatory cytokines in both states	Acute inflammatory response leads to chronic and robust anti-inflammatory response
Neuroplasticity	Chronic antidepressant administration increases new neurons in hippocampus; chronic treatment with lithium and valproic acid activates rat frontal cortex and hippocampus	Enhanced hippocampal neurogenesis; growth of blood vessels in the hippocampus, cortex, and cerebellum; increased BDNF in multiple brain regions including hippocampus

Source: Adapted from Alsuwaidan et al. (2009).

Figure 9.3 Schematic representation of the role of exercise in depression and bipolar disease.

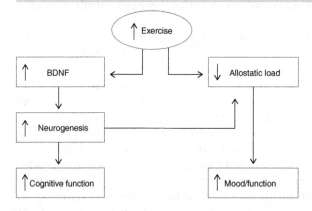

Legend: Flow chart of possible ways through which exercise can influence allostatic load and cause neurogenesis. Modified from Sylvia, Ametrano, & Nierenberg (2010).

which can then stimulate neurogenesis and help alleviate chronic stress (allostatic load). Exercise also works directly to decrease stress load, with the overall result of improving mood and brain function in general (Sylvia, Ametrano, & Nierenberg 2010).

Elder Concerns—Keeping Your Wits about You

A major component/hallmark of aging is the slow (usually) decline in cognitive function. The rate of decline is attributed mainly to physical inactivity, chronic inflammation, improperly controlled stress response, and poor antioxidant defense. Nonpathological aging involves key regions of the brain vital for cognitive function. Decline in memory, attention, speed of processing, and executive function may result in mild disability prior to the onset of dementia. Drug therapy options are limited, so lifestyle factors such as physical activity, optimizing nutrition, and engagement in cognitive stimulation can maintain and improve neuronal plasticity and resilience of the brain (reviewed in Phillips 2017b). Neuronal plasticity is the process where neurons alter and strengthen connections continuously for learning and memory. It depends on membrane depolarization of neurons and stimulus-induced synaptic activity, leading to changes in dendritic morphology and connections. Mental engagement and dietary factors also improve neurotrophic signaling, neurogenesis, inflammation, stress response, and antioxidant defense mechanisms, similar to those implicated in the cognitive response to physical activity (Phillips 2017b).

Adult neurogenesis adds new neurons to existing circuits providing another form of synaptic plasticity. Increases in hippocampal size correlate with increases in spatial memory performance in both healthy adults and persons with mild cognitive impairment. For example, aerobic or resistance training significantly increased hippocampal volume in older women with probable mild cognitive impairment (ten Brinke, Bolandzadeh, Nagamatsu, et al. 2015). Several meta-analyses show that elderly aerobic exercisers exhibited improvements in attention, processing speed, memory, and executive function. Age-related declines in cortical tissue density in the frontal, temporal, and parietal cortices were significantly reduced as a function of cardiovascular fitness, supporting the idea that physical activity may prevent age-related anatomical and physiological deterioration in the brain. A systematic analysis of 38 animal and human studies reported that physical activity attenuates Alzheimer-related neuropathology, particularly when undertaken early in the disease process (Phillips, Baktir, Das, et al. 2015).

Chronic inflammation is mechanistically linked to cognitive impairment, mood disorders, cardiovascular diseases, and neurodegenerative disorders. Long-term physical activity upregulates anti-inflammatory processes, such as fewer viral and bacterial infections and a reduced incidence of systemic low-grade inflammation. Regular exercise can be used to mitigate age-related changes in immune senescence and preserve cognitive function with aging. Persistent activation of the HPA as a result of chronic stress can cause damage to key areas of the brain. Persistently elevated levels of glucocorticoids can be neurotoxic with neuronal atrophy and loss of plasticity in the hippocampus. Voluntary exercise mitigates an overactive stress response. The ability of regular exercise to attenuate rises in cortisol levels may be especially important for preventing hippocampal atrophy and bolster physiological resilience by optimizing the stress response during aging.

Aerobic exercise decreases overall levels of reactive oxygen species (ROS) and increases adaptations to ROS-induced lipid peroxidation, in part by increasing antioxidant gene expression. Nutrition has the potential to modulate brain structure and function, as the brain consumes 20% of the total nutrient-derived energy available, though it only comprises 2% of total body weight. Dietary factors can modulate inflammation, antioxidant defense mechanisms, and energy metabolism—all important for neuroplasticity. Dietary interventions tend to be safer and more easily integrated into lifestyle changes than conventional pharmacotherapeutics, and extensive research on diet and supplements concerning brain health is ongoing. Nutrition and supplements are covered in Chapter 13.

Engagement in mental activity also conveys neuroprotective and neuroplastic benefits during aging. Leisure activities that have demonstrated pro-cognitive effects include reading, solving puzzles, discussion groups, playing musical instruments, learning a second language, and participation in card and board games. Social activities that can improve cognition include traveling, dancing, attending art-related events, participating in social organizations, and spending time with family.

Regular exercise is beneficial for people with Parkinson's disorder, multiple sclerosis, mood disorders, posttraumatic stress disorder, and schizophrenia. How does physical activity do all this? The ability of physical activity to enhance BDNF release and function contributes to neuroplasticity and neurogenesis. Regular exercise improves the ability to maintain, repair, and reorganize circuits damaged during aging and disease. Other mechanisms include reduced inflammation, reduced stress response, improved gut biome activity, improved sleep, and improved antioxidant defense mechanisms (Phillips 2017b).

Health Risks

Phenothiazine-related drugs (typical antipsychotics) can cause serious muscle movement disorders, fast heartbeat, difficulty breathing, increased sweating, and loss of bladder control. They can add to the effects of alcohol and other central nervous system depressants (antihistamines, sedatives, prescription pain medicine, muscle relaxants, etc.). Atypical antipsychotics, such as olanzapine, can cause drowsiness, increased appetite, and weight gain. They can worsen diabetes and increase blood cholesterol, increasing the risk of heart disease. Side effects of benzodiazepines are related to their ability to cause muscle relaxation and sedation. Decreased alertness, concentration, and lack of coordination may result in injuries or driving impairment, particularly for the elderly. Discontinuation of benzodiazepines may result in a withdrawal syndrome that can include insomnia, agitation, tremors, and muscle spasms. Discontinuation can also cause a rebound effect where symptoms return, sometimes worse than the original condition.

In terms of the antidepressant drugs, the efficacy and relative safety of the SSRI and SSNRI compared to monoamine oxidase inhibitors and tricyclic antidepressants are the main reasons the older drugs are rarely prescribed. The SSRI and SSNRI can cause decreased sexual desire and ability. Other rare conditions include dry mouth, overactive reflexes or muscle spasms, and unwanted effects on the heart.

In the case of lithium, attention to dosage and fluid intake is important, because lithium has a narrow therapeutic window. Side effects include impairment of alertness and reaction time. Patients taking lithium should avoid becoming overheated or dehydrated in hot weather or during exercise. Early signs of lithium toxicity include nausea, vomiting, diarrhea, muscle weakness, and blurred vision.

PES Watch

Generally, the psychotherapeutic drugs are not ergogenic and are not on the WADA list of banned substances. There has been debate over the use of some of these drugs, due to their calming ability, and the edge they might provide during certain types of competition. But whereas beta-blockers are banned for certain types of competition, Valium and other benzodiazepines are currently not on the WADA Prohibited List.

Conclusion

Mental illness affects a significant portion of the population, many of which also suffer from poor cardiovascular health. This raises the question whether some component of mental illness is a consequence of poor physical health. Many of the common types of mental illness respond to drug therapy. However, in many cases the improvement is nominal, as these drugs do not cure the disease. They help the afflicted individuals cope and function better. Certain drugs or exercise increase production of nerve growth factors such as BDNF. BDNF contributes to neuroplasticity of the brain by increasing synaptic activity and the overall number and health of neurons. The lack of sufficient neurogenesis and plasticity may contribute to depression, bipolar disease, and age-related decrease in brain function.

Key Concepts Review

antidepressant
antipsychotic
anxiolytic
atypical antipsychotic
benzodiazepine
bipolar disorder
brain-derived neurotrophic factor
   (BDNF)
catecholamine-derived neurotransmitter
dopamine hypothesis
generalized anxiety disorder (GAD)
lithium
major depressive disorder (MDD)
MAO inhibitor
monoamine oxidase (MAO)
mood-stabilizing drug

neurogenesis theory
neuroleptic
neuroplasticity
neurotransmitter hypothesis
non-benzodiazepine
Parkinson's disease
phenothiazine
psychosis
schizophrenia
sedative-hypnotic
selective serotonin and norepinephrine
   reuptake inhibitors (SSNRI)
selective serotonin reuptake inhibitor
   (SSRI)
tricyclic antidepressant
typical antipsychotic

Review Questions

1   Some people think exercise and physical fitness are important to one's mental state. What evidence from this chapter would support this idea?
2   What evidence links poor cardiovascular health to poor mental health?

3   What can be done to combat the weight gain seen with certain antipsychotic drugs? What are the drawbacks of such approaches?

4   What is GABA, and what does it do?

5   Valium is a common benzodiazepine. How does it cause its sedative effect?

6   What is neurogenesis? How might it be monitored in humans?

7   Depression rates are on the increase. Why should exercise be part of the therapy?

8   Exercise is being considered as an adjunct therapy in bipolar disorder. Why?

9   Explain why you think Bo, in the opening vignette, was helped by running.

References

Abi-Dargham A, Laruelle M (2005) Mechanisms of action of second generation antipsychotic drugs in schizophrenia: insights from brain imaging studies. *Eur Psychiatry* 20:15–27

Alsuwaidan MT, Kucyl A, Law CWY, McIntyre RS (2009) Exercise and bipolar disorder: a review of neurobiological mediators. *Neuromol Med* 11:328–336

Asmundson GJ, Fetzner MG, Deboer LB, Powers MB, Otto MW, Smits JA (2013) Let's get physical: a contemporary review of the anxiolytic effects of exercise for anxiety and its disorders. *Depress Anxiety* 30:362–373

Aylett E, Small N, Bower P (2018) Exercise in the treatment of clinical anxiety in general practice - a systematic review and meta-analysis. *BMC Health Serv Res* 18:559

Ballon J, Stroup TS (2013) Polypharmacy for schizophrenia. *Curr Opin Psychiatry* 26:208–213

Berenson A (2007) Mom wonders if psychosis drug helped kill son. *The New York Times*. Retrieved from www.nytimes.com/2007/01/04/business/04drug.html?_r=0

Castren E, Rantamaki T (2010) Role of brain-derived neurotrophic factor in the aetiology of depression of antidepressant drugs. *CNS Drugs* 24:1–7

Cipriani A, Furukawa TA, Salanti G, Chaimani A, Atkinson LZ, Ogawa Y, Leucht S, Ruhe HG, Turner EH, Higgins JPT, Egger M, Takeshima N, Hayasaka Y, Imai H, Shinohara K, Tajika A, Ioannidis JPA, Geddes JR (2018) Comparative efficacy and acceptability of 21 antidepressant drugs for the acute treatment of adults with major depressive disorder: a systematic review and network meta-analysis. *Lancet* 391:1357–1366

Collomp K, Fortier M, Cooper S, Long A, Ahmaidi S, Prefaut C, Wright F, Picot M, Cote MG (1994) Performance and metabolic effects of benzodiazepine during submaximal exercise. *J Appl Physiol* 77:828–833

Cooney GM, Dwan K, Greig CA, Lawlor DA, Rimer J, Waugh FR, McMurdo M, Mead GE (2013) Exercise for depression. *Cochrane Database Syst Rev* 9:CD004366

Cotman CW, Berchtold NC (2002) Exercise: a behavioral intervention to enhance brain health and plasticity. *Trends Neurosci* 25:295–301

Cross-Disorder Group of the Psychiatric Genomics Consortium (2013) Identification of risk loci with shared effects on five major psychiatric disorders: a genome-wide analysis. *Lancet* 381:1371–1379

Dauwan M, Begemann MJ, Heringa SM, Sommer IE (2016) Exercise improves clinical symptoms, quality of life, global functioning, and depression in schizophrenia: a systematic review and meta-analysis. *Schizophr Bull* 42:588–599

DSM-V: Diagnostic and Statistical Manual of Mental Disorders (2013) 5th ed., published by the American Psychiatric Association

Duman CH, Schlesinger L, Russell DS, Duman RS (2008) Voluntary exercise produces antidepressant and anxiolytic behavioral effects in mice. *Brain Res* 1199:148–158

Ernst C, Olson AK, Pinel JPJ, Lam RW, Christie BR (2006) Antidepressant effects of exercise: evidence for an adult-neurogenesis hypothesis? *J Psychiatry Neurosci* 31:84–92

Fabel K, Kempermann G (2008) Physical activity and the regulation of neurogenesis in the adult and aging brain. *Neuromol Med* 10:59–66

Firth J, Cotter J, Elliott R, French P, Yung AR (2015) A systematic review and meta-analysis of exercise interventions in schizophrenia patients. *Psychol Med* 45:1343–1361

Food and Drug Administration (2013) FDA Drug Safety Communication: FDA is investigating two deaths following injection of long-acting antipsychotic Zyprexa Relprevv (olanzapine pamoate). Retrieved from www.fda.gov/drugs/drugsafety/ucm356971.htm

Galper D, Trivedi MH, Barlow CE, Dunn AL, Kampert JB (2006) Inverse association between physical inactivity and mental health in men and women. *Med & Sci Sports & Exercise* 38:173–178

Garza AA, Ha TG, Garcia C, Chen MJ, Russo-Neustadt AA (2004) Exercise, antidepressant treatment, and BDNF mRNA expression in the aging brain. *Pharmacol Biochem Behav* 77:209–220

Goldstein BI, Birmaher B, Carlson GA, DelBello MP, Findling RL, Fristad M, Kowatch RA, Miklowitz DJ, Nery FG, Perez-Algorta G, Van Meter A, Zeni CP, Correll CU, Kim HW, Wozniak J, Chang KD, Hillegers M, Youngstrom EA (2017) The International Society for Bipolar Disorders Task Force report on pediatric bipolar disorder: knowledge to date and directions for future research. *Bipolar Disord* 19:524–543

Gordon BR, McDowell CP, Lyons M, Herring MP (2017) The effects of resistance exercise training on anxiety: a meta-analysis and meta-regression analysis of randomized controlled trials. *Sports Med* 47:2521–2532

Gordon BR, McDowell CP, Hallgren M, Meyer JD, Lyons M, Herring MP (2018) Association of efficacy of resistance exercise training with depressive symptoms: meta-analysis and meta-regression analysis of randomized clinical trials. *JAMA Psychiatry* 75:566–576

Gujral S, Aizenstein H, Reynolds CF 3rd, Butters MA, Erickson KI (2017) Exercise effects on depression: possible neural mechanisms. *Gen Hosp Psychiatry* 49:2–10

Gurusamy J, Gandhi S, Damodharan D, Ganesan V, Palaniappan M (2018) Exercise, diet and educational interventions for metabolic syndrome in persons with schizophrenia: a systematic review. *Asian J Psychiatr* 36:73–85

Holley J, Crone D, Tyson P, Lovell G (2011) The effects of physical activity on psychological well-being for those with schizophrenia: a systematic review. *Brit J Clin Psychol* 50:84–105

Keck PE, McElroy SL (2003) Bipolar disorder, obesity, and pharmacotherapy-associated weight gain. *J Clin Psychiatry* 64:1426–1435

Knable MB, Weinberger DR (1997) Dopamine, the prefrontal cortex and schizophrenia. *J Psychopharmacol* 112:123–131

Laske C, Banschbach S, Stransky E, Bosch S, Straten G, Machann J, Fritsche A, Hipp A, Niess A, Eschweiler GW (2010) Exercise-induced normalization of decreased BDNF serum concentration in elderly women with remitted major depression. *Int J Neuropsychopharmacol* 13:1–8

Law LL, Barnett F, Yau MK, Gray MA (2014) Effects of functional tasks exercise on older adults with cognitive impairment at risk of Alzheimer's disease: a randomised controlled trial. *Age Ageing* 0:1–8 doi:10.1093/ageing/afu055

Lövdén M, Xu W, Wang HX (2013) Lifestyle change and the prevention of cognitive decline and dementia: what is the evidence? *Curr Opin Psychiatry* 26:239–243

Malberg JE, Eisch AJ, Nestler EJ, Duman RS (2000) Chronic antidepressant treatment increases neurogenesis in adult rat hippocampus. *J Neurosci* 20:9104–9110

Malchow B, Keller K, Hasan A, Dörfler S, Schneider-Axmann T, Hillmer-Vogel U, Honer WG, Schulze TG, Niklas A, Wobrock T, Schmitt A, Falkai P (2015) Effects of endurance training combined with cognitive remediation on everyday functioning, symptoms, and cognition in multiepisode schizophrenia patients. *Schizophr Bull* 41:847–858

Melo MC, Daher Ede F, Albuquerque SG, de Bruin VM (2016) Exercise in bipolar patients: a systematic review. *J Affect Disord* 198:32–38

Metcalfe AW, MacIntosh BJ, Scavone A, Ou X, Korczak D, Goldstein BI (2016) Effects of acute aerobic exercise on neural correlates of attention and inhibition in adolescents with bipolar disorder. *Transl Psychiatry* 6:e814

Möhler H, Fritschy JM, Rudolph U (2002) A new benzodiazepine pharmacology. *J Pharmacol Exp Ther* 300:2–8

Moore AA, Sawyers Cl, Adkins DE, Docherty AR (2018) Opportunities for an enhanced integration of neuroscience and genomics. *Brain Imaging Behav* 12:1211–1219

Mura G, Moro MF, Patten SB, Carta MG (2014) Exercise as an add-on strategy for the treatment of major depressive disorder: a systematic review. *CNS Spectr* 19:496–508

Murri MB, Ekkekakis P, Magagnoli M, Zampogna D, Cattedra S, Capobianco L, Serafini G, Calcagno P, Zanetidou S, Amore M (2019) Physical exercise in major depression: reducing the mortality gap while improving clinical outcomes. *Front Psychiatry* 9:762

National Alliance on Mental Illness. (n.d.) Retrieved from www.nami.org/

National Institute of Mental Health. (n.d.) *Bipolar disorder.* Retrieved from www.nimh.nih.gov/health/topics/bipolar-disorder/index.shtml

National Institute of Mental Health. (n.d.) *Statistics.* Retrieved from www.nimh.nih.gov/statistics/

Penninx BWJH, Lange SMM (2018) Metabolic syndrome in psychiatric patients: overview, mechanisms, and implications. *Dialogues Clin Neurosci* 20:63–73

Perera TD, Coplan JD, Lisanby SH, Lipira CM, Arif M, Carpio C, Spitzer G, Santarelli L, Scharf B, Hen R, Rosoklija G, Sackeim HA, Dwork AJ (2007) Antidepressant-induced neurogenesis in the hippocampus of adult nonhuman primates. *J Neurosci* 27:4894–4901

Phillips C, Baktir MA, Das D, Lin B, Salehi A (2015) The link between physical activity and cognitive dysfunction in Alzheimer disease. *Phys Ther* 95:1046–1060

Phillips C (2017a) Lifestyle modulators of neuroplasticity: how physical activity, mental engagement, and diet promote cognitive health during aging. *Neural Plast* 2017:3589271

Phillips C (2017b) Physical activity modulates common neuroplasticity substrates in major depressive and bipolar disorder. *Neural Plast* 2017:7014146

Pozuelo L, Tesar G, Zhang J, Penn M, Franco K, Jiang W (2009) Depression and heart disease: what do we know, and where are we headed? *Cleve Clin J Med* 76:59–70

Rethorst CD, Trivedi MH (2013) Evidence-based recommendations for the prescription of exercise for major depressive disorder. *J Psychiatr Pract* 19:204–212

Saddichha S, Manjunatha N, Ameen S, Akhtar S (2008) Metabolic syndrome in first episode schizophrenia—A randomized double-blind controlled, short-term prospective study. *Schizophr Res* 101:266–272

Salam JN, Foxa JH, DeTroya EM, Guignona MH, Wohla DF, Falls WA (2009) Voluntary exercise in C57 mice is anxiolytic across several measures of anxiety. *Behavioral Brain Res* 197:31–40

Schmidt CW (2007) Environmental connections: a deeper look into mental illness. *Environ Health Perspect* 115:A404–A410

Shulman M, Miller A, Misher J, Tentler A (2014) Managing cardiovascular disease risk in patients treated with antipsychotics: a multidisciplinary approach. *J Multidiscip Healthc* 31:489–501

Stathopoulou G, Powers MB, Berry AC, Smits JAJ, Otto MW (2006) Exercise interventions for mental health: a quantitative and qualitative review. *Clin Psychol Sci Prac* 13:179–193

Strickland JC, Smith MA (2014) The anxiolytic effects of resistance exercise. *Front Psychol* 5:753

Stubbs B, Vancampfort D, Rosenbaum S, Firth J, Cosco T, Veronese N, Salum GA, Schuch FB (2017) An examination of the anxiolytic effects of exercise for people with anxiety and stress-related disorders: a meta-analysis. *Psychiatry Res* 249:102–108

Sylvia LG, Ametrano RM, Nierenberg AA (2010) Exercise treatment for bipolar disorder: potential mechanisms of action mediated through increased neurogenesis and decreased allostatic load. *Psychother Psychosom* 79:87–96

Taspinar B, Aslan UB, Agbuga B, Taspinar F (2014) A comparison of the effects of hatha yoga and resistance exercise on mental health and well-being in sedentary adults: a pilot study. *Complement Ther Med* 22:433–440

Tehrani MH, Tate CA, al-Dahan MI (1995) Age-related levels of GABA/benzodiazepine binding sites in cerebrum of F-344 rats: effects of exercise. *Neurobiol Aging* 16:199–204

ten Brinke LF, Bolandzadeh N, Nagamatsu LS, Hsu CL, Davis JC, Miran-Khan K, Liu-Ambrose T (2015) Aerobic exercise increases hippocampal volume in older women with probable mild cognitive impairment: a 6-month randomised controlled trial. *Br J Sports Med* 49:248–254

Tong L, Shen H, Perreau VM, Balazs R, Cotman CW (2001) Effects of exercise on gene-expression profile in the rat hippocampus. *Neurobiol Dis* 8:1046–1056

Vitetta L, Anton B, Cortizo F, Sali A (2005) Mind-body medicine: stress and its impact on overall health and longevity. *Ann N Y Acad Sci* 1057:492–505

Wu MK, Wang CK, Bai YM, Huang CY, Lee SD (2007) Outcomes of obese, clozapine-treated inpatients with schizophrenia placed on a six-month diet and physical activity program. *Psychiatr Serv* 58:544–550

10 Lipid-Modifying Agents

Abstract

One of the major risk factors for cardiovascular disease involves elevated levels of cholesterol-containing lipoproteins in the blood. Individuals who are hyperlipidemic or dyslipidemic are at a much higher risk of heart and related diseases. The atherogenic profile consists of the triad: (1) elevated LDL, (2) low HDL, and (3) elevated triglycerides. This lipid profile is also seen in patients with metabolic syndrome. The processing, distribution, and synthesis of cholesterol involve complex processes that include a host of lipoproteins. LDL, HDL, and the liver are central to maintaining cholesterol homeostasis. Genetics, diet, physical activity, and other factors are critical in maintaining a healthy lipoprotein profile. When lifestyle changes are inadequate to correct lipoprotein abnormalities, drug intervention is needed.

Four major classes of lipid-modifying agents are commonly used. Statins block HMG-CoA-reductase and decrease the production of cholesterol, ultimately decreasing the formation of LDL. The decrease in cholesterol synthesis makes cells more dependent on LDL uptake from the blood, decreasing LDL levels further. A resulting increase in reverse cholesterol transport back to the liver causes an increase in HDL levels. Niacin decreases release of VLDL from the liver. It inhibits the lipase activity in adipose tissues, decreasing free fatty acid release and slowing the formation of lipoproteins in the blood. Fibrates stimulate lipoprotein lipase in the vascular lining, leading to the breakdown of triglycerides. Fibrates also increase the oxidation of free fatty acids in liver and muscle and suppress synthetic pathways, so less VLDL and triglycerides are produced. The fourth class of agents works in the gut. These agents block dietary cholesterol uptake or bind bile acids and increase their rate of excretion. This class of agents is often used in conjunction with one of the other three classes of drugs. Exercise and diet can improve the atherogenic profile by mechanisms similar to those of the lipid-modifying agents. Maintaining a good diet and an active lifestyle can reduce the need for or required dosage of these agents.

CASE EXAMPLE

Megan's dad Bob has high cholesterol besides high blood pressure. Bob gets some exercise walking the dog, playing golf, and bowling, but nothing that qualifies as moderate or high intensity. He used to stop at the gym a couple of times a week and do the circuit of weight machines, but he has stopped going because it hurts—he has muscle aches much worse than when he was younger. Bob has his annual checkup and the doctor is pleased that his hypertension is under control. Bob's LDL (the "bad") is okay now that he is taking the statin atorvastatin (Lipitor). Bob's HDL is still on the low side of the desirable range. Part of this may be that Bob still hasn't quit smoking, his diet isn't great, he drinks too much beer, and he doesn't get any moderate or intense exercise. The Lipitor is working, and Bob's total cholesterol is under the desirable 200 mg/dL target. Dr. Casey asks Bob if he is having any muscle problems. Statins can cause **myopathy** (dysfunction of muscle fibers resulting in muscular weakness) as a side effect, and it can occur days to months after the start of treatment. Bob tells Dr. Casey about his issue doing resistance exercise. Dr. Casey decides to cut his dose by 50% and asks him to have blood work done in six months to confirm that his cholesterol levels are still okay. The goal is to take the lowest dose of statin that manages LDL levels. The lower dose may also help with managing the muscle soreness. She also cautions him that if the muscle soreness is extreme and persists, he should drink lots of fluid and call the office. They will run a blood test for creatine kinase (which indicates muscle cell damage) and determine if he has high levels of muscle protein in the blood (myoglobinuria). If the lower dose of the statin does not help, she will prescribe a different one from the many that are on the market, as the different statins vary among patients in their degree of muscle soreness. It is not uncommon for patients to try several different statins to find the one they tolerate best. In many cases, patients just stop taking the drug because of the muscle soreness—non-compliance is common with statins.

Introduction

About 600,000 people in the United States die from coronary heart disease each year (Centers for Disease Control and Prevention, 2014). Exercise can help reduce the risk, but only 25% of the adult population exercises regularly. The younger generation also has bad eating and exercise practices. **Hyperlipidemia** (elevated levels of blood lipids) is a positive risk factor for cardiovascular disease. Diet and exercise should be considered as treatment before drugs, but these often are not effective in keeping levels low, even with a high level of compliance. Some people have a genetic predisposition toward high blood lipids and require drug intervention, since diet and exercise are insufficient. Cholesterol-lowering drugs are annually in the top 10 for drug sales; Lipitor was #1 for the better part of a decade. The total accumulated sales of Lipitor globally exceeded $125 billion in 2012. A generic version became available in the United States in 2011, and Lipitor sales decreased from $9.6 billion in 2011 to $3.9 billion in 2012. Other statins remain in the top 10 for global drug sales. An estimated 25% of the U.S. population over 45 years old has been prescribed a statin, with the number expected to climb. The immense size of the global market for these drugs creates many issues for the health-care industry and its relationship to drug companies. Although the drugs are very useful for lowering blood lipids and reducing the risk of cardiovascular disease, diet and exercise are also effective and work well in conjunction with these drugs.

Cholesterol Biosynthesis

Cholesterol is a necessary component of the cell membrane and an important precursor for steroid hormone synthesis. Some of the needed cholesterol is obtained in the diet, and the remainder is synthesized, primarily in the liver. Cholesterol biosynthesis is a complex, energy-requiring process that involves many steps and several biologically important intermediates. The liver is the center for cholesterol metabolism and distribution, but most cells in the body have the capability of producing their own cholesterol. Since cholesterol production has a significant energy cost associated with it, most cells import it from the blood. The liver's role is to maintain proper lipid levels in the blood. Cholesterol is classified chemically as a steroid and is not soluble in water. When the liver produces cholesterol for export, it packages it within a spherical phospholipid particle composed of a single layer (monolayer) of phospholipids with an embedded targeting protein. The targeting protein on the surface of this lipoprotein particle is important for the interaction, maturation, and transport of the lipoprotein particles. These lipoprotein complexes stay suspended in the blood, solving the cholesterol solubility problem, because the cholesterol is packaged inside the particle and does not come in contact with aqueous environment in the blood.

However, if the blood level of these lipoprotein complexes becomes too high, they attach to arterial linings in increasing amounts, especially at sites of damage or areas of high turbulence. Scarring and inflammation result from this buildup, causing plaques to form along the wall of the vasculature. The progression of these events leads to atherosclerosis and hardening of the arteries. Arteries lose their elasticity and their ability to adapt to changes in blood pressure. For example, arteries cannot respond properly to nitric oxide to dilate and increase blood flow, as discussed in Chapter 4. The heart can then become damaged from hypoxia (low oxygen) when the demand for increased blood flow to the heart cannot be met during conditions such as increased physical activity. A ruptured plaque could also decrease blood flow to the heart, causing hypoxia or a heart attack.

Types of Lipoprotein Complexes Involved

Several types of lipoprotein complexes are involved in cholesterol transport; they share similar structure with LDL, with phospholipid monolayers and distinct targeting proteins.

The liver secretes **very low-density lipoprotein (VLDL)** into the blood (see Figure 10.1). VLDL contains cholesterol and triglycerides. The action of **lipoprotein lipase (LPL)**, an enzyme on the surface of endothelial cells lining the vasculature, releases free fatty acids (FFA) from the triglycerides in the VLDL. Adipose cells, as well as other cells such as liver and muscle, take up the free fatty acids. The remnants of VLDL (sometimes called IDL, for intermediate-density lipoprotein) are converted to **low-density lipoprotein (LDL)** following additional enzyme activity. The important point is that the liver secretes VLDL, which is ultimately converted to LDL, because some of the drugs we will discuss decrease VLDL release and subsequent LDL formation. The two most important lipoproteins involved in cholesterol transport are LDL, the "bad," and **high-density lipoprotein (HDL)**, the "good." High levels of LDL (and the cholesterol that it contains) are associated with plaque formation and atherosclerosis; hence, LDL levels correlate positively with cardiovascular disease (the more LDL, the greater chance of disease). The relationship between LDL levels and heart disease is actually a little more complicated. LDL exists in two major forms: small, dense particles and larger, more buoyant particles. The small, dense particles correlate better with arteriosclerosis and heart disease. The relationship and interconversion of the two types are not exactly clear, but the dense particles are more associated with poor diet, diabetes, and obesity. The fraction of buoyant particles increases with physical activity and healthier diets.

HDL encompasses a mixture of closely related lipoproteins, and its formation is similarly complex. It can be formed from VLDL remnants and chylomicron remnants. Chylomicrons are lipoprotein particles that distribute lipids derived from the diet (see Figure 10.1). HDL also functions in reverse cholesterol transport, moving cholesterol from tissues back to the liver. Reverse cholesterol transport is a hot area of research as it has potential to decrease blood cholesterol levels. HDL may provide anti-inflammatory activity in the arterial walls, helping to slow the atherogenic process. HDL is considered "the good cholesterol" because its level correlates inversely with cardiovascular disease (the more HDL, the less chance of disease). This observation is true to a point, as abnormally high levels are associated with cardiovascular problems—as are abnormally low levels (Moradi, Streja, & Kalantar-Zadeh 2017).

Figure 10.1 Overview of LDL and HDL formation.

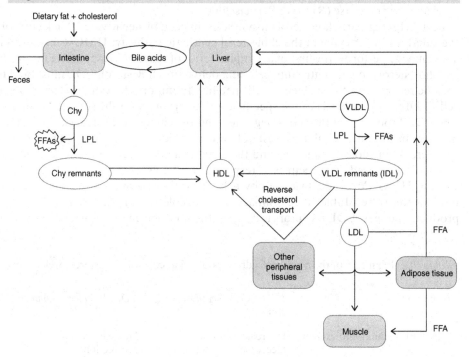

Legend: A highly schematic representation of the flow of lipid through different compartments is shown. Dietary fat is released as chylomicrons (Chy). Lipoprotein lipase (LPL) liberates free fatty acids (FFA) and other lipids from the chylomicrons and VLDL, leaving remnants behind that are incorporated into or/ captured by other lipoproteins. VLDL is released by the liver and is a precursor for other lipoproteins, such as LDL and HDL. The identity of many of these lipoproteins is attributable to the protein component, which is a detail not shown in this figure. The VLDL remnants are also called IDL (intermediate-density lipoprotein). LDL delivery to tissues is shown at the bottom, and reverse transport of HDL cholesterol to the liver is also indicated. The distribution of free fatty acids is also shown.

Table 10.1 Classification of blood levels for LDL, HDL, and triglycerides

Diagnosis	LDL cholesterol	HDL cholesterol	Total cholesterol	Triglycerides
Desirable Optimal	<130 <100	40–60	<200	<120
Borderline	130–159		200–240	120–199
High	160–189	>60	>240	200–499
Very High	>190			>500

Legend: Values shown are all expressed in mg/dL. Modified from ATP guidelines and other sources.

Assessing the risk for cardiovascular disease involves monitoring total cholesterol (the combined amount of cholesterol packaged in the different lipoproteins), as well as ratios such as LDL to HDL and total cholesterol to HDL (see Table 10.1). The evaluation and regulation of total LDL levels continue to be important in preventing arteriosclerosis and heart disease (Rizzo & Berneis 2006).

LDL helps regulate cholesterol biosynthesis, in part, by negative feedback control on the rate-limiting enzyme in the cholesterol synthetic pathway: **HMG-CoA-reductase**. This enzyme performs the first of a complex series of reactions responsible for producing cholesterol. To gain entry into cells and deliver its cholesterol, LDL must bind to a specific receptor on the surface of cells needing to import cholesterol. The importing cell's LDL receptor binds to the specific targeting protein on the surface of the LDL. The LDL brought into the cell is degraded and the cholesterol is released, causing an increase in the intracellular cholesterol concentration. HMG-CoA-reductase senses the increase in cholesterol levels, and the enzyme activity decreases, so less new cholesterol is produced. The reciprocal response is true, as well: when cholesterol levels are low, HMG-CoA-reductase activity is high, so that there is an increase in cholesterol synthesis (see Table 10.2). Similarly, when cholesterol levels are high in the cell, production of new LDL receptors is decreased, and when cholesterol levels are low the

Table 10.2 Examples of the negative feedback loops that control cholesterol level

Condition	HMG-CoA-Reductase Response	LDL Receptor Response
High intracellular cholesterol	Decrease activity Decrease cholesterol biosynthesis	Decrease receptor production Decrease LDL uptake
Low intracellular cholesterol (standard diet, regular exercise)	Increase activity Increase cholesterol biosynthesis	Increase receptor production Increase LDL uptake
Decrease intracellular cholesterol (drug treatment, such as statin)	Decrease activity Decrease cholesterol biosynthesis	Increase receptor production Increase LDL uptake

expression of new LDL receptors increases. Therefore, the cell adjusts its rate of pro-duction of cholesterol with its ability to import LDL from the blood. As we will discuss below, drugs that inhibit HMG-CoA-reductase and reduce intracellular cholesterol cause an increase in LDL-receptors at the cell surface and a reduction in circulating LDL (see Table 10.2).

If the cells' ability to import LDL is compromised, then there is a serious problem. The cells will continue to make cholesterol even though there is plenty outside the cell in the form of LDL. LDL levels in the blood rise, because the cells cannot import it. As mentioned above, high LDL levels in the blood lead to hardening of the arteries and cardiovascular disease. Genetic analysis of patients with familial hypercholesterolemia show that the defect is in the gene coding for the LDL receptor (see Box). Homozygotes (individuals with similar alleles at a particular genetic locus) for the disease allele can die from clogged arteries by the age of 10 if untreated. Heterozygotes (one normal allele and one disease allele) can have LDL levels over 250 mg/dl. Although it is clear that dietary cholesterol intake and physical activity can also affect LDL and HDL levels, one's genetic makeup contributes significantly in the case of hypercholesterolemia. In-dividuals with defective LDL receptors require drug intervention to lower their LDL levels. There is a genetic basis for other dyslipidemias. **Dyslipidemia** refers to a condition marked by an abnormal concentration of lipids or lipoproteins in the blood, such as elevated triglycerides. Prolonged elevated triglycerides can cause significant cardiovas-cular problems and also contribute to pancreatitis. Genetic makeup plays an important role in dyslipidemias, in addition to diet, physical activity, and other risk factors.

The Discovery of the Receptor for LDL and a Role for Receptor-Mediated Endocytosis

In the early 1970s, Michael Brown and Joseph Goldstein began their seminal studies in the control of cholesterol metabolism. These experiments resulted in their receiving the Nobel Prize in 1986 (Brown & Goldstein 1986). Using normal human cells (fibroblasts) grown in tissue culture, they showed that HMG-CoA-reductase activity was proportional to the concentration of LDL and VLDL in the culture medium. When they repeated the experiment with cells from patients with familial hypercholesterolemia, the HMG-CoA-reductase activity did not decrease with the addition of LDL (or VLDL), resulting in an overproduction of cholesterol. The defect was not in the LDL itself, as LDL from patients with familial hypercholesterolemia worked fine with normal fibroblasts. The defect was not with HMG-CoA-reductase, either. This result was shown in a clever experiment shown in Figure 10.2 (Brown, Dana, & Goldstein 1974). When cho-lesterol is provided in the form of LDL (solid symbols), the normal cells (circles) respond with a decrease in HMG-CoA-reductase activity. The cells from a pa-tient homozygous for the disease allele do not respond to the added LDL (closed triangles). If cholesterol is dissolved in ethanol, so that it can pass through the membrane and enter cells directly, then both the mutant cells and the normal cells respond with decreased HMG-CoA-reductase activity. Therefore, the de-fect in familial hypercholesterolemia must involve the mechanism by which LDL enters the cell and is processed into cholesterol.

Figure 10.2 Effect of cholesterol on HMG-CoA-reductase activity in cultured human fibroblasts.

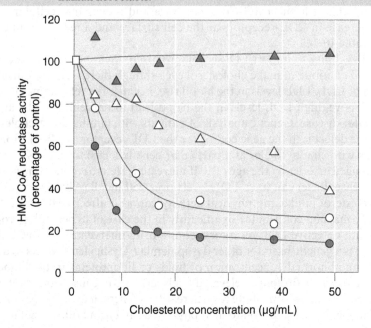

Legend: Human fibroblasts were grown for six days and were given new medium (deficient in lipoproteins) with cholesterol supplemented as LDL (closed symbols) or dissolved in ethanol (open symbols). After six hours, cells were processed to determine HMG-CoA-reductase activity. Circles represent normal fibroblasts, and triangles represent cells from patients homozygous for familial hypercholesterolemia. Note that the normal cells (open and closed circles) respond to increasing cholesterol with low HMG-CoA-reductase activity, whereas the mutant cells do not respond to cholesterol in the form of LDL (closed triangles). They respond only to cholesterol dissolved in ethanol (open triangles), showing that the defect is not with the HMG-CoA-reductase activity (Brown, Dana, & Goldstein 1974).

Back in the 1970s, not a lot was known about the process called **receptor-mediated endocytosis**, the transport of proteins and particles into a cell, of which cholesterol transport is an example. The work of Brown and Goldstein contributed significantly to our current understanding. They showed that the mutation in familial hypercholesterolemia was located in the gene for the LDL receptor. In some mutants, the receptor was not synthesized. In other mutants, the receptor was not processed correctly and never made it to the cell surface. A third class of mutant receptor made it to the cell surface but could not bind LDL.

In Brown and Goldstein's initial studies, a single example of a fourth class of mutant receptor was identified. Referred to as JD (related to the initials of the donor of the fibroblasts), this mutant receptor bound LDL at the cell surface but could not internalize it—the defect was in endocytosis (see Figure 10.3). Normally, the LDL receptor aggregates in structures on the cell surface called coated pits. The pits internalize and become cytoplasmic vesicles containing the imported LDL bound to its receptor. The vesicles fuse with lysosomes, LDL is

Figure 10.3 Internalization and degradation of radioactively labeled LDL in fibroblasts from a normal subject and a patient (JD) with familial hypercholesterolemia.

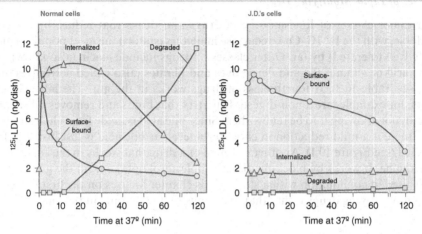

Legend: Cells were allowed to bind labeled LDL at 4° for two hours. The cells were then placed at 37° for the indicated time. Surface-bound radioactivity was distinguished from internalized radioactivity with a specific washing procedure and compared to the amount of radioactivity released from the cells as a result of protein degradation. Cells from JD are able to bind but not internalize LDL, and normal degradation and processing do not take place (Brown & Goldstein 1986).

degraded, and the cholesterol is released into the cytoplasm (Brown & Goldstein). In the case of cells from JD, LDL receptors could not enter the coated pits and, therefore, could not internalize the bound LDL (see Figure 10.3). The receptors remained dispersed on the surface of the cell. Since cells from JD cannot properly perform receptor-mediated endocytosis, the LDL is not degraded, and the cholesterol is not available to the cell. When the DNA sequence for JD's mutant gene was determined, a single point mutation was found on the relatively short cytoplasmic tail of the receptor. This single amino acid change was responsible for failure of the receptor to associate with coated pits and, ultimately, a shortened lifespan due to markedly elevated LDL levels in the blood.

The work by Brown and Goldstein was profound on many levels. They used human genetics to identify a human disease gene. They used human cells to describe the biological defect—the phenotype of the disease alleles. They studied the enzymology and biochemistry of HMG-CoA-reductase. They discovered the importance of receptor-mediated endocytosis, contributing to our understanding of this process at the cellular level. Their work provided the fundamental knowledge necessary to understand critical aspects of human health as it relates to cholesterol. They discovered that a group of previously described compounds derived from mold (the statins) were competitive inhibitors for HMG-CoA-reductase. Their basic research on the control of cholesterol synthesis led to the successful implementation of the statin class of drugs to treat dyslipidemias.

Lipid-Modifying Drugs

Classes of Lipid-Modifying Drugs

Four major classes of lipid-modifying drugs and drugs that reduce lipid levels are available, with the **HMG-CoA-reductase inhibitors (statins)** the most popular (and generally well tolerated) by far. Other classes of drugs include **niacin** (also known as **nicotinic acid** or **vitamin B$_3$**) and derivatives and **fibrates** (also called **derivatives of fibric acid**; see Table 10.3). A fourth class of drugs works in the gut. The **bile acid sequestrants**, for example, are a non-digestible matrix that binds and removes bile acid from the gut, not allowing it to be reabsorbed. Since bile acid is made from cholesterol in the liver, there is a mild reduction in cholesterol level, as bile acid is lost instead of being recycled (see Figure 10.1). Another example of a drug that works in the small intestine is **ezetimibe**. It works by blocking dietary cholesterol uptake from the gut. It is sometimes used in conjunction with a statin. This chapter focuses on the first three classes of lipid-modifying drugs rather than the drugs that work only in the gut.

How Do Lipid-Modifying Drugs Work?

Dyslipidemia encompasses a variety of lipid abnormalities. For our purposes, we will focus on the triad of abnormalities associated with the **atherogenic profile**. The three important lipid concerns that make up the profile are: (1) elevated triglycerides, (2) low HDL, and (3) high LDL (particularly the smaller, denser subfraction of LDL). Lipid-modifying agents are primarily used to decrease LDL and triglyceride levels in the blood. An increase in HDL is also a desired outcome. The different strategies include: block cholesterol synthesis, slow the release or the mobilization of lipid reserves, stimulate lipid breakdown (activate lipases; see Table 10.3), or block absorption from the gut. In conjunction with lifestyle changes, such as a diet lower in fat and regular aerobic exercise, these drugs can usually maintain blood lipids in the healthy range.

Statins

The class of drugs referred to as statins are competitive inhibitors for the rate-limiting step in cholesterol biosynthesis—HMG-CoA-reductase. Originally isolated from mold and fungi, these chemicals are substrate analogs, having a chemical structure that resembles the cellular substrate for HMG-CoA-reductase. Statins decrease

Table 10.3 Sites of action for lipid-modifying drugs

Drug	Location	Activity
HMG-CoA-reductase inhibitors statins	Liver primarily	Inhibit HMG-CoA-reductase
Niacin (nicotinic acid) derivatives Acipimox	Adipocytes, Liver	Inhibit lipolysis, decrease VLDL release
Fibrates (fibric acid derivatives) Fenofibrate	Vascular surface, liver, muscle	Stimulate lipoprotein lipase, stimulate PPARα pathway

HMG-CoA-reductase activity, causing a decrease in cellular cholesterol levels. The decrease in cholesterol levels stimulates the production of LDL receptors that are transported to the cell surface (see Table 10.2). The increase in receptors at the cell surface improves the cell's ability to import LDL, thereby decreasing LDL levels in the blood. Statins are generally well tolerated and effective at decreasing LDL. A large-scale meta-analysis found consistent evidence for a reduction in LDL and total cholesterol with at least three of the most widely used statins (Naci, Brugts, Fleurence, & Ades 2013). Whether statin-reduced cholesterol levels are associated with a reduction in morbidity has been less clear, but there is evidence that significantly lowering LDL cholesterol lowers the risk of cardiovascular events (LaRosa, Pedersen, Somatane, & Wasserman 2013; Stone, Robinson, Lichtenstein, et al. 2014).

Certain intermediates of cholesterol biosynthesis have biological activity, so inhibition of HMG-CoA-reductase can produce additional effects. These intermediates include molecules important in the attachment of sugars to proteins (formation of glycoproteins) and the modification of proteins with lipids required for protein association with membranes. However, the statins do not appear to impair these robust cellular processes significantly at recommended doses. Another intermediate of cholesterol metabolism is required for **coenzyme Q** production, an important electron carrier involved in mitochondrial ATP production. Some statin users who suffer muscle soreness find relief with supplemental coenzyme Q (discussed in Chapter 13). It is not clear if these other responses to statins are responsible for the myopathies that occur in about 15% of statin users (Bonetti, Lerman, Napoli, & Lerman 2003), but statins may negatively affect muscle cell mitochondria (Thompson & Parker 2013). Considering the typical prolonged use of statins (e.g., lifetime), cholesterol levels require regular monitoring, such as during an annual checkup (Fernandez, Spatz, Jablecki, & Phillips 2011).

Niacin Derivatives

Niacin (also called nicotinic acid or vitamin B_3) is an effective treatment for dyslipidemia. The characterization of its receptor provided insights into how it works (Vosper 2009). Niacin effectively increases HDL and decreases LDL. It does this by inhibiting lipolysis (breakdown of lipids) in adipose tissue, decreasing the release of free fatty acids. The flow of lipids between the different lipoproteins is altered, helping to generate the new lipid profile. Niacin also decreases the secretion of VLDL from the liver, which slows the generation of new LDL particles (see Figure 10.1).

Niacin elicits a variety of responses that may depend on the tissue type (Zeman, Vecka, Perlík, et al. 2016). Compliance is an issue with niacin because one of the side effects is flushing of the skin. The cause of the flushing is being sorted out (Ma, Lee, Mao, et al. 2014) and is distinct from the lipid-lowering effects (Vosper 2011). Extended-release formulations can reduce the flushing and have similar results on blood lipid profiles. Aspirin, which blocks prostaglandin synthesis (see the next chapter for more details), and potential other drugs, can also help reduce the flushing (Vosper 2011).

Acipimox is a related drug that works through the same receptor as niacin. Compared to niacin, it causes a longer sustained inhibition of lipase activity and interferes less with insulin control of sugar and lipid metabolism. It is effective at lower doses than niacin; hence, it results in fewer side effects (such as flushing) and is better tolerated than niacin (Vosper 2009).

Fibrates

The fibrates are also referred to as fibric acid derivatives. They are considered broad-spectrum lipid-lowering drugs. Fibrates effectively lower triglycerides but have less effect on lowering LDL and or increasing HDL. Fibrates stimulate the activity of lipoprotein lipase (the enzyme that hydrolyzes triglycerides in lipoproteins) and enhance catabolism of triglyceride-rich particles. Fibrates also reduce production and secretion of VLDL in the liver by altering lipid metabolism. Fibrates activate the **PPARα (peroxisome proliferator-activated receptor-α) pathway**, which alters the expression of genes involved in lipid metabolism. The PPAR-alpha pathway normally responds to lipid metabolites and unsaturated fatty acids to up-regulate lipid metabolism in liver and muscle. Activation of this pathway increases the oxidation of fatty acids and reduces triglyceride synthesis, causing a decrease in VLDL production. A new drug, Pemafibrate, is a novel selective PPARα modulator and effectively lowers triglycerides. It showed a good safety profile and efficacy in correcting lipid abnormalities in a broad range of patients, including those with chronic kidney disease (Yokote, Yamashita, Arai, et al. 2019). Interestingly, niacin may also work in part by activating PPARα and PPARγ (gamma) pathways in skeletal muscle and liver, resulting in increased expression of genes involved in lipid utilization (Tenenbaum & Fisman 2012). The activation of pathways for lipid oxidation is similar to the response observed following chronic aerobic exercise (Vosper 2011). You may remember a brief discussion of muscle fiber conversion in Chapter 2, where the PPAR pathways were mentioned. These pathways will be discussed again in Chapter 13 in connection with omega-3 fatty acids.

Exercise Pharmacology

Pharmacokinetic Concerns

The lipid-modifying agents, like many of the drugs we have discussed, do not have an extensive literature on the effect of exercise on their pharmacokinetic properties. From some of the basic pharmacokinetic data, we can infer possible interactions with exercise, especially because the liver is central to the action of these drugs. Another aspect has to do with the diurnal cycle for cholesterol biosynthesis in humans. Since cholesterol biosynthesis occurs primarily at night, many of these drugs are taken before bed. Exercise interactions affecting their pharmacokinetics are, therefore, temporally shifted. However, as we will discuss under pharmacodynamics in greater detail, these drugs are taken chronically. It can take weeks of treatment for the drugs to generate a new lipoprotein steady state. Moreover, most patients will take them for the rest of their life. As we will see, exercise can complement and enhance the lipid-modifying activity of these agents. For these patients, regular exercise is strongly recommended.

Statins

The statin class of drugs includes a wide variety of members. Some, such as lovastatin and simvastatin, are given as pro-drugs that are chemically altered in the GI-tract. Most statins are absorbed at 40% to 70% of the dose and are subjected to a high level of first-pass extraction by the liver. Only 5% to 20% is excreted by the kidneys, suggesting that a relatively small amount of the drug works in non-liver tissues. Most of the rest of the drug is excreted in the bile. As the liver is the central player in cholesterol homeostasis, statins are effective at significantly lowering LDL levels, with a modest increase in HDL and decrease in triglycerides. The serum half-lives vary for the different family members; many of the commonly used drugs have a half-life of one to three hours, and some newer drugs are in the 12-hour range. Since cholesterol biosynthesis occurs mostly at night, part of the daily dose is given after dinner or before bed, with a low-fat snack to help with absorption and effectiveness.

With the liver being of central focus for statin action, intense exercise could extend the drug's half-life, as blood flow to the liver decreases for drugs given in multiple doses a day. The myopathy associated with statins discussed earlier is related to blood concentration, so factors that potentially increase blood levels should be monitored. Myopathy results from dysfunction of muscle fibers, resulting in muscular weakness. Other symptoms of myopathy can include muscle cramps, stiffness, and spasm. Statins vary in the water solubility; more lipophilic drugs concentrate to the liver and the hydrophilic ones distribute more in the circulation giving them access to muscle cells. Besides vigorous exercise (and decreased blood flow to the liver), low body mass index and advanced age can be factors in elevating statin levels in the blood. Drug interactions and dietary factors can also alter the metabolic profile for statins and increase possible side effects. Drugs that can negatively interact with statins, such as certain antifungals, calcium channel blockers, and antibiotics, affect certain cytochrome P450 oxidases, decrease statin metabolism/elimination, and increase the risk of myopathies (Fernandez et al.). Consumption of large amounts of grapefruit or cranberry juice and excessive alcohol consumption have also been linked to possible shifts in drug metabolism and increased side effects, such as myopathies.

Niacin Derivatives

Niacin is rapidly and extensively absorbed when taken orally. It has biological activity independent of being converted to an important coenzyme in metabolism (NAD). It has a short plasma half-life (less than an hour), with 60% to 78% excreted in the urine unchanged or as metabolites. Niacin is subject to extensive first-pass metabolism in the liver, suggesting that conditions that affect liver function can alter niacin effectiveness. These factors include age, drug combinations, diet, alcohol consumption, and exercise. Because of the short half-life, controlled-release and extended-release formulations have been marketed. The extended-release formulation provides effective lipid-modifying activity, sometimes with a reduced side effect of flushing (Vosper 2009, 2011). However, it can be harder on the liver, so it is not recommended for patients with liver disease. As with the statins, niacin can be taken at bedtime with a low-fat snack. If flushing continues to be a side effect, a dose of aspirin 30 minutes before taking niacin is recommended.

Fibrates

Fibrates are often prescribed for patients with high triglyceride levels. Before drug treatment, patients may be counseled to improve their diet and lose weight. A common fibrate is fenofibrate. Taken orally, fenofibrate is a pro-drug that is converted to its active form, fenofibric acid, after it is absorbed into the body. It can be taken with or without food and reaches peak levels in six to eight hours. Fenofibric acid has a relatively long half-life of about 20 hours. It is mostly protein bound in the blood and takes about nine days to reach steady state in terms of its bioavailability. About 60% is excreted in the urine, mostly as fenofibric acid. Another 25% is excreted in feces. Metabolism of fenofibrate does not require the P450 mixed-function oxidases. Patients with renal impairment must be monitored closely, as significantly higher blood levels of the active form of the drug can be observed in them. One might predict, then, that exercise at relatively high intensities could also cause an increase in blood levels, as blood flow to the kidneys and liver decreases.

Pharmacodynamic Concerns

Exercise and the lipid-modifying agents both cause changes in the lipoprotein profiles in the blood. Diet is also a significant factor, as diets high in saturated fat, cholesterol, and caloric content contribute to the atherogenic triad of high LDL, low HDL, and high triglycerides. High fat diets are also contributors in metabolic syndrome. Generally, improvements in the lipid profile following exercise or administration of drugs occur when exercise or drugs are coupled to lifestyle changes, such as improved diet and cessation of smoking. Smoking is known to lower HDL. Obese individuals may not see much change in their lipid profile until they start losing weight, because of the quantity of their fat reserves. Even lean individuals have much more fat available than carbohydrates as an energy reserve. As an example, a 65 kg individual with 12% body fat would have over 70,000 kcal available in fat reserves, but only about 1,500 kcal in muscle and liver glycogen. Gender and race may also be factors in terms of the extent of changes observed following exercise or drug treatment, though many studies tend to use white male subjects, for the reasons discussed in Chapter 2. When measuring the percent difference following treatment, the baseline (or starting) level is an important variable. This point is particularly important when the study subjects have normal lipid profiles as opposed to dyslipidemic profiles, or are relatively lean versus overweight. This section reviews the effect of exercise on lipid profile and then compares the effects of different lipid-modifying agents. Last, it looks at some of the limited research on whether these agents increase or interfere with energy mobilization during exercise.

Exercise and Blood Lipids

There is an extensive literature on the impact of exercise on blood lipids. The majority of the studies examine the effect of chronic exercise, as regular exercise is part of a healthy lifestyle that improves the atherogenic profile. Regular exercise clearly shows a decrease in triglycerides in the blood. In addition, some very interesting studies look at changes that occur after a single bout of exercise. These experiments often probe the mechanism of the body's response, looking at the important hormones and signaling networks that are involved. Some studies examine the intensity and the total energy expenditure of the exercise component: *Is there an intensity threshold that must be reached before we see the desired changes in lipid profile? Is there a threshold in the number of calories we need to burn before meaningful changes in blood lipids occur?* In order to answer these questions, we will review the sources of energy that the body uses during exercise, with an emphasis on fat.

The body tends to use fats for low-intensity aerobic exercise and becomes more dependent on carbohydrates for high-intensity anaerobic work. As submaximal exercise progresses, the concentration of free fatty acids in the blood increases, showing the reliance on lipolysis. Fat stores are located in adipocytes, muscle, liver, and serum (as albumin-bound triglycerides). Exercise increases the activity of lipoprotein lipase, found on the endothelial lining of blood vessels; lipoprotein lipase releases free fatty acids and glycerol from serum triglycerides. The free fatty acids can then be taken up by muscle for energy or adipocytes for storage. The glycerol can be made into glucose by the liver or kidneys.

During exercise, epinephrine (through β-1 receptors) activates hormone-sensitive lipases to liberate free fatty acids from stored fat. Other hormones are involved as well. Glucagon predominates over insulin, as fats and carbohydrates are mobilized to meet energy demands instead of being stored. The changes in lipid metabolism are complex, particularly in the liver, and are related to the intensity and duration of the physical activity. Many signal transduction pathways are involved, including the PPAR family of transcription activation factors mentioned previously. To fill the energy need during exercise, genes are activated that enhance lipid oxidation and inhibit lipid synthesis. There is an increase in fatty acid transporter activity at the plasma membrane and in mitochondria, as fatty acids are used to make ATP in liver and muscle cells. The production and release of VLDL by the liver generally decreases under these conditions. In the blood, the increase in lipoprotein lipase activity causes triglyceride breakdown and can speed the clearance of VLDL. These conditions can cause an increase in HDL. There may be a slight decrease in LDL, but this decrease depends on diet and possibly percent body fat. Total cholesterol usually does not change significantly (Durstine, Grandjean, Cox, & Thompson 2002).

In a meta-analysis by Kelley, Kelley, Roberts, and Haskell (2012), exercise alone lowered only triglycerides, whereas diet and exercise caused decreases in LDL, total cholesterol, and triglycerides. The study did not show significant changes in HDL. However, in a comparison between sedentary and highly trained subjects, significant differences were found in the lipoprotein profiles (Lippi, Schena, Salvagno, et al. 2006). Sixty healthy but sedentary males were used as controls. Forty professional skiers and 102 professional cyclists had their lipid profiles determined. Compared to the sedentary controls, the professional athletes had significantly lower triglycerides, total cholesterol, and LDL. They also had significantly higher HDL and an improved total cholesterol to HDL ratio. The total cholesterol to HDL ratio is used as a predictor of cardiovascular risk. The lower total cholesterol to HDL values in the endurance athletes reinforce the evidence that regular aerobic activity improves lipid profiles. In studies where exercise improves HDL levels, the degree of change is largely dependent on weight loss, particularly a decrease in body fat mass, and the baseline (original) level of HDL. If the diet is not constrained, the increase in HDL is less. If the baseline HDL was low, an increase following exercise is greater. Genetic makeup has an influence, as certain genotypes are associated with a greater increase in HDL (Trejo-Gutierrez & Fletcher 2007).

Exercise can stimulate cholesterol flow from cells throughout the body, increasing HDL activity as it performs reverse cholesterol transport. The proportion of slow-twitch (oxidative) muscle cells increases with regular aerobic exercise. Compared to fast-twitch, slow-twitch muscle cells are more efficient users of lipid sources for energy, and they improve the lipid profile. Exercise stimulates lipoprotein lipase, increasing the breakdown of triglycerides; the breakdown products are incorporated into HDL. Similarly, lipoprotein lipase breaks down VLDL, and, as stated earlier, VLDL remnants can contribute to HDL formation. Exercise may also prolong HDL half-life. Exercise does not greatly change LDL levels, but it does cause the smaller, dense particles to become larger and more buoyant, important because the smaller, dense particles are associated with metabolic syndrome and the atherogenic profile.

The intensity of exercise may be important for changes in the lipid profile, with a possible threshold that must be exceeded for the exerciser to see the beneficial effect. Exercising for brief intervals at high intensity over relatively short time frames (e.g., HIIT protocols) can improve the lipid profile (Lira, Carnevali, Zanchi, et al. 2012). Besides intensity, exercising to a point of high energy expenditure has a greater increase in HDL when compared to low energy expenditure, suggesting a threshold must be passed for an improved lipid profile (Lira et al.). Finding the balance between intensity and energy expenditure during exercise is probably what is important in changing lipoprotein profiles. Another example includes a meta-analysis involving aquatic endurance exercise containing 10 trials and 327 subjects. Aquatic endurance exercise improved the lipid and lipoprotein levels in women and middle-aged subjects. Patients with dyslipidemia showed significant improvement (Igarashi & Nogami 2019).

Does this concept of a threshold for intensity or energy expenditure also apply to resistance training? There may a threshold that must be met to alter blood lipids following weight training (Lira et al.). To compare different lifting routines, the *volume* of exercise (the product of sets × reps × weight) can be used to standardize workload or energy expenditure. *Intensity* is usually expressed as a percentage of the one-repetition maximum (e.g., 75% 1RM). Increases in HDL were observed at moderate intensities (50% to 75% 1RM) when performed at similar volume (sets × reps × weight). Acute resistance exercise may increase the clearance of VLDL, decreasing the mean residence time that VLDL (and associated triglycerides) stay in the blood. The increase in clearance (and resulting decreased blood level of VLDL) could be the result of an increase in lipoprotein lipase activity, the interconversion of VLDL to LDL and possibly HDL, and an increase in receptor-mediated uptake of VLDL or LDL in liver and other cells. During recovery after a bout of exercise, muscle needs to replenish its energy stores. The uptake of lipoproteins from the blood occurs for several hours during recovery, and the extent of uptake is probably related to the intensity and energy expenditure of the exercise. A meta-analysis of 29 studies representing 1,329 men and women (676 exercise, 653 control) found that progressive resistance training reduces total cholesterol, LDL cholesterol, total cholesterol/HDL cholesterol, and triglycerides (Kelley & Kelley 2009). In another study, total cholesterol was significantly lower following the 12 weeks of resistance training in obese, postmenopausal women (Wooten, Phillips, Mitchell, et al. 2011). Resistance exercise, therefore, should be included in an exercise protocol to improve a lipid profile, in addition to all its other benefits.

To summarize, chronic exercise is known to increase the expression, amount, and activity of lipoprotein lipase. The increase in lipoprotein lipase causes a decrease in plasma triglycerides, a decrease in the secretion of VLDL from the liver, and an increase in the clearance of VLDL from the blood. An increase in HDL appears to be proportional to activity level. More intense activity is required to elicit reductions in LDL cholesterol. The addition of resistance training to aerobic exercise can supplement or enhance the effects on the lipid profile (Mann, Beedie, & Jimenez 2014). The net result can be an improved atherogenic lipid profile. An important meta-analysis on exercise interventions suggests that exercise and many drug interventions are potentially similar in terms of their mortality benefits in the secondary prevention of coronary heart disease, rehabilitation after stroke, treatment of heart failure, and prevention of diabetes (Naci & Ioannidis 2013).

Lipid-Modifying Agents and Exercise

As discussed above, the three major classes of lipid-modifying agents each alter the lipoprotein profile by affecting control mechanisms in ways that are similar to the effects of exercise. In some cases, the extent of alteration in lipid levels is similar between exercise and drug treatment (see Table 10.4). The statins block the production of cholesterol. In the liver, the resultant decrease in VLDL release causes a decrease in formation of LDL (see Figure 10.1). The decrease in cholesterol synthesis means that cells are more dependent on LDL uptake from the blood, also causing a decrease in LDL levels. A resulting increase in reverse cholesterol transport back to the liver causes an increase in HDL levels. Niacin also decreases transport of VLDL. It inhibits the lipase activity in adipose tissues, decreasing free fatty acid release and slowing the formation of lipoproteins in the blood. Niacin also increases reverse cholesterol transport and increases the levels of HDL. Fibrates stimulate lipoprotein lipase in the vasculature and the breakdown of triglycerides. Fibrates also increase the oxidation of free fatty acids in liver and muscle, similar to the effect of exercise. Synthetic pathways for new lipids are suppressed, so fewer VLDL and triglycerides are produced. Exercise and diet can improve the atherogenic profile. However, when genetics, metabolic syndrome, obesity, cigarette smoking, age, and perhaps race and gender conspire to make it difficult to manage lipid levels, then drugs are needed. As we have seen in these overlapping mechanisms, maintaining a good diet and an active lifestyle can decrease the need for or required dosage of these drugs.

There are limited studies on how these drugs affect exercise performance. Two older studies looked at the effect on fat oxidation as a function of exercise time at 50% VO_2max. In the first study, 24 healthy male volunteers with normal blood lipids were split into three groups of eight each (Head, Jakeman, Kendall, et al. 1993). Each group was assigned a drug from the three classes: statin (simvastatin), fibrate (gemfibrozil), and niacin (acipimox). After five days of treatment, each participant performed the exercise trial twice, once on the drug and once on placebo. The results showed no difference between placebo and statin treatment in terms of blood levels of free fatty acids during exercise. There was a trend where the fibrate treatment decreased free fatty acid levels (but the effect was not statistically significant); a significant decrease in free fatty acid mobilization was observed with acipimox, consistent with the reported

Table 10.4 Comparison between effects of exercise and three major lipid-modifying agents on lipoprotein profiles

Lipoprotein	Regular Exercise	Statins	Niacin	Fibrates
Triglycerides	Decrease 4%–37%	Decrease 7%–30%	Decrease 20%–50%	Decrease 20%–50%
LDL	Little change	Decrease 18%–55%	Decrease 5%–25%	Decrease 5%–20%[a]
HDL	Increase 4%–18%	Increase 5%–15%	Increase 15%–35%	Increase 10%–20%

[a]May increase in patients with high triglycerides.

mechanism of inhibited lipase activity in adipocytes. Similar responses were observed for total fat oxidation and glycerol concentration (no effect with statins, slight, not significant decrease by fibrate, and decreases by acipimox; Head et al.). In a second study, 16 healthy volunteers with normal blood lipids were used in a crossover study (Eagles, Kendall, & Maxwell 1996). They took one of two drugs or a placebo for 21 days before their exercise trial. There was no difference in fat oxidation between the statin (fluvastatin) and placebo treatments. However, in this case, there was a significant decrease in the amount of fat oxidation following fibrate (bezafibrate) treatment (Eagles et al.). The authors raise the question whether impaired fat metabolism could result in premature fatigue in hyperlipidemic patients taking the drug.

More recent studies focus on the potential for myopathy following statin treatment. One study looked at energy expenditure in skeletal muscle during exercise and found no effect of the drug on fatty acid oxidation rates, VO_2max, or the anaerobic threshold (Chung, Brass, Ulrich, & Hiatt 2008). However, statin therapy may interfere with training, as adherence may decrease due to muscular discomfort (Thompson & Parker 2013). Exercise intensity is important to see fitness gains and cardiovascular benefits, but high-intensity exercise while taking statins is a concern. The benefit of combining exercise and statins is significant, as a large epidemiologic trial concluded that the combination of statin treatment and increased fitness level lowers the risk of all-cause mortality more than either factor alone (Kokkinos, Faselis, Myers, et al. 2013). Many mechanisms for the statin effect on muscle have been proposed, with many suggesting an involvement of mitochondria. Statin-caused reduction of other cholesterol intermediates (mentioned above) is a possible cause for the myopathies (Bonetti et al.; Thompson & Parker). The possible involvement of coenzyme Q and mitochondrial activity will be discussed further in the chapter on supplements.

Elder Concerns

Statins lower cholesterol and help prevent heart attacks and strokes in essentially all age groups. How aggressively to treat those over 75 years of age is under debate, but nearly 45% of people aged 60 and older are prescribed a statin. Compliance can be an issue, especially in the elderly, as they sometimes rebel from taking 'too many' medications and one cannot 'feel' a reduction in cholesterol. Muscle aches, a known side effect of statin use, may be confused with the aches and pains associated with aging. Whether statins accelerate or delay aging has generated some controversy with reports of muscle problems, an increased risk of diabetes, and a negative effect of statins on certain stem cells. However, a considerable amount of research supports the health benefits associated with statin treatment, some of which are not easily traced back to inhibition of HMG-CoA reductase. In the elderly, as with younger people, the high incidence of overweight or obese individuals, with metabolic syndrome or diabetes, makes drawing clear conclusions on potential negative effects attributable to statins very difficult.

The potential benefits of statins are significant enough that some medical experts suggest that all adults should be prescribed statins, regardless of their risk for (or history) of heart disease. Statins substantially retard arterial aging and inhibit inflammation and plaque buildup. They also decrease plaque buildup on heart valves. Since statins inhibit arterial aging, statins may slow memory loss, impotence, and wrinkling of the skin, besides fewer heart attacks and strokes. In addition to lowering cholesterol and the risk of cardiovascular disease, statins lower levels of inflammation.

Inflammation is monitored by measuring the amount of C-reactive protein in the blood. Inflammation is linked to other health issues in the elderly, including diabetes, cancer, and Alzheimer's disease. Statins decrease C-reactive protein in patients following acute coronary events and ischemic stroke, leading to fewer impairments in speech and movement, with measurable improvement in future health outcomes. Exercise and treating chronic infections also reduce C-reactive protein in the blood. How statins lower C-reactive protein levels is not fully known, but the greatest benefit from taking statins is observed in individuals who start out with high levels of C-reactive protein.

Research on long-term statin use continues as the population of elderly taking statins expands. The incidence of other age-related diseases in this population can be compared to those not taking statins. For instance, statins reduce the risk of intracerebral hemorrhage (Anderson 2019). Moreover, statin use may be beneficial to cancer outcomes, such as a decrease in deaths from breast cancer (Beckwitt, Brufsky, Oltvai, & Wells 2018). Statins may also be effective in pancreatic cancer (Huang, Chang, Li, et al. 2017). Statins have antitumor, cytostatic (growth-halting), and cytotoxic (cell-killing) effects on cancer cells. Many possible mechanisms exist; inhibition of the rate-limiting step in cholesterol biosynthesis alters the metabolism of many important spin-off products dependent on cholesterol synthesis (Vallianou, Kostantinou, Kougias, & Kazazis 2014). Interestingly, statin users had higher telomerase activity and longer telomeres (discussed in Chapter 2) compared to the non-statin group, with lower telomere erosion associated with aging (Boccardi, Barbieri, Rizzo, et al. 2013). The long-term effect of statin therapy on longevity and the aging process will continue to be a very active area of research.

For healthy aging, lowering cholesterol with exercise and a healthy diet is the first step. Other risk factors should be minimized, such as smoking, high blood pressure, obesity, and diabetes. If cholesterol (and possibly C-reactive protein level) remains elevated, statin therapy may be necessary. Besides lowering cholesterol and C-reactive protein, statins have other potential ways to extend healthier lives. They are not first-line agents for cancer and other conditions, but they may be effective as adjunct therapies. Whether everyone over 60 years old should take them, as some have suggested, will probably always generate controversy, but monitoring their use in the millions of people taking them will provide insight into the aging process. Statins, however, can only do so much. Cardiovascular events still occur with statin use, emphasizing again the need for physical activity, proper diet, and weight control.

Health Risks

Muscle pain (myalgia) has been noted with use of these drugs (statins mainly), independently of intense exercise (Fernandez et al.). Large trials show that these issues usually resolve over time or with temporary suspension of use or reduced dose (LaRosa et al.). Plasma creatine kinase is a measure of muscle damage, as creatine kinase should be found inside muscle cells, not in the blood. Generally, plasma creatine kinase levels in the blood are higher in untrained than trained individuals following exercise. De-conditioned, overweight individuals starting exercise programs might be expected to show some muscle damage and soreness. For patients taking these drugs, intense exercise should be monitored. Niacin and fibrates have their own potential side effects, including myopathies, but are generally safe and well tolerated. Current practice often combines more than one drug class for improved effectiveness and lower risk of unwanted effects.

PES Watch

Lipid-modifying drugs are not ergogenic and not banned. Acipimox and fibrates may be mildly ergolytic. Statins have less impairment of fat utilization than acipimox or nicotinic acid. Older males should use caution when taking these drugs, especially if they are doing intense weight training. The benefits of exercise, especially to cardio-vascular health, outweigh possible problems.

Conclusion

The atherogenic profile consists of the triad: (1) elevated LDL, (2) low HDL, and (3) elevated triglycerides. The liver is central to maintaining cholesterol homeostasis. Genetics, diet, physical activity, and other factors are critical in maintaining a healthy lipoprotein profile. Statins block HMG-CoA-reductase, decrease the production of cholesterol, and decrease the formation of LDL. A resulting increase in reverse cholesterol transport back to the liver causes an increase in HDL levels. Niacin inhibits the lipase activity in adipose tissues, decreasing free fatty acid release and slowing the formation of lipoproteins in the blood. Fibrates stimulate lipoprotein lipase in the vascular lining, leading to the breakdown of triglycerides. Exercise and diet can improve the atherogenic profile by mechanisms similar to those of the lipid-modifying agents. Maintaining a good diet and an active lifestyle can reduce the need for or required dosage of these agents.

Key Concepts Review

acipimox
atherogenic profile
bile acid sequestrant
coenzyme Q
derivative of fibric acid
dyslipidemia
ezetimibe
fibrate
high-density lipoprotein (HDL)
HMG-CoA-reductase
HMG-CoA-reductase inhibitor

hyperlipidemia
lipoprotein lipase (LPL)
low-density lipoprotein (LDL)
niacin derivative
nicotinic acid
PPARα (peroxisome proliferator-
    activated receptor-α) pathway
receptor-mediated endocytosis
statin
very low-density lipoprotein (VLDL)
vitamin B3

Review Questions

1   Bob's neighbor, Fred, is on lovastatin to lower his blood lipids. He figures that because he is using drugs to control his blood lipids, he doesn't need to exercise or watch his diet. What advice might you give him?
2   Exercise and lipid-modifying agents cause similar changes in blood lipids. Are there common mechanisms?
3   How does LDL help regulate cholesterol homeostasis?
4   Harry has started a new exercise program and has some persistent muscle soreness. He also takes an HMG-CoA-reductase inhibitor to control his blood lipids. As his personal trainer, should you be concerned?

References

Anderson CS (2019) Reduced risk of intracerebral haemorrhage from statins: added-value of large healthcare data. *E Clin Med* 8:2–3

Beckwitt CH, Brufsky A, Oltvai ZN, Wells A (2018) Statin drugs to reduce breast cancer recurrence and mortality. *Breast Cancer Res* 20:144

Boccardi V, Barbieri M, Rizzo MR, Marfella R, Esposito A, Marano L, Paolisso G. (2013) A new pleiotropic effect of statins in elderly: modulation of telomerase activity. *FASEB J* 27:3879–3885

Bonetti PO, Lerman LO, Napoli C, Lerman A (2003) Statin effects beyond lipid lowering—are they clinically relevant? *Eur Heart J* 24:225–248

Brown MS, Dana SE, Goldstein JL (1974) Regulation of 3-hydroxy-3-methylglutaryl coenzyme A reductase activity in cultured human fibroblasts. *J Biol Chem* 249:789–796

Brown MS, Goldstein JL (1986) A receptor-mediated pathway for cholesterol homeostasis. *Science* 232:34–47

Centers for Disease Control and Prevention (CDC) (2014) *Heart disease facts*. Retrieved from www.cdc.gov/heartdisease/facts.htm

Chung J, Brass EP, Ulrich RG, Hiatt WR (2008) Effect of atorvastatin on energy expenditure and skeletal muscle oxidative metabolism at rest and during exercise. *Clin Pharmacol Ther* 83:243–245

Durstine JL, Grandjean PW, Cox CA, Thompson PD (2002) Lipids, lipoproteins, and exercise. *J Cardiopulmonary Rehab* 22:385–398

Eagles CJ, Kendall MJ, Maxwell S (1996) A comparison of the effects of fluvastatin and bezafibrate on exercise metabolism: a placebo-controlled study in healthy normolipidemic subjects. *Br J Clin Pharmacol* 41:381–387

Fernandez G, Spatz ES, Jablecki C, Phillips PS (2011) Statin myopathy: a common dilemma not reflected in clinical trials. *Cleveland Clinic J Med* 78:393–403

Head A, Jakeman PM, Kendall MJ, Cramb R, Maxwell S (1993) The impact of a short course of three lipid lowering drugs on fat oxidation during exercise in healthy volunteers. *Postgrad Med J* 69:197–203

Huang BZ, Chang JI, Li E, Xiang AH, Wu BU (2017) Influence of statins and cholesterol on mortality among patients with pancreatic cancer. *J Natl Cancer Inst* 109:djw275

Igarashi Y, Nogami Y (2019) Response of lipids and lipoproteins to regular aquatic endurance exercise: a meta-analysis of randomized controlled trials. *J Atheroscler Thromb* 26:14–30

Kelley GA, Kelley KS (2009) Impact of progressive resistance training on lipids and lipoproteins in adults: a meta-analysis of randomized controlled trials. *Prev Med* 48:9–19

Kelley GA, Kelley KS, Roberts S, Haskell W (2012) Comparison of aerobic exercise, diet or both on lipids and lipoproteins in adults: a meta-analysis of randomized controlled trials. *Clin Nutrition* 31:156–167

Kokkinos PF, Faselis C, Myers J, Panagiotakos D, Doumas M (2013) Interactive effects of fitness and statin treatment on mortality risk in veterans with dyslipidaemia: a cohort study. *Lancet* 381:394–399

LaRosa JC, Pedersen TR, Somatane R, Wasserman SM (2013) Safety and effect of very low levels of low-density lipoprotein cholesterol on cardiovascular events. *Am J Cardiol* 111:1221–1229

Lippi G, Schena F, Salvagno GL, Montagnana M, Ballestrieri F, Guidi GC (2006) Comparison of the lipid profile and lipoprotein(a) between sedentary and highly trained subjects. *Clin Chem Lab Med* 44:322–326

Lira FS, Carnevali LC, Zanchi NE, Santos RVT, Lavoie JM, Seelaender M (2012) Exercise intensity modulation of hepatic lipid metabolism. *J Nutr Metab* Epub:2012:809576

Ma L, Lee BH, Mao R, Cai A, Jia Y, Clifton H, Schaefer S, Xu L, Zheng J (2014) Nicotinic acid activates the capsaicin receptor TRPV1: potential mechanism for cutaneous flushing. *Arterioscler Thromb Vasc Biol* 34:1272–1280

Mann S, Beedie C, Jimenez A (2014) Differential effects of aerobic exercise, resistance training and combined exercise modalities on cholesterol and the lipid profile: review, synthesis and recommendations. *Sports Med* 44:211–221

Moradi H, Streja E, Kalantar-Zadeh K (2017) Serum high density lipoprotein cholesterol level and risk of death: let's avoid the extremes. *J Thorac Dis* 9:4849–4852

Naci H, Brugts JJ, Fleurence R, Ades A (2013) Dose-comparative effects of different statins on serum lipid levels: a network meta-analysis of 256,827 individuals in 181 randomized controlled trials. *Eur J Prev Cardiol* 20:658–670

Naci H, Ioannidis JP (2013) Comparative effectiveness of exercise and drug interventions on mortality outcomes: a meta epidemiological study. *BMJ* 347:f5577

Rizzo M, Berneis K (2006) Low-density lipoprotein size and cardiovascular risk assessment. *QJM* 99:1–14

Stone NJ, Robinson JG, Lichtenstein AH, Bairey Merz CN, Blum CB, Eckel RH, Goldberg AC, Gordon D, Levy D, Lloyd-Jones DM, McBride P, Schwartz JS, Shero ST, Smith SC Jr, Watson K, Wilson PW; American College of Cardiology/American Heart Association Task Force on Practice Guidelines (2014) 2013 ACC/AHA guideline on the treatment of blood cholesterol to reduce atherosclerotic cardiovascular risk in adults: a report of the American College of Cardiology/American Heart Association Task Force on Practice Guidelines. *J Am Coll Cardiol* 63:2889–2934

Tenenbaum A, Fisman EZ (2012) Fibrates are an essential part of modern antidyslipidemic arsenal: spotlight on atherogenic dyslipidemia and residual risk reduction. *Cardiovascular Diabetology* 11:125–135

Thompson PD, Parker B (2013) Statins, exercise, and exercise training. *J Am Col Cardiol* 62:715–716

Trejo-Gutierrez JF, Fletcher G (2007) Impact of exercise on blood lipids and lipoproteins. *J Clin Lipidology* 1:175–181

Vallianou NG, Kostantinou A, Kougias M, Kazazis C (2014) Statins and cancer. *Anticancer Agents Med Chem* 14:706–712

Vosper H (2009) Niacin: a re-emerging pharmaceutical for the treatment of dyslipidemia. *Br J Pharmacol* 158:429–441

Vosper H (2011) Extended release niacin-laropiprant in patients with hypercholesterolemia or mixed dyslipidemias improves clinical parameters. *Clin Med Insights Cardiol* 5:85–101

Wooten JS, Phillips MD, Mitchell JB, Patrizi R, Pleasant RN, Hein RM, Menzies RD, Barbee JJ (2011) Resistance exercise and lipoproteins in postmenopausal women. *Int J Sports Med* 32:7–13

Yokote K, Yamashita S, Arai H, Araki E, Suganami H, Ishibashi S (2019) Long-term efficacy and safety of pemafibrate, a novel selective peroxisome proliferator-activated receptor-α modulator (SPPARMα), in dyslipidemic patients with renal impairment. *Int J Mol Sci* 20:E706

Zeman M, Vecka M, Perlík F, Staňková B, Hromádka R, Tvrzická E, Širc J, Hrib J, Žák A (2016) Pleiotropic effects of niacin: current possibilities for its clinical use. *Acta Pharm* 66:449–469.

11 Analgesics and Anti-Inflammatory Drugs

Abstract

Some pain is good—it helps protect against further damage. Nociceptive and inflammatory pains are adaptive and protective. When problems develop in parts of these complex pathways, chronic pathological pain occurs. Opioids are often used for chronic pain, but they can show tolerance and have potential for addiction. They also cause respiratory depression, constipation, drowsiness, and the inability to focus. For mild to moderate pain and fever, acetaminophen is effective and is widely used for children. Its mechanism of action is still unclear and may have many different targets. The many potential mechanisms for acetaminophen may be related to a complex series of metabolites formed from the parent compound. One metabolite in particular is of interest, as it mimics actions of endogenous cannabinoids. Another metabolite, however, can cause hepatotoxicity.

Aspirin and the other NSAIDs are also commonly used for fever and mild to moderate pain. These drugs differ from acetaminophen in that they block prostaglandin synthesis and suppress portions of the inflammatory response. The traditional NSAIDs block the activity of the constitutive COX-1 and the inducible activity of COX-2. To minimize the side effects associated with blocking COX-1, COX-2 inhibitors were developed. However, safety concerns with the COX-2 inhibitors have led to their removal from the market. Although some COX-2 inhibitors have once again become available, their manufacturers give warnings about their safety. NSAIDs should probably only be taken for brief intervals. They may help decrease the severity of an injury in the first 24 to 48 hours by suppressing part of the inflammatory response; however, the inflammatory response is a normal process that works to heal and repair the damage, and extended NSAID use could be counterproductive. Prophylactic use of NSAIDs is also being questioned, as the moderate reduction in pain they provide is countered with increased markers of muscle damage. In addition, undesirable effects on the kidneys cause fluid and salt balance problems. Ice and rest sometimes are the best methods of helping the body heal.

CASE EXAMPLE

Megan is crushed. She just got off the phone with Jennifer, the Striker on her old college soccer team. Their teammate Carla died the night before from an apparent opioid overdose. Carla was their Center Back and fiercely competitive. She was a main reason they made the tournament their last two seasons. Carla was always dinged up—but she always played. The last time they had gotten together, Carla was complaining about her back. Apparently, she had been in a minor car wreck that aggravated a disc issue from her soccer days. Carla was one of her teammates that had 'connections' and was able to get prescription pain-killers. A family friend knew a Doctor—or something like that. And now she was dead like so many others who got hooked on opioids. Carla was barely breathing when they found her, and her small down first-responders did not have the opioid antagonist naloxone (Narcan). By the time they got to the emergency room, it was too late. This really hurts—something needs to be done. But for now, Megan needs to call a couple other teammates and re-arrange her schedule so she can attend the funeral.

Learning Objectives

1 Learn what causes pain.
2 Distinguish the different types of pain.
3 Learn how the opioids mimic endorphins.
4 Understand why acetaminophen is an important pain-killer.
5 Appreciate the complexities of the inflammation response.
6 Learn what causes fever.
7 Learn how NSAIDs reduce inflammation and provide pain relief.
8 Become knowledgeable about the ongoing debate on whether NSAIDs help or inhibit the healing process.
9 Appreciate the role of pain and inflammation in the healing process.
10 Consider whether the use of NSAIDs provides a competitive advantage.

Introduction

Analgesia is the deadening of pain while the person is conscious. **Analgesics**, both prescription and over the counter (OTC), are commonly called pain-killers. They are among the top-selling drugs every year. Analgesics are also distinguished by their **anti-pyretic** (fever reducing) and anti-inflammatory activities. We will concentrate on three classes of analgesics: (1) **opioids** (heroin, hydrocodone), (2) **acetaminophen** (paracetamol, Tylenol), and (3) **non-steroidal anti-inflammatory drugs (NSAIDs)**, which include salicylates (aspirin). Other types of analgesics, such as local anesthetics, will not be covered here in detail. Cannabinoids (medical marijuana) have shown promise for certain types of pain and will be discussed below and in Chapter 15. Although not a true analgesic, the nutritional supplement glucosamine (see Chapter 13) can help alleviate chronic joint pain. Glucosamine is a modified sugar used to build the ground substance of cartilage and the extracellular matrix that cushions joints. Some evidence suggests that glucosamine (and other sulfated carbohydrates, such as chondroitin and heparin) can be effective in reducing pain associated with osteoarthritis. In addition, a number of other drugs initially brought to market and prescribed for other conditions have found utility in treating chronic pain.

The Science of Pain

Pain involves peripheral terminals of sensory neurons sending signals to the spinal cord. Ascending fibers in the spinal column carry the signals to the brain. Descending pathways from the brain have a moderating function in the pain response. Pain can be classified into three major types: nociceptive, inflammatory, and pathological (Woolf 2010). The first two types are adaptive and protective, meaning the responses provide protection from further physiological damage. These types of pain are generally acute, in contrast to the third type, which is chronic, resulting from a disease associated with the nervous system.

The first type of pain is called **nociceptive pain** because it senses noxious stimuli (e.g., sharp objects, heat, cold). It is the body's early warning system to "stop and withdraw" immediately. Unpleasantness and emotional anguish are sometimes associated with this type of pain. It has a relatively high threshold, requiring an intense stimulus (burning hot vs. merely hot). It activates neuronal pathways that can become integrated into the brain with memories, mood, and level of cognitive function. A strong enough stimulus overrides most other functions, generating something like the order, "Drop it—NOW!" With some genetic defects, nociceptive pain is not felt. Individuals with these genetic abnormalities do not sense nociceptive pain and, therefore, do not respond with a stop/avoid response. They can inflict considerable damage to themselves without realizing it and present in clinics with broken bones or extreme levels of muscle/joint damage. They risk such levels of damage because they lack the ability to perceive and respond to pain.

A second kind of pain is related to recovery from damage resulting from an inflamed joint, muscle sprain, or surgery. It is called **inflammatory pain** because it results from the inflammatory response. Damaged or recovering areas are "hypersensitive" or "tender," so use of the joint is minimized or contact with the affected area is discouraged. The healing response improves as a consequence. This type of pain has a low threshold, with normally innocuous stimuli now initiating an avoidance response to lessen the pain. For example, the pain associated with a sprained ankle discourages walking.

The third type of pain is **pathological pain**. Pathological pain is maladaptive and has a low threshold; it is a disease state of the nervous system. Normal mechanisms that allow the body to adapt to stimuli or "something wrong" are defective. Common causes of pathological pain include alcoholism, amputation, diabetes, multiple sclerosis, and shingles. The problem can be in the sensing, the wiring (neuronal) circuits, or the control mechanisms; the result is that the pain becomes a chronic condition. Pathological pain is called **neuropathic pain** if nerve damage is the major cause. When no clear nerve damage or inflammation is involved, the pain is referred to as **dysfunctional pain**. Pathological pain occurs when the requirement for a noxious stimulus is uncoupled from the processing centers, or when the threshold for generating pain decreases to a point where it is easily reached. The susceptibility to become hypersensitive to pain or convert to chronic maladaptive pain may be inheritable; certain genotypes may be predisposed to this type of nerve disease (Woolf).

The Economics of Treating Pain

The availability of relatively inexpensive, effective OTC drugs for mild to moderate pain means that new drug development is not easily justified financially. For the treatment of chronic pain, however, the available drugs all have problems with their side-effect profiles. With millions of sufferers from chronic pain, drug companies are interested in advancing development of new drugs and strategies (Burgess & Williams). Better pain management is also needed for patients with arthritis, residual pain from shingles, and bone cancer.

Approaches to advancing analgesic therapy include improving the formulations and protocols for existing drugs and exploring drug combinations. Drug companies also continue to develop analgesics based on the known targets for the NSAIDs and opioids. Some drugs that were originally marketed for other purposes have potential use as analgesics. The approach requiring the greatest investment by drug companies is based on developing novel targets. As our understanding of the underlying mechanisms improves, new areas for drug design become available. Examples include the N-type calcium channel blockers or drugs related to cannabinoid pathways. Perception of pain is not hard-wired per se; it is more the consequence of a highly plastic interaction of molecules and neuronal circuits. Understanding the mechanisms involved can lead to new drug targets in the future (Burgess & Williams).

Pathological pain results from some sort of maladaptation in the complex process of peripheral terminals of sensory neurons sending signals to the spinal cord, ascending fibers in the spinal column carrying the signals to the brain, and descending pathways from the brain having a moderating function in the pain response. Analgesics can target the perception of pain in the periphery or suppress the transmission of the signals to the brain. They can also target the brain's sensitivity to these inputs. One of the tricks to pain management is to control neuropathic pain but allow some level of nociceptive and inflammatory pain to still do its job of protecting against further damage. Treating severe neuropathic pain presents a problem, in that pain suppression must not be so great as to minimize the critical nociceptive response.

Our overall understanding of the genetic, molecular, and cellular nature of pain has increased markedly in recent years. The hope is that new analgesics will be developed based on these new insights, with greater efficacy and lessened side-effect burden (Burgess & Williams 2010).

How Analgesics Work

The following sections discuss three main classifications of analgesics (opioids, acetaminophen, and NSAIDs) and how they work (see Table 11.1). The opioids are used, and frequently overused, for pathological pain, but they do not have anti-inflammatory activity. Acetaminophen also lacks anti-inflammatory activity, but it is widely used for mild to moderate pain and is effective at reducing fever. NSAIDs are effective for inflammatory pain, and we will look at inflammation in more detail to see why this is so.

Table 11.1 Classification and examples of analgesics

Drug	Class	Use/Target
Morphine	Opioid	Pain, primarily mu opioid receptor (MOR)
Codeine	Opioid	Cough, pain (MOR)
Heroin	Opioid	Pain (MOR)
Hydrocodone	Opioid	Pain (MOR)
Loperamide	Opioid	Diarrhea (MOR)
Acetaminophen (Tylenol)	Acetaminophen	Pain, fever (many possible targets)
Aspirin	NSAID	Pain, fever, inflammation (COX-1, COX-2)
Ibuprofen (Advil)	NSAID (traditional)	Pain, fever, inflammation (COX-1, COX-2)
Naproxen (Aleve)	NSAID (traditional)	Pain, fever, inflammation (COX-1, COX-2)
Celecoxib (Celebrex)	NSAID	Arthritic pain (COX-2)
Meloxicam (Mobic)	NSAID	Arthritic pain (COX-2)
Diclofenac (Voltarol)	NSAID (traditional)	Topical gel, patch (COX-1, COX-2)

Opioid Analgesics

Opium is an extract from the poppy plant; **opiates** are natural products processed from opium. Naturally occurring opiates include morphine and codeine. Synthetic derivatives, referred to as *opioids*, include heroin and hydrocodone, among many others. The **opioid analgesics** are drugs that mimic **endorphins** (*endo*genous m*orphine*), peptides that generate similar responses through the opioid receptor system. Since the discovery of the original endorphin peptide, two other peptides with endogenous opioid activity have been discovered: **enkephalin** and **dynorphin**. The term **opioid** is inclusive; it can include the opiates, the synthetics, and the endogenous peptides. The older term narcotic, derived from the Greek word *narcos* (meaning sleep or stupor), is not used much in the medical profession anymore. The lay media uses "narcotic" to describe a wide range of illicit drugs (opioids, cocaine, amphetamines, steroids, etc.). Morphine is the prototypical opioid analgesic that sets the reference point for all the others. Newer synthetic opioids such as fentanyl are much as 100 times more potent than morphine, with some fentanyl analogs estimated to be 10,000 times more potent. The influx of these potent synthetic opioids into the black market is one of the major causes for the increase in overdose deaths.

Opioids are pharmacologically complex, as the same compound can display agonist, partial agonist, and even antagonist activity with different receptor subtypes. Three related but distinct opioid receptors are mu, delta, and kappa. **Mu** is the predominant receptor and is widely distributed throughout the body. It is involved in mediating the primary opioid effects, including spinal cord analgesia, respiratory depression, decreased GI-tract motility, and modification of hormone and neurotransmitter release. The other receptors have varying degrees of involvement in these responses.

Morphine is a full agonist for the mu receptor; codeine is a partial agonist. The mu receptor predominates in the CNS and plays a major role in analgesia. Two mechanisms have been proposed for how morphine works through the mu receptor to cause analgesia. The first one involves suppression of neurotransmitter release. Mu receptor activation by morphine causes inhibition of Ca^{2+} channel activity in the pre-synaptic nerve terminal. When the action potential travels down the primary afferent fiber and reaches the synapse, less calcium enters the cell when the mu receptor has been activated by opioids. Fewer vesicles containing neurotransmitters fuse with the membrane, and there is a decrease in transmission of the signal across the synaptic cleft. As a result of this mechanism, opioids suppress transmission of pain signals up and down the spinal cord.

The second mechanism involves the post-synaptic cell, the secondary afferent fiber. Mu receptor activation by opioids in the post-synaptic cell increases K^+ channel activity, creating a greater flow of K^+ out of the cell. The resulting hyperpolarization decreases the generation of action potentials in the post-synaptic cell. Again, as a result of both of these mechanisms, opioids suppress transmission of pain signals up and down the spinal cord.

Morphine also suppresses the affective or emotional component of pain that occurs in the brain. Thus, the effectiveness of the opioids, such as morphine, is attributable to both a cerebral and a spinal effect. In addition, opioids stimulate mu receptors found in the peripheral terminals of sensory cells. By suppression of sensory cell responsiveness, opioids can inhibit nociceptive pain and provide analgesia for inflammatory pain. This property can be a double-edged sword, as reduction of nociceptive pain may help in the short term but creates problems (loss of protective mechanisms mentioned above) for long-term use of opioids in the treatment of neuropathic pain.

As discussed previously, the opioids exert their analgesic effects centrally and in the periphery. Centrally, they cause a euphoria that is experienced as "floating," with diminished feelings of anxiety or distress. Opioids can cause drowsiness and the feeling of being on the verge of falling asleep, but there is no associated amnesia. Opioids also produce respiratory depression in the brain stem, where breathing rate is controlled. The body does not respond properly to a carbon dioxide (CO_2) challenge, failing to increase the breathing rate when CO_2 levels rise, which results in a slower breathing rate and decreased oxygen availability, blackout, and even death. Suppression of respiration is a critical issue when the opioid dose is increased and in overdose emergencies.

Some opioids, such as codeine and dextromethorphan, suppress the cough reflex, making them useful in cough medications. However, prolonged suppression of this cough reflex can allow accumulation of fluids in the lungs and upper airway passages that normally are eliminated by coughing. In the eye, opioids cause contraction of the pupil (miosis), and this property does not show tolerance. An opioid abuser who increases the dose to get the same high still has the same pupillary response. Therefore, miosis is useful for diagnosing a potential overdose victim.

Opioids also act on the GI-tract by decreasing motility in the stomach and peristalsis in the large intestine. The net result is that transit time for undigested material and stool through the intestines increases, allowing more water reuptake and causing constipation. Opioids may also interfere with the normal regulation of defecation. Tolerance does not occur to this response with prolonged use, making constipation a problem in patients using opioids long term. This property was recognized a very long time ago. For centuries, opioids have been used to treat diarrhea; one of the older concoctions is called paregoric (camphorated tincture of opium). Paregoric was used to treat diarrhea, as a cough suppressant, and as an analgesic. Current formulations for diarrhea use the opioid loperamide.

The many varied responses to opioids give rise to a significant panel of side effects. Constipation, drowsiness, inability to concentrate, nausea, vomiting, and poor quality of sleep all contribute to long-term issues with the chronic use of opioids.

Endorphins and Pregnancy

The pharmacology of opioids has intrigued scientists for decades, and many have studied how these powerful and addictive drugs cause their effects. Drugs were predicted to work through receptors, and several tissue-based tests conducted in the 1970s allowed researchers to test opioids for agonist and antagonist activity. The question studied was: if these drugs work through a receptor, then what is the endogenous molecule that the opioids are mimicking? Brain extracts were fractionated and tested for opioid-like activity. When a brain fraction caused the same effect as an opioid, the extract was tested in the presence of the antagonist naloxone. If the antagonist blocked the effect, the fraction was fractionated further and the process was repeated. Finally, a peptide of 31 residues in length was purified that had true opioid activity; it was named endorphin. Endorphin is made as part of a larger peptide produced in the anterior pituitary. When the precursor peptide is processed, it produces not only endorphin but also ACTH (adrenocorticotropin). The result is that endorphin and ACTH are released from the pituitary in response to stress. The discovery of endorphin led to the question, what is the role for endorphin in the body?

One of the early discoveries was that endorphin levels are high in pregnant women and the developing fetus. The mother produces endorphin in her pituitary gland, and cells in the placenta secrete endorphin into the umbilical cord circulation. Though this research is technically challenging, endorphin levels have been monitored during pregnancy and labor. In the mother, endorphin levels become high early on, dip in the middle trimester, and then rise in the third trimester, leading to labor and delivery (Dabo, Nyberg, Zhou, et al. 2010). The newborn's level of endorphin does not seem to vary with natural birth or Cesarean section; the mother's level, however, varies with the level of stress during labor. Women undergoing natural childbirth have a five-fold increase in endorphin levels compared to women having a Cesarean section (Kofinas, Kofinas, & Tavakoli 1985). Interestingly, women who exercised during the second and third trimesters had higher levels of endorphin and less pain through labor (Varrassi, Bazzano, & Edwards 1989). Women with low levels of endorphin often required additional pain medication during labor (Dabo et al.).

The fact that pregnant women have relatively high levels of endogenous opioids for months, with a significant increase going into labor, raises an interesting question. Does the new mother undergo a withdrawal syndrome following her somewhat rapid decrease in endogenous opioid level? The answer varies greatly among women, but some argue that at least a portion of postpartum depression may be attributable to the decrease in endogenous opioids.

In the context of pregnancy, the varied properties of opioids tend to make sense. For the developing fetus, the suppression of GI-tract motility and respiration, along with a euphoric, disassociated mental state, could be useful adaptations. And for the pregnant woman, desensitization to the physical discomfort of coexisting with and then delivering a newborn infant after nine months is probably highly desired.

Acetaminophen

Acetaminophen (paracetamol, Tylenol) was developed in the 1940s and 1950s as an analgesic with less stomach irritation than aspirin. Acetaminophen has anti-pyretic and analgesic activity, but little anti-inflammatory activity, and it is not considered a NSAID. Besides being easier on the stomach, acetaminophen causes less suppression of blood clotting and fewer kidney issues than the NSAIDs. Since acetaminophen, unlike aspirin, is not associated with **Reye syndrome** (a condition that causes swelling in the liver and brain, most often affecting children and young adults), it is often prescribed for fever in children. However, acetaminophen overdose is a common diagnosis in emergency rooms and poison centers. Although acetaminophen is metabolized and cleared sufficiently at normal doses, elevated doses and certain drug interactions produce more of a hepatotoxic intermediate, which can cause serious liver damage. Alcohol consumption, for example, can induce liver enzymes that increase the amount of the toxic intermediate, increasing chances for liver toxicity.

Acetaminophen's mechanism of action remains unclear. Acetaminophen may inhibit both forms of the enzyme cyclooxygenase (COX-1 or COX-2; see details below), which are the primary targets of the NSAIDs. However, acetaminophen's activity differs from that of the NSAIDs and may involve an indirect mechanism in the central nervous system. It only weakly slows prostaglandin production. It has been postulated that acetaminophen can inhibit nitric oxide synthase activity. Nitric oxide is a powerful vasodilator, as we discussed in Chapter 4. The resulting decrease in nitric oxide attenuates nociception. Also, acetaminophen enhances serotonin activity. Serotonin has neurotransmitter and hormone-like activity. It is active in descending neuronal projections in the spinal cord. These nerve projections exert an analgesic effect by inhibiting an incoming pain signal before it moves up to the CNS. Enhancing serotonin action would, then, provide a level of analgesia. It is possible that all of these suggested roles for acetaminophen provide some portion of its analgesic effect, as none of them are fully supported by the available evidence (Toussaint, Yang, Zielinski, et al. 2010).

Acetaminophen may modulate the endogenous cannabinoid system. Cannabinoids (medical marijuana, THC—see Chapter 15) have analgesic activity and have been tested for therapeutic effect on certain types of pain. The active ingredient of cannabis, delta-9-THC, implies the existence of endogenous cannabinoids involved in memory, pain relief, the feeling of euphoria, and patterns of eating and sleeping behavior. The discovery in 1992 of anandamide, an endogenous ligand for the endocannabinoid system, has spurred progress in understanding the basic pharmacology.

Anandamide and cannabinoids work through two cannabinoid receptors (CB1 and CB2). The cannabinoid receptors are G-protein–coupled receptors. CB1 is an abundant receptor in the nervous system, where it may inhibit release of neurotransmitters. CB2 is mainly associated with immune cells in the periphery, where it may modulate cytokine release. Agonists and antagonists have been developed for both receptor subtypes (Fowler, Holt, Nilsson, et al. 2005). Agonists decrease pain associated with inflammation. They can also limit neuropathic pain and pain associated with multiple sclerosis. Cannabinoids stimulate appetite and have anti-emetic (anti-nausea and -vomiting) properties, making them particularly useful for certain cancer treatments. The receptor called TRPV1 (formerly called the vanilloid receptor) also responds to endogenous cannabinoids. It is a cation channel that opens when bound to agonists such as cannabinoids. TRPV1 is involved with pain sensation and also responds to acidic pH and elevated temperature, resulting in a burning sensation. Interestingly, it is also the receptor for capsaicin (the compound that makes chili peppers "hot"). Close association and interaction between TRPV1, CB1, and CB2 in sensory neurons may help explain the pain reduction observed with CB2 agonists (Anand, Otto, Sanchez-Herrera, et al. 2008).

Acetaminophen is metabolized to an intermediate in the brain that is responsible, in part, for its anti-nociceptive activity. This intermediate is related to the endogenous cannabinoids. Although the intermediate lacks agonist activity toward CB1 and CB2, it does activate TRPV1, as do other CB1 agonists. The acetaminophen metabolites may also block reuptake of the endogenous cannabinoids. Therefore, acetaminophen may have direct and indirect cannabinoid agonist activity.

Peripheral pain in rats was suppressed with acetaminophen. This suppression was blocked with a CB1 antagonist, suggesting that acetaminophen may work through the endocannabinoid system, at least in part (Ottani, Leone, Sandrini, et al. 2006). The CB1 receptors may reinforce the serotonergic pathways (mentioned above), involved with suppressing spinal transmission of pain (Mallet, Daulhac, Bonnefont, et al. 2008). However, CB1 antagonists do not block the anti-pyretic effects of acetaminophen, suggesting additional mechanisms are involved (Toussaint et al.). Yet another target for pain suppression has been identified for metabolites of acetaminophen and cannabinoids (Andersson, Gentry, Alenmyr, et al. 2011). The TRPA1 receptor is an ion channel involved in sensing cold, pain, and other irritants. Its activation in the spine alleviates pain, suggesting another mechanism for acetaminophen (or its metabolites), as CB1 antagonists block the receptor's action.

Clearly, we have a way to go before we fully understand how acetaminophen works. Since acetaminophen has good efficacy for a wide variety of pain, defining its molecular targets is of great importance. Once a target (or two) is known, drug screening can be done to find derivatives with improved potency. Improved potency would mean that lower doses could be used, with potentially fewer hepatotoxic effects. Since acetaminophen lacks the GI and kidney issues associated with NSAIDs and the side effects of opioids, acetaminophen derivatives show great potential for the development of safe and economical pain relievers.

Non-steroidal Anti-inflammatory Drugs

The NSAIDs are very effective analgesics with anti-pyretic activity similar to acetaminophen. Where NSAIDs differ significantly from acetaminophen and the opioids is in their anti-inflammatory action. After giving brief overviews of inflammation and fever, we will discuss the mechanism of action for NSAIDs.

The Inflammatory Response

The inflammatory response in an ancient and evolutionarily conserved response that is highly beneficial to the survival of the organism. The ability to mount a response to a wide variety of noxious agents (infection, physical injury, etc.) is essential in the face of environmental pathogens and other dangers. A blunt-force or penetrating tissue injury can initiate inflammation, as can a response to a pathogen that causes an infection. Toxins and chemical irritants can cause inflammation, as will burns, frostbite, and other injuries. The inflammation process isolates the damaged area and attracts leukocytes (white blood cells) to the site. As inflammation progresses, healing of affected tissues is promoted. In parallel, a distinct series of events called **resolution** returns the tissue back to its original state.

ACUTE INFLAMMATION

Acute inflammation is initiated by cells present in most tissues, such as resident macrophages, dendritic cells, mast cells, platelets, nerve endings, and endothelial cells. At the onset of an infection or injury, these cells undergo activation and release **inflammatory mediators** responsible for the clinical signs of inflammation (see Box). The clinical signs, also referred to as the cardinal signs, include warmth, redness, swelling, pain, and loss of function. Mechanistically, there is local vasodilation and increased capillary permeability, which allows components in the blood to leak into the spaces where the damage is located. This swelling or edema is essential for the process, as many components from the blood are now at the inflamed site. The site becomes red and warm to the touch. Some of the released molecules act as chemoattractants that draw leukocytes, neutrophils (a type of white blood cell), and other phagocytic cells to the location. As the process extends over several days, tissue degeneration and fibrosis can occur. In certain disease states, the inflammatory response can be prolonged and potentially damaging.

Mediators of Inflammation

A very large number of chemical mediators are involved in inflammation. In many cases, their action is sequential, as the process plays out and then is resolved, with the tissues returning to their initial state (see Table 11.2). Cells already present in most tissues produce early mediators that act locally at the site of inflammation. Pre-existing vesicles containing **histamine** in mast cells or **serotonin** and histamine in platelets allow quick release and get the process underway by causing arteriole dilation and increased venous permeability. **Heparin**, an anticoagulant, is secreted along with histamine and prevents the blood from clotting at the inflammation site. Leukocytes and mast cells in the inflamed tissue start producing and releasing **prostaglandins** and **leukotrienes** derived from arachidonic acid, as shown in Figure 11.1. The prostaglandins include a large number of related lipid molecules that cause vasodilation, fever, and pain. Leukotrienes mediate leukocyte adhesion and activation, allowing the white blood cells to bind the lining of the endothelium and migrate through the lining into the interstitial space. Leukotrienes are also a potent chemoattractant for neutrophils, encouraging them to the inflamed site.

   The variety of infiltrating leukocytes produce other chemical mediators that attack viral or bacterial invaders. Monocytes (a type of white blood cell) differentiate into macrophages when they leave the vasculature and enter the interstitial space. They produce **nitric oxide** to cause additional vasodilation. Many other chemical mediators released by leukocytes (interleukins and interferon are examples) aid the attraction, adhesion, and regulation of inflammation following tissue damage or microbial invasion. The liver produces protein factors that arrive at the site through the leaky vasculature and become activated by enzymes present at the inflamed site. One of these protein factors, **bradykinin**, we discussed previously in Chapter 5. Bradykinin also contributes to the vasodilation and leakiness of the vasculature at the damaged site. Additional mediators listed in Table 11.2 have an important role in chronic inflammation, where macrophages are central to the complex interaction of many cytokines and related signaling molecules. Besides a role in inflammation, tumor necrosis factor (TNF) and many of the interleukins have essential functions in regulating the immune system.

Table 11.2 A partial list of the many chemical mediators involved in inflammation, with brief descriptions of their sources and actions

Mediator	Classification	Source	Actions
Histamine	Vasoactive amine	Mast cells, platelets, basophils	Arteriole dilation, increases venous permeability
Serotonin	Neurotransmitter, vasoactive amine	Platelets	Increases vascular permeability, activates dendritic cells
Leukotriene	Eicosanoid	Leukocytes	Chemoattractant, leukocyte infiltration
Prostaglandins	Eicosanoid	Mast cells	Vasodilation, fever, and pain
Nitric oxide	Soluble gas	Macrophages, endothelial cells	Potent vasodilator, relaxes smooth muscle
Bradykinin	Peptide	Liver	Vasodilation, increases permeability
Interferon	Cytokine	T-lymphocytes	Antiviral, immunoregulatory, activates macrophages in chronic inflammation
Tumor necrosis factor (TNF), Interleukin 1 (IL-1)	Cytokines	Macrophages	Systemic effects, fever, activates connective tissue, gene expression, cytokine production, role in chronic inflammation

Many different molecules are involved in these complex activities. Histamine, serotonin, and bradykinin all play a part as inflammatory mediators, at least initially (see Table 11.2). Conversion of arachidonic acid into many different eicosanoids (biologically active lipid mediators, including prostaglandins, leukotrienes, and thromboxanes) helps generate the complex series of responses (see Figure 11.1). The infiltration of leukocytes at the inflamed site increases cyclooxygenase activity (primarily COX-2; see below) and increases the amount and types of eicosanoids. Prostaglandins and leukotrienes, along with other molecules, including ATP, serotonin, bradykinin, and H^+, increase the sensitivity of nociceptors and increase pain perception, the basis for inflammatory pain. The loss of function mentioned as a cardinal sign is probably the result of a neurological reflex in response to pain. In addition, one of the prostaglandins crosses the blood–brain barrier to stimulate the hypothalamus to increase body temperature (see discussion of fever below).

The resolution process begins early but is not fully active until after several days. The chemical mediators of resolution are called resolvins, derived from omega-3 fatty acids (discussed in Chapter 13). Under normal circumstances, tissue repair is completed and

Figure 11.1 Production of eicosanoids.

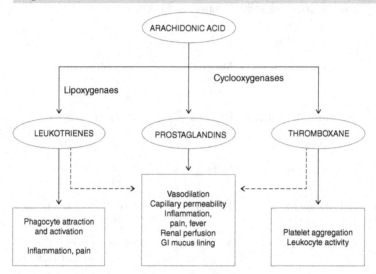

Legend: A highly schematic overview of the production and actions of the eicosanoids, including leukotrienes, thromboxane, and prostaglandins.

returned to its original state. The acute inflammatory response requires a persistent stimulus to be sustained, because the inflammatory mediators have short half-lives. They are degraded relatively quickly, so that acute inflammation ceases once the stimulus has been removed. However, if the agent causing the inflammation persists for a prolonged period of time, the inflammation becomes chronic.

CHRONIC INFLAMMATION

Inflammation can last indefinitely if the stimulus persists, even when the stimulus is a relatively harmless irritant, such as dust, pollen, or a low-grade infection. Chronic inflammation is primarily mediated by macrophages. Macrophages release several different chemical mediators, including prostaglandins, which perpetuate the pro-inflammatory response. Macrophages also engulf and digest microorganisms, dying cells, and cell debris. Lymphocytes also arrive at the site and produce antibodies that specifically target the invading microorganisms for destruction. In some cases, the body's own tissue can sustain collateral damage. Tissue damage is a hallmark of chronic inflammation. Repair of the damaged tissue can result from production of replacement cells or growth of fibrous connective tissue. The development of new blood vessels (angiogenesis) can also occur. If the body is unable to repair this damage effectively, the inflammatory cascade will continue. Chronic inflammation is abnormal and can lead to a number of disease states, such as diabetes, cancer, arthritis, neurological diseases, cardiovascular disease, and autoimmune disease. Autoimmune disease occurs when normal, healthy tissue is recognized as foreign and an inflammatory attack is launched against it.

Fever

As discussed, the inflammatory response can include fever. When bacteria or viruses invade the body and cause tissue injury, one of the immune system's responses is to raise body temperature, causing a fever. The immune system produces **cytokines**, proteins that provide communication between the various cell types that make up the immune system. The different leukocytes respond to different cues and produce and release cytokines that communicate and coordinate the functions of other cells to produce the immune response. Pyrogens are a subclass of cytokines. They increase the thermoregulatory set point in the hypothalamus, the part of the brain that regulates body temperature. The hypothalamus raises the body's temperature, causing a fever. The elevated body temperature stimulates leukocyte activity and number, helping to defend against microbial invasion.

Another critical regulator of fever is prostaglandin E_2 (PGE_2) (Dinarello 2004). PGE_2 is derived from arachidonic acid (see Figure 11.1), dependent on COX-2 activity. The brain ultimately orchestrates heat effector mechanisms via the autonomic nervous system. Increased heat production results from increased muscle tone, shivering, and hormones, such as epinephrine, that activate muscle tissue. Heat loss is reduced by vasoconstriction and decreased blood flow to the surface of the body. In infants, the autonomic nervous system can activate brown adipose tissue to produce heat (non-exercise-associated thermogenesis). In activated brown adipose tissue, the energy produced in mitochondria cannot make ATP and instead is released as heat. Increased heart rate and vasoconstriction contribute to increased blood pressure in fever. Drugs effective at reducing fever generally target the production of PGE_2. Aspirin and the NSAIDs are effective inhibitors of COX-2 and decrease the production of PGE_2, providing fever relief.

Types of NSAIDs

There many different NSAIDs, including salicylates (aspirin and derivatives), ibuprofen (Advil), and naproxen (Aleve; see Table 11.1). NSAIDs have anti-inflammatory activity, in part due to their ability to inhibit the enzyme **cyclooxygenase (COX)**, which is early in the pathway that generates prostaglandins and thromboxanes (see Figure 11.1). As stated earlier, there are two forms of cyclooxygenase: **COX-1** and **COX-2**. Aspirin and the traditional NSAIDs inhibit both forms of the enzyme. Newer NSAIDs were designed as specific COX-2 inhibitors.

The anti-pyretic activities of willow bark led to the discovery of salicylates, such as aspirin (acetylsalicylic acid), and aspirin remains the cheapest and most commonly used analgesic. Aspirin is an irreversible inhibitor of platelet COX-1, as it chemically modifies and inactivates the enzyme. By inhibiting COX-1, aspirin inhibits platelet aggregation and increases clotting time, which makes it useful in preventing heart attacks and strokes in at risk populations. It does this to a much greater degree than the other NSAIDs. Another common salicylate is methyl salicylate, which is used topically (see Box) in rubs and creams for muscle soreness (e.g., Bengay). Methyl salicylate is toxic if ingested or used in excess under conditions where absorption from the skin can increase systemic levels.

Topical Treatments for Pain

Opinions differ on the effectiveness of OTC topical pain medications. Topical treatments may have some efficacy in treating osteoarthritis in joints close to the skin's surface, such as the hands and knees. Some products work no better than placebo, although some people feel relief of their arthritis pain. Topical salicylates appear to be more effective for muscle aches, while capsaicin is more often used for pain associated with damaged nerves. Capsaicin cream causes a burning sensation that lessens over repeated use, and it may take days to provide noticeable relief from pain.

Topical pain relievers containing NSAIDs are now available in the United States. They may cause fewer instances of internal bleeding than oral NSAIDs. Topical NSAIDs include diclofenac as a gel, drops, and a patch. Patches applied to an afflicted area can release a drug for transdermal absorption lasting up to 12 hours. An older group of topical treatments is the counterirritants. Ingredients such as menthol, methyl salicylate, and camphor are called counterirritants because they create a burning or cooling sensation that distracts from or alters the sensation of pain. Doctors may also prescribe a patch containing a numbing lidocaine (a local anesthetic) to help numb joint pain. Patients who are taking blood thinners or are allergic to aspirin should consult a physician before using topical medications that contain salicylates.

There has been an increased interest in herbal remedies. For example, Arnica is an herb used in creams and ointments that many people use for muscle soreness, bruising, joint pain and swelling. Limited studies have been done, but some claim help with pain and bruising of the skin. Extracts of hemp, containing cannabidiol (commonly known as CBD oil), are also used for pain management and are covered in more detail in Chapter 15.

The other NSAIDs (e.g., ibuprofen and naproxen) are reversible inhibitors of cyclooxygenase activity. Prostaglandins and the other eicosanoids are involved in the inflammation response and take part in fever and sensitizing nerves. By blocking prostaglandin synthesis, these drugs can reduce fever and provide analgesia. As stated earlier, COX-1 is widely distributed and has constitutive activity, meaning it is usually active in cells throughout the body. It is probably important in everyday kinds of minor noxious events. For example, it plays a role in protecting the cells that line the stomach from their harsh, acidic environment. In contrast, COX-2 is inducible (activity increases in response to stimuli) and plays a greater role when the inflammatory response ramps up. The cells that arrive at the inflamed site contain more COX-2 activity and increase eicosanoid production. Salicylates and the older NSAIDs (sometimes called "traditional NSAIDs"), such as ibuprofen, inhibit both forms of cyclooxygenase.

Specific COX-2 inhibitors were developed (Vioxx, Celebrex, Mobic) with the hope that they would have fewer adverse effects, particularly on the stomach lining, than the traditional NSAIDs. The reasoning was that a specific COX-2 inhibitor could help control inflammation and pain but allow COX-1 to perform its protective function in the gut and kidneys. Inhibition of COX-2 explains most but not all of the anti-pyretic and anti-inflammatory effects of these drugs. However, an increase in cardiovascular issues caused COX-2 inhibitors to be withdrawn from the market in 2004 and 2005. Their inhibition of COX-2 and suppression of prostaglandin synthesis leads to blood clotting issues. Normally, COX-2 produces a prostaglandin (PGI_2) that suppresses platelet aggregation, while a thromboxane (TXA_2) produced by COX-1 causes platelet aggregation. When both are present sufficiently, clotting is inhibited. The lower level of the prostaglandin following COX-2 inhibition cannot compensate for the increase in thromboxane (COX-1 is not inhibited), increasing the risk of clotting and cardiovascular events. Many lawsuits resulted, and the COX-2 inhibitors were pulled from the market. A few COX-2 inhibitors are currently available, but these are required to have a warning label. Remarkably, the COX-2 inhibitors are not more potent in relieving arthritic pain, so their fast-tracking through the approval process and rapid acceptance for use in arthritis raised questions about the approval process for bringing drugs to market (Vioxx: lessons for Health Canada and the FDA 2005).

NSAIDs are used extensively for joint and muscle soreness, with millions taking the drugs for arthritis pain. At least 80% of the elderly take them (and perhaps one-third of them should not, due to GI and kidney issues—see Elder Concerns below). In the 1990s, many of these drugs became available OTC. NSAIDs and salicylates do not cause physical or psychological dependence. Because they are widely used by athletes and de-conditioned individuals, we must ask, what are their effects when taken for pain resulting from physical exertion?

Prednisone: The Anti-Inflammatory Synthetic Corticosteroid

Corticosteroids are produced in the adrenal cortex. They have many effects on the body but most often are used for their potent anti-inflammatory effects. Prednisone, a synthetic corticosteroid, is used to treat the symptoms of low corticosteroid levels. It is roughly four times more potent than the endogenous corticosteroid (hydrocortisone in humans). When prescribed at doses that exceed normal hydrocortisone levels, prednisone suppresses inflammation. It is effective in reducing swelling and redness due to inflammation following injury. Prednisone, or one of several other related synthetic corticosteroids, is used to treat diseases with an underlying inflammatory component, including certain types of arthritis, asthma, colitis, severe allergic reactions, autoimmune disease, and certain types of cancer.

At a molecular level, unbound glucocorticoids in the blood enter cells by easily crossing the cell membrane and then bind glucocorticoid receptors with high affinity. Glucocorticoid-bound receptors move to the cell nucleus, where they turn on some genes and turn off others (Coutinho & Chapman 2011). The result is the production of some new proteins and the decreased production of other proteins. Glucocorticoid-responsive cells can, then, influence the inflammation response. Possible responses include interfering with the chemical mediators that drive the inflammatory response and inhibition of leukocyte infiltration at the inflammation site. Corticosteroids activate a protein that blocks the release of the precursor arachidonic acid from membrane phospholipids (see Figure 11.1), thereby decreasing the production of prostaglandins and leukotrienes. As a result of decreased eicosanoid synthesis, there is a reduction in edema and a general suppression in the immune response. For synthetic corticosteroids, the degree of anti-inflammatory response depends on the dose administered.

Prednisone is rapidly absorbed across the gut membrane following oral administration. It is a pro-drug and requires conversion to its active form (prednisolone) by enzymes in the liver. The liver is also the primary site of its metabolism to inactive compounds. Therefore, proper liver function is important for its activity. Peak effects can be observed after one to two hours. It has relatively high levels of binding to plasma proteins, which helps to extend its biological half-life to 18 to 36 hours.

The numerous adverse effects related to synthetic corticosteroid use are related to the duration of therapy and the dose administered. Long-term use of corticosteroids can have severe consequences. Corticosteroids decrease bone formation and increase bone resorption, which can lead to osteoporosis (bone loss), particularly important in post-menopausal women. Corticosteroids can also reduce sex hormone production and slow the growth and development of children.

Exercise Pharmacology

Prolonged exercise at moderate to high intensity (heavy to difficult breathing) releases endorphins that help counteract the increasing level of discomfort associated with maintaining that workload. During recovery, many additional hormones and neurotransmitters are involved, including serotonin, epinephrine, corticosteroids, and dopamine. The physiological basis of "runner's high" has been debated, as opioid antagonists do not completely suppress the elevated mood state. It is not clear whether the endogenous opioid peptides can cross the blood–brain barrier to exert a CNS response under most conditions.

Exercise also increases the output of endogenous cannabinoids in an intensity-dependent manner (Raichlen, Foster, Seillier, et al. 2013). Cannabinoids cause a psychological state that may contribute to the runner's high (Dietrich & McDaniel 2004). Additionally, recovery from exercise involves many of the same factors involved in inflammation and pain suppression. Regular training may cause adaptation in some of these responses compared to a single acute bout of exercise. There are still many questions as to which components of recovery are important for the desired gains in strength and fitness. "No pain, no gain" is often proclaimed in the weight room, as a mantra for those wanting to build muscle.

Pharmacokinetic Concerns

Opioids

The opioid morphine is subject to significant levels of first-pass metabolism in the liver when taken orally, and increasing the dose is necessary for oral administration. Alternatively, morphine can be injected SC or IM. To avoid use of needles and the first-pass effect, morphine can also be given nasally, as a lozenge under the tongue, or as a transdermal patch. First-pass metabolism is less of an issue with codeine and oxycodone, which makes them more suitable for oral administration. Heroin (diacetylmorphine) undergoes a two-step process to be converted into morphine in the body.

Opioids distribute well to highly perfused tissues. Metabolism to water-soluble intermediates leads to most of the drug being excreted by the kidneys. For some opioids, metabolites can have increased activity. Properly functioning kidneys are, therefore, very important to clear the drug from the system while maintaining pain relief and minimizing unwanted side effects. Exercise intensity probably is not a relevant concern, as few patients (or addicts) taking morphine-like drugs will be doing much exercising at moderate or higher intensities. Some of these patients may, however, benefit from walking and stretching programs.

Acetaminophen

Acetaminophen is rapidly absorbed and reaches peak blood levels in less than an hour. It does not significantly bind to proteins in the serum. Acetaminophen crosses the blood–brain barrier, so it has a possible CNS site of action. Extensive metabolism occurs, with only about 3% excreted from the kidneys unchanged. As discussed earlier, the liver metabolites of acetaminophen may have important biological activity or cause hepatotoxicity. Therefore, liver and kidney function is important in the bioavailability and activity of acetaminophen.

NSAIDs

NSAIDs are rapidly absorbed when taken orally and reach peak blood levels relatively quickly, similar to acetaminophen. They bind serum proteins to a high extent, and this can affect their distribution kinetics. Their high degree of binding can also be an issue when they are used in drug combinations, as drugs with higher affinity for the protein sites can displace the NSAID, causing a spike in its free concentration. However, binding to serum proteins can be an advantage when serum proteins gain access to sites of inflammation, effectively delivering the drug to the site of elevated COX-2 activity. Metabolism to more water-soluble intermediates decreases activity and aids clearance by the kidneys. Only a small percentage is excreted unchanged. Given the role of liver metabolism and excretion by the kidneys, exercise would be expected to increase the serum half-life of these drugs in an intensity-dependent manner. However, the high level of bound drug probably minimizes or buffers changes in bioavailability in most cases.

Pharmacodynamic Concerns

Acetaminophen

There are limited studies on acetaminophen and exercise performance. One study showed a modest improvement in cycling time, with no difference in RPE or perception of pain (Mauger, Jones, & Williams 2010). Acetaminophen reduced the extent to which power output declined during the middle portion of the trial, with an improvement in completion time that was statistically significant in this study. Another study suggested that acetaminophen may have improved performance through the reduction of pain during repeated sprint cycling in nine male participants. For a given work rate, pain reduction may have enabled participants to exercise closer to a true physiological limit (Foster, Taylor, Chrismas, et al. 2014). Acetaminophen also increased critical torque during maximal knee extensions in 13 active males (Morgan, Bowtell, Vanhatalo, et al. 2018). Whether acetaminophen use during competition or intense training is safe or should be discouraged has generated some controversy and discussion, with evidence leaning toward discouraging its use (Esh, Mauger, Palfreeman, et al. 2017). Additional research is needed to clarify whether acetaminophen can be ergogenic and improve performance under other exercise protocols and with more diverse participants.

NSAIDs

NSAIDs are frequently used after competition or training to suppress minor symptoms of muscle and joint soreness. Soreness can peak 24 to 48 hours post-exercise; this type of soreness is distinguished as delayed-onset muscle soreness. NSAIDs are also used to treat acute musculoskeletal injuries, such as a sprained ankle. During the initial stage of an acute injury (such as a muscle strain, sudden bout of tendinopathy, or ankle sprain), NSAIDs can facilitate healing by limiting the extent of inflammation and swelling. However, when these drugs are taken for an extended time, there are questions as to whether the body's normal healing process is being retarded (Mackey, Mikkelksen, Magnusson, & Kjaer 2012). For example, evidence from animal studies suggests that COX-2 inhibition suppresses early healing of bone fractures.

Studies involving human subjects, however, have not provided convincing evidence to substantiate this concern (Kurmis, Kurmis, O'Brien, & Dalén 2012). These authors suggest that short-duration use of NSAIDs for post-fracture pain control does not significantly increase the risk of impaired healing. However, it is clear from many studies that the natural healing process is complex and dependent to some extent on the products of COX-2.

Inflammation is a protection mechanism that initiates the healing process and repairs damage. Training can create small micro-tears in muscles. The more intense the effort, the more forcefully muscles contract, creating the potential for more damage. After a hard workout or during the early stages of an injury, the injured area becomes inflamed and has increased blood flow, swelling, and inflammatory pain. By initiating the inflammatory response, these micro-tears stimulate the body to deliver resources needed to begin the healing process. When the individual takes anti-inflammatory drugs, the inflammation and healing process may be delayed (Mackey et al.). Additionally, prostaglandins have many important bodily functions under normal conditions, such as helping maintain blood flow to the kidneys and protecting the stomach lining. Inhibition of their production with the traditional NSAIDs can cause another set of problems, such as bleeding in the gut or decreased renal perfusion rates.

One line of thinking is that taking NSAIDs prophylactically (e.g., before working out) will inhibit production of inflammatory mediators and decrease muscle soreness and fatigue, ultimately shortening recovery times. In some published reports, prophylactic use was effective in pain reduction, though not in all reports. Even with pain reduction, decreases in plasma creatine kinase generally are not observed with prophylactic treatment. Plasma creatine kinase is an indicator of muscle cell damage, as it is normally found inside muscle cells, with very low levels in the serum. Following exercise or muscle injury, creatine kinase levels in the blood increase, making it a useful indicator of muscle cell damage (Clarkson, Kearns, Rouzier, et al. 2006).

Can NSAIDs be used to enhance performance for a competitive advantage? Many studies have attempted to answer this question. An older literature looked at the effects of aspirin on exercise performance. Salicylates at normal doses did not affect insulin, glucose, free fatty acid utilization, or performance. Other studies have examined whether NASIDs can enhance performance by diminishing pain before and during long endurance races or long training sessions. For example, 30% to 50% of participants in Ironman races and marathons have admitted use of NSAIDs before and during events. Are they helping their performance or putting themselves at risk (Kuster, Renner, Oppel, et al. 2013)? The evidence is mixed, with some studies suggesting these drugs may have a negative effect. In an older study, ibuprofen did not prevent delayed-onset muscle soreness or improve times during bouts of downhill running (Donnelly, Maughan, & Whiting 1990). Furthermore, the study found that known markers of muscle breakdown were elevated in the ibuprofen-treated participants, such as creatine kinase. The treatment involved two 600 mg tablets of ibuprofen or an identically appearing placebo 30 minutes before each trial (45 minutes on a decline on a treadmill) and then one 600 mg tablet (or placebo) every six hours for three days. After 10 weeks, the second trial was conducted, with the treatments reversed. The creatine kinase activity increased significantly after each downhill run, although the increase in the second period was less ($p < 0.01$). For both periods of the study, the increase in creatine kinase was significantly higher in the ibuprofen-treated group ($p < 0.01$) (Donnelly et al.).

More recently, Nieman, Henson, Dumke, and colleagues (2006) studied the influence of ibuprofen in a grueling 100-mile trail-running race. Subjects were placed in three groups: a control group and two groups taking either 600 mg or 1200 mg of ibuprofen the day before and on race day. This study did not use a double-blind or crossover protocol, due to the need for approvals/waivers by the participants. Delayed onset of pain and serum creatine kinase was the same in all groups. Race times and ratings of perceived exertion did not differ among the groups. Both groups taking ibuprofen had higher plasma levels of serum C-reactive protein, plasma cytokine, and macrophage inflammatory protein, indicating higher levels of muscle damage compared to those who did not take NSAIDs (Nieman et al.).

NSAID use during ultra distance exercise, such as an Ironman triathlon, is associated with an increased risk of exertional **hyponatremia** (abnormally low levels of sodium in the blood), which causes cells to swell (Wharam, Speedy, Noakes, et al. 2006). Issues related to altered kidney function in endurance athletes are not surprising, as these competitors deal with dehydration and salt imbalance. NSAIDs can contribute to poor fluid transport and restricted kidney function, increasing potential problems with salt and water balance. Significantly higher levels of oxidative stress were seen in runners who took ibuprofen during extreme exercise (McAnulty, Owens, McAnulty, et al. 2007). Ibuprofen administration during endurance training suppressed the adaptations in skeletal muscle that occur with training (Machida & Takemasa 2010). In this experiment, mice were used to examine the changes that occur to muscle tissue after four weeks of using an exercise wheel. Normal adaptations in muscle tissue were blunted with concurrent ibuprofen treatment. Similar results have been found in humans. For example, maximal doses of ibuprofen (1,200 mg) decreased strength and muscle hypertrophic adaptations to eight weeks of resistance training in men and women aged 18 to 35 years old (Lilja et al., 2018). The conclusions of many studies on the prophylactic or extended use of NSAIDs suggest that they may hinder muscle adaptation to training and cause significant safety concerns such that their use should be limited (Warden 2009; Warden 2010).

Elder Concerns

As patients age, the incidence and prevalence of certain pain syndromes increase (Kaye, Baluch, & Scott, 2010). Elderly patients incorrectly believe that pain is a normal process of aging leading to pain symptoms being underreported. Aging affects how patients handle medications, including those for pain. Since many pain medications are over-the-counter (OTC), they are generally thought to be 'safe.' However, this is not necessarily the case and certainly can be an issue in the elderly. The elderly often practice poly-pharmacy—they take several prescription drugs regularly. This practice can lead to more issues with side effects. As discussed in Chapter 1, the aging process changes pharmacokinetic properties. For example, elderly patients often have increased fat mass with decreased muscle mass, decreased body water, and altered drug distribution. Drug absorption may change with age as there are changes in stomach acid levels, and some have decreased saliva making swallowing difficult. The kidneys become smaller and have decreased blood flow making them less effective at drug elimination. The liver decreases in mass and blood flow, and lower metabolic rates. Keep in mind that these functional decreases in kidney and liver activity occur while the elderly patients are taking multiple medications.

To overcome these challenges, doctors often start their older patients on the lowest recommended dose and then increase the amount of medication if necessary. Elderly patients need to talk to their doctor before taking any over-the-counter medications; a lower dose should be taken than the dose recommended on the label. For elderly patients dealing with pain, a comprehensive pain assessment should be done. This assessment should include a thorough medical history and physical examination, review of pertinent laboratory results, imaging studies, and diagnostic tests.

A major issue for pain management in the elderly involves the NSAIDs. Though they are often prescribed, they are also readily available OTC. The current opioid crisis has increased the use of NSAIDs, with an estimated 30 billion OTC NSAIDs sold in the United States annually. The prevalence of NSAID use in patients over 65 years old is as high as 96% (Wongrakpanich, Wongrakpanich, Melhado, & Rangaswami, 2018). These numbers are a bit shocking because NSAIDs are not recommended for people with kidney, liver, or heart issues, and should not be taken without consulting a doctor. Other high-risk groups include those over 75 years old and those using corticosteroids, anticoagulants, or antiplatelet agents. NSAIDs are one of the leading causes of hospitalization among elderly patients admitted for adverse or side effects of medications. The elderly are more likely to suffer heart damage, strokes, and are at risk for damage to the stomach and digestive system. Many negative drug interactions are known, including (and not limited to) beta-blockers (Chapter 4), ACE inhibitors, ARBs and calcium channel blockers (Chapter 5), diuretics (Chapter 6), and SSRI (Chapter 9) (Wongrakpanich et al.).

In the elderly, NSAIDs should be used with caution at the lowest effective dose and shortest duration. Chronic use of all NSAIDs, including high dose aspirin, should be avoided because of the risk of gastrointestinal bleeding. However, large numbers of people admit to taking NSAIDs more than the recommended 21 consecutive days (Wongrakpanich et al.). One good thing is that the anti-inflammatory effect of NSAIDs may help cognitive function. Additionally, in a mouse model for Alzheimer's disease, low-dose aspirin decreased amyloid plaque pathology in both male and female mice in a PPARα-dependent fashion (Chandra, Jana, & Pahan 2018).

Health Risks

Opioids have no anti-pyretic or anti-inflammatory activity. Their euphoria and mood-change effects can lead to abuse and a high risk of addiction, dependence, tolerance, and withdrawal syndrome. In some cases the analgesic effect also shows tolerance, requiring an increase in dose. Opioids cause constipation by inhibiting gut motility, and at higher doses can suppress the respiratory rate. These effects do not show tolerance and become worse as the dose increases. Opioids are heavily prescribed and abused. Even cough syrup containing codeine or dextromethorphan is regularly abused by "syrup-heads." Many prescription opioids are combined with acetaminophen, such as Percocet. Abusers of these drugs may increase the dose to get the desired feeling, but they are also increasing the dose of acetaminophen, thereby increasing the chance for hepatotoxicity due to acetaminophen metabolites. Opioid analgesics with or without acetaminophen should not be taken with alcohol. Drowsiness, suppression of breathing rate, and potential for hepatotoxicity all increase markedly with alcohol.

The societal problems associated with prescription pain-killers containing opioids continue to escalate. Addiction to the prescription pain-killers is leading to an increase in the use of street drugs like heroin. In many communities, rates of heroin overdose continue to rise (Pradip, Muhuri, & Davies 2013). An opioid receptor antagonist called naltrexone has been used in the management of alcohol dependence and opioid dependence. Naltrexone does not stimulate the pleasure sensation associated with alcohol or opiates and can provide a buffer or safety net for recovering addicts. A once-monthly extended-release injectable formulation is marketed under the trade name Vivitrol. The treatments are expensive but are an important aid for individuals who want to combat their addiction.

Acetaminophen is generally considered relatively safe when used as directed, but acetaminophen toxicity is a significant problem. Acetaminophen overdose is a leading cause for calls to Poison Control Centers and results in over 400 deaths per year (Lee 2004). The recommended dose for an adult is 325 to 650 mg every four to six hours, primarily for acute conditions. An overdose of acetaminophen can damage the liver and be fatal. Signs of toxicity include nausea, pain in the upper stomach, itching, loss of appetite, dark urine, clay-colored stools, or jaundice (yellowing of skin or eyes). Acetaminophen is used in combination with many other prescription and OTC medicines. The cumulative dose can exceed recommended levels and lead to liver problems. Acetaminophen can interact with other drugs and dietary supplements to cause additional stress on the liver. Alcohol should be avoided when taking acetaminophen, as the liver problems can become worse.

NSAIDs cause gastropathy (stomach disease) and are potentially nephrotoxic (toxic to the kidney). Approximately 100,000 individuals in the United States are hospitalized each year because of these drugs, and an estimated 15% die annually, mostly the elderly. Nephrotoxicity from NSAIDs is well documented, especially in the elderly and people with decreased renal perfusion. Chronic renal toxicity has been observed in athletes following several months of ibuprofen, and acute renal failure has occurred following running a marathon. These drugs inhibit prostaglandin synthesis, thereby decreasing the normal vasodilatory response of prostaglandins during exercise. Combined with exercise, the augmented reduction in renal blood flow also decreases the glomerular filtration rate. For a person in a dehydrated state, ibuprofen reduces renal flow more than Tylenol. A triple impact on kidney function is seen with a combination of NSAIDs, diuretics, and ACE inhibitors. Combinations of diuretics and ACE inhibitors are used for hypertension. NSAIDs, some more than others, have an associated cardiovascular risk with their use (McGettigan & Henry 2011). The bottom line is that NSAIDs are potentially overused and overprescribed. For muscle soreness, consider ice and rest as an alternative.

Alternate Therapies for Pain

Pain can be a constant companion to those who regularly train, compete, or just do low-intensity exercise. Sometimes minor injuries can cause collateral damage, as when a pitcher in baseball ends up with shoulder soreness because of a change in mechanics following an ankle problem. As we age, joint pain, such as osteoarthritis, can become more prevalent, and sometimes back pain can be related to being sedentary and overweight. Because of the side effects from their use, people should consider choices besides drug treatment to help manage pain.

For soreness or minor injuries, early treatment and common sense often are enough to manage pain. Many follow the **RICE formula** for a muscle or joint injury:

- *Rest* the injured body part.
- *Ice* the area four times a day, for 10 to 15 minutes. Cold numbs sore areas and can reduce the pain and swelling of an arthritis flareup or joint injury. Cold may reduce inflammation by constricting blood flow to the injured area.
- *Compress* the area by wrapping it with an elastic bandage.
- *Elevate* the injured area, if possible, above the heart for a few hours a day.

These treatments should help lessen the amount of swelling. After several days and once the swelling has subsided, switching from cold to heat is recommended. Using a warm compress, heating pad, or hot-water bottle improves circulation in the affected area. Heat helps relax muscles and can decrease the sensation of pain.

Consulting a physical therapist, an athletic trainer, or other allied health professional is another alternative. These professionals can recognize when the body is out of balance and recommend strengthening exercises or stretching to bring balance back to overworked muscle groups. Strengthening relevant muscle groups and aerobic training can help reduce pain in the knee (Tanaka, Ozawa, Kito, & Moriyama 2013).

Engaging in certain physical activities is another alternative. Tai Chi can provide short-term relief from pain from osteoarthritis in the knee (Lauche, Langhorst, Dobos, & Cramer 2013). Yoga may also be useful for several pain-associated disorders. A meta-analysis showed positive effects for yoga as an intervention for back pain, arthritic pain, and migraine headaches (Bussing, Ostermann, Ludtke, & Michalsen 2012). Walking can also help with pain. A study in elderly patients with osteoarthritis in the knee showed that 12 weeks of exercise (50-minute walk three times per week) improved pain perception and increased circulating brain-derived neurotrophic factor (BDNF) levels (Gomes, Lacerda, Mendonca, et al. 2013). The increase in BDNF following physical activity may have an immunoprotective role in situations involving chronic inflammation (i.e., osteoarthritis in the knee). In Chapter 9 we saw that BDNF played a critical role in neurogenesis following physical activity. The brain is where the processing of pain input takes place. Alternate therapies target problem areas in the periphery where the pain signal is originating and may help with coping strategies in the brain.

Another alternate therapy is **acupuncture**, which has had its share of controversy. Acupuncture involves inserting needles at specific locations (called acupoints) and twisting the needle in and out to get the appropriate stimulation of afferent nerve fibers. A large-scale meta-analysis involving 17,922 patients supports acupuncture as a treatment for chronic pain (Vickers, Cronin, Maschino, et al. 2012). Negative controls for acupuncture studies include inserting needles at non-acupoint locations or inserting the needle at the acupoint but not rotating it. Imaging studies confirm that afferent fibers stimulate several regions of the brain in humans, in support of earlier animal studies (reviewed by Zhao 2008). A diverse number of molecules have been implicated in acupuncture analgesia, including adenosine, glutamate, and endorphins. The opioid peptides and all three receptors have been implicated (Zhao). A related technique call electroacupuncture pulses electric current through the needles. Interestingly, the release of opioids is frequency-dependent, with one frequency causing the release of enkephalin and another frequency causing dynorphin release.

The chemical studies, along with the brain imaging, suggest that acupuncture provides sensory input that the brain processes. In certain regions of the brain, the integration of the needle-generated "pain" and the chronic pain seems to bring the body back in balance. However acupuncture brings about pain alleviation (and much more work needs to be done to understand it fully), the result is less sensation of the pathological pain. Whether acupuncture is truly specific, with an underlying neurochemical mechanism, or just the result of sensory input, its use in alleviating pain supports the role for physical touch helping to maintain inner balance and quality of life. This concept is well known by a good massage therapist, who can provide short-term relief from aches and pains. The application of pressure and warmth changes blood flow patterns and stimulates nerves that lead to processing in the brain. Many times, a good hug and physical closeness with a loved one can relieve pain for a brief time.

Endurance exercise can cause some GI bleeding (intensity dependent), though it is subclinical in seriousness. NSAIDs cause gastropathy, but an additive effect has not been confirmed. COX-2 inhibitors may have less GI side effects but may have other issues, as mentioned previously. In a study of GI bleeding in distance runners, half of the participants had to be excluded because they were taking some form of NSAID. In general, moderate use after exercise to treat acute musculoskeletal injuries or delayed-onset muscle soreness for a short period of time is usually safe. People who have a history of gastrointestinal bleeding or kidney problems should check with their physicians before taking any NSAIDs. The goal is to balance recovery and adaptation. For a slight twinge, inflamed tendons, or delayed muscle soreness from training, NSAIDs taken for short period (one to two days) may provide relief without significant negative outcomes. Prolonged or excessive use of anti-inflammatory drugs can actually limit or cancel out the very training benefits that exercisers seek, by inhibiting adaptations to training, and such use can also lead to kidney damage.

Additionally, the use of NSAIDs to mask pain from an injury may allow an exerciser to continue training in the short term, but it can ultimately lead to a more serious and longer-lasting injury. Prophylactic use of ibuprofen by endurance athletes did not affect performance or perceived soreness, but it was associated with elevated indicators of inflammation and cell damage. As mentioned, one problem is bleeding from the gastrointestinal tract. NSAIDs can contribute to the development of hyponatremia when taken by endurance athletes during long races (Warden 2009).

In the case of salicylates, topical methyl salicylate absorption increases with exercise and temperature. Toxic episodes and death following excessive use of creams and lotions containing methyl salicylate have been reported.

PES Watch

NSAIDs are not banned. However, sometimes these drugs are combined with other drugs that are banned. NSAIDs are not ergogenic. They have potential toxicity. GI bleeding and negative effects on the kidneys should limit athletes' use of these drugs. Ethanol can make the GI problems worse. Although OTC drugs are lower in dose, these drugs potentially increase the risk of nephrotoxicity. Acetaminophen is not banned. It does not have anti-inflammatory activity and has potential liver toxicity (enhanced with alcohol). Opioids are on the banned list. Cannabinoids are banned, but these drugs raise some interesting issues, which will be addressed in Chapter 15.

Conclusion

Some pain is good—it helps protect against further damage. Opioids are often used for chronic pain, but they cause respiratory depression, constipation, drowsiness, and the inability to focus. They show tolerance and increasing the dose increases the potential for addiction. For mild to moderate pain and fever, acetaminophen is effective and is widely used for children. Aspirin and the other NSAIDs are also commonly used for fever and mild to moderate pain. These drugs suppress portions of the inflammatory response. NSAIDs should only be taken for brief intervals. They may help decrease the severity of an injury in the first 24 to 48 hours by suppressing part of the inflammatory response; however, the inflammatory response is a normal process that works to heal and repair the damage, and extended NSAID use could be counterproductive. Ice and rest sometimes are the best methods of helping the body heal.

Key Concepts Review

acetaminophen

acupuncture

analgesia

analgesic

anti-pyretic

COX-1

COX-2

cyclooxygenase (COX)

cytokine

dynorphin

dysfunctional pain

endorphin

enkephalin

hyponatremia

inflammatory mediator

inflammatory pain

mu

neuropathic pain

nociceptive pain

non-steroidal anti-inflammatory drug
   (NSAID)

opiate

opioid

opioid analgesic

opium

pain

pathological pain

pyrogen

Reye syndrome

RICE formula

Review Questions

1   How are pain, inflammation, and fever linked?
2   What advantages do opioids provide for chronic pain? Disadvantages?

3   What are the advantages and drawbacks of taking Tylenol for pain? What makes Tylenol different from aspirin?

4   NSAIDs are available over the counter. What are the medical risks involved in taking them?

5   How do NSAIDs exert their biological effect? Does their action affect exercise?

References

Anand U, Otto WR, Sanchez-Herrera D, Facer P, Yiangou Y, Korchev Y, Birch R, Benham C, Bountra C, Chessell IP, Anand P (2008) Cannabinoid receptor CB2 localisation and agonist-mediated inhibition of capsaicin responses in human sensory neurons. *Pain* 138:667–680

Andersson DA, Gentry C, Alenmyr L, Killander D, Lewis SE, Andersson A, Bucher B, Galzi JL, Sterner O, Bevan S, Hogestatt ED, Zygmunt PM (2011) TRPA1 mediates spinal antinociception induced by acetaminophen and cannabinoid delta(9)-tetrahydrocannabiorcol. *Nat Commun* 22:551–555

Burgess G, Williams D (2010) The discovery and development of analgesics: new mechanisms, new modalities. *J Clin Invest* 120:3753–3759

Bussing A, Ostermann T, Ludtke R, Michalsen A (2012) Effects of yoga interventions on pain and pain-associated disability: a meta-analysis. *J Pain* 13:1–9

Chandra Sl, Jana M, Pahan K (2018) Aspirin induces lysosomal biogenesis and attenuates amyloid plaque pathology in a mouse model of Alzheimer's disease via PPARα. *J Neurosci* 38:6682–6699

Clarkson PM, Kearns AK, Rouzier P, Rubin R, Thompson PD (2006) Serum creatine kinase levels and renal function measures in exertional muscle damage. *Med Sci Sports Exerc* 38:623–627

Coutinho AE, Chapman KE (2011) The anti-inflammatory and immunosuppressive effects of glucocorticoids, recent developments and mechanistic insights. *Mol Cell Endocrinol* 335:2–13

Dabo F, Nyberg F, Zhou Q, Sundstrom-Poromaa I, Akerud H (2010) Plasma levels of beta-endorphin during pregnancy and use of labor analgesia. *Reproductive Sci* 17:742–747

Dietrich A, McDaniel WF (2004) Endocannabinoids and exercise. *Br J Sports Med* 38:536–541

Dinarello CA (2004) Infection, fever, and exogenous and endogenous pyrogens: some concepts have changed. *J Endotoxin Res* 10:201–222

Donnelly AE, Maughan RJ, Whiting PH (1990) Effects of ibuprofen on exercise-induced muscle soreness and indices of muscle damage. *Br J Sports Med* 24:191–195

Esh CJ, Mauger AR, Palfreeman RA, Al-Janubi H, Taylor L (2017) Acetaminophen (paracetamol): use beyond pain management and dose variability. *Front Physiol* 8:1092

Foster J, Taylor L, Chrismas BC, Watkins SL, Mauger AR (2014) The influence of acetaminophen on repeated sprint cycling performance. *Eur J Appl Physiol* 114:41–48

Fowler CJ, Holt S, Nilsson O, Jonsson K-O, Tiger G, Jacobsson SOP (2005) The endocannabinoid signaling system: pharmacological and therapeutic aspects. *Pharm Bioch Behav* 81:248–262

Gomes WF, Lacerda AC, Mendonca VA, Arrieiro AN, Fonseca SF, Amorim MR, Teixeira AL, Teixeira MM, Miranda AS, Coimbra CC, Brito-Melo GE (2013) Effect of exercise on the plasma BDNF levels in elderly women with knee osteoarthritis. *Rheumatol Int* vol: pages (ePub ahead of print) doi:10.1007/s00296-013-2786-0

Kaye AD, Baluch A, Scott JT (2010) Pain management in the elderly population: a review. *Ochsner J* 10:179–187

Kofinas GD, Kofinas AD, Tavakoli FM (1985) Maternal and fetal beta-endorphin release in response to the stress of labor and delivery. *Am J Obstet Gynecol* 152:56–59

Kurmis AP, Kurmis TP, O'Brien JX, Dalén T (2012) The effect of nonsteroidal anti-inflammatory drug administration on acute phase fracture-healing: a review. *J Bone Joint Surg Am* 94:815–823

Kuster M, Renner B, Oppel P, Niederweis U, Brune K (2013) Consumption of analgesics before a marathon and the incidence of cardiovascular, gastrointestinal and renal problems: a cohort study. *BMJ Open* 3:2002090

Lauche R, Langhorst J, Dobos G, Cramer H (2013) A systematic review and meta-analysis of Tai Chi for osteoarthritis of the knee. *Complementary Therapies Med* 21:396–406

Lee WM (2004) Acetaminophen and the U.S. Acute Liver Failure Study Group: lowering the risks of hepatic failure. *Hepatology* 40:6–9

Lilja M, Mandić M, Apró W, Melin M, Olsson K, Rosenborg S, Gustafsson T, Lundberg TR (2018) High doses of anti-inflammatory drugs compromise muscle strength and hypertrophic adaptations to resistance training in young adults. *Acta Physiol (Oxf)* 222:e12948

Machida M, Takemasa T (2010) Ibuprofen administration during endurance training cancels running-distance-dependent adaptations of skeletal muscle in mice. *J Physiol Pharm* 61:559–563

Mackey AL, Mikkelksen UR, Magnusson SP, Kjaer M (2012) Rehabilitation of muscle after injury—the role for anti-inflammatory drugs. *Scand J Med Sci Sports* 22:E8-E14

Mallet C, Daulhac L, Bonnefont J, Ledent C, Etienne M, Chapuy E, Libert F, Eschalier A (2008) Endocannabinoid and serotonergic systems are needed for acetaminophen-induced analgesia. *Pain* 139:190–200

Mauger AR, Jones AM, Williams CA (2010) Influence of acetaminophen on performance during time trial cycling. *J Appl Physiol* 108:98–104

McAnulty SR, Owens JT, McAnulty LS, Nieman DC, Morrow JD, Dumke CL, Milne GL (2007) Ibuprofen use during extreme exercise: effects on oxidative stress and PGE2. *Med Sci Sports Exerc* 39:1075–1079

McGettigan P, Henry D (2011) Cardiovascular risk with non-steroidal anti-inflammatory drugs: systematic review of population-based controlled observational studies. *PLoS Med* 8: e1001098

Morgan P, Bowtell JL, Vanhatalo A, Jones AM, Bailey SJ (2018) Acute acetaminophen ingestion improves performance and muscle activation during maximal intermittent knee extensor exercise. *Eur J Appl Physiol* 118:595–605

Nieman DC, Henson DA, Dumke CL, Oley K, McAnulty SR, Davis M, Murphy EA, Utter AC, Lind RH, McAnulty LS, Morrow JD (2006) Ibuprofen use, endotoxemia, inflammation, and plasma cytokines during ultramarathon competition. *Brain Behav Immun* 20:578–584

Ottani A, Leone S, Sandrini M, Ferrari A, Bertolini A (2006) The analgesic activity of paracetamol is prevented by the blockade of cannabinoid CB1 receptors. *Eur J Pharmacol* 531:280–281

Pradip K, Muhuri J, Davies M (2013) Associations of nonmedical pain reliever use and initiation of heroin use in the United States. Center for Behavioral Health Statistics and Quality Data Review. SAMHSA. Retrieved from www.samhsa.gov/data/2k13/DataReview/DR006/nonmedical-pain-reliever-use-2013.htm

Raichlen DA, Foster AD, Seillier A, Giuffrida A, Gerdeman GL (2013) Exercise-induced endocannabinoid signaling is modulated by intensity. *Eur J Appl Physiol* 113:869–875

Tanaka R, Ozawa J, Kito N, Moriyama H (2013) Efficacy of strengthening or aerobic exercise on pain relief in people with knee osteoarthritis: a systematic review and meta-analysis of randomized controlled trials. *Clin Rehabil* vol: pages (ePub ahead of print) doi:10.1177/0269215513488898

Toussaint K, Yang XC, Zielinski MA, Reigle KL, Sacavage SD, Naga S, Raffa RB (2010) What do we (not) know about how paracetamol (acetaminophen) works? *J Clin Pharm Therapeutics* 35:617–638

Varrassi G, Bazzano C, Edwards WT (1989) Effects of physical activity on maternal plasma beta-endorphin levels and perception of labor pain. *Am J Obstet Gynecol* 160:707–712

Vickers AJ, Cronin AM, Maschino AC, Lewith G, MacPherson H, Foster NE, Sherman KJ, Witt CM, Linde K (2012) Acupuncture for chronic pain: individual patient data meta-analysis. *Arch Intern Med* 172:1444–1453

Vioxx: lessons for Health Canada and the FDA. (2005) *CMAJ* 175:5

Warden SJ (2009) Prophylactic misuse and recommended use of non-steroidal anti-inflammatory drugs by athletes. *Br J Sports Med* 43:548–549

Warden SJ (2010) Prophylactic use of NSAIDs by athletes: a risk/benefit assessment. *Physician Sportsmed* 38:132–138

Wharam PC, Speedy DB, Noakes TD, Thompson JM, Reid SA, Holtzhausen LM (2006) NSAID use increases the risk of developing hyponatremia during an Ironman triathlon. *Med Sci Sports Exerc* 38:618–622

Wongrakpanich S, Wongrakpanich A, Melhado K, Rangaswami J (2018) A comprehensive review of non-steroidal anti-inflammatory drug use in the elderly. *Aging Dis* 9:143–150

Woolf CJ (2010) What is this thing called pain? *J Clin Invest* 120:3742–3744

Zhao ZQ (2008) Neural mechanism underlying acupuncture analgesia. *Prog Neurobiol* 85:355–375

12 Antidiabetic and Antiobesity Drugs

Abstract

Diabetes and obesity have reached epidemic proportions throughout the world. The costs associated with quality of life and the toll on health-care systems is staggering. Type 1 diabetes results from loss of pancreatic beta cells and can occur early in life. Individuals with Type 1 diabetes require insulin injections to live. Type 2 diabetes generally occurs later in life, and obesity is a significant contributor to this type of diabetes. As visceral abdominal fat increases, low-grade inflammation results in many metabolically sensitive tissues, including adipocytes, liver, and muscle. Insulin resistance develops, as cells become less effective at taking up glucose. The resulting hyperglycemia leads to additional problems, including pancreatic beta cell dysfunction. Glucose intolerance develops, leading to Type 2 diabetes. Over time, chronic hyperglycemia can cause pancreatic beta cells to fail, and insulin replacement treatment becomes necessary.

Maintenance of blood glucose levels (euglycemia) is essential for good health. Insulin, glucagon, and several other hormones all play critical roles in the postabsorptive (fasting) and postprandial (fed) states. Lack of beta cell function and insulin can stress the normal homeostatic mechanisms, as can excessive intake of calories. Eating and drinking contributes the caloric energy; physical activity helps burn energy. When energy intake exceeds utilization, weight is gained. A healthy lifestyle plan should include a proper diet and exercise to help maintain a metabolically optimal weight. Exercise training can improve cardiovascular health significantly in individuals who are obese or prediabetic.

For individuals with diabetes, exercise requires additional attention to blood sugar levels. Hypoglycemia is the major concern, because if blood glucose levels get too low, the brain will shut down. Hyperglycemia is also a concern but is less critical in the short term. Prolonged bouts of hyperglycemia can induce diabetic ketoacidosis, which is also a medical emergency. Young people with Type 1 diabetes should be encouraged to participate fully in sports and physical activity; however, they need to monitor their blood glucose levels carefully, adjust their insulin and carbohydrate intake, and pay attention to the time of day. Exercise that includes high-intensity intervals and resistance training seems to minimize the chance for hypoglycemia. Interval and resistance training is also effective with people who have Type 2 diabetes. Low- to moderate-intensity exercise is good at improving HbA1c levels, which provide a measure of average glucose levels over the previous two to three months. High-intensity interval training and weight lifting improve insulin sensitivity.

Maintenance of or increase in muscle mass is a desired outcome of training, as muscle contributes a significant amount of energy utilization, both when a person is working out and when at rest.

Insulin is on the WADA prohibited substance list. It has abuse potential because it has anabolic properties (it stimulates production of protein and other macromolecules) that enhance the effect of anabolic steroids. Drugs used to treat Type 2 diabetes are not prohibited, although related compounds not approved as drugs are on the banned list (GW1516 and AICAR).

CASE EXAMPLE

Megan's aunt, Bernice, has Type 2 diabetes. She has a lot of trouble managing her blood sugar. She has always been overweight, at least as long as Megan can remember. Megan always likes to visit Aunt Bernice around the holidays, because there is always lots of great food and treats. That is part of the problem. Bernice likes to bake and eat. Her job at the bank keeps her sitting at a desk all day. She sits and watches her shows on TV every night. Bernice, like the 70% of the population that is either overweight or obese, has trouble making the necessary lifestyle changes. Obesity and diabetes are becoming epidemics and a major burden on the health-care system. Bernice now has to take insulin to keep her blood sugar in check. The fact she now takes insulin has been a bit of a wake-up call. She wants to make time for a walking program and try to limit the sweet desserts as a start.

Learning Objectives

1 Appreciate the seriousness of the obesity and diabetes epidemics.
2 Distinguish among the different types of diabetes.
3 Learn how multiple hormones are involved in blood sugar control.
4 Understand the concepts of glucose appearance and disappearance.
5 Learn the difference between the postabsorptive and postprandial states.
6 Learn how drugs for Type 2 diabetes work
7 Appreciate the different types of fat tissue and their role in obesity and diabetes.
8 Understand the issues in developing antiobesity medications.
9 Appreciate the role of exercise in improving insulin sensitivity and controlling blood sugar levels.

Introduction

Obesity rates for children and adults have grown steadily during the last 20 years (Diabetes Prevention Program n.d., Robert Wood Johnson Foundation 2014, Trust for America's Health and Robert Wood Johnson Foundation 2014). Though the rate of increase may have slowed in recent years, the percentage of obese individuals in the United States remains around 33% to 35% (Flegal, Kruszon-Moran, Carroll, et al. 2016). Worldwide in 2016, 39% of adults were overweight and 13% were obese, with over 340 million children and adolescents aged 5 to 19 considered overweight or obese. The body mass index (BMI) is a measure of body fat derived from one's height and weight. A person's weight in kilograms is divided by the square of his or her height in meters. An individual is considered to be overweight if he or she has a BMI between

25 and 29.9. A person with a BMI over 30 is considered obese. The combined percentages of the U.S. population that are overweight and obese approach 70%. Clearly, even though the rate of increase in obesity may have slowed in recent years, the extent of this problem is staggering when we consider the health consequences to over two-thirds of the population. A significant portion of our nation's health-care costs are related to health problems associated with being overweight and diabetes. Obesity costs the U.S. health-care system about $150 billion a year (Kim & Basu 2016); diabetes costs the health-care system at least $237 billion. Obesity is associated with significant morbidity and mortality, often with multisystem involvement. It is linked to dyslipidemia (e.g., high blood levels of total cholesterol or triglycerides), liver and gallbladder disease, and increased incidence of diabetes.

Diabetes is a chronic disease that results from elevated levels of glucose in the blood, sometimes referred to as **blood sugar.** Glucose levels increase in the blood after a person has eaten and when glucose stored as glycogen (a polymer of glucose) is mobilized and released into the blood, primarily from stores in the liver. The pancreas responds to elevated glucose levels by releasing the polypeptide hormone insulin into the bloodstream. Insulin stimulates cells to import glucose, thereby meeting the cells' metabolic needs. The brain, in particular, is highly dependent on blood glucose for energy. Glucose and insulin in the blood return to homeostatic levels over time.

This chapter discusses the pathophysiology of diabetes and obesity, the therapeutic approach for treatment, and the benefits of physical activity. The role of diet and nutrition, and what we chose to eat, is covered in the next chapter.

Diabetes

As stated above, the hallmark for diabetes is an elevated level of blood glucose. Glucose is a central component of metabolism. Produced by photosynthetic organisms, such as plants, glucose is used metabolically in most, if not all, organisms on the planet. Glucose also has regulatory functions. It can regulate gene expression, cause hormone secretion, regulate enzyme activity, and affect the activity of glucoregulatory neurons (Thorens & Mueckler 2010). Glucose regulates insulin secretion in the pancreas. In the brain, glucose-sensitive neurons are grouped in certain regions, and their activity is sensitive to changes in glucose concentration. These regions of the brain contribute to control of energy expenditure, feeding behavior, and overall glucose homeostasis.

For individuals with diabetes, defects in glucose regulatory mechanisms cause the concentration of glucose to exceed its relatively narrow limits. Normal glucose concentrations range between 4.0 mM and 9.0 mM, despite wide-ranging demands, such as exercise or a big meal (Gerich 2000). **Insulin** and other hormones play crucial roles in maintaining blood glucose levels. Insulin is a small protein consisting of two polypeptides and a total of 51 amino acids. It is made, processed, and stored in secretory granules in pancreatic **beta cells**; it is secreted into the circulation at a low, basal rate (a sufficient amount to manage resting blood glucose). When stimulated, the beta cells significantly increase the release of insulin. Stimuli include glucose, certain amino acids, elevated free fatty acids, and beta-adrenergic input. Certain **incretins** (gut peptides; see below) can also increase insulin release in response to food intake. Insulin binds its receptor on the surface of target cells (primarily liver, muscle, and adipose tissues) and stimulates glucose uptake, utilization, and storage. Insulin is cleared from the system rapidly, with less than a five-minute half-life in the blood, primarily by the liver and the kidneys. Diabetes primarily results from defects in insulin production or insulin action.

In the early 1900s, the discovery of insulin helped provide the basis for the understanding and treatment of diabetes. The discovery in the mid-1900s of **glucagon**, a peptide of 29 amino acids, filled in more details and led to a bihormonal definition for diabetes (Aronoff, Berkowitz, Shreiner, & Want 2004). Both insulin and glucagon are produced in the pancreas, which contains more than one million islets of Langerhans, each with distinct cell types with different secretory properties. Two of the major types are the **alpha cells** and the previously mentioned beta cells. Alpha cells produce glucagon, somatostatin (a universal regulator of secretory cells), and gastrin (which stimulates gastric acid secretion). Beta cells produce insulin and amylin (more later). The opposing actions of insulin and glucagon explain much of the basis for glucose regulation. However, the control of blood sugar levels is quite complex and involves several additional hormones and **adipokines** (hormones secreted by adipose tissue), providing strong evidence for a multihormonal model for understanding and treating diabetes (Aronoff et al.). Insulin, however, is still considered the key player and is the focal point for therapy.

Types of Diabetes and Related Conditions

There are several types of diabetes, and the term diabetes usually is used to refer to the whole group of diseases.

Type 1 Diabetes

Type 1 diabetes, which involves the inability to make or release insulin from the pancreas in response to elevated blood glucose, includes forms of diabetes previously called insulin-dependent diabetes mellitus or juvenile-onset diabetes. It results from the loss of pancreatic beta cells, the only cells in the body that make insulin. The death of pancreatic beta cells can result from autoimmune disease, viral infection, or other environmental factors, and can have an inherited component. Insulin function is essential for life, so patients with Type 1 diabetes must receive insulin by either injection or a pump. Type 1 diabetes accounts for only about 5% to 10% of the total cases of diabetes.

Type 2 Diabetes

Type 2 diabetes, also called non–insulin-dependent diabetes mellitus and previously referred to as adult-onset diabetes, accounts for the vast majority of diabetes cases. First acknowledged as a problem in affluent countries, Type 2 diabetes is a growing problem in developing countries, as well. Many causes have been suggested, such as urbanization, an aging population, and a decrease in physical activity. But the most significant correlation is with obesity: 70% to 90% of cases of Type 2 diabetes are associated with individuals who are obese (Hu 2011).

Type 2 diabetes results from inadequate insulin production or loss of responsiveness to insulin's action. In individuals with this disease, the beta cells are alive but unhealthy, and insulin production can be altered. Even though insulin is present in these patients, target cells do not respond correctly—a condition referred to as **insulin resistance**. The cells do not respond to insulin's signal to increase glucose uptake, so glucose levels remain elevated. Chronic elevated glucose levels overstimulate the pancreatic beta cells. They fail to turn off insulin production and can secrete an inactive form of insulin that has not been fully processed. As the disease progresses, eventually beta cells lose the ability to make more insulin, and insulin replacement therapy is needed. Type 2 diabetes is associated with obesity, age, physical inactivity, race/ethnicity, family history, and impaired glucose metabolism.

Symptoms of Type 2 diabetes, which may take years to develop, include frequent urination, thirst, and fatigue. Over time, other symptoms may become pronounced, such as blurred vision (retinopathy) and pain or numbness in the hands or feet (neuropathy). The decrease in insulin function and hyperglycemia cause frequent urination due to glucose excretion (with the associated water) in the kidney. Diagnosis of Type 2 diabetes is based on a fasting blood glucose measurement over 7.0 mM and a glucose tolerance test (blood glucose two hours after a bolus of glucose) that exceeds 11.1 mM. The diagnosis is confirmed with an HbA1c test (see Box) over 6.5 (see Table 12.1).

Metabolic syndrome is also increasing at alarming rates, as it is often considered a transitional state between obesity and Type 2 diabetes. The disorder called metabolic syndrome, previously termed syndrome X or insulin resistance syndrome, is a cluster of risk factors associated with an increased risk for cardiovascular disease and Type 2 diabetes. It involves a complex interaction among genetic, metabolic, and environmental factors. Dietary habits are a major environmental factor, along with smoking and a sedentary lifestyle. "Healthy" diets are likely protective against metabolic syndrome. These diets include low levels of saturated and trans fats, balanced carbohydrates rich in dietary fiber (i.e., fruits and vegetables), and low-fat dairy products. Individuals who are overweight, have high blood pressure, are sedentary, and eat diets with high levels of fat and refined sugar (e.g., high fructose corn syrup) are at risk for metabolic syndrome. The numbers in the United States are significant, as 24% of adults may qualify as candidates for metabolic syndrome.

Certain medications prescribed for hypertension may actually increase the risk of metabolic syndrome. The widely prescribed class of drugs called beta-blockers (see Chapter 4) can inhibit lipid and glucose metabolism and may promote weight gain. Certain antipsychotic drugs (see Chapter 9) can cause weight gain and may also contribute to metabolic syndrome and diabetes. Diet and smoking will be discussed in Chapter 13 and Chapter 15.

Diabetes Tests

Diabetes can be confirmed through several blood tests. Blood sugar levels can vary significantly over the course of the day. For practical reasons, most lab tests are done following at least an eight-hour fast, so that blood glucose can be measured in the postabsorptive (fasted) state. Another test used to confirm diabetes is the glucose tolerance test. In this test, the patient is given a bolus of glucose and the blood sugar level is monitored after two hours. An additional blood test, the

HbA1c (also referred to as the A1c) **test**, is considered much more accurate and better able to diagnose prediabetes (and metabolic syndrome), Type 1 diabetes, and Type 2 diabetes. The HbA1c test indicates the average level of glucose in the blood over the previous two to three months. The test is based on the fact that the predominant protein in red blood cells, hemoglobin, becomes modified with the addition of glucose molecules by a process called glycation. The percentage of modified hemoglobin (HbA1c) of the total hemoglobin depends on the level of blood glucose. A normal HbA1c for healthy people ranges from 4.5% to 6% (see Table 12.1). A person with uncontrolled diabetes may have an HbA1c over 8%. Values on two successive tests that exceed 6.5% suggest a diagnosis of diabetes. Prediabetes is the diagnosis for levels ranging from 5.7% to 6.4%. Individuals who are under treatment for diabetes may have a target of around 7%, though this can vary with the patient. As levels increase over 7%, the risk increases for complications related to hyperglycemia and diabetes. Table 12.1 provides a comparison of blood sugar levels, giving different units of concentration and hemoglobin A1c levels for normal and diabetic conditions. This test is also very useful for monitoring how well the treatment for diabetes is progressing (see Table 12.2).

Table 12.1 Range of blood glucose and HbA1c levels for normal and diabetic conditions

Condition	Fasting mM^a [mg/dL]	Post meal (2 hrs) mM^a [mg/dL]	HbA1c (%)
Normal	4–6 [72–106]	7–8 [126–145]	4.6–6
Prediabetic	>5.5 [100]	>8 [145]	5.7–6.4
Diabetic	5–7 [90–126]	<10 [180]	>6.5

a   mM = millimoles per liter, sometimes notated as millimol/L or mmol/L.

Table 12.2 Range of HbA1c percentages and average glucose levels for previous two to three months

HbA1c Level	Estimated Glucose	
5%	5.4 mM	97 mg/dL
5.5%	6.6 mM	112 mg/dL
6%	7.0 mM	126 mg/dL
6.5%	7.8 mM	140 mg/dL
7%	8.5 mM	154 mg/dL
8%	10.2 mM	183 mg/dL
9%	11.8 mM	212 mg/dL

Type 3 and Type 4 Diabetes

Type 3 diabetes is linked to Alzheimer's disease. Alzheimer's disease represents a form of diabetes that selectively involves the brain and has molecular and biochemical features that overlap with both Type 1 and Type 2 diabetes, including insulin deficiency and insulin resistance as mediators of neurodegeneration (de la Monte & Wands 2008). **Type 4 diabetes** includes gestational diabetes; 7% of women develop insulin resistance during pregnancy and for most it goes away soon after childbirth. If it persists, it is considered Type 2. All forms of diabetes result in problems regulating glucose levels in the blood, leading to hyperglycemia.

Hyperglycemia and Hypoglycemia

Hyperglycemia causes many problems. People with persistent elevated blood sugar have a much higher risk for developing cardiovascular disease, nephropathy, retinopathy, and neuropathy. **Hypoglycemia**, or low blood sugar, is also dangerous; it can injure the brain, because glucose is the primary source of energy for the brain. Alternate fuels, such as free fatty acids, do not cross the blood–brain barrier very well. The brain does not store or produce glucose, so it depends on blood glucose for proper function and, ultimately, for its survival. During fasting, the brain can use **ketone bodies** to supplement its energy needs. Ketone bodies are water-soluble breakdown products of fatty acids (acetoacetic acid and beta-hydroxybutyric acid) produced in the liver that the heart and brain use as a source of energy during periods of fasting.

A drop in blood glucose levels (under about 3.8 mM) triggers the release of glucagon and catecholamines; cortisol and growth hormone are also released, but these work over a longer time frame. The release of these factors antagonizes the action of insulin, causing mobilization and an increase in glucose in the circulation. In addition, when blood sugar levels drop, insulin release is suppressed (Gerich). The result is that blood glucose levels are brought back into the normal range (**euglycemia**).

Glucose Homeostasis

Glucose homeostasis is the process by which the body maintains a blood glucose within a narrow concentration range under various conditions. The glucose concentration in the circulation is a function of two competing rates. The first rate is the rate of glucose appearance (Ra)—the rate that glucose enters the circulation. The second rate is the rate of glucose disappearance (Rd)—the rate that glucose is removed from the circulation.

Glucose Appearance

There are three main sources of glucose entering the system and contributing to Ra. The first source is gastric emptying and intestinal absorption following feeding. The other two sources of glucose in the blood (glycogenolysis and gluconeogenesis) primarily result from metabolic activity in the liver, though the kidneys can contribute up to 20% of the metabolic glucose released into blood (Gerich). See Figure 12.1 for a schematic of the metabolic pathways discussed in this chapter.

GASTRIC EMPTYING AND INTESTINAL ABSORPTION

Although many factors contribute to the rate of glucose absorption and its appearance in the circulation in the fed state, a major determinant (and target for regulation) is the

Figure 12.1 Metabolic pathways discussed in this chapter.

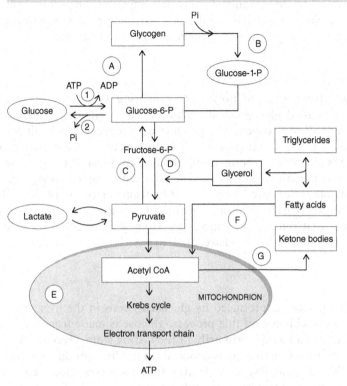

Legend: A highly schematic view of metabolism, with major pathways labeled. More than one arrow signifies multiple steps, not shown.

1 = hexokinase; 2 = glucose-6-phosphatase.

A: Glycogenesis, B: Glycogenolysis, C: Gluconeogenesis, D: Glycolysis, E: Mitochondrial: includes Krebs (citric acid) cycle, electron transport chain, and oxidative phosphorylation, F: Beta-oxidation, G: Ketosis.

rate of gastric emptying (the emptying of the stomach to the small intestine). The rate of gastric emptying depends on the nutrient density of the meal. The stomach initially relaxes to accommodate a meal. The meal is ground to a small particle size, creating the chyme (a semifluid mass of party digested food). The chyme is pumped to the small intestine in a pulsating manner. The rate of emptying is regulated primarily by inhibitory feedback arising from the interaction of nutrients with the small intestine. If the ingested food is rich in certain nutrients, such as fat or certain amino acids, the rate of gastric emptying will be considerably slowed. Simple carbohydrate–rich foods empty faster, giving rise to a quicker increase in blood sugar. Nutrient density sensed in the small intestine is relayed to the stomach as inhibitory neural and hormonal messages (i.e., the incretins discussed below) that delay emptying by slowing gastric motility. The magnitude of the small intestine's inhibitory feedback depends on the nutrient load. For example, when the fat has been absorbed in the small intestine, the inhibitory stimulus is removed, and productive gastric motility resumes.

Gastric emptying can vary with the individual and his or her state of health. Gastric emptying accounts for about 35% of the variance in the **glycemic response** (change in blood sugar levels) to carbohydrate-containing meals. Slowing gastric emptying slows the movement of glucose to the small intestine and slows the appearance of glucose in the blood.

Acceleration of gastric emptying speeds absorption and increases the likelihood of elevated blood glucose levels. Therefore, regulation of gastric emptying is important in maintaining glycemic control. Nutritional quality of the diet, activity level, and drug treatment can all affect blood sugar level through altering the rate of gastric emptying.

GLYCOGENOLYSIS

Glucose is stored as **glycogen**, large polymers containing thousands of glucose molecules. The process called **glycogenolysis**, which occurs primarily in the liver, releases the glucose stored in glycogen. The product of glycogenolysis is glucose-1-phosphate, and glucose-1-phosphate then is rapidly converted to glucose-6-phosphate. Glucose-6-phosphate is a central component of metabolism; most of the glucose inside cells is in the form of glucose-6-phosphate. The attached phosphate is significant, because glucose in the phosphorylated form cannot be transported out of the cell by the glucose transporter. Only liver cells and certain kidney cells express the enzyme (**glucose-6-phosphatase**) that removes the phosphate from glucose, allowing it to be transported out of cells and into the bloodstream.

GLUCONEOGENESIS

Besides glycogenolysis, glucose is produced by **gluconeogenesis** in the liver and to a more limited extent in the kidneys. In this process, glucose is made from lactate or breakdown products of amino acids, primarily in the fasting state. Over shorter periods of time (8 to 12 hours) of fasting, glycogenolysis in the liver produces sufficient glucose to maintain blood sugar levels. As fasting time increases, gluconeogenesis contributes more, as glycogen stores become depleted (usually within 24 hours). Kidney cells that contain glucose-6-phosphatase make glucose by gluconeogenesis and contribute up to 20% of the blood glucose during fasting. Curiously, kidney cells that contain glycogen do not contain glucose-6-phosphatase, so glycogenolysis in the kidney does not contribute to plasma glucose. Therefore, the rate of glucose appearance in the circulation depends on food intake and absorption from the gut, glycogenolysis in the liver, and gluconeogenesis in the liver and kidneys.

Glucose Disappearance

The rate of glucose disappearance from the blood depends on uptake of glucose by cells for a source of energy. As mentioned above, the brain uses blood glucose as its primary energy source. Blood cells and most of the internal organs, excluding the heart (which prefers free fatty acids), also take up glucose proportional to demand. As tissues use glucose metabolically and intracellular levels drop, glucose from the blood enters the cells by mass action, as the glucose concentration in the blood is greater than inside the cells. In a process referred to as **facilitated diffusion**, transport is mediated by glucose transporters in the plasma membrane. **Glucose transporters** (abbreviated **GLUTs**) are members of a complex gene family with 14 members found in the human genome. Four of the isoforms (GLUT1 through GLUT4) are well characterized and have distinct regulatory and kinetic roles in maintaining glucose homeostasis. Expression of different glucose transporters contributes to different glucose transport properties in different tissues (see Box).

The direction of the concentration gradient determines the direction of net glucose flow. In this case, where cells are actively utilizing glucose and there is normal glucose concentration in the blood, the net movement will be from the blood into the cells. For the liver and kidney cells mentioned above, the action of glucose-6-phosphatase generates elevated intracellular levels of glucose, so the glucose transporters transport glucose out of these cells into the bloodstream. Glucose uptake is proportional to glucose utilization for the brain, blood cells, and most internal organs; uptake into these tissues does not require insulin. Glucose uptake is sensitive to insulin for skeletal muscle, liver, and adipose tissue.

The GLUTs: Glucose Transporters

Glucose uptake into cells depends on glucose transporters (GLUTs). The GLUT gene family has 14 related members in the human genome. These genes are related to a widely distributed gene family of membrane transporters found throughout nature. Half of GLUT family members are well characterized, while the other half have relatively unknown function. The multiple isoforms allow for diverse specificity (e.g., some prefer fructose or urate, the salt of uric acid) and different kinetic properties, expression patterns, and roles in signal transduction.

GLUT1 was originally described in red blood cell membranes and was the first GLUT cloned and sequenced. It has 12 transmembrane helices but has been difficult to crystallize, so its 3D structure is not known. It is expressed in most cells and is responsible for basal levels of glucose uptake.

GLUT2 has a relatively low affinity for glucose and is expressed in high levels in pancreatic beta cells. The result is that glucose levels can rapidly equilibrate across the beta cell membrane, providing the cell with the necessary information on blood glucose concentration to regulate insulin secretion. Similarly, GLUT2 and glucose-sensing activity in alpha cells regulate glucagon secretion. GLUT2 is also expressed in the intestines, where it increases glucose absorption. In the liver, glucose uptake induces glycolytic and lipogenic gene expression. In the CNS, GLUT2 expression in glucose-sensing cells contributes to feeding behavior and other aspects of glucose homeostasis.

GLUT3 is the major CNS glucose transporter. It has high affinity and fast kinetics, ensuring that the brain gets its needed glucose. It is also expressed in certain immune and inflammatory cells, where it is recruited to the membrane during cell activation, helping provide the necessary energy.

GLUT4 has been extensively studied, but many of its underlying mechanism are still unclear and controversial. GLUT4-containing vesicles are translocated to the cell membrane of muscle and fat cells in response to insulin. The increased capacity of these cells to import glucose is critical in insulin's role in maintaining blood sugar levels. The loss of this capacity observed in those who are obese or diabetic is critical in understanding these diseases. Elucidating the underlying mechanism of how insulin regulates trafficking of GLUT4 to and from the cell membrane is fundamental to understanding how muscle and fat tissue become insulin insensitive and how diabetes develops.

*Key Physiological States to Understanding Glucose Appearance and
Disappearance*

To understand glucose flux and the two competing processes (glucose appearance and
disappearance in the blood), we need to distinguish between two distinct physiological
states: the **postabsorptive state** (occurring after a 10- to 16-hour fast, such as overnight)
and the **postprandial state** (the five to six hours following feeding).

THE POSTABSORPTIVE STATE

The postabsorptive state occurs when the stomach is empty and no longer contributing energy through digestion and absorption. Fasting that lasts eight hours or longer
causes changes in metabolism. Prolonged fasts (over 24 hours or lasting days) can
cause additional, dramatic changes in metabolism. Most people who sleep for eight
hours are also fasting, and when they wake up they break their fast by eating breakfast. For our purposes, we will concentrate on what most people consider a normal
daily cycle: sleeping eight hours at night and eating three times a day. It takes five to
six hours to return to the postabsorptive state after eating, so for most people who
eat three meals per day, the only "fast" is overnight. Following a good night's sleep,
blood glucose is relatively stable at 5 mM, suggesting that usually glucose appearance
is about the same as glucose disappearance at this time. However, glucose utilization
may be a bit greater than production under certain conditions. For example, if the fast
is prolonged, glucose will dip to about 4.0 to 4.5 mM after 24 hours (Gerich). In the
postabsorptive state, there is no net glucose storage. Glucose is completely oxidized to
CO_2 or released back into circulation as metabolites, such as lactate or certain amino
acids. As carbohydrate stores contain limited energy compared to fat stores, free fatty
acids provide most of the body's energy demands, with the exception of the brain.

   The production and release of glucose from the liver and kidneys in the postabsorptive state are under the control of a variety of hormones, with glucagon having the most
dramatic effect. Glucagon stimulates glycogenolysis and gluconeogenesis in the liver but
not the kidneys. Activation of glucagon receptors in the liver results in stimulation of enzymes that increase the rates of glycogenolysis and gluconeogenesis. Additional indirect
mechanisms involve increasing the availability of substrates for gluconeogenesis, such
as glycerol or metabolites of certain amino acids. Additional hormones that influence
glucose production and release include epinephrine, cortisol, and growth hormone. Epinephrine stimulates glucose release and gluconeogenesis in liver and kidneys. Both tissues are well innervated by the sympathetic nervous system, so that glucose production
and release can occur in minutes. Cortisol and growth hormone increase blood glucose
levels, but these work over a longer time frame, by affecting a tissue's sensitivity to insulin, glucagon, or epinephrine. Cortisol and growth hormone also access glycogen stores
and increase the availability of precursors for gluconeogenesis.

   As stated earlier, glycogen and insulin exhibit opposing actions (see Table 12.3). In
contrast to glycogen, insulin suppresses glucose release from both the liver and kidneys by causing the inhibition of gluconeogenesis. In the postabsorptive state, cells use
free fatty acids as a primary source for energy, except in the brain, which still depends
on glucose, as stated earlier. In this state, the lower glucose levels increase glucagon
and suppress insulin levels. Glucagon mobilizes glucose production that almost keeps
up with glucose utilization, if the fasting state does not last too long.

Table 12.3 Comparison of insulin and glucagon activities

Insulin's Activities	Glucagon's Activities
Produced in pancreatic beta cells	Produced in pancreatic alpha cells
Released if glucose levels rise to 6.5 nM	Released if glucose levels drop to 3.5 nM
Decrease gluconeogenesis	Increase gluconeogenesis
Make more glycogen (glycogenesis)	Break down glycogen (glycogenolysis)
Decrease glucose release from liver	Increase glucose release from liver
Increase glucose uptake by muscle, liver, and adipocytes	Decrease glucose uptake by muscle, liver, and adipocytes
Decrease glycolysis and lipolysis	Increase glycolysis and lipolysis

THE POSTPRANDIAL STATE

The postprandial state is characterized by physiological changes that occur after eating. Following a balanced meal of protein, carbohydrates, and fat, it takes about six hours for the body to return to the postabsorptive state. Many factors influence the rate and amount of glucose entering the blood system during the postprandial state. The rate of gastric emptying, digestion in the small intestine, and metabolism in the liver all come into play. Ultimately, the uptake, storage, and utilization of glucose by tissues downstream of the liver will largely determine how soon glucose levels return to postabsorptive levels. Glucose production and release from the liver are suppressed in the postprandial state, largely due to insulin action and suppression of glucagon. The level of physical activity since the last meal is also a factor in control of blood glucose, as recovering muscle tissue has elevated rates of glucose uptake.

Glucose entering the circulation from the gut exceeds the rate of removal for the first 80 to 100 minutes after eating, so that blood glucose levels rise. The elevated glucose concentration stimulates insulin release from beta cells and suppresses glucagon release from alpha cells. Production of glucose in the liver (i.e., glycogenolysis and gluconeogenesis) decreases 80% over the four to five hours after eating; glycogen formation is enhanced with glucose arriving from the gut. As much as 30% of the dietary glucose passing through the liver is retained (mostly becoming glycogen), with the other 70% entering the circulation. Of the glucose that enters the circulation, the brain will use about 20%, independent of insulin. Other tissues require insulin to increase glucose uptake. About 30% to 40% is taken up by skeletal muscle, 10% by the kidneys, and 5% to 10% by adipose tissue. The liver takes up another 20% in this way. The remainder of the glucose is spread among the remaining tissues (Gerich).

Insulin is essential in stimulating glucose uptake and returning blood glucose to normal levels. Insulin activates receptors in insulin-sensitive cells (primarily skeletal muscle, kidney, liver, and adipocytes) and increases glucose uptake by recruiting glucose transporters to the cell membrane. The increase in glucose transporters facilitates glucose uptake into these cells. In skeletal muscle, the incoming glucose replaces free fatty acids as a primary energy source. After about two hours, the muscle shifts to increased glycogen synthesis, and free fatty acids are again the preferred energy substrate for ATP production. The kidney, similarly, will use glucose as an energy source early after feeding and then will shift to storing glucose as glycogen and using free fatty acids as the primary energy source. Insulin stimulates formation of glycogen in liver at the same time it suppresses glycogenolysis and gluconeogenesis indirectly by inhibiting glucagon activity. The rise in blood glucose and other nutrients that triggers the release of insulin causes the suppression of lipolysis and a decrease in free fatty acids in adipocytes. Insulin also stimulates triglyceride formation and storage. In addition, insulin promotes protein synthesis in the liver and muscle. Therefore, insulin is considered an anabolic hormone, meaning it stimulates the formation of the macro-molecules glycogen (a polymer of glucose), triglycerides (composed of three fatty acids and glycerol), and proteins (polymers of amino acids).

In the postprandial state, insulin secretion from pancreatic beta cells is proportional to blood glucose concentration and occurs in two phases. The first phase is rapid, as insulin stored in secretory vesicles is secreted into the portal vein. The second phase occurs over time and requires synthesis of new insulin peptides. If glucose levels stay elevated, such as with excess nutrient consumption and lack of physical activity, chronic insulin release occurs. Cells also become resistant to insulin's activity, compounding the problem of elevated blood glucose. In some cases, inactive insulin that has not been fully processed is "rushed" into the bloodstream, making the problem worse and leading to beta cell dysfunction. The inability to control blood sugar, called **glucose intolerance**, is a significant problem in obesity, metabolic syndrome, and Type 2 diabetes.

A second neuroendocrine hormone co-expressed and co-excreted from beta cells was discovered in the late 1980s. **Amylin**, a peptide containing 37 amino acids, is re-leased following nutrient stimulation, similar to insulin. However, in contrast to insulin, amylin has several important functions decreasing glucose appearance in the circulation. It suppresses glucagon release and, therefore, decreases glucagon's ability to mobilize glucose. It slows gastric emptying and the rate at which glucose and other nutrients enter the small intestine. The result is that the rate of glucose and nutrient appearance in the bloodstream is slowed, allowing more time for insulin to work. Amylin also reduces food intake and body weight, probably by affecting appetite.

Additional hormones involved in glucose homeostasis include gut peptides called **incretins**, introduced briefly earlier. Several incretins were identified when it was shown that ingested food stimulated a greater insulin response than did glucose infused intravenously. As digested food reaches the small intestine, incretins are released into the circulation. In the postprandial state, incretins enhance insulin secretion, suppress glucagon secretion, slow gastric emptying, and promote beta cell health. There is also evidence that they can reduce food intake and body weight (Aronoff et al.). The major incretin involved in these activities is glucagon-like peptide 1 (GLP-1). Drugs based on amylin and GLP-1 activity are now used to treat Type 2 diabetes. Amylin and incretin biology is obviously fascinating and has important consequences as researchers continue to search for treatments to control diabetes and obesity.

How Do Antidiabetic Drugs Work?

Different types of diabetes require different therapeutic approaches. As discussed above, maintaining blood glucose levels within the optimal narrow range is a complex process. When insulin action is compromised, the process is even harder to regulate. Hyperglycemia causes problems when it is sustained, especially with the kidneys, vasculature, and vision. Hypoglycemia is life threatening and requires immediate attention, as the brain will shut down with an insufficient supply of glucose. The complexity is exacerbated with the distinctly different states of fasting and feeding—the postabsorptive and postprandial states discussed above. Antidiabetic drugs include insulin therapy for treating Type 1 diabetes and other drugs that work by a variety of mechanisms, including increasing the sensitivity of cells to insulin (thiazolidinediones) or inhibiting glucose synthesis (metformin) for treating Type 2 diabetes.

After briefly discussing the treatment for Type 1 diabetes—the different preparations of insulin available for insulin replacement therapy, we will consider the treatment for Type 2 diabetes—the drugs that deal with insulin resistance.

Treatment of Type 1 Diabetes

The selective death of beta cells leads to Type 1 diabetes, and, as stated earlier, the resulting insulin deficiency requires insulin replacement. Insulin replacement therapy has come a long way since the 1980s. Insulin derived from pigs was once the conventional therapy. Advances in genetic engineering and recombinant DNA techniques (laboratory methods of engineering DNA sequences) have made human insulin readily available. Although minor genetic manipulations in insulin's peptide sequence have improved its therapeutic capacity, they have not altered its immunoreactivity or receptor binding. To regulate insulin's onset of action or extend its duration, formulations have been created that cause the insulin peptides to aggregate or bind inactive molecules. The result is that many preparations of insulin are available, ranging in their speed of onset and the time they persist after injection.

Four main types of human insulin made with recombinant DNA technology are commercially available: rapid-acting, short-acting, intermediate-acting, and long-acting. **Rapid-acting insulin** has been modified slightly to allow its rapid appearance in the bloodstream after a subcutaneous injection. Slight changes in the peptide sequence alter the aggregation state of the peptides. Rapid-acting insulin can be taken before a meal, and, because it decays after four to five hours, it is less likely to cause hypoglycemia than the other types of insulin. It is often used in continuous subcutaneous infusion devices (pumps).

Short-acting insulin has a slower onset and lasts longer (five to eight hours). These properties make this preparation of insulin harder to synchronize with meals, resulting in a mismatch of timing with sugar levels in the blood. It has a greater risk of causing hypoglycemia. Although its use subcutaneously is becoming less common, it is still the preferred preparation for use IV because of its solubility properties.

Intermediate-acting insulin is complexed with a small, positively charged protein called protamine. When the complex is injected subcutaneously, the protamine is slowly digested by proteases found on the surface of cells. Insulin is slowly released, with an expected onset of about two to five hours and duration of 12 hours. Altering the dosage provides glucose control. Available preparations are Humulin N (Lilly) and Novalin N (Novo Nordisk).

Since the pharmacokinetics of the insulins discussed above are relatively variable, newer preparations of **long-acting insulin** are becoming preferred. Insulin glargine is a long-acting insulin with a slightly modified sequence that has a broad concentration plateau, meaning that its level in the blood is relatively constant for hours. It has a slow onset, taking four to six hours for its maximum effect, and the effect can last 24 hours. Other long-acting insulins are detemir and degludec. These insulins have been modified to have slow but steady duration of action, in some cases exceeding 24 hours.

The goal is to maintain tight control over glucose levels without triggering hypoglycemia. Insulin treatment has to account for basal levels of activity in the postabsorptive phase and the surge of glucose and other nutrients following a meal. Conventional therapy includes a split-dose injection of a mixture of rapid-acting and intermediate-acting insulins. Depending on the combination, some insulin preparations can be mixed and co-injected, whereas others (i.e., glargine and detemir) must be given as separate injections. Some newer premixed versions of rapid and intermediate insulins are now approved. The intermediate-acting (or long-acting, in some cases) insulin helps maintain the basal requirement, and the rapid-acting insulin deals with the surge in glucose in the postprandial state. Self-injection is often done subcutaneously, with disposable syringes and needles. Pen-style injectors contain a cartridge with multiple doses. More sophisticated approaches use continuous infusion devices, also known as insulin pumps. The rapid-acting insulin preparations are usually used in this application. Newer pumps are programmable and can help deliver basal or bolus insulin doses.

Even when these sophisticated devices are used, control of blood sugar can be difficult. Keep in mind the central role that beta cells play and that insulin is only one component of a complex interaction of glucoregulatory hormones. The loss of beta cells creates a "hole" in the regulatory network of factors involved in glucose homeostasis. For example, amylin and the incretins also play critical roles in normal beta cell activity, and amylin-like compounds are used as an adjunct treatment for Type 1 diabetes. New therapeutic approaches (and drugs) are under development to help fine-tune glucose levels in individuals with diabetes.

Managing Blood Glucose

In order to manage glucose levels effectively, it is necessary to monitor blood levels and maintain a log. Checking blood glucose levels is important for patients taking insulin and patients with low glucose levels (especially those who do not experience the usual warning signs). Monitoring blood glucose can also be important during pregnancy. To check blood glucose level, the patient washes his or her hands and then uses a lancing device (such as the newer spring-loaded types) on the side of a finger to produce a drop of blood, which is captured on a test strip. The test strip is inserted into a monitor (available in a range of cost and sophistication), which displays the glucose concentration. Target levels can vary depending on the patient's age, disease state, other associated co-morbidities, vascular complications, and other considerations. Keeping a log can reveal daily trends. And over time, the dosage and timing of injections can be modified accordingly.

Other aspects of managing glucose levels involve exercise (discussed below) and diet. The carbohydrate content of meals (or snacks) can influence the determination of insulin dosages. Some foods have a greater influence on blood sugar levels than other foods—for example, carbohydrates. The **glycemic index** is a rating of a food on its propensity to raise blood sugar levels. The index is based on a reference set at 100 for a food like pure glucose or white bread. As a general rule, dried beans, lentils, whole grains, non-starchy vegetables, and fruit have lower glycemic indexes (in the neighborhood of 50). Foods containing more heavily processed carbohydrates (such as instant rice, instant oatmeal, white bread, and crackers) have a higher glycemic index (over 80). As a rough guide, the higher the fiber content, the lower the glycemic index. A sample index is available at www. health.harvard.edu/glycemic.

In terms of carbohydrates, the glycemic index is concerned with the "type" of carbohydrate and how it can influence blood glucose, not the amount or the portion size. Carbohydrate "counting" takes into account the amount of carbohydrate consumed. For people with diabetes and those wanting to control their weight, paying attention to the amount and type of carbohydrate is important. They can create healthy and pleasurable diets by mixing low glycemic index food with high glycemic index food and paying attention to serving size.

Treatment of Type 2 Diabetes

Nutritional excess and lack of exercise contribute to numerous changes in blood chemistry. Obesity leads to hyperlipidemia, hyperglycemia, hypoxia (problems with oxygen distribution), and the resulting oxidative stress. When nutrient levels remain elevated, adipocytes (reversible energy depots) undergo hypertrophy (increase in cell size) and hyperplasia (increase in cell number). Adipose tissue becomes infiltrated with inflammatory cells in response to this stress. The continued high levels in circulating free fatty acids contribute to the use of less circulating glucose by liver and muscle. Chronically elevated glucose levels continue to have negative effects on pancreatic beta cells and energy metabolism in the liver.

Insulin resistance is related to the low-grade chronic inflammation seen in many metabolically relevant tissues, particularly adipose tissue. In addition to its roles in fat storage and metabolism, adipose tissue is very active as an endocrine tissue. The large numbers of secreted hormone-like factors have been dubbed adipokines. Examples include leptin, adiponectin, pro-inflammatory adipokines, and anti-inflammatory adipokines. The constant stimulus of excess nutrients on adipocytes causes inflammation that becomes self-generating, leading to the production of local and systemic pro-inflammatory factors. These factors are a major driving force leading to insulin resistance (Kwon & Pessin 2013). Therefore, understanding the interrelationships and mechanisms of these complex control loops of regulatory molecules is a rich source of information for drug development (see Table 12.4). Finding ways to block the chronic

Table 12.4 Possible causes of hyperglycemia

Organ	Altered Response	Comment
Pancreatic beta cells	Decreased insulin secretion	Death or overstimulation
Pancreatic alpha cells	Increased glucagon secretion	Lack of inhibition by insulin
Gut	Decreased incretin secretion	Loss of incretins' support of beta cells
Adipose tissue	Increased lipolysis	Glucagon >> insulin
Muscle	Decreased glucose uptake	Lack of insulin stimulation
Kidney	Increased glucose reabsorption	
Liver	Increased glucose production	Glucagon >> insulin

low-level inflammation and to restore insulin responsiveness will generate new classes of drugs to help fight obesity and Type 2 diabetes (Kwon & Pessin). Of course, any drug treatment should be combined with lifestyle changes involving diet and exercise.

Insulin Secretagogues

Insulin secretagogues are insulin-releasing drugs used to treat diabetes, including sulfonylureas and glinides.

SULFONYLUREAS

Sulfonylureas have been considered a traditional treatment for Type 2 diabetes for many years (see Table 12.5). They cause the release of insulin from pancreatic beta cells by binding and blocking a K^+ channel in the plasma membrane. When the efflux of K^+ is inhibited, the beta cells become depolarized. The depolarization activates a voltage-activated Ca^{2+} channel, allowing entry of Ca^{2+}, which then triggers the release of insulin (and amylin) from secretory vesicles.

Sulfonylureas range in their onset, time of action, and side-effects profile. Older drugs such as tolbutamide have a short half-life but can be advantageous in the treatment of elderly patients. The most serious side effect with sulfonylureas (and most oral antidiabetics) is hypoglycemia. Timing and size of dose are critical for matching the changes in glucose levels in the blood. Metabolism and clearance of these drugs depend on liver and kidney function; getting patients with diabetes, especially elderly ones, properly medicated to avoid hypoglycemia can be a challenge. Second-generation sulfonylureas (i.e., glyburide)

Table 12.5 Types of antidiabetic drugs

Drug Class	Examples	Mechanism

Insulin Secretagogues
  Sulfonylureas
 	
  Glinides
	Tolbutamide, glyburide
	Repaglinide
	Nateglinide
		Increase insulin release from pancreatic beta cells

Biguanides	Metformin	Decrease glucose production in the liver
Thiazolidinediones	Rosiglitazone	Decrease insulin resistance
Gliptins	Sitagliptin, saxagliptin	DPP-4 inhibitors, increase GLP-1 activity
SGLT2 inhibitors	Canagliflozin	Block glucose reuptake in kidneys
Alpha-glucosidase inhibitors	Acarbose, miglitol	Slow digestion of starch and disaccharides in gut
Bile-acid sequestrants	Colesevelam	Probably slow absorption
Incretin-based	Liraglutide Exenatide	GLP-1 receptor agonist Postprandial insulin increase and glucagon decrease
Amylin analogs	Pramlintide	Decrease postprandial glucose level, slow gastric emptying, and decrease appetite

have fewer drug interactions and adverse effects than the older drugs. However, the newer, more potent drugs require caution, as they can also increase the risk of hypoglycemia.

GLINIDES

Other insulin secretagogues include the **glinide** group of drugs, such as **repaglinide**. They can block the same K^+ channel as sulfonylureas, producing insulin release. Repaglinide has a fast onset of action and sufficient duration to be effective when taken before a meal. Hypoglycemia can occur if the meal is delayed or if the meal is low in carbohydrates. Repaglinide is metabolized primarily in the liver. It lacks sulfur, so it is useful for patients with sensitivity or allergies associated with sulfur or sulfur-containing drugs. Another newer secretagogue, **nateglinide**, also blocks the same ATP-sensitive K^+ channel. It is effective in patients with isolated postprandial hyperglycemia. Nateglinide causes a faster release of insulin than sulfonylureas, though its action does not persist. It is, therefore, useful when taken before every meal to enhance post-meal insulin production. Glinides are used in combination with drugs such as metformin to help control overnight or fasting glucose levels. Nateglinide may have the lowest chance of causing hypoglycemia and may be the safest choice for patients with renal problems.

Metabolic Regulators

BIGUANIDES

The **biguanides** are a class of oral glucose-lowering agents that work primarily by preventing the liver from breaking down glycogen and increasing glucose utilization. The drug **metformin** is an example and is considered a first-line agent for Type 2 diabetes. Its primary effect is to lower blood glucose without involvement of pancreatic beta cells. Metformin decreases gluconeogenesis in the liver, along with several other possible sites of action. In liver, metformin works by activating the AMP-activated protein kinase, a critical target involved in regulating metabolism. Stimulating AMP-activated protein kinase causes an increase in glucose uptake and fatty acid oxidation. Metformin can also increase glucose uptake in other tissues, such as muscle, as well as increasing the rate of glycolysis. Metformin is effective at lowering postabsorptive and postprandial glucose levels, with little chance of hypoglycemia. Since it does not work by increasing insulin release, it is called an "insulin sparing" agent. Metformin is used in combinations with secretagogues when monotherapy is inadequate. It is also effective in preventing Type 2 diabetes in individuals with prediabetes who are older, obese, and have impaired glucose tolerance.

THIAZOLIDINEDIONES

Patients with Type 2 diabetes develop resistance to the physiological effects of insulin. **Thiazolidinediones** decrease insulin resistance. These drugs act as ligands for one of the **peroxisome proliferator-activated receptors (PPAR)**. The PPAR are part of the superfamily of nuclear receptors that includes steroid hormone and thyroid receptors. The PPAR family modulates genes involved in fat and sugar metabolism, mitochondrial activity, and insulin signal transduction. The thiazolidinediones used for Type 2 diabetes probably target adipose tissue as their major site of action. They modulate lipid synthesis, including production of adipokines and other regulatory proteins involved in metabolism. They also promote glucose uptake and utilization. These drugs are highly efficacious and work to prevent Type 2 diabetes, but they have possible adverse effects that can be severe. These include fluid retention, weight gain, congestive heart failure, bone issues in women, and they have oncogenic potential (potential to cause cancer). Concern over the side effects has decreased their use. The drugs troglitazone (Rezulin) and pioglitazone (Actos) have been withdrawn or suspended from the U.S. and European markets. Rosiglitazone remains available in the United States, but its annual sales have plummeted.

GLIPTINS

Gliptins are inhibitors of the enzyme dipeptidyl peptidase-4 (DPP-4). Examples include sitagliptin (Januvia) and saxagliptin (Onglyza). Inhibition of DPP-4 prolongs and enhances the activity of incretins, including glucagon-like peptide 1 (GLP-1) and glucose-dependent gastric inhibitory polypeptide (GIP). Normally, DPP-4 cleaves two amino acids from the N-terminal end of these peptides, causing their inactivation. During a meal, GLP-1 and GIP are released from the small intestine into the vasculature. These peptide hormones increase insulin secretion dependent on increases in blood glucose. Besides increasing insulin production, GLP-1 inhibits glucagon secretion. Remember that glucagon increases blood glucose, so gliptin-enhanced GLP-1 activity will suppress glucose appearance into the blood. Additionally, GLP-1 slows gastric emptying (which also slows glucose entry into the blood) and can reduce appetite. Normally, GIP and GLP-1 are rapidly inactivated by DPP-4 and have extremely short plasma half-lives. DPP-4 is present in body fluids and attached to the surface of endothelial cells throughout the body. Gliptin inhibition of DPP-4 extends the half-life of GIP and GLP-1 and makes these drugs a potent class of oral hypoglycemics for Type 2 diabetes.

Reported adverse effects of gliptins (and GLP-1 agonists) include respiratory tract infections, headache, nausea, hypersensitivity, and skin reactions. There has been a debate over whether gliptins increase the chance of pancreatic cancer in rats and humans. A meta-analysis with 59,404 patients concluded there is no association between DPP-4 inhibitors and pancreatic cancer, with a small risk for acute pancreatitis that was not definitive (Pinto, Rados, Barkan, et al. 2018).

SODIUM GLUCOSE COTRANSPORTER 2 INHIBITORS

Canagliflozin (Invokana), the first in a new class of glucose-lowering drugs, is an oral inhibitor of sodium glucose cotransporter 2 (SGLT2) approved by the FDA in 2013 (U.S. Food and Drug Administration). SGLT2 is located in the proximal tubule in the kidneys and is responsible for 90% of glucose reabsorption during urine formation. Inhibition of SGLT2 leads to the loss of glucose in the urine, thereby lowering blood glucose levels. The **SGLT2 inhibitors** also cause a modest weight loss and a low risk of hypoglycemia. Their efficacy is not affected by the extent of insulin resistance or beta cell dysfunction; therefore, in principle, they can be used at any stage in the natural history of Type 2 diabetes (MacEwen, McKay, & Fisher 2012). In animal models of diabetes, SGLT2 inhibition and reduction in blood glucose reverse the toxicity observed with hyperglycemia, improve insulin sensitivity, and improve beta cell function (Rossetti, Smith, Shulman, et al. 1987).

Vaginal yeast infections and urinary tract infections are the most common side effects associated with canagliflozin. The increase in urination could lead to water and electrolyte issues. Canagliflozin use is not indicated in patients with Type 1 diabetes, those with renal impairment, those with end-stage renal disease, or those receiving dialysis. Other drugs in the SGLT2 inhibitors class include empagliflozin, dapagliflozin, ipragliflozin, and ertugliflozin. The long-term effects of these drugs are limited due to their short time on the market.

SGLT2 inhibitors provide a novel approach for treatment of Type 2 diabetes, the only indication for which they are currently approved. In conjunction with exercise and a healthy diet, they can improve glycemic control alone or in combination with other medications, including metformin, sulfonylureas, thiazolidinediones, and insulin.

ALPHA-GLUCOSIDASE INHIBITORS

The **alpha-glucosidase inhibitors** use another strategy to prevent and treat Type 2 diabetes. Drugs in this class, such as acarbose and miglitol, slow or decrease the uptake of glucose from the gut. Unlike the monosaccharides (e.g., glucose and fructose), which can be transported from the gut into the bloodstream, the polysaccharides and disaccharides must be broken down to release the monosaccharides. Carbohydrates in the diet consist of a mixture of long, complex polysaccharides (i.e., starch) that are essentially polymers of glucose. Simple sugars include the disaccharides sucrose (common table sugar) and lactose (the predominant sugar in mammalian milk). Enzymes (**glucosidases**) that break the bonds of polysaccharides and release monosaccharides (e.g., glucose, fructose, and galactose) are produced in the pancreas and found on surfaces of cells lining the gut, mainly along the upper portion of the small intestine. Acarbose and miglitol are competitive inhibitors of the intestinal glucosidases. They delay the digestion and absorption of glucose derived from starch, oligosaccharides, and disaccharides. Since absorption is delayed (or diminished), postprandial glucose load is reduced and less insulin is required, so these drugs can be considered insulin sparing. Monotherapy with these drugs, taken just before a meal, produces a modest drop in HbA1c levels. They are often used in combination with sulfonylureas.

Undigested carbohydrate that appears in the colon can cause some distress, including flatulence, abdominal pain, and diarrhea, but these symptoms can lessen over time as the lower small intestine increases expression of glucosidase activity.

BILE-ACID SEQUESTRANTS

Another agent that works in the gut is colesevelam, originally developed as a **bile-acid sequestrant** (discussed in Chapter 10) to lower cholesterol. Its mechanism isn't totally clear, but it does lower hemoglobin HbA1c by 0.5% and cholesterol by 15%. Colesevelam can also cause some lower GI complaints and interfere with absorption of other drugs and vitamins.

INCRETIN AND AMYLIN ANALOGS

Additional drugs for Type 2 diabetes are peptides or peptide analogs that mimic incretin or amylin activity. With loss of beta cell function, amylin secretion (directly) and incretin (indirectly) can be diminished following feeding, which makes it harder for insulin to do its job. Amylin analogs (pramlinitide) suppress glucagon activity, slow gastric emptying, and suppress appetite. Moreover, they have been used as supplemental therapy in Type 1 diabetes. Incretin analogs (liraglutide and exenatide) can enhance insulin release, suppress glucagon release, slow gastric emptying, and centrally suppress appetite. These drugs must be injected, and attention to timing and dose is needed to maximize their effectiveness. Their ability to suppress appetite also makes them candidates for the treatment of obesity.

Section Summary

Type 2 diabetes affects a large number of people worldwide, and the number is growing at an alarming rate. As we have seen, there are many drug choices for treating the symptoms. Each treatment has some limitations and possible adverse effects. These issues can often be minimized through the use of different drugs in combination or at different times of day to deal with either fasting or postprandial glucose levels.

Obesity

The obesity epidemic has become a worldwide problem. Obesity is a major cause of cardiovascular disease and Type 2 diabetes, and it has many other associated co-morbidities. Individuals who are obese and overweight frequently suffer from high blood pressure and coronary heart disease and have an increased risk for stroke. They also have an increased occurrence of certain types of cancer (e.g., breast, endometrial, and colon), osteoarthritis, and gynecological problems. Being obese or overweight can cause problems breathing while asleep (i.e., sleep apnea) and other respiratory issues. Overweight children are at risk for various chronic conditions in later life. They often have dyslipidemia, insulin resistance, and elevated blood pressure. Many overweight children have at least one risk factor for cardiovascular disease.

The primary cause of obesity is often simplified to the equation of excess energy consumed relative to energy expended. However, the situation is considerably more complex. Humans have highly evolved mechanisms for efficient use and storage of energy. A readily available source of energy-rich foods has meant for many people that minimum daily needs are easily met. When this is combined with a more sedentary lifestyle and an aging population, the trend of excessive weight gain is not surprising. Food deprivation initiates powerful drives in most animals. Weight loss is difficult, as metabolic activities (and capacities) are slow to change. Moreover, weight gain does not initiate compensatory actions or psychological drives. Weight gain can occur over time with little conscious acknowledgment. Fat accumulation varies greatly with the individual. Individuals differ in what is considered their metabolically normal weight. There are individuals who are thin with abnormal metabolism (and health issues) and individuals who are overweight with apparently normal metabolic activity and health. It is becoming clear that not all fat is the same from a metabolic, health, or endocrine point of view. Fat distribution may vary greatly based on diet and activity level and contribute to the ethnic differences in the prevalence of obesity-related diseases. After a brief discussion of fat metabolism and distribution, we will look at some of the drugs available to help deal with obesity.

Fat Metabolism

Most tissues are capable of fat metabolism. Quantitatively, three tissues are most important: liver, skeletal muscle, and adipose tissue. In these tissues, free fatty acids are combined to form triacylglycerol for storage and then released as needed by lipolysis (see Figure 12.1). In the liver, triacylglycerol is used in the distribution of lipoproteins. In skeletal muscle, triacylglycerol is an energy source, as released free fatty acids are oxidized for ATP production. In adipose tissue, insulin stimulates triacylglycerol formation and inhibits fat mobilization to encourage energy storage in the postprandial state.

Fat Distribution

Fat is stored in different locations in the body. **Visceral fat** fills the abdominal cavity surrounding the major organs. It contains "white" adipose tissue and is probably the source of many of the activities associated with fat tissue, including metabolic activity, immune function, and satiety. "Brown" fat is dispersed and is involved in temperature regulation.

Abdominal visceral fat that packs with the internal organs is the fat that is associated with chronic low-level inflammation and the development of insulin resistance. Visceral fat accumulation correlates with metabolic syndrome and associated lipid disorders, impaired glucose metabolism, and hypertension. One of the mechanisms underlying these problems involves **adiponectin**, an adipokine produced by adipocytes in visceral fat, which protects against diabetes, atherosclerotic vascular disease, inflammation, and hypertension. Blood levels of adiponectin decrease as visceral fat accumulation increases, providing a mechanism for how visceral fat accumulation contributes to diabetes.

People with an apple-shaped fat distribution have a large waist and a higher risk for the aforementioned conditions. Those with a pear-shaped body, where the fat distributes more to the hip and thighs and the waist is smaller, have a lower risk. Women tend to store fat around the hips and thighs (called **gluteal adipose tissue**) under the influence of estrogen. Following menopause, more fat storage occurs in the waist region. Whether gluteal fat is less of a health problem than visceral fat is debated; what isn't debated is that too much of either is not good.

The fat that you can pinch around the waist or under an arm is **subcutaneous fat**. Subcutaneous fat seems to be less physiologically active (e.g., immune response, production of adipokines) and acts primarily as an energy depot. **Intramuscular fat** is predominantly used for muscle function.

As discussed, fat distribution and its consequences are important in the development of obesity and Type 2 diabetes. The consumption of excess calories coupled with physical inactivity causes fat to accumulate subcutaneously and in the abdomen. Fat cells can increase in size significantly. However, there is a limit to this type of hypertrophic growth. Visceral adipocytes can replicate and increase in cell number. This type of hyperplastic growth is less pronounced in subcutaneous fat. As subcutaneous fat "fills" and can handle less of the load, visceral fat works to keep up with storing excess calories. The visceral fat becomes inflamed as immune cells infiltrate the tissue. Adipocytes produce adipokines in response. Eventually, visceral adipose tissue becomes resistant to insulin's signal to store more fat. Fat storage begins to spill out and involve other tissues, such as the liver and skeletal muscle. This **ectopic** (abnormally positioned) **fat** contributes to the growing insulin resistance. Normally, there is cooperation between adipose tissue, skeletal muscle, and the liver. For example, during exercise, fat is mobilized to meet the energy demand. The lack of exercise, however, contributes to the ectopic buildup of fat and the underlying low-grade inflammation that becomes self-generating: excess calories, more fat depositing, more inflammation, more insulin resistance, chronic hyperglycemia, unhealthy pancreatic beta cells, and eventually diabetes.

How Do Antiobesity Drugs Work?

Obesity and the related problems are largely attributable to an unhealthy lifestyle. Although some individuals may be able to change and maintain an optimum body weight and a healthier lifestyle, many cannot. Because of the enormity of the problem, additional intervention strategies are needed, especially for individuals who are morbidly obese. Drug treatment that can complement lifestyle changes (even if only moderate ones) could have a significant impact on quality of life for these individuals. Drugs developed to treat obesity should meet at least three goals:

1 To decrease body weight while clearly improving measures of morbidity and mortality.
2 To have a good benefit-to-risk ratio. All drugs have some associated risk, but many of the drugs brought to market for weight loss have had relatively higher associated risk. Several drugs have been pulled from the market. For individual who are morbidly obese, however, some of the risks associated with drug use may be less than the risks involved in being excessively overweight.
3 To have a low cost of treatment, as obesity and the associated health problems are disproportionately prevalent in the poor and underfunded.

Although the choices of drugs available to treat obesity are limited (see Table 12.6), this is an active area of drug development, with several possible targets for drug design. Body weight is under central control. Brain circuits control the initiation and termination of eating, as well as control the choice of what to eat. Several brain neuropeptides are involved, as well as the neurotransmitters dopamine, norepinephrine, and serotonin (5-HT). Drugs used as part of a weight-loss strategy could increase energy expenditure or reduce energy intake. Except when the patient is exercising, energy

Table 12.6 Types of antiobesity drugs

Drug	Classification	Notes
Lorcaserin	Selective serotonin agonist	Safer than discontinued fenfluramine
Phentermine	Appetite suppressant, sympathomimetic	Limited to 12 weeks due to sympathomimetic effects
Osymia	Combination of phentermine and topiramate	Low-dose phentermine and slow-release topiramate decrease side effects
Tesofensine	Neurotransmitter reuptake inhibitor	Blocks reuptake of norepinephrine, serotonin, and dopamine
Orlistat	Lipase inhibitor	Blocks absorption of fat in the gut
Amylin and incretin analogs		See Table 12.5.

expenditure is relatively constant and difficult to alter pharmacologically in a safe way. Energy intake is highly variable and depends on food consumption. **Satiation** is the process that terminates food consumption. Signals that invoke satiation could be a target for drug design. Restraint, the ability to stop eating when satiated, is also a property that could be targeted. Drugs could be targeted to decrease hunger (and the number of snacks or meals) or portion size (by reinforcing satiation signaling). Education can help with food choices and maintaining a proper diet.

Serotonin Agonists

There are many levels of behavior that control eating patterns, and several neurotransmitter-mediated pathways are involved (Adan 2013). Serotonin is involved both centrally and in the periphery in controlling appetite. Increasing serotonergic activity is one of the targets of drugs to combat obesity. Blocking reuptake with specific serotonin-selective reuptake inhibitors (SSRIs; see Chapter 9) can decrease appetite, but this can lead to stimulation of most serotonin receptors and create unwanted side effects. A selective serotonin receptor agonist called lorcaserin has been approved for treating obesity. It is selective toward one subclass of receptor (5-HT$_{2C}$), so it may not have the same potency as other indirectly acting uptake inhibitors, such as fenfluramine. Fenfluramine has serotonin-selective reuptake inhibitor activity and was a component of a preparation (Fen-Phen) that was used for obesity into the 1990s but withdrawn because of heart-related issues. Lorcaserin, as a specific agonist, has a much better side-effect profile.

Appetite Suppressants

Increasing norepinephrine activity suppresses appetite and can cause weight loss, as we saw with the centrally acting sympathomimetics in Chapter 8. Amphetamine, for example, is known for decreasing appetite and causing weight loss. Phentermine, the only member of this class of drugs prescribed for weight loss, is used exclusively for short-term treatment (less than 12 weeks). As a potent sympathomimetic, it can increase heart rate and blood pressure. Phentermine is approved for use in combination with topiramate, originally prescribed as an antiepileptic. Qsymia combines low levels of phentermine with a slow-release formulation of topiramate for an effective antiobesity drug with a lessened side-effect profile. Another drug with potential is tesofensine, an antidepressant that can cause weight loss. Tesofensine is a norepinephrine/dopamine/serotonin reuptake inhibitor that shows promise. Amylin and incretin analogs (see Table 12.5) also provide appetite suppression and may be useful for obesity and diabetes (Adan).

Lipase Inhibitors

Orlistat is a gastric and pancreatic **lipase inhibitor**. By blocking lipase activity in the gut, it prevents the release of fatty acids from triglycerides and their absorption. It is a derivative of a natural product of microbes. Orlistat is given orally with meals and can reduce dietary fat absorption by 30%. Very little of the drug is absorbed, and most is excreted unchanged in the feces. Orlistat also can lower LDL and decrease the rate of incidence for diabetes when compared to placebo. In long-term studies, it has little effect on blood pressure. Since very little is absorbed from the gut, there are few systemic toxic effects. However, a significant number (15% to 30%) of patients reported lower GI issues.

Cannabinoid Receptor Antagonists

Other drugs have been introduced in the past but withdrawn after concerns were raised about their safety. Rimonabant is a cannabinoid receptor antagonist that was released in Europe as an appetite suppressant but recalled in 2008 after reports of severe depression and potential suicidal tendencies. Other cannabinoid receptor antagonists have been patented but none have yet to be approved for treating obesity (Yadav & Murumkar 2018).

Section Summary

For successful treatment of obesity, drug choice matched with lifestyle coaching will be essential. This personalized medicine approach will be necessary, as one size certainly does not fit all. The available drugs for obesity, such as those discussed above, have modest efficacy and relatively low rates of persistence, meaning people stop taking them after a while. The goal of antiobesity treatment is to cause a 10% decrease in placebo-subtracted weight. Studies with these drugs need to continue long enough to generate meaningful results, often for a year or longer. Few, if any, studies have reached the overall goal of a 10% reduction, though some small percentage (usually less than 25%) of the participants may see that level of result.

Low-Carbohydrate Diets

Many people continually search for a miracle diet that will help them shed unwanted pounds. However, few diet plans withstand the careful scrutiny that comes from long-term studies with a large number of participants. Examples include low-fat or low-carbohydrate diets. Though the Atkins diet is now synonymous with low-carbohydrate, high-protein, high-fat diets, there has been a long history of diets with: (a) a low to very low carbohydrate content, (b) no restriction of protein and fat, and (c) unrestricted calories (AMA Council on Foods and Nutrition 1973). Ketogenic diets, as they are often referred to, create controversy as many experts have trouble with various aspects of this diet, starting with whether caloric intake is limited or the high percentage of calories from fat. Proponents of the ketogenic diet believe that low-carbohydrate diets generate sufficient ketone bodies to cause urinary losses in amounts sufficient to account for weight loss, even with high caloric intake. The ketogenic diet may help increase insulin sensitivity and reduce insulin resistance. However, experimental evidence from properly controlled studies does not support such large losses of ketones in the urine or the breath. A successful weight-reducing diet needs to incorporate a decrease in energy intake, an increase in the utilization of energy, or both.

Debate centers on whether the Atkins or ketogenic diet is a safe and effective solution to America's obesity epidemic. To assess the Atkins diet (or newer ketogenic versions) properly, a control or alternate diet must be employed for comparison. Studies on the Atkins diet often used a calorie-restricted (portion controlled) version of a typical diet with approximately 30% of the calories as fat. However, the calorie-restricted approach to weight loss has a consistent history of failure, so it may not be a valid choice for comparison. Short-term (weeks to months) studies suggest people on the Atkins diet lose more weight than do people on the calorie-restricted diet. However, after one year, the difference in weight lost is statistically insignificant (Foster, Wyatt, Hill, et al. 2003). Moreover, total serum cholesterol increased by about 3% with the Atkins diet; the conventional diet reduced cholesterol by about 5%. HDL increased by about 20% with the Atkins diet; only about a 3% increase was seen with the conventional diet (Foster et al.). The Atkins diet can raise total LDL, but a low-fat diet is more effective at reducing risk factors such as LDL (Beard, Barnard, Robbins, et al. 1996). Dropout rates are very high with both the Atkins and calorie-restricted diets. On the Atkins diet, people tend not to feel well when they are ketotic. Proponents of the ketogenic lifestyle argue that people adjust to these feelings over time. Conventional diets often fail because they make people uncomfortable with ongoing feelings of hunger and the pressure of making proper food choices.

Exercise is often not a part of the ketogenic diet research studies, because people on low-carbohydrate diets can feel like they lack sufficient energy for physical activity. The rise in popularity of ketogenic diets is attracting athletes, however, and more studies are being initiated. Some of the possible long-term effects of maintaining the ketogenic diet include higher cholesterol, blood urea nitrogen, uric acid, and free fatty acids. If the low-carbohydrate diet is maintained over many months, complications can develop that include dehydration, cardiac arrhythmias, kidney stones, and other issues with the kidneys, liver, brain, and eyes. In contrast, a true low-fat diet (less than 10% calories as fat) paired with exercise provides long-term successful weight loss (Wing & Hill 2001). The National Weight Control Registry has tracked successful dieters (loss of at least 30 kg for 5.5 years) since 1993. On average, registrants consume low-fat diets of about 1400 calories daily and expend about 400 calories/day in physical exercise.

The rationale for the ketogenic diet is that severe carbohydrate restriction will result in ketosis, the conversion of fatty acids to ketone bodies that can substitute for glucose in some tissues, such as the brain (see Figure 12.1). Under ketotic conditions, lipid oxidation (fat loss) is promoted, satiety (satisfaction of appetite) occurs, and increased energy expenditure is expected. On a low-carbohydrate diet, energy is expended to make carbohydrate for tissues that absolutely require glucose, such as the brain and red blood cells. This process is inefficient, so that extra calories are expended when ketone bodies are made from fatty acids or glucose is made from amino acid derivatives by gluconeogenesis. Gluconeogenesis is normally used to make glucose during the postabsorptive state or when fasting. Since the brain, red blood cells, and other tissues must have carbohydrate to function well, the body must call upon these mechanisms to survive.

Taxing the body's survival mechanisms to create a ketotic state can make it hard to continue the diet. Consuming diets high in meat/protein (with associated saturated fat and cholesterol) increases the risk of heart disease, stroke, and atherosclerosis; total cholesterol and LDL increase with the low-carbohydrate diet (Foster et al.). The initial weight loss seen with the low-carbohydrate diet, which may represent reduction of fatty tissue and associated water loss, does not seem sustainable. Weight loss on the ketogenic diet may be like that of other diets, where people lose their desire to eat the required food, causing an overall lower consumption of calories. Opponents of the ketogenic diet point out that the diet exaggerates consumption of the unhealthiest components of the Western diet—animal protein and fat. It also minimizes the importance of dietary fiber and a healthy microbiome (see Box in Chapter 13). However, proponents of the ketogenic diet argue that too much carbohydrate (especially refined sugars) contributes to obesity. They argue that the body adjusts to the ketotic state and significant weight loss can result. Most experts agree that too much sugar contributes to weight gain. When it comes to a healthy diet, a reasonable overall goal is to encourage people to eat balanced meals that promote both ideal body weight and health.

Exercise Pharmacology

A common element in patients suffering from diabetes and obesity is difficulty maintaining a healthy weight. Certain genetic defects can lead to these conditions, and, in the future, as each individual's genetic makeup becomes known, subtle genetic patterns may identify those with a greater disposition to become obese or diabetic. For most people, however, maintaining a healthy weight involves balancing energy in (consumed) and energy out (expended). Excess energy consumed on a daily basis is stored for later use, available should the need arise for exercise or other physical activity.

Daily exercise is important for everyone, especially individuals who are diabetic or overweight. Physical activity can increase insulin sensitivity in most tissues, particularly skeletal muscle. Lack of physical activity can decrease insulin sensitivity. However, many patients who are obese or diabetic have associated cardiovascular problems, such as high blood pressure. Therefore, initial exercise plans for these individuals should primarily be of low intensity. With intensity held low, the exercise variables that can be controlled are duration and frequency. Again, depending on the status of the patient, duration may also be limited. Frequency then becomes the most important variable in building an exercise plan. An initial plan might be to walk for 10 minutes, three times a day. Since the goal initially is to get a patient out of the chair and walking, the impact of exercise on the pharmacology of antiobesity and antidiabetic drugs will be nominal in this population. After a very brief consideration of the impact of exercise on pharmacokinetics, we will look at the role of exercise in treating diabetes and obesity. In the case of Type 1 diabetes, we will briefly cover some of the issues in terms of insulin dosing and **glycemic control**, the maintenance of glucose levels.

Pharmacokinetic Concerns

Individuals with Type 1 diabetes are insulin-dependent and must be careful about the amount and type of food that they eat. To start an exercise program, individuals with Type 1 diabetes need clearance from their doctor. They should monitor glucose levels before and after exercise and keep a journal. By keeping good records, they can understand how their bodies respond to certain types of exercise. Wearing an ID bracelet and planning to exercise with a partner are important. Those with Type 1 diabetes should also carry snacks high in carbohydrate in case they suffer from hypoglycemia. A regular exercise program is important with Type 1 diabetes because exercise uses glucose and therefore helps lower the blood glucose level, similar to insulin. The amount of insulin injected can sometimes be lowered for individuals who have Type 1 diabetes and become physically active. Timing of exercise and eating is also important and depends on the individual, the activity, and the food. Exercise provides the same benefits for these individuals as for others, including lowering blood pressure, managing body weight, improving blood lipids, and improving self-image and confidence. For substantial health benefits, the currently accepted guidelines for adults recommend moderate-intensity aerobic exercise for at least 150 minutes each week, 75 minutes of vigorous exercise each week, or some equivalent combination of the two. Muscle strengthening exercises at least twice a week are also recommended.

Oral antidiabetic and antiobesity drugs include a variety of agents with several different targets and mechanisms of action. Most of the drugs that act systemically have their own sets of unwanted side effects. Proper liver and kidney function is often critical to minimize possible toxic effects. Since patients who are diabetic or obese are often severely de-conditioned, exercise programs will start at low intensities and remain there until significant gains in cardiovascular health can be made and significant amounts of weight can be lost. Therefore, these individuals should not expect to experience significant changes in blood flow to the liver and kidneys, because their exercise will be of low to moderate intensity for relatively short durations. As an individual's conditioning level improves and the intensity and duration of the exercise increase, drug dosages and the effects of exercise should be reevaluated. There is limited information available on the effects of exercise on the pharmacokinetics of oral antidiabetic and antiobesity drugs; common sense, attention to side-effect profiles, and monitoring of blood glucose levels should suffice. For the agents that work in the GI-tract and are largely excreted in the feces unchanged (i.e., bile-acid sequestrants and orlistat), low-intensity exercise should not have a significant effect. Individuals taking these drugs may not want to stray too far from home or a bathroom facility, however, as fecal urgency is a possible side effect. The importance of the gut microbiome in obesity (Santos, Alves, Hammes, & Dall'Alba 2019) and diabetes (Aw & Fukuda 2018) is now well established. Interestingly, some drugs for diabetes interact with the gut microbiome, some with possibly positive effects. For example, metformin changed the population of bacteria and conferred improved glucose tolerance to mice via fecal transplant (Wu, Esteve, Tremaroli, et al. 2017). Additionally, acarbose significantly changed the gut community structure and increased beneficial short chain fatty acid output in a diet-dependent manner (Baxter, Lesniak, Sinani, et al. 2019). Obesity and diabetes will provide a rich environment for studies on the interaction of the gut microbiome and human health.

Pharmacodynamic Concerns

During physical activity, energy demands placed on the body are significant, as whole-body oxygen consumption increases. Skeletal muscle uses its own stores of glycogen and triglycerides; it also transports in glucose and free fatty acids from the blood. The liver is largely responsible for replenishing blood glucose, while adipose tissue breaks down triglycerides to replenish the levels of free fatty acids. Remember that the central nervous system relies on glucose, so blood levels must be maintained during exercise. Hypoglycemia rarely occurs in normal (i.e., non-diabetic) individuals. Hormones play a critical role in maintaining blood sugar levels. Pancreatic hormones, such as insulin and glucagon, are secreted into the portal vein and directly affect liver function. As exercise begins, glucose production by the liver increases due to glucagon activity. Blood glucose levels during prolonged physical activity depend primarily on glucagon and catecholamines.

In individuals with insulin deficiency, these adaptations are altered. The lack of insulin to counterbalance the glucose-mobilizing effects of glucagon and catecholamines can result in dangerously high levels of glucose and ketone bodies, possibly triggering **diabetic ketoacidosis**. Diabetic ketoacidosis is a serious medical emergency that results when free fatty acids become the dominant energy source due to low levels of insulin, diminished glycogen stores, and low intracellular glucose. Ketone bodies, a product of fatty acid metabolism, build up to toxic levels, and the result can be vomiting, dehydration, breathing problems, confusion, and even coma. Conversely, too much administered insulin can blunt glucose mobilization, and hypoglycemia may ensue. However, the benefits of an active lifestyle are significant, and with a good understanding of their condition and monitoring of glucose levels, individuals with diabetes can enjoy a wide range of activities.

Type 1 Diabetes, Exercise, and Glycemic Control

Individuals who have good metabolic control are encouraged to exercise after a thorough physical examination. Young people with Type 1 diabetics can participate in most activities. Older individuals should continue to be physically active but should use common sense. Those who have had diabetes long-term need to take precautions, depending on the status of their vision, circulation, and peripheral neuropathy (loss of protective sensations, especially in the feet). Proper attention to a warm-up and cool-down routine is highly encouraged, as is proper hydration. Identification as an individual with Type 1 diabetes is also important, either with a bracelet or a shoe tag. Weight training with high resistance and heavy weights may be acceptable for the young. For a middle-aged individual with diabetes, using lighter weights with a higher number repetitions is recommended.

Many studies have been done to understand glucose regulation in those with diabetes who exercise. Researchers have examined many variables to learn how to minimize the chance of hypoglycemia, such as intensity, duration, time of day, replenishment of carbohydrates, and type of training (aerobic and resistance). The risk of hypoglycemia during exercise depends on initial glucose levels and intensity of exercise. The contraction of working muscles causes a number of physiological changes that affect glucose utilization. Muscle contraction stimulates the recruitment of glucose transporters to the cell membrane, increasing glucose uptake capacity in an insulin-independent manner. Insulin also stimulates glucose transporter activity. There is also a significant increase in blood flow to working muscles. Regular exercise (training) regulates glucose use by increasing the number of glucose transporters and metabolic enzymes that use glucose. Exercise increases insulin sensitivity in most tissues, resulting in higher glucose uptake. During the recovery phase following exercise, skeletal muscle shifts from glucose to free fatty acids for ATP production but continues elevated glucose uptake to rebuild glycogen stores. Post-exercise hypoglycemia can be delayed 7 to 11 hours, and perhaps longer in individuals with Type 1 diabetes (Davey, Howe, Paramalingam, et al. 2013).

Nighttime hypoglycemia occurs at a higher incidence after 45 minutes of afternoon exercise compared to afternoon rest (McMahon, Ferreira, Ratnam, et al. 2007). The risk of nocturnal hypoglycemia is also related to exercise intensity. As exercise intensity increases, glucose utilization contributes more to the energy demand, since fatty acid oxidation does not keep up. This increased reliance on glucose with increasing intensity of exercise depends on catecholamines such as epinephrine. For young people with Type 1 diabetes who engage in competitive sports, delayed or nighttime hypoglycemia is an issue. Modification of insulin treatment and supplemental dietary carbohydrates may be needed to counteract the risk of hypoglycemia.

Brief high-intensity exercise protocols (e.g., HIIT from Chapter 2) show promise in providing the desired benefits with less chance for hypoglycemia. These types of protocols also roughly simulate team sports like soccer and football, where players engage in intermittent bursts of activity. Moderate exercise provides good benefits but can require higher exercise volume (i.e., extended exercise time) than many people can achieve. Brief, high-intensity exercise protocols can reach similar energy expenditures in less time. For an example using a cycle ergometer, sprint intervals totaling 2.5 minutes were done for a total of 25 minutes, including warm-up and cool-down. Brief, high-intensity exercise showed improved glycemic control for one to three days (Adams 2013). In one study, seven individuals with Type 1 diabetes were tested on separate occasions with two protocols (Guelfi, Jones, & Fournier 2005). The moderate exercise protocol was for 30 minutes at 40% VO_2max on a cycle ergometer. The intermittent high-intensity protocol was also at 40% VO_2max but with a four-second sprint every two minutes. The results indicated that blood glucose declined less with the intermittent sprint protocol, and it stabilized sooner than with the moderate exercise protocol. The intermittent sprinters had higher levels of lactate, catecholamines, and growth hormone; glucagon, insulin, cortisol, and free fatty acids did not show a significant difference between the protocols. Therefore, the decline in blood glucose is less during exercise and during recovery with intermittent sprinting.

Another study showed that sprinting can be used as a tool to prevent hypoglycemia. Sprints as short as 10 seconds can cause a sustained increase in blood glucose (Bussau, Ferreira, Jones, & Fournier 2006). Seven male participants with Type 1 diabetes had their usual morning dose of insulin and breakfast. Once their blood sugar dropped to about 11 mM, they pedaled for 20 minutes on a cycle ergometer at 40% VO_2max. At this point they either sprinted for 10 seconds or rested. The group that rested exhibited a steady decline in blood glucose, whereas the sprint group had a relatively flat response, with little decline. This result is intriguing, because the short sprint at the end of the workout helped to keep the blood glucose level from becoming hypoglycemic.

In a more recent study with eight subjects with Type 1 diabetes and eight matched normal controls, blood levels of glucose were determined following a 10-second sprint (Fahey, Paramalingam, Davey, et al. 2012). The researchers used a euglycemic-euinsulinemic clamp technique and infused labeled glucose to distinguish the rate of glucose appearance (Ra) from the rate of disappearance (Rd; Fahey et al.). Intense exercise is known to cause an increase in glucose appearance, as the liver increases glycogenolysis and gluconeogenesis. Participants sprinted on a cycle ergometer with maximum effort for 10 seconds. The short sprint caused an increase in blood glucose in the individuals both with and without diabetes, similar to the above experiment by Bussau and colleagues. Surprisingly, the increase in blood glucose was due to a decline in the rate of glucose disappearance and not to an increase in glucose appearance. In Type 1 diabetes, insulin is not released, so glucose levels may remain elevated longer. The short sprint caused a brief rise in epinephrine and norepinephrine, but not to the extent observed during prolonged intense exercise, which is usually responsible for the increase in glucose appearance in the blood. Following a 10-second sprint, Ra does not change, but Rd decreases, with a slow return to resting levels. The underlying mechanism is unclear, but the 10-sprint at the end of the workout does appear to lessen the chance of hypoglycemia in individuals with Type 1 diabetes (Fahey et al.).

Resistance exercise may have a greater effect in reducing HbA1c levels than aerobic exercise in individuals with Type 1 diabetes (Yardley, Kenny, Perkins, et al. 2013). Twelve physically active participants with Type 1 diabetes were tested on separate days doing either nothing (no-exercise control) or one of two different exercise protocols. The resistance protocol consisted of three sets of eight repetitions for seven different weight-lifting exercises, completed in 45 minutes. The aerobic protocol consisted of running 45 minutes at 60% VO_2max on a treadmill. Plasma glucose was determined at time 0 and 60 minutes post exercise. Interstitial glucose was determined continuously for 24 hours before and after, by using a continuous glucose monitor. The results are shown in Table 12.7. During exercise, the decline in glucose was steeper with aerobic exercise than with resistance exercise. During recovery, glucose climbed back after aerobic exercise but remained relatively stable after resistance exercise for the first hour. Mean glucose levels 4.5 to 6 hours post exercise were significantly lower with resistance than aerobic exercise. This decrease in post-exercise glucose following resistance exercise may account for the reduction in HbA1c reported following resistance exercise (Yardley et al.).

Resistance exercise is associated with improvements in muscular strength, higher bone mineral density, increased insulin sensitivity, and lower self-monitored blood glucose levels. It can also improve lipid profiles and cardiovascular function. Individuals with diabetes may have an increased risk of myopathy, and performing regular resistance exercise should help maintain or improve muscle mass and metabolism. Muscle mass and metabolism are also important in that they contribute to the basal metabolic rate and baseline energy utilization. More muscle mass takes up more

Table 12.7 Comparison of blood glucose levels following aerobic or resistance exercise

	Plasma Glucose (mmol/L)		
Status	*No Exercise*	*Resistance Exercise*	*Aerobic Exercise*
Start	8.4 ±2.7	8.4 ±2.7	9.2 ±3.4
45 min of exercise	8.6 ±3.8	6.8 ±2.3[a]	5.8 ±2.0[a]
60 min of recovery	No change	No change	Increase 2.2 ±0.6[b]

a   Significant difference between exercise and baseline.
b   Significant difference between aerobic exercise and other two conditions; n = 11 for resistance exercise group; n = 12 for no-exercise and aerobic exercise groups. Data derived from Yardley, Kenny, Perkins, et al. (2013).

glucose, amino acids, and free fatty acids from the blood in response to insulin. More exercise-associated glycemic fluctuation was observed with moderate levels of aerobic exercise compared to resistance exercise (Yardley et al.). Therefore, resistance exercise appears beneficial as far as glucose stability is concerned.

Exercise and Type 2 Diabetes

As Type 2 diabetes develops, insulin resistance morphs into impaired glucose tolerance, eventually becoming overt hyperglycemia. Drug intervention is then necessary, until insulin therapy becomes required. Structured physical activity can slow or even reverse this progression, especially with high levels of adherence and follow-up assessment. Individuals with uncomplicated Type 2 diabetes, prediabetes, or metabolic syndrome are candidates for exercise intervention. Physical activity increases insulin sensitivity, and a lack of physical activity contributes to insulin insensitivity.

Several studies have explored the exercise volume, intensity, and modalities needed to see the increase in insulin sensitivity. In a study with a large number of runners (33,060) and walkers (15,945), equivalent energy expenditures by walking or running produced similar risk reductions for diabetes, hypertension, and cholesterol (Williams & Thompson 2013). A reduction in Hb1Ac is the primary goal for drug and exercise treatment in Type 2 diabetes. As stated earlier, the HbA1c reflects the average glucose level in the blood over the previous two to three months. The level of HbA1c is also a strong predictor of complications associated with Type 2 diabetes. A group of 22 women with diabetes in a supervised exercise program showed an improvement in insulin sensitivity that was related to exercise intensity. A reduction in HbA1c was related mainly to exercise volume (Segerstrom, Glans, Eriksson, et al. 2010). The suggestion from this study is that to improve insulin sensitivity, exercise with a high-intensity component is recommended.

Aerobic training will reduce HbA1c, with the recommendation being 30 minutes on most days. A structured exercise-training program with or without dietary advice is more effective than providing advice alone (Umpierre, Ribeiro, Kramer, et al. 2011). In a meta-analysis of 47 randomized controlled clinical trials involving 8,538 patients, a significant decrease in HbA1c was observed for supervised aerobic and/or resistance training in patients with Type 2 diabetes (Umpierre et al.). However, HbA1c monitoring cannot track the variability that occurs in glucose levels over the course of the day. Individuals who have widely variable glucose levels may suffer related quality of life issues. For a person with diabetes, controlling blood glucose is already difficult, with medications to take, diet/food concerns, and daily stress, so adding physical activity can be too much for some patients. Advances in continuous glucose monitoring may be very helpful for those who are prone to hypoglycemia or hyperglycemia (Riddell & Perkins 2009). The goal is for individuals with diabetes who are physically active to improve their metabolic control.

Exercise can decrease abdominal visceral fat, leading to improvements in insulin sensitivity. As mentioned earlier, excessive abdominal fat triggers many of the metabolic and cardiovascular issues observed in metabolic syndrome and diabetes. A meta-analysis that included 15 studies and 852 subjects concluded that moderate- or high-intensity training reduced visceral adipose tissue in overweight males and females, in as few as 12 weeks, without incorporating hypocaloric diets (Vissers, Hens, Taeymans, et al. 2013). Long-term intervention with high-intensity interval training not only improved body composition but also decreased the prevalence of metabolic syndrome in 62 obese men and women (Gremeaux, Drigny, Nigam, et al. 2012).

Additionally, sedentary behavior is strongly and adversely associated with cardio-vascular and metabolic disease (Henson, Yates, Biddle, et al. 2013). A large number of participants at risk for diabetes were assessed from several ongoing research projects. The researchers found that sedentary behavior may be a better indicator for poor health than the amount of moderate to vigorous exercise. As the amount of time sitting increased from 9.6 hours to over 11 hours per day, blood sugar and triglyceride levels increased and HDL decreased (Henson et al.). For people with diabetes and those at risk, physical activity is essential for improving their health. Getting up and moving is a start; a structured, supervised exercise program combining endurance, resistance, and high-intensity interval training is the ultimate goal.

Exercise Effect on Antidiabetic Drugs

Over the years, many studies have looked at possible interactions between oral antidiabetics and exercise. Studies have also examined whether these medications can delay or halt the progression from prediabetes to Type 2 diabetes. For the insulin secretagogues, the question centers on the effect of exercise on the drugs' ability to cause insulin secretion. In an experiment by Larsen, Dela, Madsbad, and colleagues (1999), eight individuals with Type 2 diabetes were tested following three different protocols. In the first, they took an oral sulfonylurea, and in the second, they exercised at about 60% VO_2max for 60 minutes; the third was the combination of drug and exercise. Drug treatment and exercise both caused a decrease in blood sugar, with the hypoglycemic action enhanced when the treatments were combined. Exercise caused a decrease in insulin with or without drug treatment, though the insulin decrease in the presence of the insulin secretagogue was smaller in magnitude. The result was more insulin while the subjects took the insulin secretagogue and exercised; the additional insulin provided more suppression of hepatic glucose production, which explains the lower glucose level observed in the combined treatments (Larsen et al.).

One of the most widely used antidiabetic drugs is metformin. Metformin works in part by activating the AMP-dependent protein kinase. Exercise and certain adipokines also stimulate AMP-dependent protein kinase. Since there is a possible shared mechanism, we might ask, do exercise and metformin have an additive effect on blood sugar control in diabetics? In one study, 10 participants with Type 2 diabetes took either metformin or placebo for 28 days (Boule, Robert, Bell, et al. 2011). At the end of the treatment, they were assessed with and without exercise. Metformin increased heart rate and lactate formation during exercise. However, exercise interfered with the glucose-lowering effect of metformin after a standardized meal (Boule et al.). In another study with men and women with prediabetes, the subjects were split into four groups: placebo, metformin, exercise and placebo, and exercise and metformin (Malin, Gerber, Chipkin, & Braun 2012). Each of the three treatment groups had improved insulin sensitivity compared to the placebo control. However, the data suggested that metformin blunted the full effect obtained in the exercise group (Malin et al.). In a more recent study, 403 patients (85 metformin users, 318 non-users) were analyzed after a 12-week exercise program. Changes in HbA1c were similar for both groups and there were no between-group differences in lipid profile, quality of life, and weight. There was an improvement in the six-minute walk trial in the metformin group. Though the results are mixed, metformin does not appear to have a large additive effect on exercise, but may complement exercise in some tasks (Eltonsy et al., 2019).

Section Summary

Antidiabetic drugs have varied mechanisms of action that each attempt to lower blood glucose levels. Exercise uses glucose and stimulates the uptake of glucose from the blood, primarily in skeletal muscle, increasing the rate of disappearance. However, exercise also increases glucose appearance by stimulating hepatic production of glucose, creating a bit of a paradox. The key feature is the total energy expenditure during time exercising and the recovery time following exercise. Drugs and exercise combining to cause hypoglycemia poses a danger. Also possible is a prolonged hyperglycemic state that results from glucose mobilization and insufficient insulin activity to counter the elevated glucose levels. In the obese and prediabetic condition, exercise and caloric restriction have obvious benefit. In patients with long-term diabetes, careful attention to medications and monitoring of blood glucose levels is necessary for safe and productive exercise programs. Clearly, exercise is an important component to help these patients improve their quality of life.

Elder Concerns

Besides maintaining our posture and producing movement, skeletal muscle has many other critical roles. It is a major target of insulin, helping regulate blood glucose and providing a major site of glucose storage and utilization. Skeletal muscle secretes several polypeptide hormones, myokines, associated with coordinating whole-body metabolism. During starvation, muscle breakdown provides amino acids for gluconeogenesis in the liver.

As we age, muscle mass and power progressively decrease—the process called sarcopenia (discussed previously in Chapter 2). As age and sarcopenia progress, the risk increases for mobility disorders, falls and fractures, impaired daily activities, loss of independence, and shortened lifetime (Dhillon & Hasni 2017). These risks increase in overweight and obese individuals. Central obesity with sarcopenia is known as sarcopenic obesity. Sarcopenic obesity is associated with higher risk than simple obesity for metabolic syndrome, diabetes, atherosclerosis, and cardiovascular disease (Umegaki 2015). Conditions common in the obese, such as higher free fatty acids, increased inflammatory cytokines, increased reactive oxygen species (ROS), and decreased mitochondrial oxidative capacity, can contribute to the progression of sarcopenia. The chronic inflammation and mitochondrial dysfunction associated with obesity and diabetes negatively impacts the health of skeletal muscle.

Insulin resistance contributes to sarcopenia. Normally, insulin stimulates protein synthesis and other anabolic properties in muscle. Muscle mass depends on the balance between protein synthesis and protein degradation. Defects in insulin signaling can lead to reduced muscle mass because the synthetic rate decreases relative to the degradation rate. Other age-related decreases in sex hormones, growth hormone, and insulin-like growth factor-1 contribute to the decrease in muscle mass. In the elderly (and everyone else!), physical inactivity leads to muscle disuse and loss. A poor diet also contributes to loss of muscle mass, sometimes with an increased lipid accumulation in muscle cells. Reduced muscle mass diminishes a critical target of insulin, and can alter insulin sensitivity and blood glucose regulation.

Type 2 diabetics have increased rates of sarcopenia and frailty. Hyperglycemia (measured by HbA1c), contributes to poorer muscle quality and strength, and these effects are observed in patients in their 40s (Umegaki). Hyperglycemia might contribute to mitochondrial dysfunction, paving the way to muscle loss in older patients with Type 2 diabetes. Therefore, maintaining glucose in the normal range with drugs like metformin could slow the loss of muscle mass and strength when treated early in the process. The best, and currently only way, to maintain muscle mass is exercise. The recommendation for 150 minutes of moderate to intense exercise per week with one to two days of resistance training helps maintain muscle mass and insulin sensitivity. Muscle mass contributes to resting metabolic rate and the burning of calories. Dieting to lose weight is recommended, but weight loss can involve both fat and muscle tissue. Regular physical activity helps minimize muscle loss during reduced caloric uptake during dieting. Nutritional supplements and possible therapeutic approaches have been put forward, but with little evidence of their effectiveness to date (Dhillon & Hasni). Regular exercise, weight training, and a healthy diet are the best antidote for aging-related decrease in muscle strength and combating the onset of diabetes.

Health Risks

Diabetes and obesity are major worldwide health concerns. The control of euglycemia is a complex physiological process that is difficult to regulate with drugs. Lifestyle changes are also required, especially concerning diet and exercise. Insulin and insulin secretagogues can induce hypoglycemia when glucose appearance in the bloodstream cannot keep up with insulin-driven and/or exercise-induced glucose disappearance. Hypoglycemia is very dangerous, as brain function declines with dropping glucose levels. Unmanaged diabetes is also very dangerous. The lack of insulin or insulin responsiveness leads to hyperglycemia. Cells cannot access the glucose available in the blood. Glucagon activity proceeds unchecked, due to the lack of insulin activity. Glycogen stores in the liver become depleted. As cells turn more to fatty acids as an energy source, byproducts of fatty acid metabolism (ketone bodies) build up. The increase in ketone bodies results in ketosis; if their production continues, the condition ultimately becomes ketoacidosis when normal acid–base compensatory mechanisms become overwhelmed. Diabetic ketoacidosis can result in a diabetic coma if left untreated.

The different insulins are injected subcutaneously, requiring safe use of needles and syringes or proper use of pump technologies. The incretin and amylin analogs are also peptides requiring subcutaneous injection, requiring additional care in their handling and use.

The oral antidiabetics all have associated, unwanted side effects. Proper kidney and liver function helps minimize these problems, but people with diabetes and the morbidly obese can have impaired function, giving rise to additional problems in dosing and administering these drugs. Antidiabetic drugs have targets involved in metabolic regulation and glucose homeostasis, so their use needs regular monitoring. Antiobesity drugs have been released and then pulled from market. Newer antiobesity drugs are coming to the market and will have utility for individuals who are morbidly obese. The side-effect profiles of these drugs will probably restrict their use and exclude those who are overweight and looking for a pill to help them lose weight. Preparations containing centrally acting stimulants are prescribed only for limited lengths of time for those who are seriously obese. Perhaps the day will come when a safe pill will help people shed some pounds. However, currently, the drug treatments have risks that must be balanced with the health risks of obesity. Diet and exercise will remain necessary components of a healthy lifestyle.

PES Watch

The International Olympic Committee banned insulin in 1998. Insulins are on the WADA list of banned substances and were moved to section S4.5.a (Metabolic Modulators) in 2013, a more appropriate category based on their mechanism of action. Athletes with diabetes, whose health depends on insulin, can qualify for a therapeutic use exemption. Bodybuilders pioneered the illegal use of insulin, and abuse has now extended to other sports. Insulin works in conjunction with anabolic steroids (testosterone) to improve muscle mass; insulin also prevents muscle from being broken down. It can improve stamina by stimulating glycogen production in muscle following dosing with glucose (or regular sucrose/table sugar). The danger of an overdose of insulin in a person who does not have diabetes, resulting in severe hypoglycemia, is a very real problem. A recent case report concerned a 30-year-old male bodybuilder who presented with coma due to severe hypoglycemia from unknown cause. Subsequently they found he had been injecting insulin (Heide, Wahab, Ebadi, et al. 2019). Insulin is easily obtainable and very difficult to detect. The extent of the problem is not known, but anecdotal evidence suggests that it is becoming more common (Ip, Barnett, Tenerowicz, & Perry 2012). Other antidiabetic drugs, including incretin mimetics (exenatide and liraglutide), are not prohibited.

Included with insulin under section S4.5.a (Metabolic Modulators) is GW1516 (a PPARδ agonist), a drug not legally approved for use in humans but available through alternate sources. GW1516 activates some of the same pathways activated by exercise, including PPARδ and AMP-activated protein kinase. GW1516 was originally developed as an antiobesity drug, with potential use for diabetes, dyslipidemia, and cardiovascular disease. The high rate of cancer in animal studies caused the discontinuation of the clinical trials, and the drug was not marketed for clinical use. However, professional cyclists have been found using GW1516. WADA has issued a warning about the potential dangers of GW1516, which is also known as GW501516 or Endurobol. GW1516 is available as a supplement and is produced and sold for research. Bodybuilders and others use GW1516 to build endurance and lose weight, because of its effective use of body fat for energy. By activating the PPARδ pathway, GW1516 causes the development of slow-twitch muscle fibers. As we discussed in Chapter 2, slow-twitch fibers rely heavily on oxidation of fatty acids. GW1516 is relatively easy to detect in urine and can persist for as long as 40 days after a single dose.

Also included in section S4.5.a is AICAR (also known as ZMP), an analog of AMP that activates AMP-activated protein kinase. This drug is another example of an experimental drug that is not legal for use in humans but has been detected in athletes. One of its responses is to increase glucose uptake by skeletal muscle cells. AICAR has been used for treatment of ischemic reperfusion, where it can help protect the heart under certain conditions. AICAR may be a potential treatment for diabetes, because it increases the metabolic activity of tissues and possibly alters the composition of muscle fibers. It may also enhance physical performance. Mice given AICAR were able to run 44% farther than untreated mice. A similar enhancement was seen in mice lacking any training (Narkar, Downes, Yu, et al. 2008). AICAR has been referred to as "exercise in a pill." It is a very expensive drug and can be detected in the urine. AICAR is produced normally in the body, so baseline values in urine have been established to detect illegal use when the drug is taken as a supplement. GW1516 has a synergistic effect when combined with AICAR; the combination can significantly increase exercise endurance in animal studies compared to either compound alone (Narkar et al.). The abuse potential of these drugs in sports seems very high, as their effect on performance and muscle mass is significant. The risk of toxic side effects, including cancer, also appears to be very high, but it is not sufficient to keep these drugs from being abused.

Conclusion

Obesity is a significant contributor to Type 2 diabetes. As visceral abdominal fat increases, low-grade inflammation results in many metabolically sensitive tissues, including adipocytes, liver, and muscle. Insulin resistance develops with resulting hyperglycemia, ultimately causing pancreatic beta cell dysfunction. Maintenance of blood glucose levels is essential for good health. A healthy lifestyle plan should include a proper diet and exercise to help maintain a metabolically optimal weight. For individuals with diabetes, exercise requires additional attention to blood sugar levels. Hypoglycemia is the major concern, because if blood glucose levels get too low, the brain will shut down. Exercise that includes high-intensity intervals and resistance training seems to minimize the chance for hypoglycemia. Low- to moderate-intensity exercise is good at improving HbA1c levels, which provide a measure of average glucose levels over the previous two to three months. High-intensity interval training and weight lifting improve insulin sensitivity. Maintenance of or increase in muscle mass is a desired outcome of training, as muscle contributes a significant amount of energy utilization, both when a person is working out and when at rest. Insulin is on the WADA prohibited substance list because it has anabolic properties that enhance the effect of anabolic steroids.

Key Concepts Review

adipokines
adiponectin
alpha cells
alpha-glucosidase inhibitors
amylin
beta cells
biguanides
bile-acid sequestrant
blood sugar
diabetes
diabetic ketoacidosis
ectopic fat
euglycemia
facilitated diffusion
glinides
gliptins
glucagon
gluconeogenesis
glucose homeostasis

glucose intolerance
glucose transporters (GLUTs)
glucose-6-phosphatase
glucosidases
gluteal adipose tissue
glycemic control
glycemic index
glycemic response
glycogen
glycogenolysis
HbA1c test
hyperglycemia
incretins
insulin
insulin resistance
insulin secretagogues
intermediate-acting insulin
intramuscular fat
ketone bodies

lipase inhibitor
long-acting insulin
metabolic syndrome
nateglinide
peroxisome proliferator-activated
   receptors (PPAR)
postabsorptive state
postprandial state
rapid-acting insulin
repaglinide
satiation

SGLT2 inhibitors
short-acting insulin
subcutaneous fat
sulfonylureas
thiazolidinediones
Type 1 diabetes
Type 2 diabetes
Type 3 diabetes
Type 4 diabetes
visceral fat

Review Questions

1   Glucagon and insulin antagonize each other in regard to glucose homeostasis. Give examples of how their interplay controls glucose levels in the blood.
2   Bernice is now walking two miles each day. What changes are taking place in her body? How will this change in lifestyle help her deal with Type 2 diabetes?
3   If you skip breakfast and don't stop to eat until 1:00, how does your body compensate to keep your brain and heart functioning properly?
4   Why can it be difficult for people with Type 1 diabetes to treat themselves properly with insulin? What are some of the possible obstacles in maintaining euglycemia?
5   How does obesity contribute to Type 2 diabetes?
6   We saw in Chapter 8 how centrally acting stimulants such as amphetamine suppress appetite. How is that property being targeted in antiobesity medications?
7   How do exercise intensity, exercise duration (and volume), and resistance training help in diabetes and obesity?
8   Why is insulin on the WADA prohibited list? What would a healthy athlete gain from injecting insulin?

References

Adams OP (2013) The impact of brief high-intensity exercise on blood glucose levels. *Diabetes, Metab Syndr Obes: Targets Ther* 6:113–122
Adan RAH (2013) Mechanisms underlying current and future anti-obesity drugs. *Trends Neurosci* 36:133–140
AMA Council on Foods and Nutrition (1973) A critique of low-carbohydrate ketogenic weight reduction regimens: a review of Dr. Atkins' Diet Revolution. *JAMA* 224:1415–1419
Aronoff SL, Berkowitz K, Shreiner B, Want L (2004) Glucose metabolism and regulation: beyond insulin and glucagon. *Diabetes Spectrum* 17:183–190
Aw W, Fukuda S (2018) Understanding the role of the gut ecosystem in diabetes mellitus. *J Diabetes Investig* 9:5–12
Baxter NT, Lesniak NA, Sinani H, Schloss PD, Koropatkin NM (2019) The glucoamylase inhibitor acarbose has a diet-dependent and reversible effect on the murine gut microbiome. *mSphere* 4:1–12
Beard CM, Barnard RJ, Robbins DC, Ordovas JM, Schaefer EJ (1996) Effects of diet and exercise on qualitative and quantitative measures of LDL and its susceptibility to oxidation. *Arterioscler Thromb Vasc Biol* 16:201–207

Boule NG, Robert C, Bell GJ, Johnson ST, Bell RC, Lewanczuk RZ, Gabr RQ, Brocks DR (2011) Metformin and exercise in Type 2 diabetes. *Diabetes Care* 34:1469–1474

Bussau VA, Ferreira LD, Jones TW, Fournier PA (2006) The 10-s maximal sprint. A novel approach to counter an exercise-mediated fall in glycemia in individuals with Type 1 diabetes. *Diabetes Care* 29:601–605

Davey RJ, Howe W, Paramalingam N, Ferreira LD, Davis EA, Fournier PA, Jones TW (2013) The effect of midday moderate-intensity exercise on postexercise hypoglycemia risk in individuals with Type 1 diabetes. *J Clin Endocrinol Metab* 98:2908–2914

de la Monte SM, Wands JR (2008) Alzheimer's disease is Type 3 diabetes: evidence reviewed. *J Diabetes Sci Technol* 2:1101–1113

Dhillon RJ, Hasni S (2017) Pathogenesis and management of Sarcopenia. *Clin Geriatr Med* 33:17–26

Diabetes Prevention Program (n.d.) Diabetes prevention program outcomes study. https://dppos.bsc.gwu.edu/web/dppos

Eltonsy S, Dufour Doiron M, Simard P, Jose C, Sénéchal M, Bouchard DR, LeBlanc R, Bélanger M (2019) Effects of the combination of metformin and exercise on glycated hemoglobin, functional capacity, lipid profile, quality of life, and body weight. *J Int Med Res* 47:300060518817164. [Epub ahead of print]

Fahey AJ, Paramalingam N, Davey RJ, Davis EA, Jones TW, Fournier PA (2012) The effect of a short sprint on postexercise whole-body glucose production and utilization rates in individuals with Type 1 diabetes mellitus. *J Clin Endocrinol Metab* 97:4193–4200

Flegal KM, Kruszon-Moran D, Carroll MD, Fryar CD, Ogden CL (2016) Trends in obesity among adults in the United States, 2005 to 2014. *JAMA* 315:2284–2291

Foster GD, Wyatt HR, Hill JO, McGuckin BG, Brill C, Mohammed BS, Szapary PO, Rader DJ, Edman JS, Klein S (2003) A randomized trial of a low-carbohydrate diet for obesity. *N Engl J Med* 348:2082–2090

Gerich JE (2000) Physiology of glucose homeostasis. *Diabetes Obesity Metab* 2:345–350

Gremeaux V, Drigny J, Nigam A, Juneau M, Guilbeault V, Latour E, Gayda M (2012) Long-term lifestyle intervention with optimized high-intensity interval training improves body composition, cardiometabolic risk, and exercise parameters in patients with abdominal obesity. *Am J Phys Med Rehabil* 11:941–950

Guelfi KJ, Jones TW, Fournier PA (2005) The decline in blood glucose levels is less with intermittent high-intensity compared with moderate exercise in individuals with Type 1 diabetes. *Diabetes Care* 28:1289–1294

Heide M, Wahab AA, Ebadi V, Cogne Y, Chollet-Xemard C, Khellaf M (2019) Severe hypoglycemia due to cryptic insulin use in a bodybuilder. *J Emerg Med* 56:279–281

Henson J, Yates T, Biddle SJH, Edwardson CL, Khunti K, Wilmot EG, Gray LJ, Gorely T, Nimmo MA, Davies MJ (2013) Associations of the objectively measured sedentary behaviour and physical activity with the markers of cardiometabolic health. *Diabetologia* 56:1012–1020

Hu FB (2011) Globalization of diabetes: the role of diet, lifestyle, and genes. *Diabetes Care* 34:1249–1257

Ip, EJ, Barnett MJ, Tenerowicz MJ, Perry PJ (2012) Weightlifting's risky new trend: a case series of 41 insulin users. *Curr Sports Med Rep* 11:176–179

Kim DD, Basu A (2016) Estimating the medical care costs of obesity in the United States: systematic review, meta-analysis, and empirical analysis. *ScienceDirect* 19:602–613

Kwon H, Pessin JE (2013) Adipokines mediate inflammation and insulin resistance. *Frontiers Endocrinol* 4:1–13

Larsen JJ, Dela F, Madsbad S, Vibe-Petersen J, Galbo H (1999) Interaction of sulfonylureas and exercise on glucose homeostasis in Type 2 diabetic patients. *Diabetes Care* 22:1647–1654

MacEwen A, McKay GA, Fisher M (2012) Drugs for diabetes: part 8 SGLT2 inhibitors. *Br J Cardiol* 19:26–29

Malin SK, Gerber R, Chipkin SR, Braun B (2012) Independent and combined effects of exercise training and metformin on insulin sensitivity in individuals with prediabetes. *Diabetes Care* 35:131–136

McMahon SK, Ferreira LD, Ratnam N, Davey RJ, Youngs LM, Davis EA, Fournier PA, Jones TW (2007) *J Clin Endocrinol Metab* 92:963–968

Narkar VA, Downes M, Yu RT, Embler E, Wang Y-X, Banayo E, Mihaylova MM, Nelson MC, Zou Y, Juguilon H, Kang H, Shaw RJ, Evans RM (2008) AMPK and PPARδ are exercise mimetics. *Cell* 134:405–415

Pinto LC, Rados DV, Barkan SS, Leitão CB, Gross JL (2018) Dipeptidyl peptidase-4 inhibitors, pancreatic cancer and acute pancreatitis: a meta-analysis with trial sequential analysis. *Sci Rep* 8:782

Riddell M, Perkins BA (2009) Exercise and glucose metabolism in persons with diabetes mellitus: perspectives on the role of continuous glucose monitoring. *J Diabetes Sci Tech* 3:914–923

Robert Wood Johnson Foundation (March 3, 2014) Signs of progress on childhood obesity. www.rwjf.org/en.html

Rossetti L, Smith D, Shulman GI, Papachristou D, DeFronzo RA (1987) Correction of hyperglycemia with phlorizin normalizes tissue sensitivity to insulin in diabetic rats. *J Clin Invest* 79:1510–1515

Santos JG, Alves BC, Hammes TO, Dall'Alba V (2019) Dietary interventions, intestinal microenvironment, and obesity: a systematic review. *Nutr Rev.* doi: 10.1093/nutrit/nuz022. [Epub ahead of print]

Segerstrom AB, Glans F, Eriksson K-F, Holmback AM, Groop L, Thorsson O, Wollmer P (2010) Impact of exercise intensity and duration on insulin sensitivity in women with T2D. *Eur J Int Med* 21:404–408

Thorens B, Mueckler M (2010) Glucose transporters in the 21st century. *Am J Physiol Endocrinol Metab* 298:E141–E145

Umegaki H (2015) Sarcopenia and diabetes: hyperglycemia is a risk factor for age-associated muscle mass and functional reduction. *J Diabetes Investig* 6:623–624

Umpierre D, Ribeiro PA, Kramer CK, Leitao CB, Zucatti AT, Gross JL, Ribeiro JP, Schaan BD (2011) Physical activity advice only or structured exercise training and association with HbA1c levels in Type 2 diabetes: a systematic review and meta-analysis. *JAMA* 305:1790–1799

Vissers D, Hens W, Taeymans J, Baeyens JP, Poortmans J, Van Gall L (2013) The effect of exercise on visceral adipose tissue in overweight adults: a systematic review and meta-analysis. *PLoS One* 8: e56415

Williams PT, Thompson PD (2013) Walking versus running for hypertension, cholesterol, and diabetes mellitus risk reduction. *Arteriosclerosis, Thrombosis, Vascular Biol* 33:1085–1091

Wing R, Hill JO (2001) Successful weight loss maintenance. *Annu Rev Nutr* 21:323–341

Wu H, Esteve E, Tremaroli V, Khan MT, Caesar R, Mannerås-Holm L, Ståhlman M, Olsson LM, Serino M, Planas-Fèlix M, Xifra G, Mercader JM, Torrents D, Burcelin R, Ricart W, Perkins R, Fernàndez-Real JM, Bäckhed F (2017) Metformin alters the gut microbiome of individuals with treatment-naive Type 2 diabetes, contributing to the therapeutic effects of the drug. *Nat Med* 23:850–858

Yadav MR, Murumkar PR (2018) Advances in patented CB1 receptor antagonists for obesity. *Pharm Pat Anal* 7:169–173

Yardley JE, Kenny GP, Perkins BA, Riddell MC, Balaa N, Malcolm J, Boulay P, Khandwala F, Sigal RJ (2013) Resistance versus aerobic exercise: acute effects on glycemia in Type 1 diabetics. *Diabetes Care* 36:537–542

Section IV

Self-Medication

13 Dietary Supplements

Abstract

Sound nutrition and a healthy diet are essential for maintaining an active and healthy lifestyle. Though there are common principles, such as consumption of fruits and vegetables and controlling calorie intake, the population varies greatly in terms of individual requirements for essential nutrients. Differences in nutritional needs can vary with culture, race, gender, age, fitness level, and genotype. Supplementation of a diet may be needed in a significant portion of the population to ensure that optimal levels of all essential nutrients are met. In this case, supplementation is intended to get to "normal" levels. Some people have the attitude that if a little is good, then a lot might be even better. In the case of most vitamins and essential nutrients, the body's ability to store excessive daily intake is very limited or nonexistent. The result is that excessive nutrients end up as either urine or feces. For exercise performance, there is very little data to support any demonstrable benefit of supra-physiological doses. Besides wasting money, excessive doses can cause toxicity. High doses of supplements, 'natural' or not, expose the user to possible contaminants in the formulation.

WADA recommends extreme caution regarding supplement use. Many countries have no strict rules for the manufacturing and labeling of supplements. Dietary supplements may contain an undeclared substance that is prohibited under anti-doping regulations. A significant number of positive tests have been attributed to the misuse of supplements. A poorly labeled dietary supplement is not an adequate defense for an athlete who is caught doping. For the vast majority of the population, a healthy diet containing fresh fruits and vegetables with a balance of complex carbohydrates, protein, and healthy fats should be sufficient.

CASE EXAMPLE

Megan likes to eat. She may not be a 'Foodie' quite yet, but that may be more of a function of having two small children. She wasn't always this way. Actually, she was a bit of a pain when it came to eating when she was younger. She did not like red meat, and after seeing a report on the news, no longer would eat chicken. So Megan wasn't vegan, but her diet was light in protein. When she got to college, the dorm food did not help. Getting a scholarship and playing soccer at a big-time Division 1 program taught her some things about nutrition. Halfway through her first season, she ran out of gas. Between practice, classes, and adjusting to dorm life, she started getting sluggish on the field. Some of the other women on the team drank protein shakes and took creatine. Creatine was on the list of substances to avoid provided to her by her coaches.

She decided to try the protein shakes and skip the creatine. They seemed to help, so she started making them part of her routine. She also found that the salad bar in the dorm cafeteria had a lot of fresh options. After she graduated and entered 'The Real World,' she discovered that eating was enjoyable and became much braver about trying new foods. Her eventual husband, Brad, took her out to nice restaurants, and this became a weekly occurrence after they got married. With the kids now, the challenge is to cook something interesting and healthy that the whole family will enjoy.

Learning Objectives

1 Distinguish essential from nonessential supplements.
2 Appreciate the need for quality protein in the diet.
3 Recognize the value of good nutrition beyond just appropriate amounts of carbohydrates, fats, and protein.
4 Appreciate the variability in the human population in terms of dietary needs.
5 Learn the basics of hormonal control of appetite.
6 Understand how exercise can contribute to a healthy weight.
7 Understand when and how creatine may affect exercise performance.
8 Appreciate the critical roles played by essential fatty acids.
9 Understand how a well-maintained extracellular matrix can help a person withstand the discomfort associated with overuse and aging and the possible role supplements for joint health.
10 Recognize the issues concerning vitamin D deficiency.

Introduction

Dietary supplements encompass a wide variety of substances, including vitamins, minerals, and other nutraceuticals. The term **vitamin** is generally used for substances that cannot be made in the body in sufficient quantities, so that a dietary source is needed. *Nutraceuticals* are dietary or nutritional supplements taken to benefit general health. A nutraceutical can be a vitamin, mineral, herb or botanical, amino acid, metabolite, or some type of extract. Optimal daily requirements for vitamins likely differ from the minimum daily requirement necessary to avoid symptoms associated with deficiencies determined years ago. Individuals vary in the amounts of vitamins that they require for optimal health. Little is known about these individual variations in daily requirements, and even less is known about whether vitamin supplements benefit athletic performance.

Essential nutrients generally do not "cure" disease, but rather they prevent or cure the pathology associated with a deficiency. Obtaining necessary nutrients from a diet that includes whole (i.e., not heavily processed) foods and provides a natural source of nutrients can be better than taking a pill, even when the pill contains the specified amount of the supplement. Whole foods contain many other nutrients that alone or in combinations can contribute to health. Exercise and intense training put additional demands on the body, increasing the need for good nutrition.

Dietary supplements that are used for putative gains in performance are referred to as **nonessential nutrients.** More research is needed to validate the role of nonessential nutrients in performance gains and "boosts" in energy, as opposed to the prevention of disease resulting from deficiency of essential nutrients. In general, little evidence supports taking mega doses of supplements or vitamins to improve performance in normal, healthy individuals. For most people who eat a balanced diet and exercise regularly, nonessential supplements are probably not needed.

Essential nutrients must be consumed daily, because our bodies cannot produce sufficient quantities of them. For example, of the 20 amino acids essential for protein production, the human body can make only a dozen; the other eight are considered essential nutrients (see Table 13.1). Of the 12 amino acids generally considered nonessential, two or three may not be made in sufficient amounts in newborns or the elderly. Under these conditions, those amino acids are referred to as **conditionally essential nutrients.** The concept of conditional nutrients is important, as some people, because of

Table 13.1 Nutritional status of amino acids in humans

Amino Acid	Nutritional Status	Comment	Three-Letter Abbreviation	One-Letter Abbreviation
Alanine	Nonessential		Ala	A
Arginine	Nonessential	Conditionally essential— young and old may require dietary sources	Arg	R
Aspartic acid	Nonessential		Asp	D
Asparagine	Nonessential	Made from aspartic acid	Asn	N
Cysteine	Nonessential	Conditionally essential— young and old may require dietary sources	Cys	C
Glutamic acid	Nonessential		Glu	E
Glutamine	Nonessential	Made from glutamic acid	Gln	Q
Glycine	Nonessential		Gly	G
Histidine	Nonessential	Conditionally essential— young and old may require dietary sources	His	H
Proline	Nonessential		Pro	P
Serine	Nonessential		Ser	S
Tyrosine	Nonessential	Conditionally essential— young and old may require dietary sources	Tyr	Y
Isoleucine	Essential	Branched chain	Ile	I
Leucine	Essential	Branched chain	Leu	L
Lysine	Essential		Lys	K
Methionine	Essential		Met	M
Phenylalanine	Essential	Used to make tyrosine	Phe	F
Threonine	Essential		Thr	T
Tryptophan	Essential		Trp	W
Valine	Essential	Branched chain	Val	V

their age, genetics, or disease state, may have a higher daily requirement and may benefit from dietary supplements. Meat, egg whites, and dairy products are good sources of protein that provide essential amino acids. Vegetarians and vegans need a source of quality protein in their diet to supply these critical amino acids. For them, beans, nuts, and soy products are sources of protein.

In 1994, Congress passed the Dietary Supplement Health and Education Act, which allows distribution of nutraceuticals without a prescription. The 1994 Act created a regulatory status for nutraceuticals with the FDA under which nutraceuticals are dealt with differently from pharmaceuticals (conventional drugs) and food products (discussed in Chapter 1). The manufacturer of nutraceuticals is responsible for ensuring that the product is safe before it is marketed. The FDA's responsibilities include ensuring the accuracy of product information, such as labeling, claims, package inserts, and accompanying literature. The FDA does not test these products; however, it is responsible for taking action against any unsafe nutraceutical after it reaches the market. The Federal Trade Commission (FTC) regulates dietary supplement advertising. Manufacturers cannot claim that a nutraceutical will "cure, mitigate, treat, or prevent" a specific disease, but they can make general statements concerning benefits to overall health and well-being. Under FTC regulations, the dose, the amount of active ingredient, and the complete contents of the mixture can vary from what is stated on the label. In contrast to the FDA, NSF International (www.nsf.org; previously the National Sanitation Foundation) is an example of an independent laboratory that certifies the safety of food, water, supplements, and many other products, such as medical devices. Its seal of approval on a product ensures that the product has passed tests concerning its safety.

The general public has shown an increasing interest in nontraditional health care, and many people want to improve their appearance or performance with the help of a pill. Advertisements and endorsements by celebrities have further fueled the popularity of nutraceuticals. They are now part of a market worth about $15 billion in the United States and about $75 billion worldwide, depending on the products included in these types of analyses. For instance, "one shot" energy drinks are not included, although they can be loaded with vitamins and other supplements. An NIH report states that $32.5 billion was spent in 2012 for all dietary supplements in the United States (National Institutes of Health Office of Dietary Supplements 2013). A significant fraction of available nutraceuticals probably has no scientifically proven value for normal, healthy people. Very few of the hundreds of botanicals have been subjected to clinical trials. However, anecdotal information and word of mouth cause people to try and continue using certain supplements.

The Need for Supplements

This section first discusses nutrition, emphasizing that what we eat is important to our health. The next section addresses appetite control and its role in an individual's ability to control aspects of his or her health without medication. By considering nutrition and appetite control, we can address the question of whether dietary supplements are needed for most individuals.

Diet and Nutrition

Diet clearly involves more than calories obtained from carbohydrates, fats, and protein. Though an understanding of calories is important in maintaining a healthy weight, many other components in food contribute to good health. Many of the complex mixtures of chemicals found in food, especially fresh fruits and vegetables, help our bodies fight disease or slow the aging process. The saying "You are what you eat" has been around a long time. James Duke and other researchers have extended this concept to the "Green Pharmacy." In his book *The Green Pharmacy Guide to Healthy Foods: Proven Natural Remedies to Prevent More Than 80 Common Health Concerns*, Duke identifies active components in plants that have therapeutic potential. For example, the additive and synergistic properties of many of the components in whole grains contribute to health in ways that are only partly understood. Whole grains contain more fiber than refined or enriched grains, which contributes to feeling full and helps decrease caloric intake. Fiber also contributes to a healthy GI-tract (see Box).

The Role of Fiber in a Healthy Diet

Fiber is a critical and often overlooked component of a healthy diet. Living on fast food and other highly processed foods often results in a diet low in fiber and many unhealthy consequences. Good sources of dietary fiber include fruits, vegetables, whole grains, and legumes. Dietary fiber helps a person maintain a healthy weight, lowers the risk of diabetes and heart disease, and prevents or relieves constipation. Sufficient dietary fiber encourages growth of desirable microbes in the gut microbiome; lack of fiber allows undesirable microbes to become prevalent.

What exactly is dietary fiber? Fiber, also called roughage, is composed of parts of a plant that the body cannot digest or absorb. It passes relatively intact through the stomach, small intestine, and colon and forms a significant portion of stools. Soluble fiber can dissolve in water; insoluble fiber does not. Both types are important. Soluble fiber helps lower cholesterol and glucose levels in the blood, probably by slowing the digestive process. Soluble fiber is plentiful in oats, barley, apples, carrots, peas, and beans. Insoluble fiber promotes movement through the GI-tract, increasing stool bulk. Nuts, whole wheat flour, beans, and vegetables (e.g., broccoli, cauliflower) are good sources of insoluble fiber. Most plant-based foods contain both soluble and insoluble fiber, although the relative amounts vary. Eating a wide variety of high-fiber foods helps ensure adequate amounts of both types of fiber.

High-fiber foods usually require more chewing. This gives the body more time to signal that it is satiated, making the person less likely to overeat. High-fiber foods are usually low in their energy density, meaning they have fewer calories per volume of food. High-fiber foods can make a meal feel "larger" and extend the time until a person is hungry again. The daily recommended intake of fiber is 30 to 35 grams for men and 20 to 25 grams for women. Adding too much fiber too quickly to a diet can result in intestinal gas, bloating, and cramping. Fiber in the diet is best increased gradually, allowing the bacteria in the digestive system to adjust. Drinking enough water is also important. Fiber absorbs water. The result of enough fiber in the diet is a healthy and happy digestive system.

In addition, other components in certain foods may help promote health and prevent disease. For example, certain flavonoids (found in fruits and vegetables) have bioactivities that may offer protection against cardiovascular disease (Erlund 2004). Diet can play a role in maintaining healthy bones and preventing osteoporosis (Love 2002).

Not surprisingly, socioeconomic factors influence the quality of nutrition in an individual's diet. Fresh fruits and vegetables can be expensive, whereas high-caloric fast foods can be relatively inexpensive. People on limited incomes often have poorer diets and the associated problems of metabolic syndrome, obesity, diabetes, and cardiovascular disease. Governments and health officials may tout the benefits of a good diet, but for many people, the recommendations are not economically feasible. The obstacles to healthful nutrition contribute to burdens on the nation's healthcare system.

Nutrigenomics

One approach to the study of nutrition is the "omics" approach. We discussed in an earlier chapter the rapidly growing field of pharmacogenomics, which suggests that an individual's genotype may provide the basis for drug therapy in the near future. A similar approach to nutrition is being undertaken. A detailed genetic analysis will provide the basis for a tailored diet, with individually recommended supplementation for an elite athlete or weekend exerciser. For most nutrients, a bell-shaped dose–response curve is expected for large populations. As with drugs, people will absorb, metabolize, distribute, and excrete nutrients based on their own underlying genetics. We would expect the 67% of individuals in the middle of the bell curve to be "normal" and require daily amounts in a similar "normal" range. However, for those individuals at either extreme of the curve, health consequences may occur from taking "normal" doses. These individuals may be hypersensitive (respond to small amounts) or hyposensitive (require much larger daily doses). Nutrigenomics could play a major role in health maintenance for these people.

Nutrigenomics focuses on the genetic factors that influence the body's response to diet. It also studies how the bioactive constituents of food affect gene expression. Nutrigenomics will lead to the development of personalized diets, based on an individual's genetic makeup. This approach is becoming a reality very quickly, due to the rapid advances in proteomics (identification of specific proteins present in cells or tissues), metabolomics (sensitive measures of changes in blood chemistry), and transcriptomics (determination of which genes are expressed and in what amounts) and the availability of individuals' DNA sequence information. The hope is that personalized diets will improve quality of life and help prevent disease (Ozdemir, Motulsky, Kolker, & Godard 2009). In training programs with elite athletes, many of these approaches are being adopted.

The genetic traits that interact with diet offer possible targeted clinical interventions and preventive medicine. Individuals who are susceptible to unfavorable dietary/genomic interactions will be identified. For example, lactose intolerance—the inability to digest lactose, a component of milk—has a clear genetic component. Humans with northern European ancestry have a mutation in the gene that normally suppresses expression of the enzyme lactase after weaning. These people continue to make lactase, which allows them to digest milk and foods derived from or containing milk throughout their life. Lactase breaks the bond in the disaccharide lactose, releasing the monosaccharides glucose and galactose. People with lactose intolerance lack lactase activity in their gut, so lactose makes it to the lower gut, where it can cause undesirable effects, such as excessive gas or diarrhea.

A nutrigenomic approach to diet could also allow modifications to diet or the biochemical response to food for disease prevention. To understand how this could work, consider the rise in serum cholesterol in Japanese women who moved to the United States following World War II and adopted a "Western" diet. This population of Japanese women also saw a shift to Western/American rates of breast cancer and colon cancer. Another example is present among the Inuit people. Modernization of their lifestyle (i.e., living in heated houses and using snowmobiles for travel) while they have maintained their traditional high-fat diet has contributed to a rapid rise in obesity. Another example is that elevated levels in the blood of homocysteine, an amino acid, are related to a higher risk of cardiovascular disease. Elevated homocysteine can be caused by a genetic variant of an enzyme involved in folate metabolism. Patients with this genotype should take elevated levels of B vitamins (including folate) to decrease homocysteine levels. In the relatively near future, a nutrigenomic approach, merged with a pharmacogenetic approach, will provide physicians with a detailed plan for treating and preventing disease.

Appetite Control

In the previous chapter, we discussed the obesity and diabetes epidemic and the costs and problems associated with both for treatment under the care of a physician. In this chapter, we examine the healthful choices that individuals can make in terms of their own diet and the associated physiology that controls hunger. Appetite control has both a physical and a mental component. In past times, weight gain in the fall may have helped people survive the severe weather and limited food supply in winter. Today, however, weight gain is very often detrimental to health and survival. Many people overeat in response to emotional stress or external cues. Hunger and other triggers are part stomach, but also part brain. Controlling the mind is an important component of eating properly, and it is also involved in other healthful lifestyle choices, such as exercising regularly and getting sufficient rest.

The Role of the Hormonal Systems

Several hormonal systems are involved in controlling appetite. We saw in the previous chapter how gut peptides (incretins) and amylin respond during feeding. Other hormone systems, such as leptin, ghrelin, serotonin, and endocannabinoids, are concerned with long-term energy control and appetite.

LEPTIN

Adipocytes (fat cells) produce the hormone **leptin**. Leptin suppresses appetite and contributes to the sense of feeling full (Klok, Jakobsdottir, & Drent 2006); it is considered
a long-term regulator of energy balance. Leptin levels in the blood are proportional to
the amount of body fat—the more body fat, the more leptin in the circulation. Neurons
in specific regions of the brain have leptin receptors (see Figure 13.1). Leptin binds receptors primarily in the hypothalamus and affects the release of several neuroendocrine
factors, producing satiety, the feeling of having had enough to eat. Among the factors
suppressed by leptin are **neuropeptide Y** (performs many functions, including stimulation of appetite and storage of fat) and **orexin** (promotes wakefulness and appetite). The
suppression of neuropeptide Y also suppresses the endocannabinoid system and appetite (see Figure 13.1). Leptin increases the secretion of brain-derived neurotrophic factor, corticotropin-releasing hormone, and other anorexic (appetite decreasing) factors.

Leptin levels also depend on sleep duration. The longer a person sleeps, the more
leptin activity controls appetite (Spiegel, Leproult, Lhermite-Baleriaux, et al. 2004).
Quality sleep is essential for weight management, immune function, and many other
factors associated with good health. Lack of sleep drives leptin levels down, increases
ghrelin levels, stimulates appetite, and can give rise to binge eating, especially with
carbohydrate-dense foods.

Genetic studies of a mutant, very obese mouse (Ob) led to the discovery of the gene
that codes for leptin. Mice or humans that lack the Ob gene function (Ob⁻/Ob⁻) lack
circulating leptin and are obese. Fortunately, Ob⁻/Ob⁻ mutants in humans are very
rare, suggesting that humans who are obese have defects in the leptin response rather
than lacking circulating leptin. The Ob mouse has very high levels of circulating endocannabinoids. If leptin is injected back into Ob mice, endocannabinoid levels decrease.
Interestingly, many humans who are obese have high levels of leptin, suggesting that

Figure 13.1 Simplified scheme for different hormonal substances in the control of
hunger.

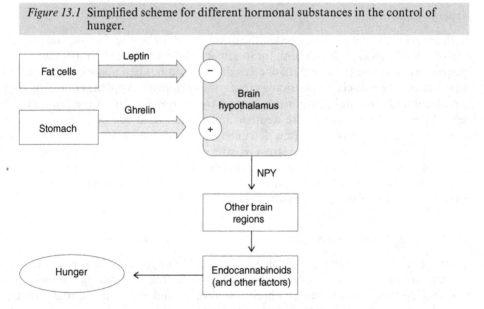

Legend: Leptin inhibits and ghrelin stimulates the release of neuropeptide Y (NPY) from sensitive
neurons in a specific area of the brain. NPY has many actions, including increasing levels of endocannabinoids and other factors/hormones that regulate hunger.

they have become resistant—similar, perhaps, to individuals with type 2 diabetes who have become insensitive to chronic high levels of insulin. Rats fed diets high in fructose develop leptin resistance, have increased plasma triglycerides, and eat more. The increased use of high fructose corn syrup in many common foods and drinks has been cited as a contributing factor to obesity, metabolic syndrome, and diabetes. Chronic fructose intake promotes white adipose tissue accumulation through activating adipogenesis (Hernández-Díazcouder, Romero-Nava, Carbó, et al. 2019).

GHRELIN

Cells in the fundus of the stomach and certain cells in the brain produce **ghrelin**. Ghrelin increases appetite, in part by indirectly decreasing leptin activity (see Table 13.2). Ghrelin activates a variety of neurons, including neuropeptide Y neurons. Neuropeptide Y stimulates feeding, by stimulating the endocannabinoid system and other orexic factors that stimulate appetite (see Figure 13.1). Injection of neuropeptide Y into regions of the rodent brain produces feeding behavior. Elimination of the neuropeptide Y system produces anorexia.

SEROTONIN

Serotonin is another hormone involved in eating behavior and mood. Its role in these processes is complex and only partly understood. Cells in the gut and in the CNS release serotonin. Serotonin that reaches the blood is taken up and stored in platelets. It suppresses appetite, and its release is sensitive to the protein and carbohydrate content in a meal. Low serotonin levels are associated with food cravings, binge behavior, lack of sleep, and depression. Dietary carbohydrate and protein can increase serotonin levels and contribute to satiety and suppression of appetite. On the other hand, candy

Table 13.2 Comparison of leptin and ghrelin activities

Leptin	Ghrelin
Produced primarily in adipocytes	Produced primarily in the gut, activated with addition of lipid group (octanoylation) to serine at position 3
Receptors located in hypothalamus and other regions of brain, vasculature, and gut, as well as red blood cells	Receptors located in hypothalamus, anterior pituitary, and other regions of the brain
Increased levels proportional to BMI, % fat	Elevated in postabsorptive state, decreased in postprandial state
Decreases following exercise	Stimulates appetite, hunger
Suppresses food intake	Increases food intake
Suppresses neuropeptide Y activity and other factors	Stimulates neuropeptide Y activity and release of growth hormone
Decreases endocannabinoids	Increases endocannabinoids
Increases corticotropin-releasing hormone	Decreases corticotropin-releasing hormone

(processed simple sugar), caffeine, and alcohol in sufficient amounts can lower serotonin levels and cause food cravings, binge behavior, and depression. Exercise increases serotonin and helps improve mood and regulate blood sugar levels, thereby helping to control cravings.

ENDOCANNABINOIDS

Endocannabinoids play a central role in appetite and energy balance. The identification of endogenous lipids that work through the same receptor systems as the active ingredient in marijuana (delta-9-THC) has provided insight into the anorexic mechanisms of leptin and orexigenic (appetite stimulating) mechanisms of ghrelin. The endocannabinoids will be discussed further in Chapter 15. Endocannabinoid levels increase during fasting and decrease during satiety (Maccarrone, Gasperi, Catani, et al. 2010). Increases in ghrelin increase the levels of endocannabinoids; conversely, increases in endocannabinoids can stimulate the release of ghrelin. Leptin decreases endocannabinoid activity (see Figure 13.1). Endocannabinoids can also increase neuropeptide Y, increasing appetite. In adipocytes and liver, endocannabinoids stimulate fatty acid and triglyceride synthesis, helping to store the incoming calories.

A dysregulated endocannabinoid signaling system is involved in eating disorders and cardiovascular disease. Endocannabinoids have both central and peripheral functions, making this whole physiological system ripe for drug development. An endocannabinoid antagonist (rimonabant) was released as an antiobesity drug, but was withdrawn because of side effects that included depression. Other cannabinoid-related drugs are in development that have agonist or antagonist activity or that target the enzymes responsible for the degradation of endocannabinoids (Maccarrone et al.).

Hedonic Eating

Consumption of food just for pleasure is called **hedonic eating**. In hedonic eating, eating occurs not simply for maintenance of energy homeostasis but rather for a gustatory reward. Endogenous reward mediators come into play, although this type of behavior is not fully understood. In an interesting preliminary study, eight satiated healthy subjects were fed either highly palatable food or unpalatable food on separate occasions (Monteleone, Piscitelli, Scognamiglio, et al. 2012). The food was of equal nutrient composition and available ad libitum, meaning the subjects could eat as much as they wanted. The consumption of the palatable food (food for pleasure) caused an increase in circulating ghrelin. Of the three different endogenous cannabinoids monitored, one of them also increased when subjects ate the highly palatable food (eating for pleasure). The other two cannabinoids progressively decreased. These results suggest that hedonic eating activates two peripheral chemical signals involved in reward behavior. Hedonic brain pathways activated by palatable food overlap with pathways activated by drugs of abuse (Allen, Baltra, Geiger, et al. 2012).

Sugar itself may be addictive. High-glycemic foods increase hunger and selectively stimulate brain regions associated with reward and craving (Lennerz, Alsop, Holsen, et al. 2013). The current food environment encourages addictive behavior.

Advertisements for food are pervasive, food scientists work to make food irresistible (e.g., Cheetos, bacon cheeseburgers, chocolate), junk food is readily available, and portion size continues to escalate. Similar to the strategy used to fight tobacco, a policy change to reclassify dietary obesity as an addictive behavior could change regulatory efforts and educational approaches (Allen et al.). This new approach to fighting the obesity epidemic could encourage the food industry and political leaders to work with the medical community to establish new awareness programs and therapeutic approaches based on scientific evidence.

Calculating Caloric Intake

Based on simplified calculations, it is easier to compute weight loss than weight gain. Weight gain involves efficiency parameters and appears to have a greater amount of individual variance. Individuals vary in activity level and how efficiently they build muscle or store energy in carbohydrate and fat. However, the general concept of calorie counting still applies. Weight loss results when an individual's daily intake of calories is less than the expenditure of calories, and weight gain occurs when the daily intake of calories exceeds expenditure.

How many calories per day are needed to maintain a target weight? What surplus or deficit of daily calorie intake must be reached in order to achieve a target weight? Health and practical concerns suggest that a person's daily caloric intake should not be more than 500 calories higher or lower than the daily intake that would maintain the person's current weight. A pound of fat contains about 3,500 calories, in this context. A 500-calorie deficit per day for one week (seven days) should result in the loss of about one pound. Successful weight-loss programs target losses of two to four pounds per month.

For women, the target number of calories per day is 10 to 11 times the target body weight. The lower number is used for less active women with a higher percent body fat. For an athletic woman who wishes to weigh 150 pounds, a reasonable target would be about 1,650 (150 × 11) calories per day. If that woman currently weighs 160 pounds, the intake that would maintain her weight is 1760 calories per day (160 × 11). Hence, she would have to reduce her daily consumption by 110 calories (1,760 to 1,650) to reach her target weight. For men, the conversion factor ranges from 12 to 14, based on activity and amount of musculature. Highly fit and muscular males should multiply their target weight by 14 to find their target number of calories per day. A 200-pound man would need about 2,800 calories per day to maintain his weight. To lose weight and achieve a new target weight, men should use the same strategy as detailed above for women. Weight gain to achieve a new, higher goal can be calculated the same way, though the results will be more variable than the results of dieting to lose weight. Exercise and training are necessary to ensure that most of the weight gain will be muscle and not fat. Moreover, exercise and weight training are necessary to ensure weight loss targets fat tissue, otherwise weight loss includes both fat and muscle tissue.

Exercise and Appetite

The effects of exercise on hunger sensations and food intake can vary with the intensity and duration of the exercise (Stensel 2010). Exercise intensity may be an important factor when a person is attempting to control appetite. Moderately vigorous exercise can decrease appetite. Prolonged treadmill exercise (120 minutes) with mixed intensity decreased ghrelin, decreased relative energy intake, and temporarily decreased hunger (Vatansever-Ozen, Tiryaki-Sonmez, Bugdayci, & Ozen 2011). Longer, very low intensity (e.g., leisure walking) exercise may have a neutral effect on appetite. Some studies also suggest that low-intensity exercise can increase ghrelin more than high-intensity exercise, but the observed changes in ghrelin were not duration dependent (Erdmann, Tahbaz, Lippl, et al. 2007). It is possible, therefore, for low-intensity exercise to stimulate appetite to the point of negating the energy burned by exercising. However, there is little evidence to support overeating in compensation of extensive exercising (Stensel). For athletes undergoing heavy training and trying to maintain their weight, overeating is not an issue. For people trying to exercise regularly and lose weight, managing hunger can be a problem. Evidence suggests that during this type of training, energy balance is only partially compensated, and a negative energy balance is possible (Stensel). Therefore, regular exercise and attention to caloric intake can help the individuals achieve or maintain a target weight.

Fasting

Fasting is an ancient tradition. Benjamin Franklin said, "The best of all medicines is resting and fasting." Starvation is involuntary—food is not available. Fasting is the voluntary withholding of food for spiritual or health reasons. Fasting may be done for portions of days or much longer. Many believe that fasting improves cognitive abilities. The practice of fasting developed independently among different religions and cultures, as something that was intrinsically beneficial for the body and spirit. Fasting is ingrained into human heritage, and as old as mankind itself.

Most of us break our overnight fast when we eat breakfast in the morning. Eating, especially a large meal, shunts blood to the digestive system leaving less blood going to the brain. What happens to our body when we eat nothing? Glucose and fat are the body's main sources of energy. If we stop eating, the body will adjust by using stored fat to make up the energy deficit, without any detrimental health effects. Periods of low food availability are part of human history and mechanisms have evolved to adapt. If food is unavailable, the human body switches from burning glucose and fat to mostly burning fat. Fat is the body's stored energy reserve for times of low food availability. The body does not breakdown muscle protein until the fat stores are diminished. Our intellect, our primary advantage against wild animals or bad neighborhoods, stays intact, or even improves, when dietary glucose and other sources of calories are limited.

The lack of dietary glucose causes changes in metabolism, including an increase production of ketone bodies. Ketone bodies are derived from fatty acids and can cross the blood–brain barrier, providing the brain with a substitute for glucose. The ketotic state is being studied now because of many potential health benefits or as a supplementary treatment of disease. Fasting causes a decrease in insulin levels. Increased adrenalin (epinephrine and norepinephrine) levels during fasting increase metabolic rate and helps find or acquire food. Cellular (muscle) protein is conserved during fasting, as increased levels of growth hormone maintain muscle mass and lean tissue. Although growth hormone secretion decreases steadily with age, fasting is one of the most potent stimuli for growth hormone secretion. Fasting, but not low-calorie diets, results in these numerous beneficial hormonal adaptations.

Can athletes benefit from the elevated growth hormone stimulated by fasting, and increase muscle mass? There is extensive literature on training in the fasted state, with results linked to desired outcomes (e.g., body composition, size, strength, power, quickness). The early proponents of training in the fasted state were bodybuilders who maintain high-intensity training with low body fat for definition. The increased adrenalin during fasting could make workouts more intense and recovery faster. The increased norepinephrine during fasting increases resting energy expenditure and increases the body's metabolism. VO_2 also increases slightly indicating a greater capacity of the body for physical exertion.

Fasting offers therapeutic flexibility. One can fast until achieving the desired effect. If you don't eat, you will lose weight. Whether for 12 hours, 16 hours, or the Warrior diet with an emphasis on natural unprocessed foods eaten only in the evening, these fasting regimens lower insulin. People still eat dinner with family and do this 24-hour fast a couple times per week. Often, as people get used to fasting, their appetite starts to decrease and they can eat to satiation at their eating time or day.

In summary, an elite athlete or healthy person, while fasting, can potentially: (1) Train harder because of increased adrenalin and improved VO_2; (2) Recover faster and build muscle because of increased growth hormone; (3) Burn fat due to the increased rate of fatty acid oxidation; or (4) Decrease insulin secretion. Note that from a safety standpoint, children should not fast—fasting is only for adults.

Diet and Appetite and the Role of Supplements

To this point, we have examined reasons why we get hungry, what we should eat, and how much. Eating a perfectly balanced diet with large amounts of fresh produce is not always feasible, however. There are many essential nutrients that are required daily in our diet, and dietary supplementation may be necessary to meet those needs. The population as a whole varies significantly in terms of individuals' genetics and nutritional needs. Our needs can also change as we age, deal with health issues, or maintain physically active lives. We will examine several dietary supplements in detail, discussing their physiological roles and whether there is evidence that they can enhance exercise performance. Finally, we will briefly review several supplements associated with potential performance improvement. Also keep in mind that supplements, especially at elevated doses, can interact with each other and with prescription drugs, causing additional problems with side effects or efficacy of the prescription drug. Many of the known interactions are updated on websites such as WebMD.

Creatine

Athletes are constantly looking for that extra increment of improvement in performance. During the 1996 Summer Olympics in Atlanta, 80% of athletes were estimated to have used creatine. Most of the body's creatine is found in skeletal muscle, but it is also found in heart muscle and the brain (Brosnan & Brosnan 2007; Cooper, Naclerio, Allgrove, & Jimenez 2012). The brain distribution of creatine overlaps with neurons that undergo periodic rapid firing rates. Tissues with a constant high level of metabolic activity, such as the liver, do not use the creatine system.

The Role of Creatine in the Body

Creatine is converted to **phosphocreatine** (sometimes called creatine phosphate) inside skeletal muscle cells, where it acts as a high-energy reservoir for ATP production. The enzyme **creatine kinase** is responsible for the phosphate transfer between ATP and creatine (see Figure 13.2). Phosphocreatine acts as a metabolic buffer to maintain ATP levels over a short timeframe. This temporal role, where phosphocreatine provides high-energy phosphates to maintain ATP levels during high-intensity activity, is essential in fast-twitch muscle fibers. In fast-twitch muscle cells, the concentration of phosphocreatine is higher in regions with myofibril activity. In slow-twitch muscle fibers, there is a spatial component to the supply of phosphocreatine. As ATP is produced in mitochondria, the high-energy phosphate is transferred to creatine to form phosphocreatine. Phosphocreatine has a faster diffusion rate than ATP (Brosnan & Brosnan), and the phosphocreatine produced in mitochondria shuttles to areas with high demand for ATP, such as near the myofibrils. After the high-energy phosphate from phosphocreatine is transferred to ADP, producing ATP, creatine diffuses back to mitochondria to be phosphorylated again (see Figure 13.2). The creatine/phosphocreatine shuttle activity helps supply energy where it is needed inside these types of cells (Brosnan & Brosnan; Wallimann, Tokarska-Schlattner, & Schlattner 2011).

Creatine kinase also acts a metabolic regulator in a variety of ways. For example, its cytoplasmic activity can help maintain the ATP to ADP ratio inside cells. The ATP/ADP ratio is important because the buildup of ADP can inhibit the activity of ATPases involved in calcium transport, muscle contraction, and many other important functions (Brosnan & Brosnan). ADP also converts to AMP, and as AMP levels increase, the extra AMP becomes degraded.

The mitochondrial version of creatine kinase is also of interest. The protein occurs as an octamer in the space between the two mitochondrial membranes. It forms attachments with both the inner and outer mitochondrial membrane. It is associated with a complex of other proteins, allowing close functional coupling of the substrates and products of the reaction (see Figure 13.2) with their movement in and out of mitochondria. Mitochondrial creatine kinase is therefore tightly coupled to ATP synthesis and transport, and the release of phosphocreatine into the cytoplasm.

Figure 13.2 Creatine kinase activity in schematic form.

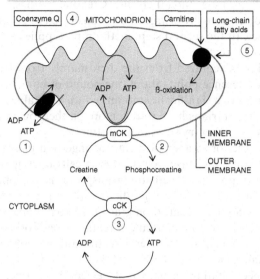

Legend: ATP production occurs in mitochondrial inner membrane through oxidative phosphorylation. (1) ATP in the mitochondrial matrix is exchanged for ADP from the cytoplasm. (2) A mitochondrial form of creatine kinase (mCK) transfers the high-energy phosphate from ATP to creatine, making phosphocreatine released into the cytoplasm. (3) The cytoplasmic form of creatine kinase (cCK) transfers the high-energy phosphate from phosphocreatine back to ADP, making ATP. ATP is used for energy-requiring processes, including muscle contraction, ions pumps, and other ATPases. Creatine kinase helps maintain ATP levels during times of intense activity. Creatine can shuttle back to mitochondria and be phosphorylated, or be phosphorylated by ATP generated by glycolysis in the cytoplasm. (4) The supplement coenzyme Q is an electron carrier that helps to produce ATP in the inner membrane of the mitochondria (discussed later). (5) Carnitine is another supplement discussed later in the chapter; it helps fatty acids enter mitochondria to undergo beta-oxidation and fuel ATP production.

Besides the role of creatine as an energy buffer, it has several other functions as a metabolic regulator. Creatine can improve brain function, particularly in those people who may be creatine deficient or who have an inborn error that affects creatine synthesis or transport. Creatine has been used therapeutically in certain neuromuscular and neurodegenerative diseases, such as Huntington's disease. It may have neuroprotective activity, and it functions as an antioxidant. Creatine has a protective effect on membranes, probably due to its antioxidant activity. Supplementation has been recommended for the elderly, pregnant mothers, newborns, and dialysis patients. There is even support for use of creatine as an additive to animal feed to decrease waste associated with feeding poultry, swine, and the aqua-farming of fish (Wallimann et al.).

Sources of Creatine

For most people, about half of the needed creatine comes from the diet, and the other half is produced by the body on a daily basis. Omnivores obtain about one gram per day from the diet and make about one gram per day. Skeletal muscle stores about 95% of the body's creatine. Creatine content can vary with muscle fiber type; fast-twitch muscle fibers have more than slow-twitch.

In humans, creatine is synthesized from three amino acids: (1) methionine, an essential amino acid (see Table 13.1), (2) arginine, and (3) glycine. Creatine synthesis is a two-step process in which the functional group from arginine is transferred to glycine, with ornithine created as a byproduct. In the second step, methionine supplies a methyl group to complete the formation of creatine.

The balance of the needed creatine is acquired from the diet, mainly from fresh meat, fish, and dairy products. As a reference point, about one pound of hamburger provides two grams of creatine (along with a significant amount of fat). Vegetables are not a source of creatine. Vegans and vegetarians have to rely more on their own production from the three amino acids than a dietary source of creatine.

Whether creatine is ingested in the diet or as a supplement, the ingestion increases plasma levels, providing available creatine for muscle cells. Muscle cells take up creatine as needed by using a specific transporter. The creatine transporter is a symport (a sodium/creatine co-transporter) that uses the sodium gradient to drive transport of creatine into muscle cells against the creatine concentration gradient. Two Na^+ and one Cl^- are transported with the entry of each creatine molecule. Creatine is reabsorbed in the kidneys through a Na^+ and Cl^-–dependent transporter. Creatine and phosphocreatine spontaneously degrade to **creatinine**. One to two percent of the total body's pool of creatine is lost as creatinine per day, necessitating the daily replacement of creatine. An average 70-kilogram young male has a creatine pool of about 120 to 140 grams (Cooper et al.), so about two grams are needed daily to maintain the pool size.

Exercise Pharmacology

The Russians first explored creatine as a performance enhancer in the 1970s, and in the 1980s creatine acquired cult status. In the 1990s, several well-known athletes admitted using it, including sprinter Linford Christie and baseball player Mark McGwire as he pursued Babe Ruth's home-run record in 1998. Creatine use has sparked considerable debate and research on its effectiveness and safety. Results from these studies range from no significant effect to large ergogenic responses. In an updated position statement, the International Society of Sports Nutrition supports the effectiveness and safety of creatine supplements (Kreider, Kalman, Antonio, et al. 2017). They argue that creatine is an effective ergogenic supplement and that its use is not detrimental when it is used appropriately in healthy individuals. Creatine supplementation, in conjunction with resistance training, improves anaerobic capacity, strength, and lean body mass. Creatine supplementation may also provide protection and recovery from injury (Kreider et al.).

The intramuscular concentration of phosphocreatine is about three times higher than that of ATP, but stores can be depleted in 15 seconds of intense exercise (see Figure 13.3). Performance correlates with tissue levels of phosphocreatine (i.e., low levels of phosphocreatine tested more poorly). The total creatine pool size in skeletal muscle is approximately 60% to 70% phosphocreatine and 30% to 40% creatine (Kreider et al.; Cooper et al.). Rough estimates suggest that 10% to 40% can be gained in total muscle creatine. Responders with lower initial levels of total muscle creatine content and greater populations of type II fibers have a higher potential to improve performance in response to creatine supplementation (Cooper et al.).

The following discussion begins with dosing strategies and then examines some of the evidence for the ergogenic effects of creatine.

Figure 13.3 Relative changes to phosphocreatine and ATP during maximal-intensity exercise.

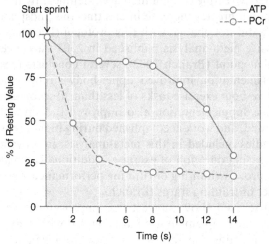

Legend: A hypothetical time course is shown where phosphocreatine is used to maintain ATP levels during maximal burst activity lasting 15 seconds. ATP: solid line; phosphocreatine: dashed line.

Dosing

Athletes looking to gain an advantage with creatine use a "loading" strategy. For example, an athlete might take 20 grams over the course of the day as four 5-gram doses, often in carbohydrate-containing drinks. Although there are many different creatine preparations on the market (usually differing in the associated salt or counter-ion present), creatine hydrate is the most widely used and the least expensive, and it has comparable activity in most cases. After five days of loading, the athlete will usually adopt a maintenance plan of two to five grams per day. Muscle uptake increases over the first two days, though the amount will depend largely on the starting amount of creatine inside the muscle cells. Newer recommendations decrease the amount needed to load to about 0.1 gram per kilogram body weight for three days (Cooper et al.).

An alternate strategy that provides a gradual increase is to ingest 3 g/day for 28 days, so that performance gains may take closer to a month. The goal is to max out muscle phosphocreatine and then maintain that level with lower doses on following days. The concentration of muscle phosphocreatine is slow to rise and then slow to fall. Ergogenic effects can persist for a week after treatment is discontinued.

Ergogenic Effects

The increase in creatine depends on the level of resistance training. Training optimizes muscle content of creatine to meet demand (with some limit or ceiling), although a protein-rich diet or supplementation may be needed to make up the shortfall if endogenous synthesis cannot keep up, particularly in an elite athlete. Exercise increased creatine levels in a series of experiments (Harris, Söderlund, & Hultman 1992). First, researchers showed that to increase the total creatine content in leg muscle (determined from punch biopsies), at least five grams of creatine were needed in multiple doses per day. In an experiment with a stationary bike used over multiple sessions, one leg worked and while the other leg rested. Creatine content increased significantly in both legs; the exercising leg, however, saw a greater increase in creatine and phosphocreatine. ATP pools in the leg muscle did not change with this protocol (Harris et al.; Brosnan & Brosnan). In an extensive meta-analysis published in 2003 that covered most creatine-related studies to that point (Branch 2003), several conclusions were drawn. Short-term creatine supplementation improved upper-body strength more than lower-body, improved repetitive-bout exercise tasks of less than 30 seconds, and improved lean body mass. Creatine supplementation also improved the amount of mass lifted, force and power generated, and work accomplished during high-intensity, short-duration exercise. In the studies included in this meta-analysis, improvement in performance declined with increasing duration of exercise. Additionally, creatine supplementation did not clearly improve swimming or running performance, nor was there support for an effect of gender or training status (Branch).

Conclusions from the studies discussed above suggest that improvements in exercise measures observed with creatine supplementation are coupled with heavy resistance training. Heavy resistance training may increase creatine storage in muscle. The increased muscle cell volume that results from water intake following creatine intake could also allow for increased glycogen storage, increased rate of protein synthesis, or a decreased rate of muscle protein degradation. These changes could contribute to improved muscle mass and anaerobic capacity. A related supposition is that creatine supplementation helps maintain a higher workout intensity, which, over time, improves the quality of workouts during a training period. With this reasoning, the improved performance attributable to creatine is indirect: the effects on muscle result from better workouts. Other research suggests that creatine supplementation increases expression of certain genes, including GLUT-4 (a glucose transporter; see Chapter 12) and insulin-like growth factor 1 (IGF-1). IGF-1 can increase muscle cell protein content and cause hypertrophy. The increased gene activity, particularly IGF-1 expression, could be due to the creatine supplementation or to the higher intensity of the workout achieved with supplementation. Another theory suggests that if the enhanced phosphocreatine pool helps maintain ATP levels better, then one benefit could be to the calcium pump (ATPase) responsible for calcium reuptake following muscle contraction. A more vibrant calcium pump returns cytoplasmic free calcium to resting levels quicker, causing the detachment of the bridge between actin and myosin; hence, the muscle can contract again faster. Another possible benefit of creatine supplementation is related to creatine's antioxidant and membrane-protecting activities. Supplementation could help attenuate muscle damage following a long endurance-training session or an intense resistance-training protocol (Cooper et al.; Wallimann et al.).

In summary, generally, the longer the duration of the exercise, the less significant the result, although results from lab testing are variable. The biggest enhancement of performance with supplemental creatine is observed in the 15- to 30-second range with intense bursts of activity. Variable results with creatine supplementation could be attributable to several factors. Diets vary in their amount of animal protein: a vegetarian may see a more pronounced effect with a creatine supplement. Carbohydrate and other nutrient loading may augment the beneficial effects of creatine supplements. When creatine was given in a sugar solution, muscle creatine levels were higher (Steenge,

Simpson, & Greenhaff 2000). Improved stores of muscle glycogen could also help with performance gains. Creatine supplementation does not affect resting or exercise heart rate. No direct short-term effect on VO_2max is expected, although an indirect effect might occur if the individual trains harder on creatine. An increase in body mass was observed in bodybuilders but not elite runners. Some increase in body mass can be attributed to an increase in intracellular water. Another variable may be caffeine. Caffeine at 5 mg/kg/day (about three cups of coffee) decreased the beneficial performance from creatine on repetitive leg extensions (Vandenberghe, Gillis, Van Leemputte, et al. 1996). However, muscle phosphocreatine levels did not show a caffeine effect. Other studies have not shown a negative effect of caffeine on creatine loading; caffeine taken after loading and prior to exercise can enhance performance (Lee, Lin, & Cheng 2011). With creatine supplementation, untrained individuals may see a larger gain in performance than trained exercisers. Exercise augments creatine uptake, but a saturation point can be reached. Trained athletes may have augmented this pathway relative to the untrained. Therefore, to evaluate an effect of creatine supplementation, the training level of the subjects, diet, dose, type of exercise, and type of study (lab vs. field) are important variables.

Health Risks

Most studies on creatine supplementation suggest that it is safe when proper protocols are carefully followed; however, long-term studies on the effects of supplementation are limited. The major concern with creatine supplementation is that the nitrogen load on the kidneys increases because the unabsorbed creatine is added to the metabolic breakdown product creatinine. However, most results to date have not seen this effect. High-protein diets and amino acid supplements also add to the nitrogen load and excretion of urea. Excess amino acids and creatine in the diet are not stored in the body. Therefore, greatly exceeding the daily requirement does little for the body, but it can make very expensive urine. Note that any contaminate in the commercial product also increases when a person takes mega doses and during loading. Short-term use of reasonable doses (3 g/day) is probably safe. Caution should also be taken with NSAIDs, since they also put strain on the kidneys. Cramps following creatine loading may be more likely on hot and humid days. The take-home message: excess protein and creatine in the diet can be expensive, potentially has negative effects on the kidneys, and provides very little, if any, competitive edge in well-trained and well-fed athletes.

Creatine has many different effects, and supplementation may be recommended for a variety of conditions (Wallimann et al.; Keider et al.). Several genetic errors of metabolism affect creatine production and transport, so individuals with these problems have a higher daily requirement that must be met with supplementation. Patients on kidney dialysis also benefit from supplementation. Certain myopathies that result from poor mitochondrial function may improve with creatine supplementation. Changes in diet, lower activity level, and other metabolic issues occur as we age and can contribute to creatine deficiency. In the elderly, creatine supplementation improves cognitive function, improves strength, enhances fatigue resistance, and improves performance of basic daily activities (Rawson & Venezia 2011; Keider et al.). The improved cognitive function from creatine supplementation and reported neuroprotection activity has led to supplementation experiments in animal models for Alzheimer's disease,

Parkinson's disease, and Huntington's disease. Supplementation in humans is considered a safe and cost-effective option that could extend and improve the quality of life for these patients (Kreider et al.; Cooper et al.).

PES Watch

Creatine is not on the WADA Prohibited List. Although it may not be banned, its use can raise some ethical questions. Abnormally high doses of a physiological substance, such as 30 grams a day, are considered doping by some sport organizations like the IOC. Aggressive training coupled to creatine and protein supplementation can help increase lean muscle mass. The effect will decay if the protocol is not maintained. Following this protocol may provide a competitive advantage, even if creatine is not banned. Although it is not banned, sports governing bodies may still maintain policies that do not endorse or support creatine use at high doses.

Determining the Value of Using a Supplement

Here is a basic approach for anyone interested in supplements:

- For many supplements, buy the smallest-size container and take the supplement for a month or until you have used up the contents. Ask yourself whether it has had any noticeable effect.
- If you are not sure, discontinue use and see if the effect is lost (e.g., pain returns or your energy is once again lagging).
- If so, retake the supplement for another month.
- If you are convinced that the supplement is helping and provides a reasonable cost-to-benefit ratio, then continue its use.
- If not, discontinue its use and save your money for trips to the local farmers market for fresh local produce.

For athletes, particularly competitors that are subject to drug testing, individuals should follow the decision tree provided in the National Athletic Trainers' Association position statement (Buell, Franks, Ransone, et al. 2013). In this case, the first question is whether the athlete's diet is consistent with their performance goals. It then tracks legality, eligibility, and safety issues before making recommendations.

Essential Fatty Acids

Fatty acids are more than a source of energy. They are incorporated into membrane phospholipids and have many roles in transduction of signals involved in inflammation, cell growth, aging, and neurological function. The variation in their length (12 to 24 carbons) and number of double bonds (0 to 6) provides tremendous diversity in their

Figure 13.4 Pathway for production of essential fatty acids.

Alpha-linolenic acid | Eicosapentaenoic acid | Docosapentaenoic acid | Docosahexaenoic acid
(ALA) (18:3n-3) → → → (EPA) (20:5n-3) ⟶ (DPA) (22:5n-3) ⟶ (DHA) (22:6n-3)

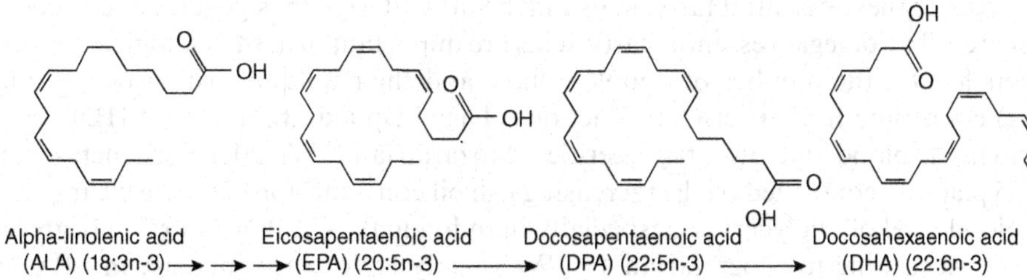

Legend: Starting with ALA, three enzymatic steps are needed (the two intermediates are not shown) to form EPA, which is two carbons longer and has two additional double bonds. EPA is elongated by two carbons to form DPA. DPA adds another double bond to form DHA.

structure and function. In humans, certain fatty acids are considered essential nutrients. In particular, the **omega-3** (also called n-3) **fatty acids** play many critical roles. The three significant types of omega-3 fatty acids in humans are alpha-linolenic acid (ALA), eicosapentaenoic acid (EPA), and docosahexaenoic acid (DHA). ALA has 18 carbons and 3 double bonds and is designated 18:3 (see Figure 13.4). ALA has a double bond at the third carbon from the methyl end (opposite the fatty acid end), making it an n-3 or omega-3 fatty acid (see Figure 13.4). Humans (and most animals) lack the enzyme activity to insert double bonds at this location efficiently, making ALA an essential nutrient. ALA then forms EPA (20:5, eicosapentaenoic acid) and DHA (22:6, docosahexaenoic acid), but the metabolic pathway in humans shown in Figure 13.4 is not efficient. The formation of EPA and DHA from ALA is so slow that these two fatty acids are also considered essential nutrients and required in the diet.

Omega-6 fatty acids have a double bond six bonds from the methyl end of the molecule and are also considered essential fatty acids. They are precursors for the synthesis of arachidonic acid (20:4, n-6), often found in membrane phospholipids involved in cell signaling. Arachidonic acid is at the head of at least 20 signaling pathways (Figure 11.1), many of which play an important role in inflammation and pain.

Sources of Essential Fatty Acids

ALA is largely obtained from leafy greens and seeds in the diet; flax seeds are a good source of ALA. Seafood, particularly cold-water fish (sometimes called oily fish), is a good dietary source for EPA and DHA. Fish that are a good source include anchovies, Atlantic herring, and salmon. Fish acquire these fatty acids by filter feeding on plankton, which are the primary producers of these fatty acids. The polyunsaturated fats become concentrated in the fish and help their membranes maintain fluidity at low temperatures. Because mercury or PCB/dioxin contamination can occur in fish, many people prefer to take fish oil supplements, which supply sufficient levels of essential fatty acids for those who do not choose to eat fish or do not have access to them.

The Role of Essential Fatty Acids

The role of these essential fatty acids in a healthy lifestyle has generated considerable research. The omega-3 essential fatty acids are important in many biological processes. Their length, the number of double bonds, and their unique structures (see Figure 13.4) contribute to their critical functions. They help maintain a good HDL to LDL ratio in the blood and lower triglycerides (Mozaffarian & Wu 2011). In a meta-analysis of 55 placebo-controlled trials, increasing fish oil consumption caused a clear decrease in blood level of triglycerides, especially in individuals with high starting triglyceride levels. According to Mozaffarian and Wu's analysis, for each increase in EPA/DHA consumption of 1 gram per day, blood triglycerides were lowered by almost 6 mg/dL (Mozaffarian & Wu). These essential fatty acids also contribute to cognitive development, learning, and visual function (Calder 2012). They improve conditions associated with vascular and cardiac function, thrombosis (the formation of blood clots), and arrhythmia (Mozaffarian & Wu; Calder 2012).

The omega-3 fatty acids also promote anti-inflammatory activity, as well as other activities associated with anti-aging and good health. For example, omega-3 fats are necessary for formation of **resolvins**, which return tissues back to normal after an inflammatory event. The E-series resolvins are derived from EPA, and aspirin enhances their production. The D-series resolvins are derived from DHA. Resolvins can suppress the inducible (activity increases in response to a stimulus) form of cyclooxygenase (COX-2; see Chapter 11) and are an essential component of the resolution of inflammatory responses. Many health organizations in countries around the world are recommending consumption of fish at least twice per week or supplementation with fish oil to get the recommended amounts of EPA and DHA. Similarly, there are also dietary recommendations for ALA consumption (Mozaffarian & Wu).

Omega-3 fatty acids are involved in other functions, as well. They are incorporated into membrane phospholipids and can affect membrane structure, fluidity, and function. The omega-3 lipids modify the eicosanoid pathways by incorporating and displacing omega-6 fatty acids (more details below). They or molecules derived from them are involved in a myriad of signal transduction pathways. The omega-3 fatty acids also affect gene transcription through two different mechanisms, including the family of regulatory proteins *peroxisome proliferator-activated receptors* (PPARs), which we encountered in previous chapters (Deckelbaum, Worgall, & Seo 2006). Exercise, diet, and other signals also activate the PPARs to regulate metabolic processes, particularly mitochondrial genes involved in oxidative metabolism. PPARs regulate the pathways that coordinate increases in mitochondrial activity and associated changes in slow-twitch fibers. Activation of these pathways by exercise or diet increases the relative amounts of slow-twitch muscle fibers. The resulting change in overall metabolic profile helps protect against insulin resistance and obesity (Demmig-Adams & Carter 2007). Omega-3 fatty acids play an important role in membrane fluidity and make up a higher percentage of the membrane phospholipids in the Type I and IIa fiber types than the Type IIb. Dietary ALA altered muscle cell plasma membrane composition and increased rate of lipid uptake (Chorner, Barbeau, Castellani, et al. 2016). Possible mechanisms on how omega-3 fatty acids influence the exercise and nutritional response of skeletal muscle are reviewed in Jeromson, Gallagher, Galloway, and Hamilton (2015).

The health-supporting activities of essential fatty acids depend on a high ratio of omega-3 fats to omega-6 fats. Omega-3 and omega-6 fatty acids are linked biochemically; their interaction leads to various physiological responses that depend on the ratio of omega-3 to omega-6. The omega-3 fatty acids are part of pathways that produce cytokines with anti-inflammatory activity, while the derivatives of omega-6 fatty acids, such as arachidonic acid, are involved in inflammation. As stated earlier, arachidonic acid is at the head of at least 20 signaling pathways, many of which play an important role in inflammation and pain. Eicosanoids are the family of signaling molecules resulting from these pathways; they include prostaglandins, thromboxanes, and leukotrienes. Cyclooxygenase activity leads to prostaglandin synthesis and thromboxanes. Alternatively, lipoxygenase activity leads to formation of leukotrienes (discussed earlier in Chapters 7 and 11; see Figure 11.1). Supplementation of the diet with EPA/DHA increases their rate of substitution for arachidonic acid in membrane phospholipids. Upon activation of inflammatory pathways, the resulting eicosanoids made from EPA/DHA (instead of arachidonic acid) are less potent or have shorter duration.

Over the past 100 years, changes in human diet (more heavily processed foods) and in agriculture (farming of commercial crops, such as corn, on an industrial scale) have led to a ratio greatly favoring omega-6 fats (Simopoulos 2002). The extensive literature that has analyzed the significant, potentially beneficial effects of increasing the omega-3 to omega-6 ratio is reviewed by Calder (2013). Diets with a low omega-3 to omega-6 ratio are associated with inflammation-related diseases and other "diseases of modern civilization." Cardiovascular disease, diabetes, asthma, cancer, and depression all have an inflammatory component. Increasing dietary omega-3 fats ameliorates some of these diseases and the associated inflammation; omega-3 fat supplementation may ease symptoms in psychiatric disorders (De Caterina & Basta 2001). Insufficient omega-3 fats are associated with memory impairment. Adequate dietary intake of these fats can slow the age-related cognitive decline and may help prevent brain deterioration, including senile dementia (Denis, Potier, Vancassel, et al. 2013). The activation of PPARγ by omega-3 fats has cancer-fighting potential. PPAR activation can inhibit cell proliferation and induce cell death in cancer cells. Dietary intake of these fatty acids is associated with a reduced risk of certain types of cancers in animal studies and human populations (Edwards & O'Flaherty 2008), possibly by decreasing chronic inflammation (Gu, Shan, Chen, & Chen 2015).

Exercise Pharmacology

One of the important results of a favorable omega-3 to omega-6 ratio concerns muscle fiber subtype. The three major muscle fiber types differ in their preferred energy source and their role in exercise performance. Endurance runners have a higher proportion of slow-twitch (oxidative, Type I) fibers relative to sprinters, who have a higher proportion of fast-twitch (glycolytic, Type IIx) fibers. An additional type of fast-twitch (oxidative, Type IIa) fiber is intermediate in their amount of glycogen and mitochondria, compared to Type I and Type IIx fibers. Slow-twitch fibers are more sensitive to insulin. The relative amounts of different fiber types correlate with diseases such as diabetes (see Chapter 12), with more slow-twitch fibers correlating with a lower incidence of diabetes. PPAR family members differ in their expression in different fiber types (Kramer, Ahlsen, Norrbom, et al. 2006). Endurance training leads to fiber type–specific increases in PPARα and PPARγ activity that may play a role in increasing muscle mitochondria content, oxidative phenotype, and sensitivity to insulin (Russell, Feilchenfeldt, Schreiber, et al. 2003). The PPAR family, with its associated co-activators, coordinates lipogenesis, lipid accumulation, and substrate oxidation in skeletal muscle (Summermatter, Baum, Santos, et al. 2010). The role for essential long-chain fatty acids in affecting gene expression and muscle fiber type alteration is intriguing and requires further investigation (Deckelbaum et al.; Demmig-Adams & Carter).

In a study with elderly women, fish oil supplementation enhanced strength training (Rodacki, Rodacki, Pereira, et al. 2012). In this study, 45 women around the age of 64 were split into three groups. One group did just the strength training for 90 days (ST). A second group took fish oil (about 400 mg EPA and 300 mg DHA per day) with their major meals during the training period (ST90). The third group started taking the fish oil supplements 60 days in advance of the 90-day training session (ST150). There was no difference in strength testing in the base test (60 days out) or pretest for the three groups (see Figure 13.5). Peak torque (shown in Figure 13.5) and other measures of

Figure 13.5 Effect of fish oil on strength training in older women.

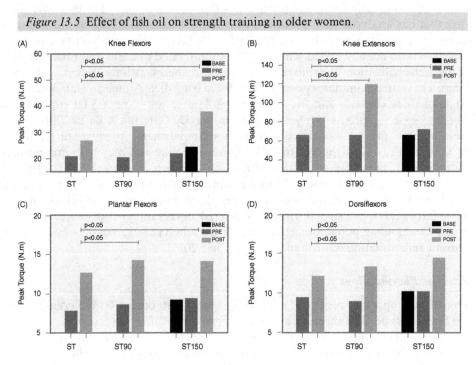

Mean (± SD) peak torque of lower limb joints [knee flexor (A), knee extensor (B), plantar flexor (C), and dorsiflexor (D) muscles] before and after strength training (ST) in the ST ($n = 15$), ST90 ($n = 15$), and ST150 ($n = 15$) groups. *$p < 0.01$ compared with pre-training. Two-factor ANOVA for repeated measures was used to identify differences between factors (groups and times), and the Bonferroni-corrected t-test was applied to determine where differences occurred. There was no difference between baseline (pre-supplementation) and pretest in the ST150 group. BASE, baseline (refers to data collected 60 days before initiating training period); PRE, pre-training (refers to data collected immediately before starting the training program); POST, post-training (refers to data collected after the end of the training program). ST, strength-training group; ST90, strength-training group supplemented with fish oil for 90 days; ST150, strength-training group supplemented with fish oil for 150 days.

Source: Rodacki CLN, Rodacki ALF, Pereira G, Naliwaiko, Coelho, Pequito D, Fernandes LC (2012) Fish-oil supplementation enhances the effects of strength training in elderly women. *Am J Clin Nutr* 95:428–436. Used with permission.

muscle development, however, showed an increase with training, and the increase was significantly greater statistically with fish oil treatment. However, there was no benefit seen with the longer treatment (ST150 vs. ST90; Rodacki et al.).

In another study, omega-3 fatty acid supplementation was shown to relieve inflammation following eccentric strength exercise. In 11 healthy volunteers, supplementation for one week decreased the severe localized soreness from doing eccentric bicep curls (Jouris, McDaniel, & Weiss 2011). Other results from a variety of studies have differed in terms of the degree that omega-3 fatty acids can decrease delayed-onset muscle soreness. Variables include the dose and type of fatty acid supplement, the type of exercise, the training status of the subjects, and how soreness, inflammation, and muscle damage are measured. Additional studies will be needed to clarify this possible effect, as well as others concerning benefits of omega-3 fatty acid supplementation and exercise. More information is available in a review by Gammone, Riccioni, Parrinello, and D'Orazio (2018), including their anti-inflammatory and antioxidant activity providing improved performance during training.

Health Risks

Fish oil supplementation has been found to be relatively safe. Quality supplements that ensure purity can be safer than diets with large quantities of fish, as fish can bioconcentrate potential toxins and metals, such as mercury. Discomfort from taking fish oil capsules can be minimized when they are taken with or following meals. Fish oil supplements taken at recommended doses do not significantly add caloric content to the diet.

PES Watch

Essential fatty acids are not on the WADA list of banned substances. They are not banned by any governing body associated with sports.

Glucosamine and Related Supplements Used for Joint Health

There has been rapid growth in the use of supplements for relief of joint pain. Aches and pains associated with aging are common, and many people choose to take nutritional supplements instead of pain medication such as NSAIDs or prescription drugs. For chronic overuse joint pain, glucosamine as a nutritional supplement may be helpful. **Glucosamine** is an amino sugar used in the ground substance in the body that is a component of the **extracellular matrix.** The extracellular matrix is the complex material found between cells, which varies greatly in different tissue types.

Supplements containing glucosamine and **chondroitin sulfate** comprise a $700 million dollar (and growing) industry. The benefits were first observed by veterinarians; supplementation with ground cartilage gave some relief to old dogs with joint issues. Ground shark cartilage has been replaced by products of large-scale synthesis and manufacturing. Hyaluronic acid has been added to some products, as well as **methylsulfonylmethane (MSM)**, a source of sulfur and methyl groups needed for the production of glycosaminoglycans (see below). Many products contain additional components, such as vitamin C and Mn^{2+}. Glucosamine is usually taken as a pill to supplement the diet, but it can be injected as part of a more intensive therapy. Glucosamine taken in combination with other supplements, such as chondroitin, has recommended doses of around 1500 mg per day (500 mg three times a day taken with food).

Some evidence suggests that supplements containing glucosamine can be as effective as ibuprofen in reducing pain associated with osteoarthritis of the knee (discussed below). Additional clinical trials have examined glucosamine and related supplements for the treatment of osteoarthritis, with mixed results. **Osteoarthritis** is the most common form of arthritis. It is sometimes called the "wear and tear" arthritis, to distinguish it from other types that have an autoimmune basis, such as **rheumatoid arthritis**. The connective tissue and cartilage that protects the ends of the bones deteriorate over time, leading to inflammation, swelling, and pain. Normally, cartilage is well lubricated and permits nearly frictionless joint motion. Eventually, the cartilage wears down and becomes rough, causing friction and pain. Ultimately, bone may be rubbing on bone. Osteoarthritis can affect knees, hips, shoulders, neck, and hands. There is no cure for osteoarthritis, but treatments can slow the progression of the condition. Risk factors include age, obesity, other diseases, occupations with repetitive tasks or stress on certain joints, and old injuries. Osteoarthritis is more common in women. Treatments include drugs (analgesics; see Chapter 11), supplements such as glucosamine, physical therapy, and exercise to relieve pain and/or swelling. In extreme cases, cortisone shots, lubrication injections, or joint replacement may be required. To understand better how supplementation with glucosamine and related compounds might work, we need to examine the role of the extracellular matrix in joint health.

The Extracellular Matrix

The extracellular matrix is a complex network of secreted proteins and carbohydrates that fills spaces between cells. It is important in cell attachment and tissue structure, and it provides a lattice through which cells move, especially during differentiation and development. In skeletal muscle, the extracellular matrix supports the repair and regeneration process, helps regulate satellite cell function, aids growth of blood vessels, and supports innervation of newly formed muscle fibers (Prüller, Mannhardt, Eschenhagen, et al. 2018). The matrix contains tough fibrous proteins embedded in a gel-like ground substance composed of polysaccharides. It can vary greatly throughout the body; examples include loose connective tissue in organs, the glomerulus in the kidney, and even bone and fingernails. Cells in different parts of the body secrete the molecules that make up the extracellular matrix; they are specialized for that tissue's function. The major components of the extracellular matrix include the fibrous collagen proteins, proteoglycans (a carbohydrate component that includes glycosaminoglycans bound to proteins), hyaluronate (a very large, charged polysaccharide of many thousand disaccharides in length), and multi-adhesive glycoproteins.

Different cell types secrete different multi-adhesive glycoproteins, providing matrix-specific functions. Cells have specific surface receptors called **integrins** that bind the multi-adhesive glycoproteins (see Figure 13.6). Properly bound integrins signal the cell nucleus to express genes appropriate for that cell's local environment. The integrins also link to the cell's cytoskeleton, providing tissue strength. Therefore, cells self-identify and function based on their location and attachment to the components in the extracellular matrix.

Figure 13.6 Simplified diagram of the extracellular matrix.

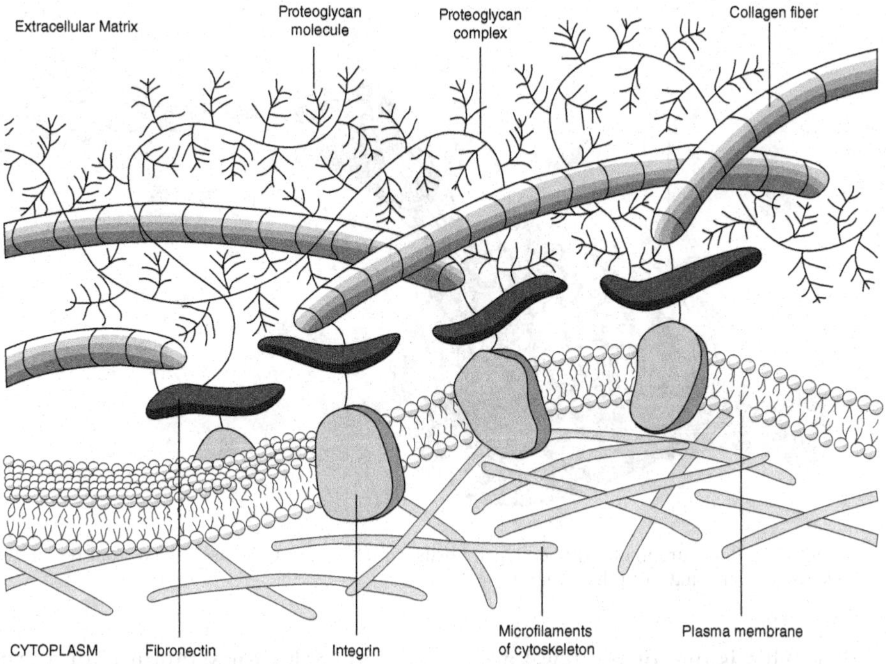

Legend: Integrins are proteins in the plasma membrane that bind to specific proteins in the extracellular matrix, such as fibronectin in this example. The integrins play a critical role in connecting the underlying cytoskeleton to the cell's exterior. The tough, fibrous collagen proteins are shown embedded in the gel-like ground substance composed of proteoglycan.

Source: Copyright © Pearon/Benjamin Cumming, Adapted with permission.

Collagen

Collagen, a major component of the extracellular matrix, is the most abundant animal protein in the world. Collagen contains three peptide chains that form a triple helix (see Figure 13.7). There are many members of the collagen gene family, and expression of the different family members varies with cellular location and function. Once secreted out of the cell, collagen undergoes further modification and self-associates into collagen fibrils that are chemically cross-linked for greater stability. Many fibrils associate into collagen fibers, which contain thousands of copies of collagen in cross-section. These collagen fibers provide the tough, fibrous structure essential for extracellular matrix function. Dense connective tissue found in bone, cartilage, and tendon contains large amounts of specialized collagen fibers. The triple helix constructed from the original proteins, as well as the association into fibers, requires a primary protein sequence with certain amino acids used over and over. More than half of the collagen sequence is constructed from glycine and proline. Moreover, much of the proline is converted to hydroxyproline after the protein has been synthesized. Proline conversion to hydroxyproline requires **ascorbate** (vitamin C) and O_2. Hydroxyproline is necessary for triple helix and collagen fiber

Figure 13.7 Structure of collagen.

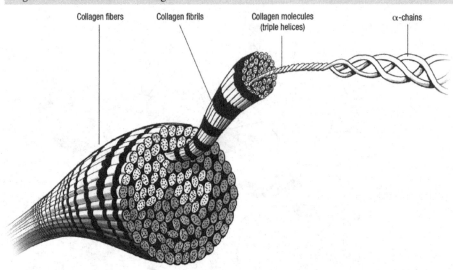

Legend: The fibers are made from collagen fibrils, which are, in turn, assembled from the individual collagen proteins that form the initial triple helix.

stability. This is one of the few known bona fide roles for vitamin C in a crucial metabolic process. A lack of vitamin C in the diet leads to the disease **scurvy,** characterized by saggy skin and a loss of teeth, nails, and hair—all symptoms of defective collagen and poor extracellular matrix. Vitamin C is a common component in supplements marketed for joint health.

Proteoglycans and Hyaluronate

Another major component of the extracellular matrix is the family of **proteoglycans,** formed from a protein with many attached chains of glycosaminoglycans, of which glucosamine is a fundamental building block. These gigantic complexes of protein and carbohydrate create the gel-like properties associated with the ground substance (see Figure 13.8A). At the core of one of these complexes is **hyaluronate,** a negatively charged polysaccharide with a repeating disaccharide (glucuronic acid-ß, N-acetylglucosamine); it can extend 50,000 molecules in length. Other glycosaminoglycans are also composed of repeating disaccharides, some of which are sulfated (see Figure 13.8B). Examples include chondroitin sulfate (glucuronic acid, N-acetylgalactosamine), keratan sulfate (galactose, N-acetylglucosamine), and heparin (also called heparan sulfate; iduronic acid, N-acetylglucosamine). The charged polysaccharides bind divalent cations (Ca^{2+}, Mg^{2+}, Mn^{2+}, etc.) and lots of water— up to 50 times their weight—creating the hydrated gel-like matrix. The resulting gel has high viscosity and low compressibility, making an ideal lubricating fluid in joints. Overuse, dehydration, or aspects of osteoarthritis can impair joint function and lead to pain and inflammation. Joint care supplements usually contain some mixture of glucosamine, chondroitin sulfate, and hyaluronate to help maintain the carbohydrate component of the ground substance.

The functioning of healthy extracellular matrix depends on vitamin C (for good collagen), quality sleep (rehydration of joints occurs while a person is horizontal at rest), exercise (which maintains good blood flow), and water. The sources of sulfated or amino carbohydrates are limited in the diet. These modified carbohydrates, found in ground substance in such large amounts, can be made from glucose. However, their rates of synthesis may be insufficient, especially as we age or if we are physically active.

Figure 13.8 Proteoglycan structure in cartilage.

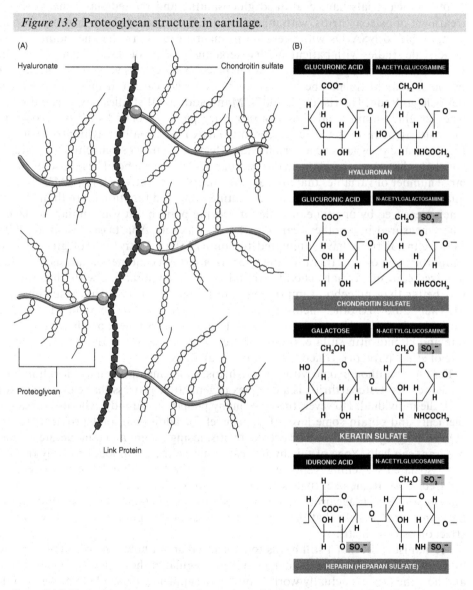

Legend: (A) The long hyaluronate molecule associates with the indicated molecules to form the ground substance that is the basis for the gel-like character of the extracellular matrix component of cartilage and other structures. (B) The major types of glycosaminoglycans are shown. The repeating disaccharide units often contain sulfate; an exception is the disaccharide hyaluronan, which makes up hyaluronate.

For the large number of people who buy supplements for joint care, such products probably provide some level of pain relief.

Health Effects

Do joint care supplements work? The underlying biology is sound. The proper functioning of joints, cartilage, and the extracellular matrix in general may be compromised if adequate amounts of the building block molecules are not available. Many clinical trials have examined glucosamine and related supplements for the treatment of osteoarthritis, with mixed results. Some studies have shown pain relief comparable to NSAIDs with these supplements, usually in the knee joint. Several large-scale studies with patients with osteoarthritis did not show a significant effect versus placebo, though in some cases the placebo effect was very high. The severity of the osteoarthritis may be a factor, as more severe cases did show some pain relief (Clegg, Reda, Harris, et al. 2006). Many additional studies have been done on whether glucosamine and chondroitin reduce pain associated with osteoarthritis. For osteoarthritis in the knee, glucosamine may reduce pain, may improve physical function, and does not cause serious side effects (e.g., upset stomach). Other studies conclude that glucosamine provides similar relief as placebo. These studies have a large number of variables that are hard to control (age, activity level, BMI, diet, and quantifying pain). For example, glucosamine improved function more than placebo when measured by one type of scale for scoring pain, but it was similar to placebo when measured by another scale (Towheed, Maxwell, Anastassiades, et al. 2005). Many clinical trials have attempted to confirm the effectiveness of glucosamine/chondroitin on osteoarthritis of the knee. In a more recent meta-analysis of 43 randomized controlled trials, chondroitin (alone or in combination with glucosamine) was better than placebo in improving pain (Singh, Noorbaloochi, MacDonald, & Maxwell, 2015). Another meta-analysis using 47 trials (22,037 patients) focused on those that had over 12-months of follow-up found improvement by glucosamine sulfate and chondroitin sulfate, though there was uncertainty in the estimates of the size of effect (Gregori, Giacovelli, Minto, et al. 2018).

For the 27 million people with osteoarthritis, supplementation may yield limited or mixed results. Osteoarthritis is a complex degenerative process that can vary greatly with the individual. However, there are many people, apparently, who use these supplements and obtain some level of pain relief for additional joint problems associated with aging or overuse. For osteoarthritis, losing weight and a moderate exercise program can help. Yoga or tai chi also can improve the condition, probably through the associated stretching, gentle exercises, improved breathing, improved sleep, and reduced stress. Remember that extracellular matrix is important throughout the body, not just where cartilage protects against bone-to-bone contact. Supplementation may have an overall benefit that people appreciate, even though it does not have a large effect on osteoarthritis.

Mechanistically, much still needs to be learned about how cells with the responsibility of building the extracellular matrix are regulated, how they change with age, and how the process actually works. Joint care supplements may help make up a deficiency, but they may be very inefficient in building good cartilage or other related structures. Additional factors or therapies could possibly improve the efficiency of getting these supplements into a targeted area. In the near future, designer extracellular matrix precursors may be constructed containing modified stem cells for implantation into the proper joint or other location. The carefully selected components in the gel matrix would help program the embedded stem cells. After implantation, these cells would divide and differentiate into the cells required to reconstruct the damaged tissue. Although these therapies may seem like science fiction, rapid advances in skin replacement for burn victims and a host of other plastic surgery techniques are built on similar principles.

Health Risks

These types of supplements are generally well tolerated. When they are taken with food, the likelihood of stomach issues is reduced. Newer products contain less extracted material and more chemically synthesized compounds, minimizing allergic reactions.

PES Watch

Glucosamine and related substances are not deemed ergogenic and are not banned by WADA or sports governing bodies.

Vitamin D

Numerous studies show that vitamin D deficiency exists worldwide. Additional epidemiological evidence links vitamin D deficiency to many different disease states (see Table 13.3). However, an Institute of Medicine report published in 2010 supported vitamin D supplementation for musculoskeletal health but did not support supplementation for other indications (Haines & Park 2012). The report suggested that most North Americans receive sufficient vitamin D from sun exposure and diet. However, these recommendations have created some controversy. In recent years, studies have continued to examine the consequences of vitamin D deficiency (Lavie, Lee, & Milani 2011).

Many different factors can contribute to problems maintaining proper levels of vitamin D (see Table 13.4). Blood levels of vitamin D can be monitored to determine the

Table 13.3 Various physiological effects and pathological consequences of vitamin D deficiency

Physiological Effects	Physiological Consequences	Pathological Conditions
Elevated parathyroid hormone	Atherosclerosis	Cardiovascular disease
Activation of the renin-angiotensin-aldosterone system	Hypertension	Cancer
	Systemic inflammation	Autoimmune disease
Increased insulin resistance	Left ventricular hypertrophy	Depression
Decreased calcium uptake	Metabolic syndrome	Dementia
Calcium homeostasis issues	Type 2 diabetes	Musculoskeletal decline
Phosphate homeostasis issues	Asthma	Infectious diseases
Bone resorption	Fertility problems	Rickets/osteomalacia

status of an individual (see Table 13.5). People who are deficient cannot maintain bone health and may experience some of the physiological effects listed in Table 13.3 in addition to bone problems. Most of the controversy surrounds the range of blood levels needed for optimal health in the majority of the population. Many epidemiological studies have compared vitamin D status in large populations with different diseases or conditions. Correlations between disease state and vitamin D status generate the list found in Table 13.3 (Pludowski, Holick, Pilz, et al. 2013). Since the majority of the data is correlative—meaning that a certain percentage of a given population with a vitamin D level below some threshold has a higher chance of having the condition measured—there is considerable room for argument. One conclusion that can be drawn is that vitamin D plays many crucial roles that are only partly understood. The next section defines what vitamin D is and then examines some of the possible roles it plays.

Table 13.4 Factors that contribute to vitamin D deficiency

Insufficient Sunlight	
Winter season Being housebound/institutionalized Sunscreen or clothing (little exposed area)	Darkly pigmented skin Living far from the equator Air pollution
Lifestyle Factors	
Physical inactivity Smoking	Diet Aging
Genetics and Disease	
Malabsorption Defects in transport and metabolism Renal disease	Liver disease Obesity
Medication Side Effects	
Glucocorticoids Certain anti-inflammatory and antiviral drugs	

Table 13.5 Definition of vitamin D status based on blood levels

Condition	*Level of 25-Hydroxyvitamin D*	
Deficiency	<20 ng/mL	<50 nmol/L
Insufficiency	20–29 ng/mL	50–75 nmol/L
Sufficiency	30–60 ng/mL	75–150 nmol/L
Range with conflicting data	50–150 ng/mL	125–375 nmol/L
Toxicity	>150 ng/mL	>375 nmol/L

Note: Blood levels are described as nanograms per milliliter (ng/mL) or nanomoles per liter (nmol/L nM), where 0.4 ng/mL = 1 nmol/L.

The Role of Vitamin D

The active form of vitamin D (**calcitriol**) is important in regulating calcium and phosphate levels in the body, particularly in the mineralization of bone. Moreover, calcitriol has endocrine function and works as a steroid hormone. Receptors for vitamin D are present in a wide variety of cells, providing evidence that its biological effects extend beyond calcium and phosphate homeostasis. The term **vitamin D** refers to members of a group of modified steroid molecules derived from cholesterol, with one of the rings opened (see Figure 13.9).

Vitamin D is not a true vitamin, in that sufficient amounts can be generated with adequate exposure to sunlight. (As stated previously, the term vitamin is usually used for substances that cannot be made in the body in sufficient quantities, so that a dietary source is needed.) Vitamin D, as either D_2 or D_3, does not have significant biological activity. Vitamin D_2 (**ergosterol**) is primarily found in plants and mushrooms. Vitamin D_3 (**cholecalciferol**) is generated in the skin when sunlight (UVB) is absorbed by an inactive precursor. Dietary sources of vitamin D_3 include fish (i.e., oily fish, such as salmon or mackerel), egg yolk, and dairy products, which are often fortified with additional D_3. Natural diets typically have inadequate quantities of either source of vitamin D. Individuals with adequate exposure to sunlight do not require dietary supplementation. Exposure to bright, outdoor sunshine for 15 minutes three times a week

Figure 13.9 Pathway for production of vitamin D.

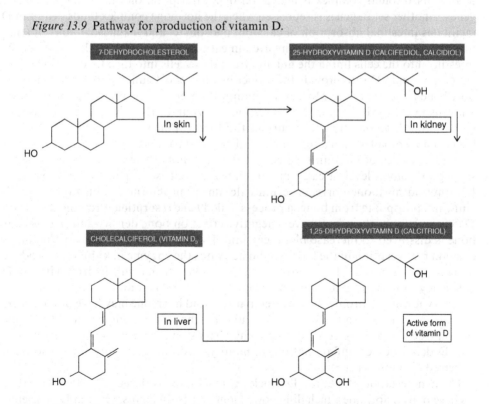

Legend: The critical steps in the formation of active vitamin D are shown, including the steps that occur in the skin (due to sunlight), liver, and kidney. 25-Hydroxyvitamin D (calcifediol) is the form of vitamin D monitored in the blood to determine vitamin D status.

should be enough to produce the body's requirement of vitamin D. The sun needs to shine on the skin of the face, arms, back, or legs. Apparently, a significant percentage of the world's population is deficient and needs some type of supplementation. Exposure to sunlight or consumption of foods supplemented with vitamin D (dairy products, orange juice, etc.) is necessary to prevent a vitamin D deficiency.

The hormonally active form of vitamin D (calcitriol) is transformed from D_3 in two steps, the first in the liver and the second in the kidney (see Figure 13.9). The product of the reaction in the liver is **25-hydroxyvitamin D** (also called **calcifediol** or **calcidiol**). Blood levels of 25-hydroxyvitamin D are used as an indicator of vitamin D status. It has a serum half-life of several weeks. In the kidney, conversion of 25-hydroxyvitamin D to the biologically active 1,25-dihydroxyvitamin D (calcitriol) is tightly regulated. The primary regulator of its production in the kidney is parathyroid hormone. Low calcium or phosphate levels in the blood stimulate an increase in calcitriol. The half-life of calcitriol is only a few hours. Each of the varieties of vitamin D mentioned above is hydrophobic (relatively insoluble in water) and is transported in blood bound to a carrier protein called vitamin D–binding protein.

The vitamin D receptor has hormone-binding and DNA-binding domains similar to other steroid hormone receptors. Upon binding of the calcitriol, the vitamin D receptor forms a complex with another intracellular receptor, the retinoid-X receptor, and that heterodimer binds DNA at specific sequences. The most common response to the DNA-bound complex is activation of transcription of vitamin D–responsive genes. Another set of genes is repressed when the hormone complex binds. Vitamin D facilitates intestinal absorption of calcium, phosphate, and magnesium ions. It stimulates the expression of proteins involved in calcium transport from the lumen of the intestine into the cells lining the gut and from these cells into the blood. The primary effect of vitamin D is to provide the proper balance of calcium and phosphate to support bone mineralization. Moreover, vitamin D receptors are present in most, if not all, cells in the body. Cultured cells respond to vitamin D with potent responses of growth and differentiation. The current thinking is that vitamin D has physiologic effects much broader than a role in mineral homeostasis and bone function.

In the absence of vitamin D, dietary calcium is not efficiently absorbed. The resulting low blood level of calcium stimulates the release of parathyroid hormone. Parathyroid hormone corrects serum calcium by promoting mobilization of calcium and phosphate from bone, a process called **bone resorption**. Prolonged vitamin D deficiency can, therefore, have a negative effect on bone density and strength, as bone is dissolved to increase blood calcium. Parathyroid hormone also stimulates calcium reabsorption in the kidneys and activates the enzyme in kidneys to produce more active vitamin D. The relative hyperparathyroidism resulting from vitamin D deficiency can lead to pancreatic beta cell dysfunction, insulin resistance, and metabolic syndrome. Chronically elevated parathyroid hormone may have other effects on cardiovascular health, such as stimulating the renin-angiotensin-aldosterone system (see Chapter 5), contributing to hypertension (Lavie et al.). Effects of vitamin D deficiency on inflammation, immunity, and autoimmunity have also been reviewed (Pludowski et al.).

The manifestation of vitamin D deficiency in children is **rickets**. Children with rickets have bony deformities, including bowed long bones. In adults, vitamin D deficiency leads to the condition called **osteomalacia**, indicated by the softening of the bones, bending of the spine, bowing of the legs, muscle weakness, bone fragility, and increased risk for fractures. Both rickets and osteomalacia reflect impaired mineralization of bone matrix, and both can result in reduced bone density (**osteoporosis**). Vitamin D plays a central role in the complex hormonal control of calcium and phosphate homeostasis. Insufficient vitamin D disrupts the hormonal control loops and can be damaging for bone and, probably, muscle. Also, keep in mind that calcium itself is a critically important ion with many extracellular and intracellular functions. Therefore, it is not surprising that vitamin D research is a very hot area. Vitamin D touches on virtually every cell type and organ system in the body and is involved in many medical conditions.

Vitamin D deficiency or insufficiency can occur for a variety of reasons (see Table 13.4). Mutations have been identified in humans that lead to hereditary vitamin D resistance. Severe liver or kidney disease can interfere with generation of active vitamin D. Insufficient exposure to sunlight is another potential cause. Sunscreens, widely used to minimize skin cancer, effectively block synthesis of vitamin D in the skin. Elderly people who stay indoors and have poor diets can have subclinical deficiency. Vitamin D deficiency tracks away from the equator and correlates with less exposure to sunlight. Americans who live north of the 42nd parallel do not get adequate sunshine during the winter months. Moreover, low vitamin D levels are also seen in hot, sunny countries, where people cover themselves for protection from the sun or their culture dictates that they (mostly women) wear covering veils when outdoors in public. Excessive exposure to sunlight does not lead to overproduction of vitamin D. Vitamin D toxicity can, however, result from ingestion of excessive (milligram) quantities of vitamin D over periods of weeks or months. In rodenticides, large quantities of vitamin D are used effectively as bait.

Dosing

Vitamin D supplementation improves musculoskeletal health (e.g., reduces the rate of fractures in adults over age 65), in those people who are vitamin D deficient. In patients with documented vitamin D deficiency, a cumulative dose of at least 600,000 IU administered over several weeks is needed to replenish vitamin D stores (see Table 13.6).

Exercise Pharmacology

Few studies exist on vitamin D supplementation and exercise performance, although that may change, as there is currently great interest in vitamin D research. Physical

Table 13.6 Recommended daily allowance for vitamin D

Age	Recommended Daily Allowance	Upper Limit
Infants	400 IU (10 mcg/day)	1,000 to 1,500 IU/day
Children	600 IU (15 mcg/day)	2,500 to 3,000 IU/day
Adults	600 IU (15 mcg/day)	4,000 IU/day
Adults over 70	800 IU (20 mcg/day)	4,000 IU/day
Pregnant and breast-feeding women	600 IU (15 mcg/day)	4,000 IU/day

Note: One microgram (mcg) of cholecalciferol (D3) is the same as 40 IU of vitamin D.

activity, particularly resistance training, improved bone mineral density in young females deficient in vitamin D (Constantini, Dubnov-Raz, Chodick, et al. 2010). These results suggest that regular exercise might counteract the detrimental effect of vitamin D deficiency on bone mass. The prevalence of vitamin D deficiency in athletes is prominent, with concerns about increased injury risk due to the condition. In a meta-analysis of 23 studies and 2,323 athletes, 44% to 67% had vitamin D inadequacy. The risk was higher in winter and spring seasons and indoor sports (Farrokhyar, Tabasinejad, Dao, et al. 2015). In a separate analysis, 13 randomized control studies on vitamin D supplementation showed athletes achieved vitamin D sufficiency, but there was no significant increase in performance measures in the seven trials that measured it (Farrokhyar, Sivakumar, Savage, et al. 2017). Clearly, more research is needed to assess vitamin D status with performance level and risk of injury for different sports, latitudes, and ethnicities.

Health Risks

The decision by adults to take vitamin D in doses of 2,000 IU/day or lower is unlikely to cause harm. Blood levels of 25-hydroxyvitamin D that exceed 150 ng/ml are considered toxic. As with most supplements, taking sufficient amounts to correct for diet or other potential deficiency makes sense, as part of a healthy lifestyle. Taking excessive amounts does not seem to provide any additional value and, in the case of vitamin D, can cause a toxic response. Keep in mind that calcitriol is actually a steroid hormone, and steroid hormones are extremely potent, with many possible and diverse effects.

PES Watch

Vitamin D supplementation does not provide documented ergogenic activity and is not prohibited by WADA or other sports governing bodies.

Miscellaneous Supplements (Abbreviated List)

As mentioned in the introduction to this chapter, literally hundreds of supplements are available on the market claiming to improve quality of life or performance without actually claiming to treat disease. The many essential nutrients and vitamins should be obtained in the diet, but the quality of diets and the specific needs of individuals vary greatly. Below are brief descriptions of additional supplements for which a developing body of research supports their consideration as a dietary supplement in some people. In some cases, gains in performance are claimed. Another approach gaining popularity is called multi-ingredient pre-workout supplements. Taken prior to exercise as a blend, the expectation is that there is a synergistic effect on acute exercise performance and subsequent training adaptations. Ingredients such as caffeine (next chapter), creatine, beta-alanine, amino acids, and nitric oxide agents are combined to provide an ergolytic lift (Harty, Zabriskie, Erickson, et al. 2018). Many in the field of sports and performance nutrition, however, like to share the saying: "If it works, it is banned. If it isn't banned, it doesn't work." A comprehensive list of supplements and associated research is at Examine.com.

Amino Acids

The importance of quality protein in the diet has been covered. Protein is digested into the 20 amino acids found in Table 13.1. Other amino acids found in nature have a variety of roles in cell metabolism. Amino acid supplements either provide essential amino acids to correct dietary deficiencies or provide other modified amino acids to optimize their levels. For example, *branch chained amino acid* (leucine, iso-leucine, valine—see Table 13. 1) supplementation can promote muscle protein synthesis and increase muscle growth in those with protein deficient diets. Leucine is central in the pathways that control protein synthesis. *Beta-alanine* is a modified version of the amino acid alanine and may enhance muscular endurance if taken in sufficient quantities. It is a precursor to carnosine, a dipeptide. Carnosine acts as an intramuscular buffer. Heavily working muscle can become acidic and carnosine re-lease helps buffer and minimize this effect. *Trimethylglycine* (also known as *Betaine*) is a derivative of the amino acid glycine. It may act as a methyl-donor in a number of metabolic pathways, including creatine and nitric oxide. At sufficient doses, some studies show enhanced repetitions to fatigue and total volume load completed dur-ing resistance exercise (Harty et al.). *D-aspartic acid* (L-aspartic acid is naturally found in proteins) may act as a testosterone booster for infertile men, and by athletes as a temporary booster, as testosterone levels soon return to normal. It may work in the brain to release pituitary hormones and in the testes to slightly increase testos-terone production (Examine.com).

Carnitine

Carnitine is the generic term for a number of compounds that include L-carnitine, acetyl-L-carnitine, and propionyl-L-carnitine. Animal products such as meat, fish, poultry, and milk are the best dietary sources. All three forms are available over the counter as supplements. L-carnitine is the most common and least expensive. Acetyl-L-carnitine is sometimes recommended because it is better absorbed from the small intestine than L-carnitine. It also crosses the blood–brain barrier more ef-ficiently, making it preferred for studies on Alzheimer's disease and mood disorders. Propionyl-L-carnitine has been used in studies for heart disease and vascular disease. Note that the D-form of carnitine is inactive and can possibly block some functions of L-carnitine.

Healthy children and adults generally do not need carnitine from food or supple-ments. Daily needs are met by production of carnitine from the amino acids lysine and methionine, primarily in the liver and kidneys. However, note that both lysine and methionine are essential amino acids (see Table 13.1), so a diet with quality pro-tein is needed. Because most humans make sufficient amounts of carnitine, it is not considered an essential nutrient. Carnitine can be a conditionally essential nutrient for genetic or medical reasons, as some individuals cannot make enough (i.e., pre-term infants). Biological effects of low carnitine levels may not be clinically significant until the level reaches 10% to 20% of normal. Carnitine plays an essential role in the transfer of long-chain fatty acids into the mitochondria for beta-oxidation (refer back to Figure 13.2). It also transports potentially toxic compounds out of mitochondria, preventing their accumulation. Carnitine is concentrated in tissues that utilize fatty acids as fuel, such as skeletal and cardiac muscle.

Carnitine has been studied extensively because it is important to energy production and is a well-tolerated and generally safe therapeutic agent. Carnitine is promoted as an aid for weight loss, to enhance a sense of well-being, and to improve exercise performance. There is little consistent evidence, however, that carnitine supplements improve exercise performance in healthy subjects; no available studies use sizable doses over extended times. Carnitine supplements do not significantly or consistently increase carnitine content in skeletal muscle or improve VO_2max. A decline in mitochondrial function may contribute to the aging process. The concentration of carnitine can decrease with age and might contribute to the problems associated with mitochondria. Supplemental carnitine may help manage cardiac ischemia (restriction of blood flow to the heart) and peripheral arterial disease, conditions where carnitine levels may be in decline. In certain studies, carnitine supplementation for one year benefited the cardiovascular system. A more recent meta-analysis suggests that L-carnitine is cardioprotective (DiNicolantonio, Lavie, Fares, et al. 2013). However, other studies show that intestinal microbes metabolize L-carnitine into a molecule that has atherogenic activity. Interestingly, vegetarians and vegans, when given carnitine, make less of this molecule (trimethylamine-N-oxide, abbreviated TMAO and sometimes called TMA), due to differences in intestinal bacteria composition. Omnivores produced more TMAO following consumption of L-carnitine. This finding could partly explain the link between consumption of red meat and increased cardiovascular disease risk (Koeth, Wang, Levison, et al. 2013). It also raises the concern of over-supplementation of carnitine in normal, healthy individuals, as this side reaction could contribute to cardiovascular disease.

Chromium

Trivalent chromium is an essential micronutrient, sometimes called a trace element. Hexavalent chromium is toxic. No chromium-containing biomolecules are known, but deficiency has been documented, particularly in hospital-bound patients fed IV. Exercise may speed its depletion. A role in maintenance of blood sugar and insulin action has been suggested. How many individuals may be deficient is also debated. Daily needs are about 50 to 100 micrograms per day, obtained mostly from fruits and vegetables. Supplementation over daily needs shows no effect in healthy people.

Coenzyme Q

Coenzyme Q (also called Q-10) is an intermediate in the electron transport chain in mitochondria, playing an important role in oxidative phosphorylation and ATP production (see Figure 13.2). People with certain diseases may have lower levels of coenzyme Q. These diseases include hypertension, congestive heart failure, certain muscular diseases, Parkinson's disease, and AIDS. Coenzyme Q supplementation may benefit patients with heart disease or patients undergoing cancer chemotherapy. Its production shares intermediates with cholesterol biosynthesis, and patients taking statins have reduced serum levels of coenzyme Q. They may benefit from supplementation to relieve muscle aches and pains that can be a side effect of statin use. Coenzyme Q has possible antioxidant activity. Supplementation with coenzyme Q has been tried for inherited or acquired mitochondrial disorders that limit energy production. The limited studies that exist are inconclusive about whether coenzyme Q improves exercise performance, with most results showing moderate, if any, effect.

Elder Concerns

The supplements discussed in this chapter all have anti-aging properties. Creatine supplementation may help fight against aging as its source in the daily diet may be insufficient. Creatine may have indications for certain age-related neurological conditions (Kreider et al.). Omega-3 fatty acids also help slow age-related deterioration (and inflammation) in many tissues including the brain and heart. Glucosamine/chondroitin helps with the joints that are wearing out. Vitamin-D helps maintain bone and muscle. Physical activity slows sarcopenia. But what about our skin and wrinkles and our appearance?

Very few vitamin-enhanced or expensive skin creams are actually effective in preventing or reversing skin damage and aging. The main problem is the possible active ingredients are not well absorbed by the skin—remember that the skin functions to keep foreign matter out of our bodies. The skin is bombarded with environmental chemicals and sunlight (particularly UV light) every day; free radicals are generated in the deeper skin layers. Free radicals can react with cell membranes and cause cell damage. Application of anti-oxidant creams should therefore help minimize the damage from free radicals if applied in timely fashion and the ingredients are sufficiently absorbed by the skin. Some of the antioxidants known to help the skin recover from the damaging effects of the sun and environment are selenium, vitamin E, and vitamin C.

Selenium, a mineral, has anti-cancer activity, preserves tissue elasticity, and slows the toughening of tissues associated with aging and accumulated oxidative damage. Dietary sources of selenium include seafood, eggs, garlic, and whole grains. Vitamin E protects cell membranes by inactivating free radicals, making them less likely to cause damage. Vitamin E is found in vegetable oils, grains, nuts, and dairy products. Vitamin E creams help the skin repair damage, such as that caused by sun exposure. Oral vitamin E supplements (400 milligrams a day) reduce sun damage, wrinkles, and improve skin texture. Vitamin C is the most common antioxidant located in the skin. Topical application is not effective as it is sensitive to UV light and ozone (common during the summer in urban areas). Besides having antioxidant activity and fighting free radicals, vitamin C is important in collagen structure and the health of the extracellular matrix. A healthy extracellular matrix underlying the skin can contribute to a healthier and younger appearance. The best sources of vitamin C are citrus fruits and vegetables. Vitamin A also is important in the growth and differentiation of skin cells. Zinc is another mineral that helps maintain the integrity skin tissue and has antioxidant activity (www.webmd.com/beauty/nutrients-for-healthy-skin#2).

The common thread is that diets rich in fresh fruits, vegetables, fatty fish, and nuts provide vitamin and mineral support for healthy skin. Besides *feeling good* as one ages, doesn't one want to *look good*, too?

Conclusion

Differences in nutritional needs can vary with culture, race, gender, age, fitness level, and genotype. Supplementation of a diet may be needed in a significant portion of the population to ensure that optimal levels of all essential nutrients are met. In the case of most vitamins and essential nutrients, the body's ability to store excessive daily intake is very limited or nonexistent. For exercise performance, there is very little data to support any demonstrable benefit of supra-physiological doses. For the vast majority of the population, a healthy diet containing a balance of complex carbohydrates, protein, and healthy fats should be sufficient. Limit the intake of highly processed food, and include fresh fruits and vegetables whenever possible. Take a multivitamin for insurance. Snack smart: consider nuts and vegetables. Avoid sugar when possible. Drink water. Exercise regularly.

Key Concepts Review

25-hydroxyvitamin D	integrins
ascorbate	leptin
bone resorption	methylsulfonylmethane (MSM)
calcidiol	neuropeptide Y
calcitriol	nonessential supplement
carnitine	nutrigenomics
cholecalciferol	omega-3 fatty acids
chondroitin sulfate	omega-6 fatty acids
collagen	orexin
conditionally essential nutrient	osteoarthritis
creatine kinase	osteomalacia
creatinine	osteoporosis
dietary supplement	phosphocreatine
ergosterol	proteoglycans
essential nutrient	resolvins
essential supplement	rheumatoid arthritis
extracellular matrix	rickets
ghrelin	scurvy
glucosamine	serotonin
hedonic eating	vitamin
hyaluronate	vitamin D

Review Questions

1   Wally eats a lot of beef and potatoes and plays a lot of soccer. He takes fairly high levels of creatine in hopes of improving his endurance and performance for the full 90 minutes of action. Is he gaining any benefit? Why or why not?

2   Holly is a sprinter on the track team and is a vegetarian. Would creatine supplements help her? What does creatine do?

3   Your little sister returned home for the summer after her first year away at college. She was always a little pudgy, but she has put on another 15 to 20 pounds. She asks you for advice. She wants to lose that weight during summer break and seems serious this time. What kind of plan should you put her on? Is her goal realistic?

4   What are omega-3 fatty acids? Why is fish oil recommended as a supplement?

5   Iain, an aging rugby player, has started refereeing as a way to keep up with the lads. However, his knees are bothering him. He tries Joint-Aid (with glucosamine, vitamin C, MSM, and chondroitin) for a couple of weeks and has started jogging again. He actually feels pretty good. Is it the pills?

6   Vitamin D isn't actually a vitamin. Why not? Yet it seems that vitamin D deficiency is starting to be recognized as a big problem. How can vitamin D be associated with so many different health problems?

References

Allen PJ, Baltra P, Geiger BM, Wommack T, Gilhooly C, Pothos EN (2012) Rationale and consequences of reclassifying obesity as an addictive disorder: neurobiology, food environment and social policy perspectives. *Physiol Behav* 107:126–137

Branch JD (2003) Effect of creatine supplementation on body composition and performance: a meta-analysis. *Int J Sport Nutr Exercise Metab* 13:198–226

Brosnan JT, Brosnan ME (2007) Creatine: endogenous metabolite, dietary, and therapeutic supplement. *Annu Rev Nutr* 27:241–261

Buell JL, Franks R, Ransone J, Powers ME, Laquale KM, Carlson-Phillips A; National Athletic Trainers' Association (2013) National Athletic Trainers' Association position statement: evaluation of dietary supplements for performance nutrition. *J Athl Train* 48:124–136

Calder PC (2012) Mechanisms of action of (n-3) fatty acids. *J Nutr* 142:592S–599S

Calder PC (2013) Omega-3 polyunsaturated fatty acids and inflammatory processes: nutrition or pharmacology? *Br J Clin Pharmacol* 75:645–662

Chorner Z, Barbeau PA, Castellani L, Wright DC, Chabowski A, Holloway GP (2016) Dietary α-linolenic acid supplementation alters skeletal muscle plasma membrane lipid composition, sarcolemmal FAT/CD36 abundance, and palmitate transport rates. *Am J Physiol Regul Integr Comp Physiol* 311:R1234–R1242

Clegg DO, Reda DJ, Harris CL, Klein MA, O'Dell JR, Hooper MM, Bradley JD, Bingham CO, Weisman MH, Jackson CG, Lane NE, Cush JJ, Moreland LW, Schumacher HR, Oddis CV, Wolfe F, Molitor JA, Yocum DE, Schnitzer TJ, Furst DE, Sawitzke AD, Shi H, Brandt KD, Moskowitz RW, Williams HJ (2006) Glucosamine, chondroitin sulfate, and the two in combination for painful knee osteoarthritis. *N Engl J Med* 354:795–808

Constantini NW, Dubnov-Raz G, Chodick G, Rozen GS, Giladi A, Ish-Shalom S (2010) Physical activity and bone mineral density in adolescents with vitamin D deficiency. *Med Sci Sports Exerc* 42:646–650

Cooper R, Naclerio F, Allgrove J, Jimenez A (2012) Creatine supplementation with specific view to exercise/sports performance: an update. *J Int Soc Sports Nutr* 9:33–44

De Caterina R, Basta G (2001) n-3 fatty acids and the inflammatory response—biological background. *Eur Heart J Suppl* 3(*Supplement D*):D42–D49

Deckelbaum RJ, Worgall TS, Seo T (2006) n-3 fatty acids and gene expression. *Am J Clin Nutr* 83(suppl):1520S–1525S

Demmig-Adams B, Carter J (2007) Interaction among diet, genes, and exercise affects athletic performance and risk for chronic disease. *Nutrition Food Sci* 37:306–312

Denis I, Potier B, Vancassel S, Herberden C, Lavialle M (2013) Omega-3 fatty acids and brain resistance to aging and stress: body of evidence and possible mechanisms. *Ageing Res Rev* 12:579–594

DiNicolantonio JJ, Lavie CJ, Fares H, Menezes AR, O'Keefe JH (2013) L-carnitine in the secondary prevention of cardiovascular disease: systematic review and meta-analysis. *Mayo Clin Proc* 88:544–551

Edwards IJ, O'Flaherty JT (2008) Omega-3 fatty acids and PPAR-gamma in cancer. *PPAR Res* 2008:article 358052. doi:10.1155/2008/358052

Erdmann J, Tahbaz R, Lippl F, Wagenpfeil S, Schusdziarra V (2007) Plasma ghrelin levels during exercise—effects of intensity and duration. *Regul Pept* 143:127–135

Erlund I (2004) Review of the flavonoids quercetin, hesperetin, and naringenin. Dietary sources, bioactivities, bioavailability, and epidemiology. *Nutr Res* 24:851–874

Farrokhyar F, Tabasinejad R, Dao D, Peterson D, Ayeni OR, Hadioonzadeh R, Bhandari M (2015) Prevalence of vitamin D inadequacy in athletes: a systematic-review and meta-analysis. *Sports Med* 45:365–378.

Farrokhyar F, Sivakumar G, Savage K, Koziarz A, Jamshidi S, Ayeni OR, Peterson D, Bhandari M (2017) Effects of vitamin D supplementation on Serum 25-Hydroxyvitamin D concentrations and physical performance in athletes: a systematic review and meta-analysis of randomized controlled trials. *Sports Med* 47:2323–2339.

Gammone MA, Riccioni G, Parrinello G, D'Orazio N (2018) Omega-3 polyunsaturated fatty acids: benefits and endpoints in sport. *Nutrients* 11:E46.

Gregori D, Giacovelli G, Minto C, Barbetta B, Gualtieri F, Azzolina D, Vaghi P, Rovati LC (2018) Association of pharmacological treatments with long-term pain control in patients with knee osteoarthritis: a systematic review and meta-analysis. *JAMA* 320:2564–2579.

Gu Z, Shan K, Chen H, Chen YQ (2015) n-3 polyunsaturated fatty acids and their role in cancer chemoprevention. *Curr Pharmacol Rep* 1:283–294

Haines ST, Park SK (2012) Vitamin D supplementation: what's known, what to do, and what's needed. *Pharmacotherapy* 332:354–382

Harris RC, Söderlund K, Hultman E (1992) Elevation of creatine in resting and exercised muscle of normal subjects by creatine supplementation. *Clin Sci (Lond)* 83:367–374

Harty PS, Zabriskie HA, Erickson JL, Molling PE, Kerksick CM, Jagim AR (2018) Multi-ingredient pre-workout supplements, safety implications, and performance outcomes: a brief review. *J Int Soc Sports Nutr* 15:41

Hernández-Díazcouder A, Romero-Nava R, Carbó R, Sánchez-Lozada LG, Sánchez-Muñoz F (2019) High fructose intake and adipogenesis. *Int J Mol Sci* 20: E2787

Jeromson S, Gallagher IJ, Galloway SDR, Hamilton DL (2015) Omega-3 fatty acids and skeletal muscle health. *Mar. Drugs* 13 6977–7004

Jouris KB, McDaniel JL, Weiss EP (2011) The effect of omega-3 fatty acid supplementation on the inflammatory response to eccentric strength exercise. *J Sports Sci Med* 10:432–438

Klok MD, Jakobsdottir S, Drent ML (2006) The role of leptin and ghrelin in regulation of food intake and body weight in humans: a review. *Obesity Reviews* 8:21–34

Koeth RA, Wang Z, Levison BS, Buffa JA, Org E, Sheehy BT, Britt EB, Fu X, Wu Y, Li L, Smith JD, DiDonato JA, Chen J, Li H, Wu GD, Lewis JD, Warrier M, Brown JM, Krauss RM, Tang WH, Bushman FD, Lusis AJ, Hazen SL (2013) Intestinal microbiota metabolism of L-carnitine, a nutrient in red meat, promotes atherosclerosis. *Nat Med* 19:576–585

Kramer DK, Ahlsen M, Norrbom J, Jansson E, Hjeltnes N, Gustafsson T, Krook A (2006) Human skeletal muscle fiber type variations correlate with PPAR alpha, PPAR delta and PPAR PGC-1 alpha mRNA. *Acta Physiol (Oxf)* 188:206–216

Kreider RB, Kalman DS, Antonio J, Ziegenfuss TN, Wildman R, Collins R, Candow DG, Kleiner SM, Almada AL, Lopez HL (2017) International Society of Sports Nutrition position stand: safety and efficacy of creatine supplementation in exercise, sport, and medicine. *J Int Soc Sports Nutr* 14:18.

Lavie CJ, Lee JH, Milani RV (2011) Vitamin D and cardiovascular disease. Will it live up to its hype? *J Am Col Cardiol* 58:1547–1556

Lee CL, Lin JC, Cheng CF (2011) Effect of caffeine ingestion after creatine supplementation on intermittent high-intensity sprint performance. *Eur J Appl Physiol* 111:1669–1677

Lennerz BS, Alsop DC, Holsen LM, Stern E, Rojas R, Ebbeling CB, Goldstein JM, Ludwig DS (2013) Effects of dietary glycemic index on brain regions related to reward and craving in men. *Am J Clin Nutr* 98:641–647

Love C (2002) The role of diet in the prevention of osteoporosis. *J Orthopoedic Nursing* 6:101–110

Maccarrone M, Gasperi V, Catani MV, Diep TA, Dainese E, Hansen HS, Avigliano L (2010) The endocannabinoid system and its relevance for nutrition. *Annu Rev Nutr* 30:423–440

Monteleone P, Piscitelli F, Scognamiglio P, Monteleone AM, Canestrelli B, Di Marzo V, Maj M (2012) Hedonic eating is associated with increased peripheral levels of ghrelin and the endocannabinoid 2-arachidonoyl-glycerol in healthy humans: a pilot study. *J Clin Endocrinol Metab* 97: E917–E924

Mozaffarian D, Wu JHY (2011) Omega-3 fatty acids and cardiovascular disease. *J Am Col Cardiol* 58:2047–2067

National Institutes of Health Office of Dietary Supplements (January 7, 2013) Multivitamin/mineral supplements. http://ods.od.nih.gov/factsheets/MVMS-HealthProfessional/

Ozdemir V, Motulsky AG, Kolker E, Godard B (2009) Genome–environment interactions and prospective technology assessment: evolution from pharmacogenomics to nutrigenomics and ecogenomics. *OMICS* 13:1–6

Pludowski P, Holick MF, Pilz S, Wagner CL, Hollis BW, Grant WB, Shoenfeld Y, Lerchbaum E, Llewellyn DJ, Kienreich K, Soni M (2013) Vitamin D effects on musculoskeletal health, immunity, autoimmunity, cardiovascular disease, cancer, fertility, pregnancy, dementia, and mortality—a review of recent evidence. *Autoimmunity Rev* 12:976–989

Prüller J, Mannhardt I, Eschenhagen T, Zammit PS, Figeac N (2018) Satellite cells delivered in their niche efficiently generate functional myotubes in three-dimensional cell culture. *PLoS One* 13:e0202574.

Rawson ES, Venezia AC (2011) Use of creatine in the elderly and the evidence for effects on cognitive function in young and old. *Amino Acids* 40:1349–1362

Rodacki CLN, Rodacki ALF, Pereira G, Naliwaiko K, Coelho I, Pequito D, Fernandes LC (2012) Fish-oil supplementation enhances the effects of strength training in elderly women. *Am J Clin Nutr* 95:428–436

Russell AP, Feilchenfeldt J, Schreiber S, Praz M, Crettenand A, Gobelet C, Meier CA, Bell DR, Kralli A, Giacobino JP, Deriaz O (2003) Endurance training in humans leads to fiber type-specific increases in levels of peroxisome proliferator-activated receptor-gamma coactivator-1 and peroxisome proliferator-activated receptor-alpha in skeletal muscle. *Diabetes* 52:2874–2881

Simopoulos AP (2002) The importance of the ration of omega-6/omega-3 essential fatty acids. *Biomed Pharmacother* 56:365–379

Singh JA, Noorbaloochi S, MacDonald R, Maxwell L (2015) Chondroitin for osteoarthritis. *Cochrane Database Syst Rev* 1:CD005614

Spiegel K, Leproult R, Lhermite-Baleriaux M, Copinschi G, Penev PD, Van Cauter E (2004) Leptin levels are dependent on sleep duration: relationships with sympathovagal balance, carbohydrate regulation, cortisol, and thyrotropin. *J Clin Endocrinol Metab* 89:5762–5771

Steenge G, Simpson E, Greenhaff P(2000) Protein- and carbohydrate-induced augmentation of whole body creatine retention in humans. *J Appl Physiol* 89:1165–1171

Stensel D (2010) Exercise, appetite, and appetite-regulating hormones: implications for food intake and weight control. *Ann Nutr Metab* 57(suppl 2):36–42

Summermatter S, Baum O, Santos G, Hoppeler H, Handschin C (2010) Peroxisome proliferator-activated receptor-gamma coactivator 1 alpha promotes skeletal lipid refueling in vivo by activating de novo lipogenesis and the pentose phosphate pathway. *J Biol Chem* 285:32793–32800

Towheed TE, Maxwell L, Anastassiades TP, Shea B, Houpt J, Robinson V, Hochberg MC, Wells G (2005) Glucosamine therapy for treating osteoarthritis. *Cochrane Database Syst Rev* 2005(2):CD002946. [PubMed:15846645]

Vandenberghe K, Gillis N, Van Leemputte M, Van Hecke P, Vanstapel P (1996) Caffeine counteracts the ergogenic action of muscle creatine loading. *J Appl Physiol (1985)* 80:452–457

Vatansever-Ozen S, Tiryaki-Sonmez G, Bugdayci G, Ozen G (2011) The effects of exercise on food intake and hunger: relationship with acylated ghrelin and leptin. *J Sports Sci Med* 10:283–291

Wallimann T, Tokarska-Schlattner M, Schlattner U (2011) The creatine kinase system and pleiotropic effects of creatine. *Amino Acids* 40:1271–1296

webmd.com/beauty/nutrients-for-healthy-skin#2

14 Caffeine

Abstract

Although many biological mechanisms are attributed to caffeine, most of the effects from normal consumption probably are attributable to caffeine's action as an adenosine antagonist. By blocking adenosine's inhibitory effect on nerve activity, many neurotransmitter activities are elevated. Caffeine has ergogenic properties for a variety of exercise protocols, including endurance and resistance training. Tolerance develops over time, so caffeine's ergogenic effect may diminish with regular use. Abrupt cessation of caffeine use has a withdrawal syndrome that can last several days and include disrupted sleep, nausea, and headaches.

CASE EXAMPLE

A couple of years ago, Megan was desperate. She had started a new job soon after her second child, and the lack of sleep was getting to her. One morning, after a long sleepless night dealing with a child's earache, she needed something to make it through her morning presentation. She grabbed one of those little bottles promising 'Energy' at the counter of the convenience store on her way to work. She made it through the morning, but felt kind of nauseous. It reminded her of her soccer days when a teammate convinced her to try caffeine pills as an extra boost before the game. Maybe they helped, but it didn't matter because she felt sick to her stomach after an hour or so and she never tried it again—just like she didn't try the Energy Drink again. Her husband Brad, a coffee connoisseur, bought a fully automated expresso machine last year and now she has her morning latte with a double shot…the current problem is getting the kids out of bed every morning.

Learning Objectives

1 Appreciate the prevalence of caffeine in our diet and our society.
2 Learn how caffeine exerts its effect on the body.
3 Recognize the ergogenic effects of caffeine on endurance and strength performance.
4 Understand the possible negative effects of too much caffeine use.

Introduction

Caffeine is the most widely used drug in the world. Coffee is the world's most popular beverage, and caffeine is also found in many other beverages, in OTC headache pills, and in anti-drowsiness remedies. The physiological response to caffeine differs from the response to coffee, probably due to the hundreds of other chemicals present in coffee (and it is usually only about 2% caffeine). **Caffeine** is a xanthine alkaloid derived from the seeds, leaves, and fruits of certain plants where it can reward pollinators or can act as a natural pesticide, paralyzing insects that feed on the plant. Theophylline is a related xanthine alkaloid found in tea leaves.

The Effect of Caffeine on the Body

Xanthine alkaloids cross the blood–brain barrier, exerting a central effect, in addition to systemic responses. One target for their activity is **phosphodiesterase**, the enzyme responsible for degradation of cyclic AMP, a very important intracellular messenger. The inhibition of phosphodiesterase increases cyclic AMP levels, contributing to the diverse responses caused by caffeine and related drugs. Another target is a subclass of calcium channels, resulting in an increase in intracellular calcium. However, some researchers argue that these two targets of caffeine require relatively high concentrations and may not come into play after just one or two cups of coffee (Riksen, Smits, & Rongen 2011). See Table 14.1 for caffeine levels in widely used products.

Caffeine is an effective adenosine receptor antagonist at blood levels consistent with normal consumption. The structures for caffeine and adenosine are compared in Figure 14.1. Adenosine is part of the nucleotide ATP and deoxy-ATP (DNA), having many critical functions in genetics and metabolism. Adenosine also has neurotransmitter activity, though not in the classical sense: it is not stored in secretory vesicles like transmitters involved in synaptic transmission. Rather, neurons in the brain and the periphery express adenosine receptors, and adenosine slows the firing rate of these neurons. Adenosine receptors are often classified as purinergic (adenine is a purine) receptors and their pharmacology is complex (Sachdeva & Gupta 2013). For our purposes, adenosine activation of A1 receptors promotes muscle relaxation and sleepiness and activation of A2A receptors interferes with the release of neurotransmitters such

Table 14.1 Approximate caffeine levels in popular beverages and other widely used products

Beverage	Amount (mg)	Other Products	Amount (mg)
Coffee, 8 oz.	100–150	NoDoz caplet	200
Coffee, decaffeinated, 8 oz.	2–20	Vivarin caplet	200
Tea, 5 oz., brewed	20–110	Excedrin tablet	65
Coca-Cola (or Diet), 12 oz.	45	Midol caplet	60
Pepsi (or Diet), 12 oz.	38		
Mountain Dew, 12 oz.	55		
5-hour Energy, 2 oz	200		
Red Bull 8.4 oz.	80		

Figure 14.1 Comparison of the structures of caffeine and adenosine.

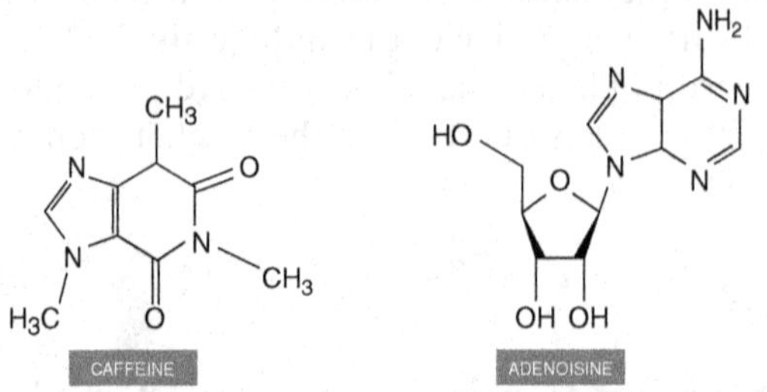

as glutamate and dopamine. Other adenosine receptors are involved in bronchospasm, smooth muscle contraction, and cardiac muscle relaxation.

Adenosine plays a part in the body's response to stressful conditions and helps provide a neuroprotective function. Under certain stressful conditions, such as low oxygen levels, adenosine slows nerve action to minimize negative consequences or damage. Adenosine is also involved in the sleep/awake cycle (Huang, Zhang, & Qu 2014). During a normal day, physical labor and mental activity stimulate glucose and fatty acid utilization to make ATP. ATP fuels the daily activities and adenosine accumulates as a metabolic breakdown product. In the evening, increased adenosine levels promote muscle relaxation and non-REM sleep. During sleep, adenosine is reutilized or metabolized and the body rebuilds its stores of glycogen. Adenosine levels are low in the morning, favoring awakening. The morning cup of coffee helps clear the remaining adenosine from its receptors, aiding the waking up process. Lack of sleep means that adenosine levels remain high, the brain's glucose levels stay low, and caffeine levels may need to be maintained to compete and fight off drowsiness. Ghrelin levels are elevated with insufficient sleep, stimulating the craving for sugary foods.

When caffeine antagonizes adenosine activity, the increased neuronal activity can stimulate the pituitary gland. The resulting activation of the HPA (hypothalamus–pituitary–adrenal) axis (see Chapter 3) causes symptoms similar to the fight or flight response or stress. Increased caffeine consumption increases circulating epinephrine and cortisol, although the underlying mechanisms are not completely understood. When the inhibitory effect of adenosine is blocked by caffeine, there is an increase in nerve activity utilizing many other neurotransmitters. For example, caffeine increases dopamine levels and feelings of well-being, probably contributing to the addictive nature of caffeine. Serotonin activity is also enhanced, as caffeine increases serotonin levels and the sensitivity of serotonin receptors. GABA and acetylcholine signaling are also affected. Therefore, caffeine and related drugs have many diverse and complex effects on the body through several direct and indirect mechanisms. Natural products, such as the xanthine alkaloids, often have many diverse targets. Modern drug designers use structure and activity relationships to design derivatives that have more specific targets.

Exercise Pharmacology

Caffeine use is universal and legal during competition, within specified limits. Its effect on individuals is complex and varied. The literature on the ergogenic properties of caffeine is extensive and continues to grow. We will cover only a fraction of the evidence that supports caffeine's ergogenic properties.

Caffeine is 99% bioavailable, with blood values peaking 15 to 75 minutes after ingestion; other physiological effects occur hours later. The mixed-function oxidases in the liver are responsible for most caffeine metabolism; only about 2% of the drug is excreted unchanged in the urine. Therefore, caffeine would be expected to be flow-limited during intense exercise. At 30% VO_2max, little change was seen in the elimination rate, but sustained exercise at 50% VO_2max decreased the elimination rate significantly (Duthel, Vallon, Martin, et al. 1991).

Serum half-life for caffeine is three to seven hours, depending on physical activity, obesity, and gender. Caffeine and theophylline are both cardiovascular stimulants, probably by causing the release of catecholamines from the adrenergic nerve terminals in the heart and adrenal medulla. Both drugs increase the force (positive inotropic effect) and rate (chronotropic effect) of heartbeats. As discussed in Chapter 3, the release of epinephrine can increase blood flow to muscles and increase glucose release from the liver.

In muscle cells, caffeine may increase fat utilization and decrease glycogen utilization. Caffeine mobilizes free fatty acids, and their availability can help spare muscle glycogen breakdown, thereby enhancing endurance performance. Mechanistically, caffeine may increase activity of hormone-sensitive lipase (see Chapter 10) and decrease the activity of glycogen phosphorylase (reviewed by Pesta, Angadi, Burtscher, & Roberts 2013). Theophylline has a stronger effect on the cardiovascular system; caffeine is stronger in the CNS. Caffeine taken as a capsule may cause different responses than coffee, although the results in individuals vary (Pesta et al.). Higher doses of caffeine can cause "the jitters," restlessness, and tachycardia. Exercise also increases release of epinephrine. Therefore, an exaggerated pressor response may occur when an individual takes caffeine and exercises strenuously.

Tolerance to caffeine develops with daily use, so studies on exercise performance often use caffeine-"naive" subjects. This property can confuse the results of studies, as the level of tolerance can vary with the person and the effect that is being measured. It also makes chronic treatment studies harder to interpret. Acute treatment of caffeine in naive subjects increases resting heart rate and has variable effects on exercise heart rate. It probably does not affect cardiac output or stroke volume. Caffeine does increase blood pressure in both normotensive and hypertensive subjects. Caffeine can increase blood pressure during maximal exercise (Sung, Lovallo, Pincomb, & Wilson 1990).

Caffeine causes mild diuresis, particularly in people who are not very active. This property suggests that caffeine could be ergolytic and that attention to salt and water balance is important, especially for endurance activities under demanding weather conditions. However, most of the research suggests that caffeine does not have diuretic activity during exercise under normal or extreme conditions. In an extensive review of the literature, Armstrong concluded that caffeine stimulates a mild diuresis, similar to water, but without a fluid–electrolyte imbalance; tolerance to caffeine probably reduces the likelihood that a fluid–electrolyte imbalance will occur (Armstrong 2002). For example, Wemple, Lamb, and McKeever compared the effects of caffeinated versus noncaffeinated carbohydrate electrolyte drinks in six subjects (1997). They measured urine volume, osmolality, and water clearance during four hours of rest or one hour of rest followed by three hours of cycling at 60% VO_2max. At rest, mean urinary volume was significantly greater for caffeine than placebo. During exercise, the difference between caffeine and placebo was not significant, suggesting that caffeine consumed in electrolyte-containing drinks does not compromise hydration status during moderate endurance exercise.

Caffeine does not affect the body's ability to thermoregulate. In one study, seven trained male subjects exercised at 70% to 75% VO_2max to exhaustion on a treadmill at room temperature and 50% humidity (Falk, Burstein, Rosenblum, et al. 1990). Subjects exercised after caffeine and placebo, in a double-blind crossover design. Caffeine was given at both 5 mg/kg two hours before exercise and 2.5 mg/kg 30 minutes before exercise. No significant differences were observed in total water loss, sweat rate, or rise in rectal temperature following caffeine ingestion, suggesting caffeine does not disturb body fluid balance or affect thermoregulation during physical activity (Falk et al., 1990). In another study, nine heat-adapted male runners ran at 70% VO_2max on a treadmill in a heat-controlled laboratory (Ping, Keong, & Bandyopadhyay 2010). Caffeine (5 mg/kg) increased running time to exhaustion but did not significantly change heart rate, core body temperature, oxygen uptake, or RPE, suggesting caffeine did not affect cardiorespiratory parameters under hot and humid conditions. Therefore, during exercise, caffeine does not augment fluid loss or significantly change kidney function, probably because of the exercise-induced decrease in renal activity.

Caffeine causes the release of catecholamines, which stimulate lipolysis and, to some degree, glycogenolysis. During a 40-kilometer march, caffeine caused an increase in lactate and a lower RPE, suggesting a greater reliance on carbohydrate stores (Falk, Burstein, Ashkenazi, et al. 1989). However, epinephrine levels do not reliably reflect caffeine dose. Therefore, caffeine's metabolic effects do not correlate well with epinephrine levels, so additional factors are in play. Caffeine generally does not change VO_2 of exercisers. Caffeine and theophylline have bronchodilatory effects, increasing tidal volume and ventilation during walking in acute or chronic treatment (Brown, Knowlton, Sullivan, & Sanjabi 1991). They are not used for exercise-induced bronchoconstriction, although theophylline has been used for asthma (see Chapter 7).

Caffeine can reduce reaction time on simple muscle tasks, but it can also be detrimental on tasks requiring fine motor control. Caffeine exerts metabolic, CNS, and musculoskeletal effects that can augment performance. Caffeine can delay fatigue. Acute treatment increased time to exhaustion in cyclists. Lower doses (5 mg/kg vs. 9 to 13 mg/kg) were also ergogenic when subjects cycled to exhaustion at 80% VO_2max (Pasman, van Baak, Jeukendrup, & de Haan 1995). Caffeine decreases the level of perceived exertion. A meta-analysis of 21 studies supported a significant decrease in RPE and increase in exercise performance (Doherty & Smith 2005). Caffeine, when given with carbohydrate, increased post-exercise glycogen replacement compared to carbohydrate alone (Pedersen, Lessard, Coffey, et al. 2008). An increase in treadmill performance is documented with caffeine but not with coffee at a similar dose (Graham, Hibbert, & Sathasivam 1998). However, another study, with a different exercise, saw an effect with coffee versus decaffeinated coffee (Hodgson, Randell, & Jeukengrup 2013). In this case, there was a significant decrease in finishing time during a cycling time trial. The coffee versus caffeine debate will probably continue as coffee is a complex mixture with variable caffeine levels and different exercise tests may respond differently.

Caffeine also improves performance in field trials. Eight competitive male distance runners ran an eight-kilometer race on a standard synthetic track. They raced against one another to obtain their fastest possible times under three conditions. The first was without treatment (control), and the following two trials were with either caffeine

(3 mg/kg) or placebo, in a double-blind protocol. Caffeine ingestion one hour before running led to a significant 23.8-second improvement compared to the placebo and control trials. In addition, caffeine caused a significantly higher blood lactate concentration three minutes after completion of the race (Bridge & Jones, 2006).

The effect of caffeine on endurance is well documented. However, its effect on anaerobic performance is less clear (Astorino & Roberson 2010). Studies with trained subjects and protocols of intermittent high-intensity exercise have shown ergogenic effects by caffeine (Davis & Green 2009). Examples include sprints lasting 60 to 180 seconds and intermittent bursts of high-intensity exercise lasting four to six seconds (mimicking sport/game activity). Aerobic enhancement by caffeine is thought to result from epinephrine's increasing the oxidation of fatty acids and sparing glycogen. The ergogenic effect on anaerobic performance probably has a CNS site of action involving the antagonism of adenosine receptors. The dampening of pain and blunting of perceived exertion could indirectly increase anaerobic performance (Davis & Green). Experimental evidence supports these theories. In a study with 11 trained subjects, the number of repetitions to failure was measured, along with the RPE and pain perception (Duncan, Stanley, Parkhouse, et al. 2013). Caffeine at 5 mg/kg was given one hour before a series of weightlifting exercises at 60% of the subject's one-lift maximum. Caffeine caused a significant increase in the number of repetitions to failure and decreased perception of exertion and pain (Duncan et al.). In another study, improvement in cycling performance by caffeine was repeatable when it was performed on two separate days (Astorino, Cottrell, Lozano, et al. 2012), suggesting the riders overcame the soreness and fatigue from the previous session. Though more research is necessary, caffeine does appear to have ergogenic effects on anaerobic performance. The suppression of pain and perceived exertion that occurs centrally due to antagonism of adenosine allows an increased generation of force, particularly in lower-body exercises (Duncan et al.).

For an ergogenic effect from caffeine, the recommendation is ingestion of 3 to 9 mg/kg approximately 60 min prior to exercise. However, there is extensive inter-individual response ranging from significant ergogenic effects to ergolytic effects. Part of the variation is due to usual factors such as age, gender, training level, previous caffeine use, temperature, etc., but with caffeine there is also a genetic component. Common polymorphisms within two genes, one involved in caffeine metabolism (CYP1A2) and the other an adenosine receptor (ADORA2A), are important in how different individuals respond to caffeine (Pickering & Kiely 2018). Getting the dosing right is important, because high caffeine doses produce gastrointestinal upset, nervousness, inability to focus, and disturbed sleep. A reduced caffeine dose (around 3 mg/kg) can still produce ergogenic effects with less change in exercise heart rate, levels of catecholamines, lactate, and free fatty acids, suggesting that the ergogenic effect of caffeine is mediated through the central nervous system (Spriet 2014). Optimization of dose, based in part on an individual's genotype, will be personalized in elite athletes and eventually everyone else looking to improve performance.

Elder Concerns

There has been a long, ongoing saga concerning the health benefits or disadvantages associated with coffee consumption. At various times in recent history, coffee drinking was associated with an increased chance of cancer or cardiovascular disease. However, many of these studies were attacked as being flawed or having insufficient statistical power to draw any meaningful conclusions. A comprehensive review published in 2018, based on extensive new research, seems to have settled most of the debate (O'Keefe, DiNicolantonio, & Lavie 2018). Habitual intake of three to four cups of coffee a day is considered safe and is associated with the most robust beneficial effects. Though many of these large-scale studies are observational (not randomized controlled trials), their size and scope support many broad-reaching, positive effects of coffee consumption.

The evidence supports an inverse association between coffee consumption and all-cause mortality, meaning coffee drinkers live longer than non-coffee drinkers. Regular coffee consumption has a lower risk of death from cardiovascular disease, including congestive heart failure and stroke. Coffee consumption had a neutral effect on ar-rhythmias and hypertension. It lowered the chances of obesity and type 2 diabetes, and improved control of asthma. Coffee drinkers had lower risks for liver disease and cancer. It lowered the risk for depression and some neurodegenerative diseases. There are potential risks from high coffee consumption, including anxiety, insomnia, and headaches. People can become shaky and have heart palpitations. Overall, however, coffee consumption can be considered part of a healthy lifestyle.

In women, coffee may have some effects that differ somewhat. Coffee contains a complex mixture of estrogenic compounds. These compounds can include estrogen agonists, antagonists, mixed, or they can act as endocrine disrupters. However, the health benefits associated with estrogenic coffee constituents include bone protection, cancer prevention, cardio-protection, neuroprotection, and the improvement of menopausal syndromes (Kiyama 2019). A final note that may not be an Elder Concern, during pregnancy, coffee consumption should be limited, as it increases the risk for low birth weight and preterm labor, possibly due to these estrogenic compounds.

Health Risks

To maximize the ergogenic effect of taking caffeine, athletes should avoid routine use, due to tolerance effects. Caffeine can increase the pressor response. Individuals with high blood pressure or other cardiovascular problems should monitor themselves carefully. However, a meta-analysis assessed the dose–response relationship of long-term coffee consumption with cardiovascular disease to address the ongoing controversy (Ding, Bhupathiraju, Satija, et al. 2014). Thirty-six studies were included, with 1,279,804 participants and 36,352 cases of cardiovascular disease. A nonlinear association was observed between coffee consumption and cardiovascular disease risk. Moderate coffee consumption was inversely associated, with three to five cups per day having the lowest risk for cardiovascular disease. Heavy coffee consumption was not associated with elevated risk (Ding et al.).

Caffeine use when the individual lacks sleep can create an ongoing unhealthy cycle. Several hours after caffeine ingestion, the increased epinephrine diminishes and fatigue and depression occur. The individual sometimes responds by taking more caffeine. Additional caffeine increases the stress response, and the individual may become "jumpy," irritable, and short-tempered. Disruption of normal sleep patterns contributes to the overall state of exhaustion. With a six-hour half-life, a 200-mg dose of caffeine taken at five o'clock p.m. means the equivalent of 100 mg is still in the system at eleven o'clock; some people avoid caffeine after two in the afternoon to get a restful night's sleep. Caffeine also has a significant withdrawal syndrome for those who consume significant amounts daily. Nausea and GI-tract problems are common upon cessation. The withdrawal syndrome following cessation can cause poorer overall performance and sleep problems for several days. As caffeine leaves the system, adenosine has access to its receptors, and the resulting dilation of blood vessels in the brain can lead to serious headaches. Cutting back over several weeks can help minimize the withdrawal symptoms.

PES Watch

In 2004, WADA removed caffeine from the Prohibited List; however, its use is monitored. Caffeine is considered an ergogenic agent and is described as such in the position statement of the International Society of Sports Nutrition (Goldstein, Ziegenfuss, Kalman, et al. 2010). It is considered a restricted substance, in that organizations have set an allowable amount that may be detected in urine without penalty. Urine levels are affected by exercise, dietary uptake, and gender. The NCAA limit is 15 µg/ml of urine. About 10 mg/kg would probably be below the limit, so a 60-kilogram person could take 600 mg (about five cups of coffee).

Conclusion

Coffee may or may not have similar effects to caffeine, as coffee is a complex mixture resulting from a hot-water extract of roasted coffee beans. By blocking adenosine's inhibitory effect on nerve activity, many neurotransmitter activities are elevated. Caffeine has ergogenic properties on endurance and resistance training. Tolerance develops over time, so caffeine's ergogenic effect may diminish with regular use. Abrupt cessation of caffeine use has a withdrawal syndrome that can last several days and include disrupted sleep, nausea, and headaches.

Key Concepts Review

adenosine receptor
caffeine

phosphodiesterase
xanthine alkaloid

Review Questions

1 Is caffeine ergogenic, ergolytic, or both? Why?
2 Are drinking coffee and taking caffeine pills the same when it comes to athletics?
3 How does antagonism of adenosine signaling contribute to caffeine's effect?
4 What is the effect of caffeine on muscle tasks?
5 What is the effect of caffeine on endurance performance?

References

Armstrong LE (2002) Caffeine, body fluid-electrolyte balance, and exercise performance. *Int J Sport Nutr Exerc Metab* 12:189–206
Astorino TA, Roberson DW (2010) Efficacy of acute caffeine ingestion for short-term high-intensity exercise performance: a systematic review. *J Strength Cond Res* 24:257–265

Astorino TA, Cottrell T, Lozano AT, Abruto-Pratt K, Duhon J (2012) Increases in cycling performance in response to caffeine ingestion are repeatable. Nutr Res 32:78–84

Bridge CA, Jones MA (2006) The effect of caffeine ingestion on 8 km run performance in a field setting. *J Sports Sci* 24:433–439

Brown DD, Knowlton RG, Sullivan JJ, Sanjabi PB (1991) Effect of caffeine ingestion on alveolar ventilation during moderate exercise. *Aviat Space Environ Med* 62:860–864

Davis JK, Green JM (2009) Caffeine and anaerobic performance: ergogenic value and mechanisms of action. *Sports Med* 39:813–832

Ding M, Bhupathiraju SN, Satija A, van Dam RM, Hu FB (2014) Long-term coffee consumption and risk of cardiovascular disease: a systematic review and a dose-response meta-analysis of prospective cohort studies. *Circulation* 129:643–659

Doherty M, Smith PM (2005) Effects of caffeine ingestion on rating of perceived exertion during and after exercise: a meta-analysis. *Scand J Med Sci Sports* 15:69–78

Duncan MJ, Stanley M, Parkhouse N, Cook K, Smith M (2013) Acute caffeine ingestion enhances strength performance and reduces perceived exertion and muscle pain perception during resistance exercise. *Eur J Sport Sci* 13:392–399

Duthel JM, Vallon JJ, Martin G, Ferret JM, Mathieu R, Videman R (1991) Caffeine and sport: role of physical exercise upon elimination. *Med Sci Sports Exerc* 23:980–985

Falk B, Burstein R, Ashkenazi I, Spilberg O, Alter J, Zylber-Katz E, Rubenstein A, Bashan N, Shapiro Y (1989) The effect of caffeine ingestion on physical performance after prolonged exercise. *Eur J Appl Physiol* 59:168–173

Falk B, Burstein R, Rosenblum J, Shapiro Y, Zylber-Katz E, Bashan N (1990) Effects of caffeine ingestion on body fluid balance and thermoregulation during exercise. *Can J Physiol Pharmacol* 68:889–892

Goldstein ER, Ziegenfuss T, Kalman D, Kreider R, Campbell B, Wilborn C, Taylor L, Willoughby D, Stout J, Graves BS, Wildman R, Ivy JL, Spano M, Smith AE, Antonio J (2010) International society of sports nutrition position stand: caffeine and performance. *J Int Soc Sports Nutr* 7:5–20

Graham TE, Hibbert E, Sathasivam P (1998) Metabolic and exercise endurance effects of coffee and caffeine ingestion. *J Appl Physiol* 85:883–889

Hodgson AB, Randell RK, Jeukengrup AE (2013) The metabolic and performance effects of caffeine compared to coffee during endurance exercise. *PLoS One* 8:e59561

Huang ZL, Zhang Z, Qu WM (2014) Roles of adenosine and its receptors in sleep-wake regulation. *Int Rev Neurobiol* 119:349–371

Kiyama R (2019) Estrogenic activity of coffee constituents. *Nutrients* 11:E1401

O'Keefe JH, DiNicolantonio JJ, Lavie CJ (2018) Coffee for cardioprotection and longevity. *Prog Cardiovasc Dis* 61:38–42

Pasman WJ, van Baak MA, Jeukendrup AE, de Haan A (1995) The effect of different doses of caffeine on endurance performance time. *Int J Sports Med* 16:225–230

Pedersen DJ, Lessard SJ, Coffey VG, Churchley EG, Wootton AM, Ng T, Watt MJ, Hawley JA (2008) High rates of muscle glycogen resynthesis after exhaustive exercise when carbohydrate is coingested with caffeine. *J Appl Physiol* 105:7–13

Pesta DH, Angadi SS, Burtscher M, Roberts CK (2013) The effects of caffeine, nicotine, ethanol, and tetrahydrocannabinol on exercise performance. *Nutr Metabol* 10:71–86

Pickering C, Kiely J (2018) Are the current guidelines on caffeine use in sport optimal for everyone? inter-individual variation in caffeine ergogenicity, and a move towards personalised sports nutrition. *Sports Med* 48:7–16

Ping WC, Keong CC, Bandyopadhyay A (2010) Effects of acute supplementation of caffeine on cardiorespiratory responses during endurance running in a hot & humid climate. *Indian J Med Res* 132:36–41

Riksen NP, Smits P, Rongen GA (2011) The cardiovascular effects of methylxanthines. Methylxanthines, *Handb Exp Pharmacol*. (BB Fredholm ed.) 200:413–437

Sachdeva S, Gupta M (2013) Adenosine and its receptors as therapeutic targets: an overview. *Saudi Pharm J* 21:245–253

Spriet LL (2014) Exercise and sport performance with low doses of caffeine. *Sports Med* 44(Suppl 2):175–184

Sung BH, Lovallo WR, Pincomb GA, Wilson MF (1990) Effects of caffeine on blood pressure response during exercise in normotensive healthy young men. *Am J Cardiol* 65:909–913

Wemple RD, Lamb DR, McKeever KH (1997) Caffeine versus caffeine-free sports drink: effects on urine production at rest and during prolonged exercise. *Int J Sport Nutr* 4:120–131

15 Ethanol, Nicotine, and Cannabis

Abstract

Drinking in moderation may actually have some health benefits, but defining moderation can be the key. Some people can be very sensitive to the effects of alcohol, while others can consume significant amounts with few outward signs. Excess alcohol can affect the liver and most organ systems to some degree. Ethanol is ergolytic, with negative effects on metabolism and the cardiovascular system, particularly when the individual is exercising. Alcohol can contribute to a negative water and salt balance. Judgment, coordination, and motivation can all be negatively affected by alcohol.

Cigarette smoking is a major health problem for everyone who comes in contact with it—the smoker, those who breathe the secondhand smoke, and those who come into contact with surfaces contaminated by cigarette smoke. The many chemicals in cigarette smoke can lead to poor health and death in many different ways.

Marijuana smoking also has negative consequences, particularly for heavy smokers. For occasional users, the ergolytic effects and lack of motivation can negatively affect exercise performance. However, the pain suppression and appetite stimulation make marijuana a useful adjuvant therapy in certain types of diseases, such as cancer. In the United States, many states have voted to reduce the penalty for the sale or possession of marijuana. Derivatives or extracts of cannabis, such as CBD, may have health benefits without the high associated with smoking pot.

CASE EXAMPLE

Brad knows wine. Growing up, wine was part of his everyday life and culture. His grandparents had made wine in the old country. His Dad worked for a major wine importer and distributor. Brad has slowly converted Megan. Megan typically drank light beer and an occasional gin and tonic. They actually met at a 'kegger' hosted by Brad's fraternity her junior year in college. Most weekends in college, it was easy to find a frat or sorority (or some other group) that was hosting a party. Some of her teammates were regulars at these events, but she only went occasionally—and luckily met Brad at one of them. Her soccer mates were not like the women's rugby team that was closely associated with the men's rugby team. Those guys drank and some of their parties were legendary. But nowadays, splitting a nice bottle of wine paired with a dinner made from local produce makes for a much more pleasant evening.

Learning Objectives

1 Recognize the impact of drinking and smoking on our health and society.
2 Learn how ethanol exerts its effect on the body and affects behavior.
3 Recognize the significant negative impact of cigarette smoking on public health.
4 Appreciate the complexities of the ongoing debate over the use of cannabis.
5 Learn how drugs designed to regulate cannabinoid-dependent physiological processes may be important in the near future.

Introduction

On the surface, this chapter may appear to include an odd collection of topics. However, all three of these subjects concern the exposure of a large fraction of the world's population to powerful drugs that significantly affect physiological and psychological processes. All three may have addictive properties. The use and misuse of ethanol, nicotine, and cannabis lead to many important medical conditions, with an enormous economic impact on societies around the world. About one in six U.S. adults binge drink about four times per month (CDC). Worldwide, three million deaths every year result from harmful use of alcohol, about 5% of all deaths (WHO). Almost 30 alcohol-impaired–driving fatalities occur every day in the United States, about one-third of all driving fatalities. In 2010, alcohol misuse problems cost the United States $249 billion, with almost three-quarters of the total cost related to binge drinking (CDC).

In the case of nicotine, the negative impact on society caused by cigarette smoking cannot be overstated. Cigarette smoking can damage every organ system in the body and is directly responsible for 480,000 deaths per year in the United States alone, including 41,000 from secondhand smoke (CDC). This rate is about 20% of all deaths annually, or about 1,300 deaths every day. Smoking cannabis is prevalent in certain cultures and portions of Western society. Up to 16% of young adults admit use in the previous month, in both Europe and the United States. Estimates from 2017 say one in seven adults used marijuana during the year, usually by smoking. Currently, 38 states allow some form of marijuana use with only 12 states where its use is considered illegal.

Curiously, moderate use of ethanol may actually provide health benefits, and cannabis (or new related drugs) may have therapeutic potential. Nicotine gum or patch may have ergogenic properties. Drinking and smoking cigarettes or cannabis exert negative effects on exercise performance, implying that use by competitive athletes should be avoided. Yet, it is often famous athletes who make the news after an incident involving alcohol or marijuana. We will briefly cover the main pharmacological effects of these drugs and examine some of the limited literature available on their effects on exercise.

Ethanol

Ethanol is produced as a byproduct during fermentation when yeasts have an ample supply of nutrients but have limited oxygen. Unlike muscle cells, which produce lactate from pyruvate when oxygen is lacking (see Figure 15.1), yeasts use pyruvate to produce the two-carbon alcohol ethanol and CO_2 (carbon dioxide), which is given off as a gas. The result can be beer or wine, depending on the starting material. The ethanol can be distilled, possibly aged in wood barrels, and then bottled as a spirit or liquor such as vodka or whiskey.

How Ethanol Works

Ethanol is readily absorbed through the GI-tract. It is converted to acetaldehyde in the liver (see Figure 15.1). Acetaldehyde is rapidly converted to acetate and then converted to acetyl-CoA. Each oxidation step (ethanol to acetaldehyde and acetaldehyde to acetate) uses NAD+ as the electron acceptor, making the reduced form NADH. Glycolysis requires NAD+, making NADH and ATP in the cytoplasm. If NAD+ is limiting, it is regenerated from NADH by lactate dehydrogenase converting pyruvate to lactate (see Figure 15.1). In mitochondria, acetyl-CoA can make ATP via oxidative phosphorylation, or it can be used to make fatty acids. In mitochondria, the production of ATP from acetyl-CoA requires NAD+. However, since alcohol oxidation uses NAD+, the accumulation of NADH and decrease in NAD+ depresses oxidative phosphorylation. The depressed production of ATP shunts more acetyl-CoA conversion to fatty acids. Alcoholics often suffer from a "fatty liver," and they can die from the resulting liver disease.

Many studies have looked at the health-related effects of moderate alcohol consumption. For moderate drinking, the Centers for Disease Control and Prevention (CDC November 7, 2014) recommends one drink per day for women and two drinks per day for men. Ethanol blood levels peak higher in females, probably because ethanol is excluded from fat stores and women generally have a higher percent body fat than males. Women may also have faster uptake from the GI-tract. The body's maximum rate to metabolize ethanol is one "drink" per hour. Very little can be done to accelerate alcohol metabolism. A standard drink is equal to:

Beer: 12 ounces (355 ml), 4% to 6% alcohol
Wine: 5 ounces (150 ml), 12% to 14% alcohol
Spirits: 1.5 ounces (45 ml), 40% alcohol for 80-proof liquor

Figure 15.1 Ethanol metabolism.

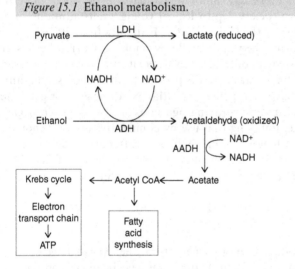

Legend: A schematic is shown for the oxidation of ethanol to acetaldehyde by alcohol dehydrogenase (ADH). NAD+ accepts the electrons and becomes reduced as NADH. Lactate can be a byproduct as the NADH is oxidized back to NAD+ so that it can participate in glycolysis, by the enzyme lactate dehydrogenase (LDH). The acetaldehyde is rapidly oxidized further to acetate by acetaldehyde dehydrogenase (AADH), also producing NADH. Acetate is converted to acetyl-CoA in mitochondria. Acetyl-CoA can be used to make ATP. However, it requires NAD+ for this process, and NAD+ is being used for ethanol metabolism. When ATP is not in demand or NAD+ levels are low, acetyl-CoA is converted into fatty acids.

The ethanol content of a standard drink is 0.6 ounces (14.0 grams or 1.2 tablespoon). In a strict interpretation of the CDC recommendation, this amount of drinking is the daily limit and is not a value that is averaged over several days or a week. The reason for this interpretation is that elevated **blood alcohol content (BAC)** creates the possible negative consequences of drinking.

However, there is a social component to drinking, as well as the difference associated with a weekend night versus a weeknight. A broader interpretation of the CDC guidelines would suggest that "moderate drinking" consists of no more than eight drinks per week for women and 12 to 14 for men, with no more than three to four standard drinks per drinking episode (Moderatedrinking.com 2014). To define moderate drinking, we must also include a time component and consider how quickly the drinks are consumed. The desired result is to maintain the BAC below 0.055, despite the higher limit of 0.08% for driving in the United States (see Table 15.1). One way of looking at moderate drinking is that alcohol consumption should be significantly less than the amount needed to become intoxicated. Excessive drinking is defined as greater than four drinks during a single occasion for a woman (or greater than eight drinks per week) and five drinks for a man (or greater than fifteen drinks per week). Binge drinking is defined as five or more drinks for men, and four or more for women, in about two hours.

Pregnant women and people under 21 years of age should avoid alcohol consumption altogether. Note, however, that when statistics are gathered regarding drinking, the researchers often consider an adult to be any subject over 18. When consumed in moderate amounts, ethanol may have beneficial effects on the cardiovascular system in some individuals. Red wine may benefit those with a poor lipid/cardiovascular profile. Consumption of red wine may explain the "French paradox," the low incidence of coronary artery disease in individuals who consume a diet rich in saturated fats, although this is just one potential explanation. For people who exercise regularly and are fit, little benefit is expected, since the exercise contribution outweighs the weaker cardiovascular effect of drinking red wine (Scribbans, Ma, Edgett, et al. 2014). A chemical called resveratrol is one of many possible active components found in the skins of red grapes. Resveratrol is turning out to be a very interesting chemical with multiple properties, including anti-aging and anti-cancer activities.

From a population or statistical viewpoint, moderate drinking does not have significant negative consequences and may have slight benefits. Light to moderate alcohol use is associated with a reduced risk of dementia and Alzheimer's disease, and it possibly has a protective effect on cognitive decline and pre-dementia syndromes during aging (Panza, Frisardi, Seripa, et al. 2012). Wine consumption may be more healthful than consumption of beer or spirits, although this is not conclusive (Panza, Capurso, D'Introno, et al. 2009). It is not possible to specify the age to start drinking or the level of alcohol intake that might be protective for cognitive function and dementia (Panza et al. 2012).

High rates of binge drinking are a major public health concern. Most college campuses actively try to educate young people about the problems associated with binge drinking, especially in athletes. Binge drinking leads to inappropriate behavior and serious accidents. Table 15.1 shows the physiological effects of increasing BAC. Compared to many other countries, the United States' legal limit of 0.08 BAC for driving is quite high. Some countries have zero tolerance: if you drink, you do not drive (Drinkdriving.org 2015).

Exercise Pharmacology

Limited data show a slight increase in ethanol clearance with exercise. In rats, aerobic activity can increase the clearance rate of ethanol. Acute alcohol intake causes cutaneous vessels to dilate and increases heat radiation (causing the flushed look, with red cheeks, often observed). It increases resting heart rate. Most effects of alcohol on the CNS and peripheral nervous system are ergolytic. Ethanol stimulates postganglionic fibers in the sympathetic nervous system, causing a rise in heart rate and blood pressure. As a diuretic, it causes negative water balance and electrolyte loss. Note that these diuretic effects can add to exercise effects on salt and water balance. Rehydration with water or sport drinks may help during recovery or decrease the hangover effect.

Table 15.1 Changes in behavior at different levels of blood alcohol content

Blood Alcohol Content (% by volume)	Behavior
0.02–0.03	No loss of coordination; slight euphoria and loss of shyness. Mildly relaxed and maybe a little lightheaded.
0.04–0.06	Feeling of well-being, relaxation, sensation of warmth. Judgment is slightly impaired, along with reasoning and memory. Less cautious. Behavior may become exaggerated and emotions intensified.
0.07–0.09	Impairment present in everyone, including impairment of balance, speech, and hearing. Feelings of euphoria in some. Self-control and caution are reduced. Riskier behaviors displayed. Judgment, reason, and memory suffer. You are not functioning as well as you think.
	Driving skills, such as vision, steering, lane changing, and reaction time, are impaired. A BAC of 0.08 is the legal limit for driving.
0.10–0.125	Significant impairment of motor coordination, balance, vision, reaction time, and hearing. Loss of good judgment, and speech may be slurred.
0.13–0.15	Gross motor impairment, blurred vision, and loss of balance. Euphoria is replaced by dysphoria (anxiety, restlessness). Judgment and perception are severely impaired. Vomiting is common.
0.16–0.19	Dysphoria and nausea; the person becomes incapacitated.
0.20	The person requires help to stand or walk and may not feel pain if injured. The gag reflex is impaired, and the person can choke if he or she does vomit. Blackouts are likely, memory of the event unlikely.
0.25	All functions are severely impaired; there is near total loss of motor function control. Serious injury is possible from falls or other accidents. Increased risk of asphyxiation from choking on vomit.
0.30–0.40	The person becomes unconscious or has little comprehension of the surroundings. This is at the level of surgical anesthesia. Coma and death are possible.

Legend: The effects of alcohol are greatly influenced by individual variations among users, including gender, body weight and BMI, activity level, and stomach contents. Some users may show a behavior at a much lower BAC.
Source: Preeti Dalawari, Chief Editor, Eric B Staros (2014). Ethanol level. Medscape http://emedicine.medscape.com/article/2090019-overview

Ethanol suppresses inhibitions, is a CNS depressant, and may de-motivate athletes from extra effort. Ethanol suppresses ventilatory adaptation. At 3,000 meters altitude, blood pO_2 decreased while pCO_2 increased significantly after ingestion of 50 grams of alcohol, probably due to a decreased respiratory rate (Roeggla, Roeggla, Roeggla, et al. 1995). Most studies with ethanol show impairment in automobile drivers and pilots. Navy pilots showed significantly poorer performance on flight simulators 14 hours after having a blood alcohol level of 0.1%, compared to pilots who had no alcohol for 48 hours (Yesavage & Leirer 1986).

Ethanol acutely impairs aerobic performance. In rugby players, an 11.4% decrease in VO_2max was observed following alcohol ingestion. Anaerobic performance was not affected to the same degree (O'Brien 1993). These results are consistent with the metabolic effects discussed above—ethanol can suppress oxygen-dependent mitochondrial production of ATP. Ethanol slows times in sprinting and middle distances and impairs maximum work during cycle ergometry. The exerciser may feel that reflex time has improved, but often it has declined. Ethanol decreases hand–eye coordination, arm steadiness, and reaction time. The negative effects of alcohol on the heart and capillary density in skeletal muscle are blunted with regular exercise (Pesta, Angadi, Burtscher, & Roberts 2013). Most effects of alcohol are ergolytic, even though drinking involves ingesting fluids and calories. Beer and most drinks are a source of carbohydrates (about 12 grams in a regular beer and 5 grams in a light beer). The euphoria wears off, and the diuretic effects defeat any possible performance benefits from the consumption of alcohol.

Health Risks

The short-term effects of drinking in moderation are minimal for most people. Moderate drinking may actually enhance longevity and cardiovascular health. However, the calories add up when drinking; most drinks are over 100 calories and some craft beers or sweet cocktails can easily be 300 calories. The body uses the calories in alcohol before using glucose or fatty acids, contributing to weight gain. For individuals with sensitivity to alcohol or the inability to metabolize ethanol normally, it is best to avoid drinking. Binge behavior creates many risks besides the direct effects on organs such as the liver and heart. Poor choices related to binge drinking behavior could affect or ruin a lifetime.

To summarize the diverse effects of ethanol consumption in humans:

- *Cardiovascular*: dehydration, electrolyte loss, cutaneous vasodilation and potential heat loss, cardiac arrhythmias ("holiday heart syndrome").
- *Neurological*: impaired judgment, coordination, and reaction time.
- *Metabolic*: impaired aerobic metabolism, dehydration, fatty liver.
- *Nutritional imbalances*: alcoholics often have dietary deficiencies (vitamins C and B complex, potassium, magnesium), liver problems, and GI blood loss.
- *Drug interactions*: drowsiness with antihistamines and other drugs with sedative activity, GI problems with NSAIDs (including aspirin), liver toxicity with acetaminophen.

Dependency on alcohol creates its own serious set of health concerns. Physical and psychological dependence can become all consuming. The seriousness of the withdrawal syndrome often requires hospitalization or use of a treatment center. Drugs can be given to discourage alcohol consumption. Alcoholics who clean up and get sober often need a strong support system at home (or work) for help and encouragement.

Alcoholism

Alcoholism is a form of alcohol dependence. It involves excessive or maladaptive alcohol use. Tolerance can develop, requiring that the alcoholic use more alcohol to achieve the desired effect. Alcoholics lose control over the amount and length of time they drink and are unable to cut back or stop. They give up important social, occupational, or recreational activities and continue to drink despite knowing alcohol is causing them serious problems. One of the reasons they continue to drink is the unpleasantness of the withdrawal symptoms. When they reduce or stop drinking, they can suffer from rapid pulse, tremors, nausea, vomiting, agitation, anxiety, insomnia, hallucinations, and possible life-threatening seizures. The result is that they start drinking in the morning and continue throughout the day.

There may be a genetic predisposition for alcoholism. Close relatives of an alcoholic are more likely to abuse alcohol than the general population. One of the candidate genes is a variant dopamine receptor that increases a person's chance of developing alcoholism, but alcoholism is more complex and is not attributable to a single gene. Twice as many men than women are alcohol dependent, and individuals who start drinking before age 21 are more likely to develop dependence. Social factors (e.g., family or peers) and psychological factors (e.g., stress or inadequate coping mechanisms) can contribute to alcohol abuse. Once the disease develops, the original factors may become less important as the physical dependence becomes dominant.

PES Watch

Alcohol is prohibited in competition. It is banned in certain sports (anything involving driving, boating, flying, archery, or karate). The NCAA bans the use of ethanol. The USOC reserves the right to test for it. Ethanol has no ergogenic benefit before, during, or after a competition. For serious competitors, alcohol should be avoided for 24 to 48 hours before a competition. Alcohol decreases psychomotor skills and recovery from injury. Nutrient deficiencies are a problem in heavy drinkers. The diuretic action of alcohol can make salt and water loss important.

Nicotine

Nicotine is a powerful drug with complex pharmacological activities, as well as a potent poison (used to kill pests), acting as an acetylcholine receptor agonist. Nicotine is just one of hundreds of chemicals present in cigarette smoke, and cigarettes can contain a range of nicotine concentrations, from 8 to 20 mg per cigarette. About 1 mg is absorbed per smoked cigarette, which starts reaching the brain in 7–15 seconds. There is enough pure nicotine in about five cigarettes to be lethal. It has about a 60-minute half-life.

How Nicotine Works

Nicotine causes the release of epinephrine, which can speed the resting heart rate, raise the basal metabolic rate, block insulin activity, and increase blood sugar. In the brain, nicotine acts as an acetylcholine agonist and may cause the release of dopamine from dopaminergic neurons. The dopamine release is part of the "reward" circuit that contributes to "feeling good." Nicotine may also cause the release of glutamate, which is involved in memory; glutamate release could help reinforce the good feelings associated with the dopamine activity. However, tolerance develops to many of these effects, requiring higher doses of nicotine to get the same level of pleasure. Given the combination of tolerance with nicotine's 60-minute half-life, smokers tend to crave another cigarette more frequently over time.

Exercise Pharmacology

For several decades, smoking's negative impact on exercise performance has been documented. Inhaled smoke has particulates that negatively affect air exchange, increase mucous, and increase airway resistance. The most dominant negative effect, though, probably results from the presence of carbon monoxide in smoke. Carbon monoxide has higher affinity for hemoglobin than O_2. To distribute sufficient O_2 in the presence of carbon monoxide, the heart works harder. As a result, smokers have a higher resting heart rate and decreased VO_2max. Carbon monoxide also competes for O_2 binding to myoglobin in muscle cells, decreasing O_2 availability for ATP production. The lactic acid threshold decreases, and increased lactate production occurs at comparable intensity levels, leading to more rapid muscle fatigue in smokers. The negative effects of carbon monoxide can be as pronounced in nonsmokers exposed to secondhand smoke.

Other documented negative effects of cigarette smoking (and smoke) include diminished benefits from training and decreased muscle strength and flexibility. Smokers are more likely to suffer from sleep disturbances. Smokers suffer from shortness of breath at three times the rate of nonsmokers. They have an increased risk of injury, and they heal more slowly. Young smokers have altered developmental and growth rates. Smokers (and smoke) can alter platelet activity, cause atherosclerotic lesions, and cause cardiac infarct.

The role of pure nicotine, without the complication of the complex mixture of chemicals in cigarette smoke, has been tested in experimental animals and in humans. Animals can be treated with nicotine at regular intervals to mimic the dosing seen with smoking. Human studies use nicotine-containing nasal spray, chewing gum, or patches as sources of the drug. The gum and patches are commercially available to help wean smokers away from their nicotine addiction. Though patches and gums are intended as aids to quitting, nicotine delivered in these ways may have ergogenic properties. Nicotine administration can increase heart rate and blood pressure with no effect on ventilation during light physical activity. Nicotine has little effect on RPE, but it does increase circulating levels of epinephrine and norepinephrine. Blood levels of free fatty acids and lactate also increase. However, at high exercise intensity, these effects may be overshadowed by the endogenous sympathetic response. A review of ten studies showed the difficulty in these experiments, with differences reported in individual responses, tolerance to nicotine, the nicotine delivery system used and problems with experimental design. The intervention of nicotine or smokeless tobacco on muscular strength and power, maximal endurance, and high-intensity exercise produced mixed results. Most of the studies reported little effect; two studies observed an ergogenic effect and one had an ergolytic effect (Mündel 2017).

Nicotine and smoking certainly have central effects, as well, including improved alertness and positive mood changes. By increasing dopamine release in certain regions of the brain involved with the reward response, nicotine could enhance motivation during prolonged exercise. A similar activity may be shared by caffeine, which has ergogenic properties. In one study on the effects of nicotine, 10 of 12 healthy males significantly increased their time on a cycle ergometer, without significant differences in RPE, plasma glucose, lactate, or free fatty acids. Results like these support a centrally acting mechanism by nicotine (Mundel & Jones 2006).

Some smokers are regular exercisers. They may think that by exercising, they are reducing the harm associated with smoking. Some may use smoking and exercise as part of a weight-reduction strategy, as smoking does suppress appetite. Smokers with good exercise habits have other behaviors (better diet, seatbelt use, attitudes toward illegal drugs, etc.) that are similar to exercising nonsmokers, and they may be, as a group, more amenable to cessation of smoking than non-exercising smokers (Shephard 1989). Smokers who are not physically active have proportionally higher levels of behaviors associated with health risk.

Exercise can help people quit smoking. Vigorous exercise may decrease withdrawal symptoms and craving from quitting smoking. Women who quit smoking and followed a 12-week exercise program showed increased time to exhaustion and an improved VO$_2$max (Albrecht, Marcus, Roberts, et al. 1998). Quitting smoking, however it is accomplished, is a worthy goal for any smoker, and the attempt should be encouraged and supported by all who care about that person.

Health Risks

The negative health effects of nicotine have been known for decades. Smoking is a major contributor to death by cancer, coronary heart disease, stroke, peripheral vascular disease, and chronic obstructive pulmonary disease. Smoking is the cause of one in five deaths in the United States. Estimates are that one in three of all cancer cases are directly related to cigarette smoke, including 80% to 90% of all lung cancer cases. From an economic standpoint, smoking costs the country close to $300 billion annually. About half of that cost is for direct medical care and about half is the lost productivity of smokers with poor health (CDC).

The risks of **secondhand smoke** (environmental tobacco smoke) have also been documented. Secondhand smoke contains at least 250 chemicals with documented toxicity; 50 of these chemicals can cause cancer. There is no risk-free level of secondhand smoke. Brief exposure can be dangerous, especially for children and other at-risk populations, such as the elderly. Nonsmokers exposed to secondhand smoke at home or work have increased risk of disease, including cancer and heart disease. There are also health problems from **thirdhand smoke** (Martins-Green, Adhami, Frankos, et al. 2014). Thirdhand smoke is the term for the oily residue that covers surface areas in places where people smoke. The complex chemical residue that coats surfaces has significant toxic activity, especially when it comes into direct contact with the skin.

Laws limiting smoking in public places have decreased the detectable levels of nicotine in nonsmokers. Increases in the price of cigarettes correlate with decreased rates of smoking in certain subpopulations. However, the fact that 20% of the U.S. population still smokes fuels the massive negative health consequences in the United States and around the world (CDC April 24, 2014). Quitting the habit is very difficult, due to the addictive nature of nicotine and the unpleasant withdrawal syndrome. Withdrawal symptoms include anxiety, irritability, anger issues, restlessness, insomnia, difficulty concentrating, and weight gain. Most smokers have triggers that cause them to fail in their efforts to quit. Understanding and dealing with those triggers can help, whether they are emotional or associated with certain social settings. Nicotine substitutes may help some people, and electronic cigarettes provide an acceptable alternative for some, but regardless of the difficulty or mode of quitting, the need to quit is critical to a healthy lifestyle for the smoker and those around them. The body does respond fairly quickly following cessation of smoking, in terms of certain respiratory and cardiovascular issues. Long-term effects, such as cancer, however, are age-related and may not become apparent for many years.

Electronic Cigarettes: Novelty or the Next Public Health Menace?

Electronic cigarettes (E-cigarettes, also called vaporizers) were initially marketed as a way to curb the nicotine addiction and stop smoking. However, the surge in their popularity, especially among young people, suggests that their use as a drug-delivery mechanism may be creating many new problems.

E-cigarettes contain synthetic nicotine and no tobacco products. They come in many shapes and sizes. The user inhales through a mouthpiece that triggers a sensor that, in turn, activates a battery-powered heater. The heater vaporizes the synthetic liquid nicotine in a small cartridge. The cartridges come in many different flavors with or without nicotine. The cartridge also contains propylene glycol (PEG), a compound used to make theatrical smoke. When the heater activates, the user gets a puff of hot gas that feels a lot like tobacco smoke. The heater also activates a light at the "lit" end of the e-cigarette. When the user exhales, the e-cigarette produces a cloud of PEG vapor that looks like smoke. The vapor quickly dissipates. Each cartridge is good for several uses.

E-cigarettes have raised concerns among the health community, pharmaceutical industry, regulators, and governments, with some jurisdictions now regulating their use in public spaces. Legislation and public health investigations are currently pending in many countries. In 2014, the FDA and the European Parliament passed regulations requiring standardization and quality control for vaporizers and the liquids contained in the cartridges. In 2019, the FDA outlined new potential e-cigarette policies and guidelines. A number of states and local governments have taken steps to restrict e-cigarette use. Many states have raised the age for purchasing tobacco products and e-cigarettes to 21. Additionally, many states are banning flavored vaporizers after a sharp increase in the number of serious lung injuries in habitual users.

PES Watch

The potential of nicotine as an ergogenic agent is sufficiently documented, and WADA has begun a monitoring program. Whereas smoking is mostly ergolytic, alternative sources of nicotine are readily available. Tobacco products that are chewed or placed under the gums are examples. Nicotine gum and transdermal patches, intended to help smokers quit, are additional sources of nicotine. Nicotine is a sympathetic nervous system stimulant that acts centrally and in the periphery. Nicotine delays feeling of fatigue centrally, similar in some ways to caffeine (Pesta et al.). WADA's monitoring program for nicotine began in 2013 with in-competition testing. A significant number of positive urine tests for nicotine could result in tighter rules governing its use. The use of transdermal patches requires attention, as increased rates of absorption occur during exercise, and nicotine-related toxicity is possible.

Cannabis

Cannabis, derived from hemp plants, is usually smoked as a resin (hashish) or as leaves and flowers (marijuana). It can also be consumed orally in baked goods. Alternatively, it can be extracted with heated vegetable oil, as most of the active ingredients at lipid-soluble and many are heat activated. Hundreds of potentially active compounds exist in the variety of cannabis plants found around the world. As we discussed earlier in the context of medicinal marijuana for treatment of pain (Chapter 11), smoking marijuana by athletes raises a series of questions besides legality. The primary question is whether smoking "pot" is ergogenic or ergolytic. Although there is not a lot of research on the effect of cannabis on exercise performance, the general belief is that cannabis use is ergolytic. It is on most lists of banned substances because of its illegality (as a Schedule 1 narcotic); there continues to be debate whether it is a potential performance-enhancing substance.

How Cannabis Works

There are two major types of cannabis plants commonly referred to as marijuana or pot. *Sativa* is a taller and slimmer plant with longer leaves. Upon smoking, it provides the 'high' that many find uplifting and euphoric. Some feel more energetic, alert, and creative after smoking it. *Indica* is a shorter and bushier plant. After smoking, it is relaxing, stimulates the appetite, provides pain relief, and aids sleep. These differences reinforce the complexity of plant-based medicinals and the hundred or so active compounds they produce. In addition, cannabis types are capable of cross-breeding to produce fertile progeny. The result is a profusion of cannabis varieties available through the legal and black markets. It makes generalizations on the actions of marijuana difficult because of the degree of variation in plant product, let alone the variation in the human population.

   The main active ingredients of cannabis, delta9-tetrahydrocannabinol (THC) and cannabidiol (CDB), implied the existence of endogenous cannabinoids involved in memory, pain relief, euphoria, and patterns of eating and sleeping behavior. An endogenous ligand for the endocannabinoid system, **anandamide**, was discovered in 1992. Several additional derivatives of lipids with endogenous cannabinoid activity have been described since the discovery of anandamide (Battista, DiTommaso, Bari, &

Maccarrone 2012). Two of these additional cannabinoids are shown in Figure 15.2. Two cannabinoid receptors (CB1 and CB2) are known, in addition to the vanilloid receptor, now called TRPV1. TRPV1 is an ion-gated channel that responds to acidic pH and high temperatures. It is involved with pain sensation and is also the receptor for capsaicin (found in hot pepers). An additional receptor, the TRPA1 receptor, responds to cannabinoids. It is an ion channel involved in sensing cold, pain, and other irritants. Its activation in the spine alleviates pain, suggesting another mechanism for cannabinoids, as CB1 antagonists block this activation. Exercise increases the output of endogenous cannabinoids and may contribute to the runner's high, in association with the endogenous opiate/endorphins and other hormones.

Anandamide and the other cannabinoids primarily work through the CB1 and CB2 receptors. Agonists and antagonists have been developed for both receptor subtypes (Fowler, Holt, Nilsson, et al. 2005). Agonists decrease pain associated with inflammation. They also relieve neuropathic pain and pain associated with multiple sclerosis (see Chapter 11). They can stimulate appetite, and they have anti-emetic properties, making them particularly useful for certain cancer treatments. CB1 antagonists are being developed for appetite control (see Chapter 12). The cannabinoid receptors are G-protein–coupled receptors. CB1 is an abundant receptor in the nervous system, where it may inhibit release of neurotransmitters. These receptors may provide reinforcement of the serotonergic pathways, involved with suppressing spinal transmission of pain (Mallet, Daulhac, Bonnefont, et al. 2008). The CB1-related pathways are probably involved in the psychotropic effects associated with cannabinoids. CB2 is mainly associated with immune cells in the periphery, where it may modulate cytokine release. Cytokines are hormone-like factors that mediate inflammation and immunity. The CB2 receptors are more likely involved with the analgesic and anti-inflammatory properties of cannabinoids.

Figure 15.2 Structures for THC and endogenous cannabinoids.

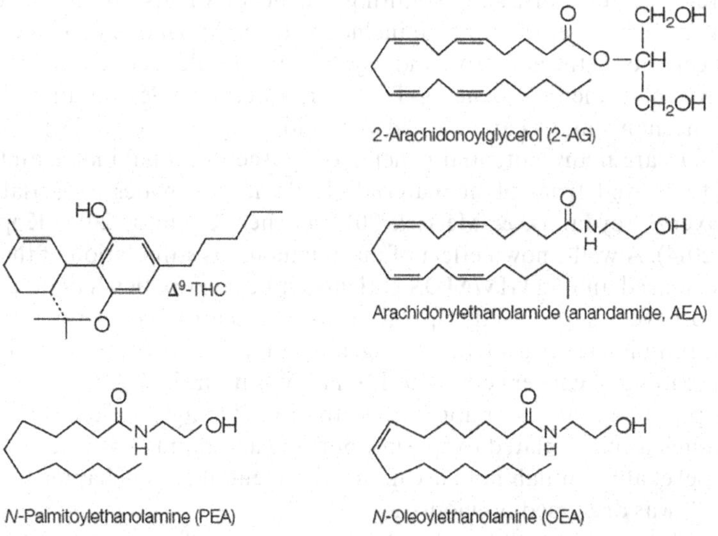

Legend: The psychoactive ingredient in marijuana, THC, is compared to the non-psychoactive but therapeutically important cannabinoids. Two of the endogenous cannabinoids (2-AG and AEA) are shown. Note that anandamide is related to the critical fatty acid arachidonic acid, mentioned in Chapters 7 and 11.

Because pain suppression and appetite stimulation make marijuana a useful adjuvant therapy in certain types of disease, several states have legalized medical marijuana. In 2014, Washington and Colorado voted to legalize and regulate the sale and possession of recreational marijuana; other states have followed suit. In 2019, recreational use was legal in eight states with some form of medical use permitted in another 30 states. Twelve states were still aligned with the federal laws making possession and use illegal. At the federal level, decriminalizing the sale of marijuana or its possession has been debated, as marijuana sales in states where it is legal have added an additional revenue stream from taxation. Moreover, legalization should lessen the burden in our correctional institutions, since a sizable portion of that population is doing time for pot-related offences.

Medicinal Use of Cannabis

The medicinal use of cannabis can be traced back to ancient physicians who prescribed marijuana for pain relief, digestive problems, and psychological disorders. Cannabis was used in ancient China, and Hindu sects used it for pain and stress relief. In early America, medical journals recommended hemp for the treatment of skin inflammation and loss of bladder control (Earleywine 2002). By 1937, marijuana use was banned in most states, and a change in tax laws made its sale and distribution cost-prohibitive.

Medical marijuana is available in several different forms. It can be smoked, ingested as an oil or added to foods, or taken as a pill or capsule. Cannabis contains about 60 active cannabinoids (referred to as phytocannabinoids when derived from plant material), with THC having strong psychoactive properties. In contrast, **cannabidiol** (CBD) is a non-psychoactive component that has therapeutic benefits without producing feelings of euphoria. Synthetic CB1 and CB2 agonists and antagonists are also available. Two FDA-approved cannabis-based drugs, dronabinol and nabilone, reduce chemotherapy-related nausea and vomiting in cancer patients. Additional cannabinoid drugs at various stages of approval include Sativex, Marinol, and Cesamet.

In the past, concerns over the addictive and psychoactive qualities of cannabis limited research on potential medical benefits. However, a better understanding of the pharmacological mechanisms of cannabinoid physiology has led to rapid progress in many areas. There are many potential benefits of synthetic cannabinoids and the phytocannabinoids derived from plant material. Table 15.2 provides a partial list (Greydanus, Hawver, Greydanus, & Merrick 2013; Pacher & Kunos 2013; Koppel, Brust, Fife, et al. 2014). A well-known effect of marijuana use is stimulation of the appetite, so it has been used among HIV/AIDS patients and cancer patients undergoing chemotherapy who have a suppressed appetite. Cancer research has also identified cannabinoids that inhibit cancer growth, angiogenesis (new blood vessel formation), and metastasis (spreading of cancer cells to additional sites in the body). In the case of multiple sclerosis, pills and oral sprays appear effective in reducing muscle spasms and easing symptoms such as pain related to spasms, burning and numbness, and overactive bladder (Koppel et al.). Cannabinoid use in the treatment of pain (Chapter 11) and obesity (Chapter 12) was discussed previously.

California became the first state to allow the medical use of marijuana in 1996. Almost half the states and the District of Columbia have public medical marijuana and cannabis programs. Medical marijuana cannot be prescribed, due to federal

Table 15.2 Some of the potential indications for cannabinoid-based therapy

Atherosclerosis	Epilepsy	Nausea and emesis in HIV
Anorexia in AIDS patients	Glaucoma	and cancer patients
Anxiety disorders, post-	Huntington's	Neuropathic pain
traumatic stress disorders,	disease	Obesity/metabolic
panic disorder, and obsessive-	Hypertension	syndrome
compulsive disorder	Inflammation and	Post-stroke neuroprotection
Cancer	wound healing	Rheumatoid arthritis
Crohn's disease	Multiple sclerosis	

laws, so physicians make *recommendations* or *referrals*. In most states, in order to receive marijuana for medical use legally from a dispensary, patients need to provide identification, fill out an application, and pay a fee to get some type of identification card. The application may require treatment information from the consulting physician.

CBD has become easily available, in part because hemp was reclassified from a Schedule 1 narcotic to an agricultural commodity in 2018. However, its legality and classification as a supplement are still getting sorted out at the federal and state levels. The purity of CBD on the market can vary greatly as it is in a regulation grey area. CBD comes in topical ointments, consumable oils, or baked goods and candy such as Gummy Bears. It is used for pain, anxiety, depression, and sleep disorders (Crippa, Guimarães, Campos, & Zuardi 2018). It is probably anti-inflammatory and may benefit children with certain types of epilepsy and autism. Similar oils derived from marijuana are effective against certain types of cancer, according to advocates on the internet. Since CBD has greatly reduced THC, side effects associated with smoking pot are not an issue, such as mind-altered states, altered judgment, impaired memory, and impaired coordination (Iffland & Grotenhermen 2017). Unwanted effects are relatively minor and depend on the dose and route of administration (topical application or ingested). They include fatigue, decreased appetite, and diarrhea. Long-term effects of heavy usage are not known at this time. CBD appears to be safer than other treatments for chronic pain and anxiety (Romero-Sandoval, Fincham, Kolano, et al. 2018).

CBD does not seem to work through CB1 and CB2 receptors. It may work through the TRPV1 receptor and possibly others including the adenosine A2A receptor (Chapter 14). However, pure CBD may be less effective than medical cannabis for managing many of these conditions, as the combination of many cannabinoids (including THC) produce a more robust stimulation of appetite and actions associated with medical marijuana. This combination effect is sometimes called an *entourage* effect, as the combination of compounds may be more effective than the sum of the individual parts. The recommendation for using CBD oil (or any plant-based material) is to start with a low dose and wait a couple of hours before taking more. The amount on the label may not be accurate and it can take time for the active ingredients to reach peak blood levels and distribute to the brain or other tissues. With so little basic research available, and such great variation from source to source, normal dosing and long-term effects are generally unknown.

Exercise Pharmacology

There is little research available that supports a direct ergogenic effect of cannabis. Indirect benefits that have been suggested include relaxation, euphoria, better sleep, and reduced stress associated with competition (Pesta et al.). Benefit to athletes may come after the game, as they unwind from the adrenaline rush of competition. However, these effects are very hard to quantify. Some users can have an opposite effect; bouts of paranoia, severe anxiety, and panic disorders have been reported. Most of marijuana's physiological responses are potentially ergolytic. These responses include impaired cognition, psychomotor activity, and exercise performance. Occasional or low cumulative marijuana smoking was not associated with adverse effects on pulmonary function (Pletcher, Vittinghoff, Kalhan, et al. 2012). Older literature suggests that inexperienced users occasionally have an elevated heart rate. There has been debate over whether smoking marijuana increases the chance of a cardiovascular event, particularly in individuals with a pre-existing condition or the elderly. A "marijuana paradox" has been suggested—that inhalation of marijuana may be linked to precipitation of acute coronary syndrome, but modulation of the endocannabinoid system by a non-inhalation route may help against the development of atherosclerosis (Singla, Sachdeva, & Mehta 2012).

The changing legality of cannabis creates the need for more research to inform policy on its use, particularly the effect of recreational cannabis on exercise and general health (Gillman, Hutchison, & Bryan 2015). A common perception is that cannabis decreases motivation, including motivation to exercise. However, there is anecdotal evidence of cannabis use prior to athletic activity. WADA includes cannabis as a prohibited substance in sport, partly because it is believed that it may enhance sports performance. Athletes that use cannabis as an anti-anxiety aid and to improve sleep may think their performance improves, but this is very hard to measure. There is limited scientific evidence for positive or negative effects on motivation, exercise performance, and recovery. Older studies from the 1970s and 1980s used less potent cannabis compared to what is available today (Gillman et al.). Different strains of cannabis and different delivery mechanisms cloud the field. Sativa probably differs from Indica when smoked (or ingested) prior to evaluation of exercise performance. Peak blood levels occur within minutes when smoking, but hours after taken orally. Previously, much of the literature concentrated on finding negative health consequences of cannabis use. Currently, research is trying to confirm the medical benefits of its use, such as decreasing pain and inflammation. If or when cannabis is legal at the federal and international level, then controlled research studies will be more common and the results more informative.

Health Risks

Marijuana, as a plant, is difficult to test for efficacy and safety because of the large variation in active chemicals. Marijuana does have side effects, such as problems with attention, judgment, and balance. Marijuana suppresses the immune system, which can be helpful in some patients suffering from chronic inflammation but can create problems in others who may be susceptible to infection. It is still not clear whether heavy smoking marijuana carries a significant cancer risk; occasional use apparently does not. The sedative effect can be compounded with ingestion of alcohol or other drugs. The ability to drive a car or pilot an airplane can be compromised. Research continues on the seriousness of dependence, withdrawal syndrome, and other aspects of long-term moderate to heavy use of cannabis. Clinical trials of cannabinoid-derived drugs have introduced unexpected complexities, suggesting that a better understanding of the endocannabinoid system will be necessary for clinically successful treatments (Pacher & Kunos) when cannabis is used for medicinal purposes. A major concern involves younger, regular users who may succumb to the negative effects that compromise concentration, motivation, and training intensity.

PES Watch

The active ingredient THC and its metabolites are detectable in urine tests. In 2013, WADA raised its threshold value to 150 ng/ml for a positive test during competition to minimize a positive test resulting from passive smoke or eating foods containing hemp-derived products. For many governing agencies, testing is limited to in-competition testing. In sporadic smokers, THC metabolites can be detected for three to five days after smoking. Regular smokers may require ten days before the level is below the limit of detection. Sport federations vary in their enforcement of cannabis testing. Professional football (soccer in the United States) players have been cautioned because the drug can be detected several days after partaking. Some leagues and competitions may not consider a positive test for cannabis grounds for suspension, whereas other leagues, such as the National Football League, have a stricter limit (raised from 15 ng/ml to 35 ng/ml in 2014). As laws governing the legalized use of cannabis change around the world, sport-governing bodies may have to reconsider the penalty associated with cannabis use. Moreover, some player associations and unions have argued for relaxing penalties for marijuana use in the current legal climate. They claim that the pain relief from cannabis is safer than the opioids provided by team doctors.

Elder Concerns

The use of medical marijuana is becoming more prevalent among senior citizens, especially as the Baby Boomers age. In states where it is legal, dispensaries often provide sativa or indica varieties. Sativa provides a little energy boost during the day that may help with the chores like cleaning, laundry, and cooking. It helps with appetite and can alleviate nausea from chemotherapy. It is also useful for headaches and can improve the mood of seniors who are suffering from chronic pain and terminal illness, often increasing laughter, talkativeness, and enhanced perception of music with visual effects. Indica provides relaxation in the evening and helps those that have trouble sleeping. It is more useful as a pain suppressant and muscle relaxant. It increases appetite and can therefore help prevent weight loss, muscle wasting, and frailty. Medical marijuana dispensaries may sell hybrids in addition to sativa or indica. In general, THC has the stimulating effect generating the "high" in marijuana, while CBD has more of the 'body' effect with anti-epileptic and anti-anxiety properties.

Medical marijuana does not need to be smoked. For example, CBD can be delivered with a vaporizer (similar to an e-cigarette), topical cream, ingestible tinctures, or edibles.

CBD extracts deliver many of benefits of marijuana without making the user high. The positive effects of CBD can help with many of the problems the aging population suffers and, in some cases, decrease the dependence on prescription drugs (NSAIDs, opioids, sleeping pills etc.). Reasons why seniors should consider CBD include:

- Pain Relief—creams can aid arthritis and nerve pain, as can ingested forms.
- Insomnia and Sleep Issues—CBD helps with deep sleep (a problem in seniors).
- Anti-aging—CBD may be a stronger antioxidant than Vitamin C and Vitamin E.
- Stimulates Appetite—seniors with loss of appetite have significant health issues.
- Bone Health—CBD can help heal fractures and support healthier bones.
- Fights Glaucoma—CBD may decrease intraocular pressure at higher dosage.
- Alzheimer's and Dementia—CBD may reduce inflammation, help the brain repair.

Before taking CBD, seniors should consult their physician. In the elderly, some of the side effects may be more pronounced and require attention or monitoring. Dizziness, low blood pressure, abnormal heartbeat, drowsiness, and other interactions are possible. In a small percentage of users, there is an increase in liver enzymes. CBD is being produced without regulation, resulting in products that vary widely in quality and quantity of active ingredients. Possession of marijuana is illegal in several states.

Conclusion

Drinking in moderation may actually have some health benefits. Excess alcohol can affect the liver and most organ systems to some degree. Alcohol is ergolytic and can negatively impact judgment, coordination, and motivation. Cigarette smoking is a major health problem for everyone who comes in contact with it—the smoker, those who breathe the secondhand smoke, and those who come into contact with surfaces contaminated by cigarette smoke. The many chemicals in cigarette smoke can kill in many different ways.

In many countries and states in the United States, cannabis use and possession has been decriminalized. Derivatives or extracts of cannabis, such as CBD, may have health benefits without the high associated with smoking pot.

Key Concepts Review

anandamide	ethanol
blood alcohol content (BAC)	nicotine
cannabidiol (CBD)	secondhand smoke
cannabis	thirdhand smoke
electronic cigarettes	

Review Questions

1 You are training with an elite athlete who likes to go out for beers, often. How is this behavior affecting her performance? What reasons could you give her to back off a little?

2　Your roommate smokes, and it is driving you crazy. He tries to keep it outside, but he smells like an ashtray. He recently has talked about quitting, but he doesn't think it is that big a deal. How can you help convince him to quit, and what can you do to help?

3　A competitive swimmer just tested positive for marijuana. Did he gain a competitive advantage?

4　You just found out your grandmother has gummy bears with CBD. Should you be concerned?

References

Albrecht AE, Marcus BH, Roberts M, Forman DE, Parisi AF (1998) Effect of smoking cessation on exercise performance in female smokers participating in exercise training. *Am J Cardiol* 82:950–955

Battista N, DiTommaso M, Bari M, Maccarrone M (2012) The endocannabinoid system: an overview. *Front Behav Neurosci* 6:9. doi: 10.3389/fnbeh.2012.00009

Centers for Disease Control and Prevention Excessive drinking costs U.S. $223.5 billion. www.cdc.gov/features/alcoholconsumption/

Centers for Disease Control and Prevention Fact sheets – Binge drinking. www.cdc.gov/alcohol/fact-sheets/binge-drinking.htm

Centers for Disease Control and Prevention Smoking and tobacco use. www.cdc.gov/tobacco/data_statistics/fact_sheets/fast_facts/index.htm

Crippa JA, Guimarães FS, Campos AC, Zuardi AW (2018) Translational investigation of the therapeutic potential of cannabidiol (CBD): toward a new age. *Front Immunol* 9:2009

Dalawari P (2014) Ethanol level. http://emedicine.medscape.com/article/2090019-overview

Drinkdriving.org (2015) Worldwide blood alcohol concentration (BAC) limits. www.drinkdriving.org/worldwide_drink_driving_limits.php

Earleywine M (2002) *Understanding Marijuana: A New Look at the Scientific Evidence.* New York: Oxford University Press

Fowler CJ, Holt S, Nilsson O, Jonsson K-O, Tiger G, Jacobsson SOP (2005) The endocannabinoid signaling system: pharmacological and therapeutic aspects. *Pharm Bioch Behav* 81:248–262

Gillman AS, Hutchison KE, Bryan AD (2015) Cannabis and exercise science: a commentary on existing studies and suggestions for future directions. *Sports Med* 45:1357–63.

Greydanus DE, Hawver EK, Greydanus MM, Merrick J (2013) Marijuana: current concepts. *Front Public Health* 1:42:1–12

Iffland K, Grotenhermen F (2017) An update on safety and side effects of cannabidiol: a review of clinical data and relevant animal studies. *Cannabis Cannabinoid Res* 2:139–154

Koppel BS, Brust JC, Fife T, Bronstein J, Youssof S, Gronseth G, Gloss D (2014) Systematic review: efficacy and safety of medical marijuana in selected neurologic disorders: report of the Guideline Development Subcommittee of the American Academy of Neurology. *Neurology* 82:1556–1563

Mallet C, Daulhac L, Bonnefont J, Ledent C, Etienne M, Chapuy E, Libert F, Eschalier A (2008) Endocannabinoid and serotonergic systems are needed for acetaminophen-induced analgesia. *Pain* 139:190–200

Martins-Green M, Adhami N, Frankos M, Valdez M, Goodwin B, Lyubovitsky J, Curras-Collazo M (2014) Cigarette smoke toxins deposited on surfaces: implications for human health. *PLoS One*, 9(1):e86391. doi:10.1371/journal.pone.0086391

Moderatedrinking.com (December 31, 2014) Welcome. www.moderatedrinking.com/

Mundel T, Jones DA (2006) Effect of transdermal nicotine administration on exercise endurance in men. *Exp Physiol* 91:705–713

Mündel T (2017) Nicotine: sporting friend or foe? a review of athlete use, performance consequences and other considerations. *Sports Med* 47: 2497–2506

O'Brien CP (1993) Alcohol and sport: impact of social drinking on recreational and competitive sports performance. *Sports Med* 15:71–77

Pacher P, Kunos G (2013) Modulating the endocannabinoid system in human health and disease—successes and failures. *FEBS J* 280:1918–1943

Panza F, Capurso C, D'Introno A, Colacicco AM, Frisardi V, Lorusso M, Santamato A, Seripa D, Pilotto A, Scafato E, Vendemiale G, Capurso A, Solfrizzi V (2009) Alcohol drinking, cognitive functions in older age, predementia, and dementia syndromes. *J Alzheimers Dis* 17:7–31

Panza F, Frisardi V, Seripa D, Logroscino G, Santamato A, Imbimbo BP, Scafato E, Pilotto A, Solfrizzi V (2012) Alcohol consumption in mild cognitive impairment and dementia: harmful or neuroprotective? *Int J Geriatr Psychiatry* 27:1218–1238

Pesta DH, Angadi SS, Burtscher M, Roberts CK (2013) The effects of caffeine, nicotine, ethanol, and tetrahydrocannabinol on exercise performance. *Nutr Metabol* 10:71–86

Pletcher MJ, Vittinghoff E, Kalhan R, Richman J, Safford M, Sidney S, Lin F, Kertesz S (2012) Association between marijuana exposure and pulmonary function over 20 years. *JAMA* 307(2):173–181

Romero-Sandoval EA, Fincham JE, Kolano AL, Sharpe BN, Alvarado-Vázquez PA (2018) Cannabis for chronic pain: challenges and considerations. *Pharmacotherapy* 38:651–662.

Roeggla G, Roeggla H, Roeggla M, Binder M, Laggner AN (1995) Effect of alcohol on acute ventilatory adaptation to mild hypoxia at moderate altitude. *Ann Intern Med* 122:925–927

Scribbans TD, Ma JK, Edgett BA, Vorobej KA, Mitchell AS, Zelt JG, Simpson CA, Quadrilatero J, Gurd BJ (2014) Resveratrol supplementation does not augment performance adaptations or fibre-type-specific responses to high-intensity interval training in humans. *Appl Physiol Nutr Metab* 39:1305–1313

Shephard RJ (1989) Adolphe Abrahams memorial lecture, 1988. Exercise and lifestyle change. *Br J Sports Med* 23:11–22

Singla S, Sachdeva R, Mehta JL (2012) Cannabinoids and atherosclerotic coronary heart disease. *Clin Cardiol* 35:329–335

Yesavage JA, Leirer VO (1986) Hangover effects on aircraft pilots 14 hours after alcohol ingestion: a preliminary report. *Am J Psychiatry* 143:1546–1550

Abstract

The search continues for ways to improve athletic performance. In earlier times, athletes consumed strychnine and brandy or concoctions containing heroin and cocaine for a perceived competitive edge or to delay fatigue and pain. Athletes today may be more sophisticated—or not, as reports surfaced in 2013 about extracts from deer antlers being used as a spray to provide insulin-like growth factor-1. When Lance Armstrong finally admitted to using banned substances in 2012/13, it became clear that he had avoided detection for years, until his story unraveled, with many of his former associates and team members providing important evidence that allowed investigators to make their case.

Anabolic steroids clearly can increase muscle cell size, muscle mass, and strength, especially in conjunction with a vigorous training program. Human growth hormone stimulates cell division and an increase in cell number. It increases levels of insulin-like growth factor-1, another powerful hormone involved in growth. Human growth hormone use probably speeds tissue repair and recovery, a very attractive property for professional athletes, who have intense training and game/competition schedules. Erythropoietin increases the oxygen-carrying capacity of the blood, a major factor in maximizing oxygen utilization—a key part of exercise performance. All three of these agents have therapeutic value for individuals who suffer from a deficiency in their production. All three of these hormones are prototypes for performance-enhancing substances: they allow athletes to get bigger and faster, recover faster, and increase VO_2max. Future athletes will likely continue to look for the edge, whether or not the means are legal and ethical. Keeping sport clean will require a significant cultural change, as appreciation for the benefits of participation, inclusion, and enjoyment must overcome the attitude of winning at all costs.

CASE EXAMPLE

Megan has been thinking of her friend and teammate Carla, the one that passed away from an opioid overdose. The more she thinks about her, the less she is surprised. Carla was a great teammate—she had great drive and enthusiasm that was contagious. But she also had a darker side. Megan first ran into Carla when they played against each other on the Select Team circuit. It was great they ended up teammates in college. But Carla was one of the girls she wondered about. Megan and some of her closer friends on the select team would speculate as to who they thought used testosterone cream.

It probably wasn't fair, but they did it anyway. Some girls just got bigger and stronger faster than others. Sometimes acne and the way their voice sounded were giveaways. On her various teams over those years, there seemed like a distinction between the girls that just loved the sport and competition, and those that were driven to excel and hoped to play for the National Team and have a pro career. Those girls, and the women they became, often had that darker, unhappier side. Their (and/or their parents'?) high expectations seemed to leave them unhappy and depressed a lot. Megan wondered if some of their problems weren't associated with the drugs they used. Not all the driven ones were users, but many of the users were driven ones. Megan was blessed with good foot speed and stamina and never really considered juicing. She misses her teammates and the games, but not the training and the rules. Maybe it is a good time for a run…

Learning Objectives

1   Learn how anabolic steroids are both masculinizing and growth stimulating.
2   Appreciate the effectiveness and the negative consequences of steroid use.
3   Recognize the impact of human growth hormone on professional sports.
4   Learn how blood doping works.
5   Appreciate the issues associated with maintaining drug-free sports.

Introduction

Historically, evidence of widespread cheating involving the use of PES has been un-covered in many sports (including cycling, baseball, football, and track and field). A PES is defined as any drug, supplement, or method that is identified by the World Anti-doping Agency (WADA) and placed on their Prohibited List (found at www.wada-ama. org/en). The Prohibited List includes the substances and methods that are prohibited in and out of competition for particular sports. These substances and methods are classified into different categories (e.g., stimulants, anabolic agents, beta-2 agonists, and so forth).

Performance-enhancing substances are found at practically all levels of competition. The Olympic Games usually present a scandal or two involving PES. High school ath-letes feel pressured to compete for college scholarships. College athletes want to be rec-ognized by pro scouts. Young professional athletes know that big money is possible if they excel. Older athletes look for ways to stay competitive with their younger counter-parts and keep their jobs (or their names in the highlights). Older athletes still want to win at Masters events or the Senior Olympics. Even weekend duffers want to stay com-petitive (Bird, Goebel, Burke, & Greaves 2016). Most professional and collegiate sports now have drug testing. Some testing is announced (e.g., at a competition or bowl game). Other testing can be random and occur year-round, not just during the season. But test-ing is expensive which limits many agencies and organizations from thorough sampling. The tests have to be sanctioned, especially if they lead to enforceable penalties. However, the sometimes vast income and the desire for a competitive edge continue to drive the development, distribution, and availability of PES. Successful testing programs tend to lag behind the rapidly emerging ways to cheat (Vlad, Hancu, Popescu, & Lungu 2018).

In this chapter, we will examine three different hormonal agents that athletes use to enhance their performance. All three have therapeutic value in patients who are deficient in their production. However, athletes have used these hormones to gain a competitive advantage, usually without a prescription or direct supervision of a physician. It is the propensity to self-administer these substances that leads us to consider them in this section of the text. The ways in which athletes illegally try to improve their performance is a vast field of research, and this chapter covers only a select few substances for which extensive research is available. Each chapter to this point has indicated the potential performance-enhancing capability of the drugs under discussion. In this chapter, we will first discuss how anabolic steroids and human growth hormone can increase muscle mass and its oxygen-utilizing capacity. We will then look at the history of blood doping and athletes' efforts to increase the oxygen-carrying capacity of their blood.

Anabolic Steroids

Anabolic steroids, sometimes called androgenic-anabolic steroids, are derivatives of the steroid hormone testosterone. They also have many names in street slang such as Roids or Juice. Anabolic steroids produce both masculinizing (**androgenic**) and tissue-building (**anabolic**) effects. None of the synthesized derivatives of testosterone have purely anabolic properties, although chemists have tried for years to synthesize such steroids. When athletes refer to "steroids," they generally mean anabolic steroids. Physicians who prescribe "steroids" usually are referring to corticosteroids. In the context of PES, the term steroids means anabolic steroids, which include testosterone and related chemicals. In earlier chapters, when we used the term steroids, we were discussing the treatment of asthma and inflammation; these steroids include corticosteroids and related compounds. To be clear, when discussing PES, we will use the term anabolic steroids.

Anabolic steroids enhance muscular mass and strength with little direct effect on aerobic exercise performance. Improved muscle strength contributes to performance in events such as the 100-meter dash. Anabolic steroids can also allow an athlete to train longer and harder. Assessment of the effects of anabolic steroids is difficult, primarily because individuals who regularly use them take them at very high doses. It is unethical to administer these dosages in research trials in males or to administer anabolic steroids at any dose to females. To complicate the issue further, the individuals who use the drugs for performance-enhancing effects often take additional drugs to compensate for or mask the use of anabolic steroids.

Following the isolation and synthesis of testosterone in the 1930s, chemists have unsuccessfully tried to derive a purely anabolic form, although derivatives have been made that are longer acting and more suitable for oral treatment. German troops used anabolic steroids in World War II to increase their strength and aggressiveness. Soviet Union athletes used anabolic steroids in the early 1950s, with noticeable results in the 1956 Olympics in Melbourne. In the 1960s and 1970s, officials studied the effects of anabolic steroids on performance. A urine test became available in the 1970s, and the IOC included anabolic steroids on the first list of banned substances. Seven athletes tested positive for anabolic steroids in the 1983 Pan Am Games. Ben Johnson set the world record in the 100-meter dash in the 1988 Seoul Olympics; however, his urine test was positive for stanozolol. As a result, he received no medal, and his time was not recognized as a world record. To what extent was his performance attributable to the drugs? The question is difficult to answer directly, but we do know that steroids improve strength and power, as we will discuss below. Ben Johnson tested positive again in 1993 and received a lifetime ban from international competition.

As discussed in Chapter 1, in the United States, the FDA and the DEA enforce the Controlled Substances Act. Five Schedules (i.e., classifications) list drugs based on criteria related to their potential for abuse, their usefulness for medical treatment, and agreements with other countries. In 1990, the United States reclassified anabolic steroids as a Schedule III drug to better control distribution, and rigorous testing has probably led to a decline in their use. Over the years, various sources have suggested an incidence of use at 3% to 12% for males and 1% to 5% for females in high school, 14% for collegiate athletes, and up to 75% for competitive bodybuilders (before testing was instituted in some competitions). In the early 1990s, studies showed that 9% of football players, 30% of "workout warriors" (non-elite athletes), and as many as 1 million people in the United States admitted current or previous use of anabolic steroids (Yesalis, Kennedy, Kopstein, & Bahrke 1993). Additionally, significant numbers of young people, including women, use anabolic steroids to achieve a certain athletic appearance (Kersey, Elliot, Goldberg, et al. 2012). This level of use has remained relatively constant.

Millions of dollars are spent annually on anabolic steroids, of which only a small fraction is for legal prescriptions. Anabolic steroids are used legally for hypogonadism, breast cancer, angioneurotic edema, and AIDS-related cachexia (wasting disease). Given the adverse effects, costs, and risks of anabolic steroid use, what are the potential gains in performance?

How Anabolic Steroids Work

Anabolic steroids bind the androgen receptor in the cytoplasm in responsive cells. The bound form of the receptor rapidly translocates to the cell nucleus, where it binds DNA at specific sequences and controls the expression of a variety of genes. One of the many genes induced by anabolic steroids is **insulin-like growth factor-1 (IGF-1)**, which is involved in metabolic control and different types of growth responses. Other genes expressed after steroid exposure contribute to the anabolic and androgenic properties of testosterone. The effects on gene expression can play out over several days following steroid treatment. Anabolic steroids are short-lived compounds, though their effects can persist for longer than their half-life suggests. Injected testosterone has a half-life of only minutes; one of its metabolites, dihydrotestosterone, retains activity and persists a little longer. The synthetic fluoxymesterone has a 9.2-hour half-life and can be taken orally. Other forms are available in creams or for injection IM. Most anabolic steroids are metabolized in the liver and are probably flow limited with exercise. Estrogen is a metabolite of testosterone (see Figure 16.1). With super-high doses of testosterone, levels of estrogen can become significant in males, causing changes in voice and gynecomastia (breast enlargement).

Exercise Pharmacology

Whether exercise causes the production and release of testosterone is controversial, with many conflicting reports. Exercise does not seem to change plasma testosterone levels when changes in volume (due to exercise) are taken into account. Problems also exist in interpreting the ergogenic properties of anabolic steroids, because of the large doses that athletes and bodybuilders take. The steroids have to bind their receptors to exert a physiological effect. Once the available receptors are saturated, excess steroid is probably metabolized and cleared, so taking 10 times the recommended dosage does not seem productive, since the receptor number is rate limiting.

Figure 16.1 Major pathways for steroid biosynthesis.

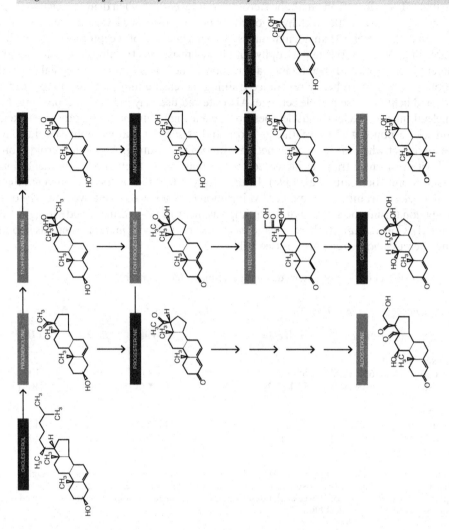

Legend: The close relationships among DHEA, androstenedione, testosterone, and estrogen are shown. Also shown are pathways to other important steroid hormones, such as aldosterone and cortisone.

Anabolic steroids can increase blood pressure, but they do not increase resting or exercise heart rate. Effects on VO_2max are variable and are not reliable indicators of endurance capacity following anabolic steroid use, so the effects on aerobic performance are uncertain. Anabolic steroids generally do not cause significant metabolic changes during exercise. With lean body mass, there does appear to be a dose–response relationship (Forbes 1985). The dose–response curve suggests a maximal effect, indicating saturation of the testosterone-mediated pathway. However, with muscle strength, the dose–response relationship is not as clear. No clear relationship exists between muscle strength gains and the dose, potency, or duration of use of anabolic steroids. Therefore, other factors, such as training regimen, diet, type of measurement, and initial hormone status also probably contribute. The effects from anabolic steroids slowly wear off when drug use ceases.

Females, as well as males with hypogonadism (low testosterone levels), are more responsive to anabolic steroids than normal males, perhaps because of receptor availability. It is possible that forced muscle hypertrophy with heavy resistance training could increase the number of receptors and thereby increase responsiveness to supra-physiological doses of anabolic steroids. With heavy resistance training increasing muscle mass, anabolic steroids could help increase muscle cell size. Also, steroid use may increase receptor number in skeletal muscle. Skeletal muscle does not have a high density of receptors, yet skeletal muscle responds well to treatment. Most studies suggest that anabolic steroids have a greater effect when taken in conjunction with weight training. Anabolic steroids combined with resistance training increased muscle mass more than either treatment alone (Bhasin, Storer, Berman, et al. 1996). In this study, 6,000 mg of testosterone enanthate over 10 weeks of training (600 mg per IM injection once a week, about five times the dose for hypogonadism) showed a significant improvement in fat-free mass and strength (see Table 16.1). Concomitantly, there was increased muscle size with anabolic steroids in both the no-exercise and exercise groups (see Table 16.2).

Table 16.1 Effect of anabolic steroids on fat-free mass and strength

Treatment	Fat-Free Mass		Bench Press		Squat	
	Baseline	10 Weeks	Baseline	10 Weeks	Baseline	10 Weeks
No exercise						
Placebo	65.1 (2.5)	65.9 (2.7)	88 (5)	88 (5)	102 (6)	105 (6)
Testosterone	69.9 (1.3)	73.1 (2.2)	96 (8)	105* (8)	103 (8)	116* (5)
Exercise						
Placebo	72.1 (2.3)	74.1*(2.2)	109 (12)	119* (11)	126 (13)	151* (13)
Testosterone	65.3 (1.8)	71.4*(1.8)	97 (6)	119* (6)	102 (5)	140* (5)

Legend: Values are mean (± standard error) weights in kilograms for fat-free mass and the weight lifted for bench-press and squatting exercises after 10 weeks of treatment. The asterisks indicate $P < 0.05$ for the comparison between means for 10 weeks and baseline for each treatment condition. Data are derived from Bhasin, Storer, Berman, et al. (1996).

Table 16.2 Effect of anabolic steroids on muscle size

Treatment	Triceps Area		Quadriceps Area	
	Baseline	10 Weeks	Baseline	10 Weeks
No exercise				
Placebo	3,621 (213)	3,539 (226)	8,796 (561)	8,665 (481)
Testosterone	3,579 (260)	4,003* (229)	9,067 (398)	9,674* (472)
Exercise				
Placebo	4,052 (262)	4,109 (230)	9,920 (569)	10,454 (474)
Testosterone	3,483 (217)	3,984* (239)	8,550 (353)	9,724* (348)

Legend: Values are mean (± standard error) areas in square millimeters for measurement of triceps and quadriceps area after 10 weeks of treatment. The asterisks indicate $P < 0.05$ for the comparison between means for 10 weeks and baseline for each treatment condition. Data are derived from Bhasin, Storer, Berman, et al. (1996).

Even after decades of research, questions concerning the effectiveness of anabolic steroids on performance remain unresolved. Inconsistent results probably reflect issues with subjects (age, fitness level), study design (diet, training methods, drug administration), dose, and length of study. Many studies support the finding that anabolic steroids increase strength if the anabolic steroids are taken in conjunction with intensive weight training and a high-protein diet. The measure of strength gain is more likely significant if it uses the same exercise that was used during training. For example, testing using the bench press may not show significant improvement if the training used squats. Resistance training increases release of growth hormone, and some of the effect of weight training could be secondary to the release of growth hormone. Also, some of the long-term effects could be indirectly attributable to release of IGF-1 following training and steroid use. Individuals taking anabolic steroids also report feeling good and powerful and having increased energy, with demonstrated increases in aggressiveness. These psychological benefits may contribute to improved performance, but this relationship is very hard to document. Similarly, it is also difficult to quantify the assertion that anabolic steroids help increase the intensity of regular workouts and speed recovery.

Steroid Enhancers and Mimics

The Dietary Supplement Health and Education Act (discussed in Chapter 13), passed by Congress in 1994, allows dietary supplements, whether vitamins, herbs, or botanical extracts, to be distributed and sold without a prescription and places supplements outside the normal regulatory domain of the FDA. Many nutraceuticals (as opposed to the tightly regulated pharmaceuticals) claiming anabolic activity are available on the market and are not banned by the IOC or the NCAA. In many cases, good experimental evidence is lacking on the efficacy of these agents. These preparations usually contain a mixture of chemicals or extracts that have reported anabolic activities. Other compounds in the mixture are supposed to increase absorption and enhance bioavailability of endogenous steroids. An example is a chemical that displaces testosterone from protein binding sites, causing an increase in free testosterone.

With the ban on steroid use, the nutraceutical industry has worked to provide alternatives. **Dehydroepiandrosterone (DHEA)** and **androstenedione** (often referred to as "Andro") are prohormones. DHEA is converted to androstenedione, which can be converted to testosterone (or estrogen in females) (Figure 16.1). DHEA, made in the adrenal glands, has weak and variable physiological activity of its own, depending on the status of the individual. Androstenedione is converted to testosterone in the circulation and can contribute to most circulating testosterone in females (but only a small percentage of the testosterone in males). DHEA was banned for suspected hepatotoxicity, but after the law changed in 1994 was once again available as a nutraceutical. As an androgenic steroid hormone, it is considered weak, due to its low potency and high rate of hepatic clearance. There is little evidence to support increased performance by androstenedione.

Baseball player Mark McGuire acknowledged the use of androstenedione during his record-breaking season of 1998 (70 home runs), bringing considerable attention to its use. He was also suspected of using anabolic steroids in that era. Several years later, MLB and WADA banned use of DHEA and androstenedione. Androstenedione is currently a Schedule III controlled substance due to changes made in the Anabolic Steroid Control Act of 2004; DHEA was exempted from this act.

Research has examined whether these nutraceuticals are effective as ergogenic or anabolic agents. In one study, no change in body composition was observed in subjects taking 300 mg/day androstenedione over eight weeks (King, Sharp, Vukovich, et al. 1999). In other studies, Welle, Jozefowicz, and Statt (1990) found that males who used DHEA (1600 mg/day) for four weeks showed no change in lean body weight, while Nestler, Barlascini, Clore, and Blackard (1988) found that males showed an increase with a similar dose.

Androstenedione did not cause a significant increase in testosterone in males when combined with resistance training (King et al.), although an increase in estradiol (a form of estrogen) was observed (see Figure 16.1). DHEA supplementation, in limited studies, does not show a large increase in testosterone, though a small fraction of DHEA has been detected in urine samples as having been converted to testosterone. In females, DHEA or androstenedione can increase serum testosterone within about two hours (based on old studies). In summary, there is little strong evidence that these two compounds enhance testosterone or its activity.

Health Risks

Physiological problems result from supra-physiological doses of anabolic steroids. Some of the anabolic steroids are very hepatotoxic. DHEA causes hepatotoxicity in animal studies. Anabolic steroids can directly oppose the beneficial cardiovascular effects of exercise. For example, overuse of anabolic steroids can lead to left ventricular hypertrophy, which can result in sudden death syndrome. Anabolic steroids also cause poor HDL and LDL ratios. Exogenous anabolic steroids at high levels cause negative feedback in the brain to decrease endogenous testosterone release. This response can affect sex drive and other issues. Abusers of anabolic steroids take other drugs to counteract many of the adverse side effects, including anti-estrogens. A variety of psychological problems (including aggression and depression) are also associated with the use of anabolic steroids.

The promotion of nutraceuticals as safe ways to increase testosterone can be very confusing for athletes, since these substances are available OTC but are banned in many sports. In 1998, before the change in its status in 2004, GNC, a nutritional supplement retailer, stopped selling androstenedione because of safety concerns. Increases in estrogen levels in males can have unwanted effects. Androstenedione may block testosterone receptors (a weak agonist could act like an antagonist). It could also suppress testosterone production by working as a weak agonist and activating the negative feedback loop that suppresses additional testosterone production.

PES Watch

Anabolic steroids are classified as Schedule III drugs, with distribution a felony and possession a misdemeanor. Anabolic steroids are banned by all sport organizations, including the NCAA, USOC, IOC, NFL, US Powerlifting Federation, and MLB. Use is unethical, illegal, and potentially dangerous. Not all of the effects disappear when the drug is discontinued.

Dosing regimens in the off season, however, can go undetected, especially in sports that lack year-round random testing. Use of testosterone cream in limited but frequent applications (a type of micro-dosing) can be very difficult to detect. Moreover, new derivatives can escape detection. The anabolic steroid called THG, of Bay Area Laboratory Co-operative (BALCO) fame, is an example of an anabolic steroid that was undetectable for years. The sprinter Marion Jones "never tested positive," but records show that she obtained and used THG. She ultimately lost her Olympic medals and went to jail. Elite athletes are still getting caught. Floyd Landis, the winner of the 2007 Tour de France, tested positive for anabolic steroids during the race (he had a skewed ratio of metabolites in his urine). In 2008, a number of baseball players, including Roger Clemens and Barry Bonds, were in trouble because of their alleged use of anabolic steroids and other PES. Numerous former All-Star baseball players are being overlooked during voting for the National Baseball Hall of Fame because the general perception that they abused PES during the era when there was no testing in Major League Baseball.

As for the nutraceuticals for which anabolic activity is claimed, in 1997, the IOC banned DHEA and androstenedione. Rodney Barnes missed the 1992 Olympics after testing positive for androstenedione, and swimmer Michelle Smith has been banned for life since her positive test for androstenedione. DHEA and androstenedione are banned by the NCAA, USOC, NFL, ITF, ATP, MLB (2004), and NBA. Even so, as nutraceuticals, they could be purchased by anyone, including minors. Androstenedione sale was banned in 2004 when it was added to the list of controlled substances.

THG and the BALCO Scandal

The Bay Area Laboratory Co-Operative (BALCO) distributed substances used in a treatment cycle that could go relatively undetected by drug testing. Mineral supplements were enhanced with erythropoietin, human growth hormone, modafinil (a central stimulant; see Chapter 8), testosterone cream, and tetrahydrogestrinone (THG; Fainaru-Wada & Williams 2006). Topical testosterone application (often called "The Cream") does not cause a significant rise in normal testosterone levels under normal drug testing. Similarly, topical application of testosterone is not nearly as effective as IM injection. THG was called "The Clear," because users' urine would test clear even on the same day it was injected. BALCO sold these substances without regulatory attention from 1988 to 2002, when the federal investigation began. Parallel with this investigation, the U.S. Anti-doping Agency (USADA) began its own investigation after a tip from an anonymous source.

In the summer of 2003, a filled syringe sent to the USADA was forwarded to Don Catlin, founder and then-director of the UCLA Olympic Analytical Laboratory. He was able to detect a previously undetectable designer steroid, tetrahydrogestrinone. The sender of the syringe was later identified as Trevor Graham, the former coach of runners Tim Montgomery and Marion Jones. Caitlin developed a new testing process for THG, as the previously used protocols caused THG to degrade and escape detection. With this new procedure, he retested 550 existing samples from athletes, of which 20 were positive for THG. These included samples from numerous track and field athletes, baseball players, and other prominent athletes. Marion Jones was sentenced to six months in prison and two years of probation for lying to federal prosecutors. Barry Bonds testified that he used a substance given to him by his trainer but that he did not know it contained steroids (ESPN 2006). Bonds was eventually convicted of one count of obstruction of justice. The *San Francisco Chronicle* ran a series of stories detailing BALCO's activities, and the reporters, Mark Fainaru-Wada and Lance Williams, turned the story into the book *Game of Shadows: Barry Bonds, BALCO, and the Steroid Scandal That Rocked Professional Sports* (2006).

Human Growth Hormone

Growth hormone, also called somatotropin, is a peptide hormone (191 amino acids long) secreted from the anterior pituitary at a rate of about 0.4 to 1.0 mg per day in males, with higher values in women and adolescents. The original source of growth hormone used as a therapeutic agent was cadavers, but a viral disease (Creutzfeldt-Jakob disease) was linked to these preparations. **Human growth hormone** (HGH) is made through bioengineering and goes by trade names such as Somatrem and Somatropin. HGH has limited clinical use, where it is prescribed for individuals with an insufficiency, but it is highly sought after by athletes, even with a $10,000 to $30,000/year price tag. Since many of the sources of HGH are from the black market, the actual contents can be suspect. HGH affects all body systems, and studies have looked at potential benefits in the elderly (such as improved muscle strength, bone density, and body composition). Some consider it a true "anti-aging" drug, although its effect on lifespan is more complicated and may provide significant risks (Junnila, List, Berryman, et al. 2013).

How Human Growth Hormone Works

Human growth hormone use causes hyperplasia (increased cell number), whereas anabolic steroids cause hypertrophy (increase in cell size) of some tissues. Its actions persist (the increase in cell number), whereas anabolic steroids' hypertrophic effects wear off over time. HGH increases amino acid uptake by cells and increases rates of protein synthesis. It can increase calcium retention and mineralization of bone. HGH also promotes lipolysis and gluconeogenesis in the liver, and it stimulates the release of IGF-1 (insulin-like growth factor-1) from the liver. IGF-1 stimulates growth in many different cell types and may represent a primary mechanism for growth hormone activity (Laron 2001).

Exercise Pharmacology

Exercise stimulates the release of growth hormone acutely, in females and males, after resistance training (Kraemer, Gordon, Fleck, et al. 1991) and aerobic exercise (Bunt, Boileau, Bahr, & Nelson 1986). Following heavy resistance training, there is a steady rise in blood levels of growth hormone, as shown in Figure 16.2 (Kraemer, Kilgore, Kraemer, & Castracane 1992). Its release may be related to the type of exercise protocol: in males and females, training with higher repetitions and lower weights stimulated greater growth hormone release than fewer repetitions and higher weights (Kraemer et al. 1991). Release of growth hormone may be lower in the elderly and obese, but one study showed an increase in release in elderly men immediately following resistance exercise (Nicklas, Ryan, Treuth, et al. 1995). A variety of other drugs and hormones can affect growth hormone release. One of the downstream effects of HGH includes release of IGF-1; IGF-1 also increases with resistance training, usually after several hours.

Limited evidence suggests that growth hormone increases lean body mass, but it does not improve strength (Liu, Bravata, Olkin, et al. 2008). Growth hormone increases fat-free mass and decreases body fat in weightlifters (Crist, Peake, Egan, & Waters 1988). It may have similar effects on the elderly and other growth hormone–deficient subjects. Other studies suggest no additional benefit in body composition with HGH supplementation over weight training alone. In power athletes on a weight-training program, HGH did not augment protein synthesis rates. Most enhancements resulting from HGH are in deficient

Figure 16.2 Effects of resistance training on growth hormone levels.

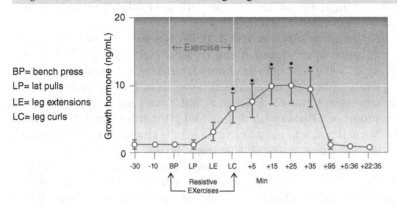

BP= bench press
LP= lat pulls
LE= leg extensions
LC= leg curls

Legend: Alteration of growth hormone concentrations before, during, and after resistance exercise, corrected for volume change. Data are mean ± SEM; $n = 8$; $p < 0.05$ compared with the −10 minute value.

individuals, including muscle mass, strength, and performance. HGH does not increase muscle strength in individuals with normal levels of growth hormone (Yarasheski, Campbell, Smith, et al. 1992). Regardless of the subjects' level of fitness, studies show that HGH did not provide improvements in muscle strength over weight training alone (Liu et al.). HGH produces a generalized anabolic action on many tissues, largely dependent on existing growth hormone status and amount of body fat.

If HGH helps speed recovery after intensive training or the wear and tear of competition (e.g., 115 pitches in a baseball game, back-to-back game days, 21 days of cycling in the mountains), then it may not test as an ergogenic agent, but it certainly can provide a competitive edge. Shoulders, elbows, knees, and so forth are subjected to considerable stress, and HGH could help in their repair and return to normal function. HGH also reportedly improves eyesight and fat utilization. It may also speed recovery from injury or surgery. Hence, testing recommended doses in a placebo-controlled study on how much weight can be bench-pressed might not demonstrate the true performance-enhancing capability of HGH. Its true value may be in extending the competitive life of older professional athletes who can afford the price tag to keep their bodies relatively young.

The Use of Deer Antler Spray

Deer or elk antler velvet and base have been used in traditional Chinese medicine for thousands of years (Wu, Li, Jin, et al. 2013). Deer antler spray is derived from deer antler velvet that is clipped from the tips of live antlers. Rapid growth of antlers suggests the presence of growth factors that stimulate that growth. IGF-1, like HGH, plays a role in growing children during their rapid growth. The FDA considers deer antler velvet a dietary supplement. Oral treatment would likely not be effective, as polypeptide hormones such as IGF-1 and HGH would be degraded in the digestive system, much like insulin. However, sublingual application may allow some absorption of peptides and would bypass the digestive system and first-pass metabolism in the liver. Even if IGF-1 makes it into the bloodstream, we might ask whether any properly controlled studies support the claims made by supplement manufacturers.

An extensive literature exists on IGF-1. IGF-1 is a potent growth factor, and studies in transgenic mice suggest it can repair muscle damage (Rabinovsky, Gelir, Gelir, et al. 2003). The data are limited, however, on whether deer or elk antler spray can significantly raise circulating levels of IGF-1. Studies of antler extracts in humans are limited. Elk velvet antler does not effectively manage residual symptoms in patients with rheumatoid arthritis (Allen, Oberle, Grace, et al. 2008). Normal males found no advantage in taking deer velvet to enhance sexual function (Conaglen, Suttie, & Conaglen 2003).

The World Anti-doping Agency lifted a ban on deer antler spray, although it recommends that athletes be vigilant with this supplement, because it could lead to a positive test for IGF-1 (World Anti-doping Agency 2013). If newer formulations can significantly raise circulating levels of IGF-1, as mentioned earlier, then WADA presumably will revisit a ban on its use, and this could influence anti-doping tests. IGF-1 is on the WADA Prohibited List under heading S2.4 of the List of Prohibited Substances and Methods, and it is banned by many professional sports leagues, including the NFL and MLB. WADA's restriction on deer antler spray was overturned because it contained trivial amounts of IGF-1. However, a significant number of professional athletes use the spray (Erskine 2013), and some prominent football players and golfers have also been identified as users. Athletes use it as an alternative to anabolic steroids to improve muscle strength, recover from injury, or boost energy. The industry claims many benefits from its use, but there are good reasons to be skeptical.

Health Risks

Acromegaly is a disease that results from overproduction of growth hormone. The disease symptoms include increased size of the left ventricle and many other organs, as well as reduced exercise capacity. Acromegaly is not reversible. Excess HGH could also cause changes to the skeleton, heart, or metabolism, or cause sexual dysfunction. Individuals overusing HGH have reported carpal tunnel syndrome. Other side effects include diabetes, fluid retention, joint stiffness, muscle pain, and high blood pressure.

HGH is a peptide and is injected, which creates another set of problems, such as infection. (A new aerosol spray may be available.) Another source of problems is the fact that, since a lot of HGH sales are on the "black market," quality control is lacking. As athletes and others continue use of supra-physiological doses of HGH, symptoms similar to acromegaly, as well as other problems, may develop.

PES Watch

With improvement in the detection of steroids, human growth hormone became the drug of choice among athletes to enhance performance, and the 1996 Olympics held in Atlanta became known as the "Growth Hormone Games." Human growth hormone has anabolic properties. It is considered ergogenic and is banned by most sport associations, leagues, and governing bodies. HGH is a prescription drug; otherwise, its use is illegal. Irreversible side effects are possible. However, HGH is not detectable in urine samples and only relatively recently can be detected in blood samples. Before these tests became available, law enforcement and sport governing agencies tracked the sale and distribution of HGH. For example, tracking the sales of HGH led to much of the evidence cited in the Mitchell Report commissioned by Major League Baseball. Testing for recombinant HGH is possible using blood samples. Two tests exist and when both are available, provide complimentary information. The Isoforms Test, after years of validation, was first used during the 2008 European Football Championship and the 2008 Summer Olympic Games. Currently, all WADA accredited laboratories test for HGH using the Isoforms Test. It detects recombinant HGH up to 24 to 48 hours after injection. The HGH Biomarkers Test is finalizing validation. It measures the increased synthesis of two biological markers of HGH bioactivity, IGF-I and P-III-NP, which persist longer than the period covered by the Isoforms Test (WADA website).

Blood Doping and Erythropoietin

In 1972, blood doping was achieved with reinfusion of red blood cells (**erythrocytes**), causing a 9% increase in VO_2max and a 23% increase in running performance (Ekblom, Goldbarg, & Gullbring 1972). Experiments published in 1945 showed that transfusion of 450 ml of blood on four consecutive days decreased exercise heart rate under hypoxic conditions, suggesting that exercise performance could be increased (Pace, Consolazio, & Lozner 1945). An **autologous transfusion** involves reinfusion of blood or blood components into the same individual who originally donated them. In a **homologous transfusion**, blood from another human donor is used; usually, it is withdrawn in advance and stored for later transfusion.

Remember that exercise capacity is dependent on oxygen delivery and oxygen utilization. The successful blood-doping experiment confirmed these principles. By increasing the concentration of red blood cells in the circulation by reinfusion of packed red blood cells into the athlete, the researchers obtained a significant increase in performance. Training at high altitudes also increases the oxygen-carrying capacity of the blood, as the athlete adjusts to the lower oxygen levels in the atmosphere. Removing a portion of the athlete's blood after high-altitude training and then reinfusing the packed red blood cells before a sport competition became a common practice, which initially was not banned. However, blood doping, or blood packing, as it is sometimes called, was outlawed by the IOC in 1986.

How Blood Doping and Erythropoietin Work

Hematinic agents are agents that stimulate erythrocyte formation or increase the amount of hemoglobin in red blood cells. Hematinic agents can increase the hematocrit, increase the oxygen-carrying capacity of blood, and improve athletic endurance and performance. Increasing the oxygen-carrying capacity of blood can decrease blood lactate following exercise, suggesting improved aerobic metabolism. **Erythropoietin**, a naturally occurring hormone produced by the kidneys, is a hematinic agent that stimulates red blood cell formation. It is a single peptide chain of 165 amino acid residues with glycans (short oligosaccharides) attached at four different residues. Erythropoietin is produced in response to hypoxia (low oxygen) or other conditions that result in low hemoglobin (Jelkmann 2013). Normally, erythropoietin levels depend on the hemoglobin concentration in the blood. Cells in the kidney sense hemoglobin levels indirectly by sensing oxygen levels; low oxygen stimulates erythropoietin production. At high workloads (supra-maximal exercise for three minutes), oxygen saturation of hemoglobin decreases sufficiently to stimulate erythropoietin release (Roberts & Smith 1999).

Erythropoietin works by decreasing apoptosis (cell death) in cells destined to become red blood cells in the bone marrow. These progenitor cells eventually become reticulocytes (precursors of erythrocytes) before maturing into erythrocytes. When the survival rate of reticulocytes increases, the number of mature erythrocytes increases. In the bone marrow, 2.5 million reticulocytes are produced every second to replace erythrocytes that are removed from the circulation because they have reached their life expectancy of 120 days. Erythropoietin increases the number of reticulocytes that successfully become mature red blood cells. The gene for erythropoietin was cloned in the late 1980s, and the production of recombinant protein soon followed. The first bioengineered form was called epoetin alfa. Many derivatives, as well as agents that stimulate erythropoietin production, are now on the market (Jelkmann).

Sports Anemia

Hematinic agents, such as erythropoietin and its related agents, are used clinically to treat anemia patients with chronic renal disease. Some athletes may justify taking erythropoietin because they are anemic. **Anemia** is the state where there is a low mass of red blood cells (low hematocrit) or the concentration of hemoglobin is low. Many athletes are pseudo-anemic; their hemoglobin concentration decreases due to plasma volume expansion. This condition is called **sports anemia** to distinguish it from the condition of anemic patients who are suffering from such maladies as renal disease. GI bleeding occurs in marathon runners and other endurance athletes who undertake long training regimens. The incidence of sports anemia is related to exercise intensity and is independent of age, iron supplementation, and gender. Sports anemia does not seem to affect performance, whereas real anemia does negatively impact performance. Why does sports anemia occur? One theory involves NSAIDs and their contribution to gastropathy (bleeding in the stomach). Another theory considers foot-strike hemolysis: the constant pounding of the feet on the pavement might cause loss or turnover of erythrocytes. However, significant blood loss through this mechanism is not supported (Lippi, Schena, Salvagno, et al. 2012).

Another contributor to sports anemia may be iron status. In some cases, iron deficiency can also cause decreased performance. Iron is required by all cells but especially by red blood cells, due to their high concentration of hemoglobin—an iron-containing protein. Iron is stored primarily in liver cells and macrophages, bound to the iron storage protein called ferritin. Iron is transported in blood bound to the transport protein called transferrin (apotransferrin if iron is not bound). Though ferritin is primarily an intracellular protein, serum ferritin levels are determined as a measure of iron status. Low ferritin levels and iron levels occur in both males and females and may contribute to sports anemia, particularly in endurance sports (Garza, Shrier, Kohl, et al. 1997). Iron status, particularly in women in their reproductive years, can be an issue in terms of peak performance (Latunde-Dada 2012). Iron supplementation may be advisable, depending on an individual's intensity of training and quality of diet.

Exercise Pharmacology

During competition, cardiac output, heart rate, and ATP production are not easily manipulated—they are based on the athlete's level of fitness. However, the oxygen-carrying capacity of the blood can be manipulated, with an increase in red blood cells and hemoglobin. Erythropoietin treatment significantly increases the hematocrit, with increases over 10% reported in normal subjects. In anemic patients, erythropoietin can increase hematocrits even more, even as much as 35%. In these patients, the increased hematocrit improves VO_2max 17% and decreases the perception of fatigue (Robertson, Haley, Guthrie, et al. 1990). Muscle strength and muscle performance improve in anemic individuals with erythropoietin treatment (Guthrie, Cardenas, Eschbach, et al. 1993). Erythropoietin given subcutaneously has peak blood levels in about 12 to 18 hours, with about 30% bioavailability. The half-life of the different preparations on the market can vary greatly, with estimated values ranging from 12 hours to over 40 hours (Jelkmann). In an interesting study that used preoperative patients, erythropoietin was given with the goal of increasing blood cell formation, in anticipation of blood loss during surgery. However, repeated administration of erythropoietin blunted the normal release of endogenous erythropoietin in the post-operative patients, resulting in the opposite of the desired outcome (Tasaki, Ohto, Hashimoto, et al. 1992).

After erythropoietin became available for study, research showed that it produced an increase in red blood cell mass, an increase in the oxygen-carrying capacity of the blood, and an increase in aerobic power. More recent studies have looked at lower doses and submaximal exercise performance. For example, the effects of erythropoietin on performance were measured with ergometer cycling for 20 to 30 minutes at 80% of maximal workload (Thomsen, Rentsch, Robach, et al. 2007). Eight subjects initially received either 5,000 IU or placebo every second day for 14 days. Subsequently, a single dose or placebo was given weekly for another 10 weeks. Exercise performance was evaluated before treatment and after 4 and 11 weeks of treatment. Erythropoietin administration increased VO_2max by about 12% and prolonged submaximal exercise performance by about 54% (Thomsen et al.).

In another study, erythropoietin increased hemoglobin mass and maximal oxygen uptake following four weeks of administration (Durussel, Daskalaki, Anderson, et al. 2013). Nineteen trained men received injections of 50 IU per kg body mass every two days for four weeks. Hemoglobin mass was determined each week, including four weeks after administration stopped. Performance on a three-kilometer run improved following four weeks of erythropoietin and remained improved four weeks after administration compared to baseline (see Table 16.3). These field performance effects correlated with increased hemoglobin mass and VO_2max (Durussel et al.). The increase in hemoglobin mass is shown in Table 16.4, expressed relative to blood volume or body weight. Therefore, the improvement in running time and oxygen utilization correlates with an increase in hemoglobin content following treatment with erythropoietin.

Very strong anecdotal information suggests that athletes perceive that erythropoietin helps recovery from heavy training or endurance events, such as Le Tour de France. Improved oxygen delivery keeps muscles from depending on anaerobic metabolism, decreases the buildup of lactate, and could be glycogen sparing. An individual's VO_2max has a genetic basis that depends on muscle oxygen utilization, as well as the hematocrit and hemoglobin concentration (reflective of erythropoietin levels). VO_2max can be improved by training, again based on the individual's genetic and physical makeup. Injecting erythropoietin allows the users to "cheat" genetics, as they

Table 16.3 Running times for 3,000-meter trial and maximal oxygen uptake following erythropoietin treatment

Measure	Group 1			Group 2		
	Baseline	End of Treatment	End of Study	Baseline	End of Treatment	End of Study
3,000-m run (minutes)	10:12 (0.42)	9:40* (0.37)	9:53* (0.43)	12:05 (0.55)	11:19* (0.53)	11:39* (0.58)
RPE	18.0 (1.7)	18.4 (0.9)	19.0 (1.2)	17.7 (2.2)	18.4 (1.6)	18.6 (1.4)
VO$_2$max (ml × min^{-1} × kg^{-1})	60.3 (5.0)	64.4* (3.9)	61.8 (3.9)	51.6 (3.5)	57.0* (5.1)	54.2* (4.7)

Legend: Group 1 ($n = 9$) included subjects who had a history of running, and Group 2 ($n = 9$) included the subjects who were involved in other activities. Values are means (standard deviation). Significant differences ($p < 0.05$) compared to baseline values are indicated by *. RPE: Borg's rating of perceived exertion. Treatment with recombinant human erythropoietin was every other day for four weeks. The end of the study was an additional four weeks later. Data derived from Durussel, Daskalaki, Anderson, et al. (2013).

Table 16.4 Hemoglobin and hematocrit changes after treatment with erythropoietin

Measure	Baseline	End of Treatment	End of Study
Hematocrit	41.9 (1.8)	49.2* (2.0)	45.1* (1.7)
Hemoglobin mass (g)	947 (109)	1,131* (131)	1,023* (132)
Hemoglobin (g/dL)	14.4 (0.7)	16.7* (0.9)	15.6* (0.7)
Hemoglobin (g/kg)	12.7 (1.2)	15.2* (1.5)	13.7* (1.1)

Legend: Values are means (standard deviation) for $n = 19$. Significant difference ($p < 0.05$) compared to baseline values indicated by *. The mass of hemoglobin is shown relative to blood volume and body weight. Treatment with recombinant human erythropoietin was every other day for four weeks. The end of the study was an additional four weeks later. Data derived from Durussel, Daskalaki, Anderson, et al. (2013).

bump their hematocrit up to just below the 50% limit. They improve their VO$_2$max by artificial means, and their training and performance reflect their illegal blood doping.

Low iron stores compromise the effectiveness of erythropoietin. Other than some loss of iron in the GI-tract, exercise does not significantly affect the pharmacology or pharmacokinetics of iron. Normal females had no change in post-exercise lactate levels with iron supplements. Females with low hemoglobin at the start of the study showed a decrease in post-exercise lactate with iron supplements. Otherwise, iron supplements had little effect on exercise performance. Supplemental iron also had little effect on sports anemia or VO$_2$max in female distance runners. Experimental animals were raised on a diet deficient in iron and then received a diet that included iron. They showed an increase in VO$_2$max but not in endurance following the iron supplementation. Endurance may be more of a function of the oxidative capacity of skeletal muscle. This result was not reproduced in humans, where iron stores are probably not as limiting as in the diet-controlled rat experiment. Iron supplements can correct an iron deficiency, but they do not produce ergogenic responses in normal individuals.

Health Risks

Erythropoietin increases hematocrit and blood viscosity. The more viscous blood (with a higher percentage of red blood cells) combined with dehydration following endurance activity can be fatal. There have been numerous reports of competitive cyclists dying in their sleep. Use of erythropoietin combined with anabolic steroids may cause kidney problems. Eating a balanced diet is important in maintaining hemoglobin, as vitamin C improves iron uptake. Taking some types of antacids and drinking tea can decrease iron uptake.

PES Watch

Erythropoietin use without a prescription is illegal, and erythropoietin is a banned substance. WADA defines blood doping broadly to include techniques or substances that increase red blood cell mass. Prohibited procedures include transfusion of red blood cells and synthetic oxygen carriers, infusion of hemoglobin, and the artificial stimulation of erythropoiesis (formation of erythrocytes in the bone marrow).

The practice of blood doping developed as athletes reasoned that erythropoietin could be as effective as high-altitude training or autologous transfusions in terms of increasing the oxygen-carrying capacity of their blood. In 1998, the Festina cycling team was found with 400 vials of erythropoietin in their support vehicle and were ejected from the Tour de France, without the cyclists' testing positive. Over the subsequent years, many cyclists have tested positive (or died) after using erythropoietin. For example, evidence of misuse was uncovered during the 2008 Tour de France. Lance Armstrong admitted to using erythropoietin and other drugs throughout his racing career, but he did not test positive during the competitions. Although some cyclists and other athletes still are caught, clearly there are ways to avoid detection.

A **hematocrit test** is used to test for blood doping, as it measures the percentage of volume of whole blood composed of red blood cells. The normal range for men is about 38% to 50%, and for women it is about 35% to 44.5%. WADA recommends that a hematocrit value of 50% or more be considered a positive test for blood doping in males; the limit is 48% for females. In athletes, a measure of hemoglobin mass is a more reliable predictor of VO_2max than is hemoglobin concentration, as blood volume expansion occurs with training; total hemoglobin mass can actually increase among athletes (Jelkmann & Lundby 2011). Once a hematocrit over 50% was established as the basis for disqualification, male cheaters would titrate themselves with enough erythropoietin to reach 49%.

A urine test can distinguish recombinant erythropoietin from endogenous erythropoietin, and tests are now available for exogenous recombinant erythropoietin. Erythropoietin is normally secreted as a glycoprotein. Genetically engineered erythropoietin is produced by non-human cells and has different sugars attached. The recombinant protein can be distinguished from the person's erythropoietin using gel electrophoresis prepared from urine samples. Detectable levels of subcutaneously injected erythropoietin last only about two days in the urine. Newer derivatives with a longer half-life are detectable slightly longer. The gel electrophoresis technique used for urine sample has been modified for blood samples. However, the effects of erythropoietin on blood cell formation can persist for weeks after cessation of the injection protocol. Moreover, users can micro-dose to maintain an elevated level of hemoglobin; detection of micro-doses has to occur within 8 to 12 hours following injection. Other tests, including analysis of immature reticulocytes in the blood, have been used to determine erythropoietin use (Jelkmann & Lundby). Although erythropoietin is a very expensive drug, its use and abuse are widespread. This may be changing with the availability of recombinant erythropoietin detection.

In addition, WADA is developing an extensive blood panel of tests to detect blood doping, called the "Biologic Passport." Each athlete is tracked over time to determine any irregularities, and blood doping can be detected weeks after the doping occurs. Blood testing, however, is much more expensive and time consuming than urine testing. Moreover, many new types of erythropoietin have been created with slight genetic differences, which complicate detection (Jelkmann & Lundby). The blood panel is used with evidence from urine samples to confirm a positive test. Professional cycling now endorses and uses the Passport system and other sports are moving in that direction.

The Fall of Lance Armstrong

In 2012, faced with a deadline for responding to allegations by the USADA, Lance Armstrong finally decided to avoid arbitration and accept the agency's punishment for using and distributing PES during his competitive cycling career (USADA 2012). USADA revoked all seven of Armstrong's Tour de France titles and banned him from competitive cycling for life. The USADA had evidence that Armstrong, starting in 1999, led a conspiracy that encouraged doping among certain cycling teams. Two former members of Armstrong's cycling teams confessed to doping and told the USADA that Armstrong used banned substances during his Tour victories. At the time, however, Armstrong refused to admit his use of PES publicly and reiterated that he had always passed his drug tests. The public pressure for him to admit the use continued to build until Armstrong admitted in an interview with Oprah Winfrey that aired January 17 and 18, 2013, that he used erythropoietin, human growth hormone, and blood doping during his seven Tour wins.

The USADA allegations implicated Armstrong, teammates, trainers, and physicians in the delivery and cover-up of a highly sophisticated illegal doping protocol. Erythropoietin was given as micro-doses or IV (with a faster clearance time) to help avoid detection. Infusions of saline, plasma, or glycerol were other strategies that worked to prevent detection of an illegal hematocrit or erythropoietin use. Multiple riders testified that Armstrong was observed having blood reinfused during the Tour de France and that he had blood-doping equipment at his residence. The USADA also found evidence that Armstrong administered a testosterone–olive oil mixture to himself and other riders. This mixture (technically an emulsion) apparently improves absorption into the lymphatic system, bypassing first-pass metabolism in the liver. There was also considerable evidence that team doctors provided HGH to Armstrong and team members. Team doctors and trainers also improperly provided corticosteroids to enhance recovery and performance and provide an energy boost.

In following the World Anti-doping Agency regulations, the USADA can test athletes during competitions and at any time afterward. Samples are kept for eight years, and the agency can retest samples as screening technology for detecting banned substances or new performance-enhancing drugs improves. These powers allowed the USADA to build the case against Armstrong. Testing for erythropoietin significantly improved between 1999 and 2012. As the evidence mounted, associates of Armstrong began to testify against him, and the whole story emerged. Ultimately, Armstrong was guilty of having used, possessed, trafficked, and administered PES and to have assisted, aided, covered up, and been complicit in one or more anti-doping rule violations.

Elder Concerns

Throughout this book, attention has been paid to aging and aging well. In this chapter, three hormones that are used by athletes to illegally improve performance and recovery were discussed in detail. In the case of androgenic steroids and HGH, levels decline with age, and some age-related decline in health may result. The question becomes whether hormone replacement can extend healthy lifetimes. Or is the declining hormone level a protection mechanism against age-related diseases such as cancer? Some physicians feel replacement therapy results in younger-looking and younger-feeling clients or patients. Others look at available research in humans and experimental animals and suggest using caution (Bartke & Darcy 2017). HGH stimulates cell replication and uncontrolled cell replication is a hallmark of cancer and other diseases. Interestingly, there is now interest in developing HGH antagonists (Lu, Flanagan, Langley, et al. 2019). Testosterone has many diverse effects, and as with most hormones, supplementation may uncouple the body's fine-tuned feedback control loops. Estrogen replacement in post-menopausal women may be similar in some ways. The relatively rapid decrease in estrogen (compared to the decrease in testosterone in males) initiates many biological changes, many of which are unpleasant. Hormone replacement therapy, with estrogen and possibly progesterone, was quite the new thing years ago. It relieves or postpones many of the symptoms of menopause, but comes with increased risks of stroke, heart attack, and cancer. It is no longer considered a long-term treatment option for most women.

As people age, they will consider some of these hormone treatment options. In most cases, it will depend on income level. Most patients are not covered by health insurance for off-label use of HGH or other hormones in otherwise healthy people. HGH can cost about $5,000 a month for daily injections. Testosterone creams are considerably less expensive and generally easier to obtain. The choice, assuming one can find an anti-aging doctor to write the prescriptions, is up to the individual and their retirement plan. The alternative costs less but takes more effort and time. As we have discussed throughout the book, attention to diet and regular exercise provides the safest and most effective anti-aging strategy. Get quality sleep. Take care of your skin. Avoid sugar and fast food. Eat fresh foods. Lift weights (it can help produce your own HGH). Walk whenever you can. Stay connected to people face-to-face. Learn a musical instrument or foreign language. Find something creative like oil painting. Live long and prosper.

Conclusion

Anabolic steroids clearly can increase muscle cell size, muscle mass, and strength, especially in conjunction with a vigorous training program. Human growth hormone stimulates cell division and an increase in cell number, related to its stimulation of insulin-like growth factor-1, another powerful hormone involved in growth. HGH use probably speeds tissue repair and recovery. Erythropoietin increases the oxygen-carrying capacity of the blood, a major factor in maximizing oxygen utilization—a key part of exercise performance. All three of these hormones are prototypes for performance-enhancing substances: they allow athletes to get bigger and faster, recover faster, and increase VO_2max. Keeping sport clean will require a significant cultural change, as appreciation for the benefits of participation, inclusion, and enjoyment must overcome the attitude of winning at all costs.

Key Concepts Review

acromegaly

anabolic

anabolic steroids

androgenic

androstenedione

anemia

autologous transfusion

dehydroepiandrosterone (DHEA)

erythrocyte

erythropoietin

erythropoietin

growth hormone

hematinic agent

hematocrit test

homologous transfusion

human growth hormone (HGH)

insulin-like growth factor-1 (IGF-1)

performance-enhancing substances
   (PES)

sports anemia

Review Questions

1   What hormone are anabolic steroids derived from? Why is it difficult for researchers to determine accurately the effectiveness of these agents on performance?

2   Estimates are that 50% to 85% of Major League Baseball players took steroids in the 1990s, and a similar number may take them today. Is this fair? What should be done? What are the risks to the ballplayers?

3   Many drugs or supplements are available over the Internet that claim to increase testosterone levels "naturally." Even if they work, should they be legal in terms of competition and testing?

4   What are hematinic agents? What physiological role might they play that would aid in exercise performance? Does blood doping work?

5   What is exercise-induced anemia? Can it be cured with iron supplements?

6   Racers in the Tour de France may have passed their drug test in 2004, but drug use that occurred in 2004 may still be detected in 2011. How might that work?

7   Why is taking human growth hormone a bad idea? Is there a benefit to injecting it into an individual with a normal level? When might taking HGH be a good idea?

8   Some baseball players were accused of taking HGH, yet there was no positive blood test. How was the use detected? How might players or other users of HGH be detected in the future?

References

Allen M, Oberle K, Grace M, Russell A, Adewale AJ (2008) A randomized clinical trial of elk velvet antler in rheumatoid arthritis. *Biol Res Nurs* 9:254–261

Bartke A, Darcy J (2017) GH and ageing: Pitfalls and new insights. *Best Pract Res Clin Endocrinol Metab* 31:113–125

Bhasin S, Storer TW, Berman N, Callegari C, Clevenger B, Phillips J, Bunnell TJ, Tricker R, Shirazi A, Casaburi R (1996) The effects of supraphysiological doses of testosterone on muscle size and strength in normal men. *N Engl J Med* 335:1–7

Bird SR, Goebel C, Burke LM, Greaves RF (2016) Doping in sport and exercise: anabolic, ergogenic, health and clinical issues. *Ann Clin Biochem* 53:196–221

Bunt JC, Boileau RA, Bahr JM, Nelson RA (1986) Sex and training differences in human growth hormone levels during prolonged exercise. *J Appl Physiol* 61:1796–1801

Conaglen HM, Suttie JM, Conaglen JV (2003) Effect of deer velvet on sexual function in men and their partners: a double-blind, placebo-controlled study. *Arch Sex Behav* 32:271–278

Crist DM, Peake GT, Egan PA, Waters DL (1988) Body composition response to exogenous GH during training in highly conditioned adults. *J Appl Physiol* 65:579–584

Durussel J, Daskalaki E, Anderson M, Chatterji T, Wondimu DH, Padmanabhan N, Patel RK, McClure JD, Pitsiladis YP (2013) Haemoglobin mass and running time trial performance after recombinant human erythropoietin administration in trained men. *PLoS One* 8:e56151 doi:10.1371

Ekblom B, Goldbarg AN, Gullbring B (1972) Response to exercise after blood loss and reinfusion. *J Appl Physiol* 33:175–180

Erskine C (February 2, 2013) Take two spritzes of deer antler spray and call me in the morning. *Los Angeles Times.* http://articles.latimes.com/2013/feb/02/sports/la-sp-erskine-super-bowl-20130203

ESPN (March 8, 2006) Book details Bonds' steroid regimen. http://sports.espn.go.com/mlb/news/story?id=2358236

Fainaru-Wada M, Williams L (2006) *Game of Shadows: Barry Bonds, BALCO, and the Steroids Scandal that Rocked Professional Sports.* New York: Gotham Books

Forbes GB (1985) The effect of anabolic steroids on lean body mass: the dose response curve. *Metabolism* 34:571–573

Garza D, Shrier I, Kohl HW 3rd, Ford P, Brown M, Matheson GO (1997) The clinical value of serum ferritin tests in endurance athletes. *Clin J Sport Med* 7:46–53

Guthrie M, Cardenas D, Eschbach JW, Haley NR, Robertson HT (1993) Effects of erythropoietin on strength and functional status of patients on hemodialysis. *Clin Nephrol* 39:97–102

Jelkmann W (2013) Physiology and pharmacology of erythropoietin. *Tranfus Med Hemother* 40:302–309

Jelkmann W, Lundby C (2011) Blood doping and its detection. *Blood* 118:2395–2404

Junnila RK, List EO, Berryman DE, Murrey JW, Kopchick JJ (2013) The GH/IGF-1 axis in ageing and longevity. *Nat Rev Endocrinol* 9:366–376

Kersey RD, Elliot DL, Goldberg L, Kanayama G, Leone JE, Pavlovich M, Pope HG Jr; National Athletic Trainers' Association (2012) National Athletic Trainers' Association position statement: anabolic-androgenic steroids. *J Athl Train* 47:567–588

King DS, Sharp RL, Vukovich MD, Brown GA, Reifenrath TA, Uhl NI, Parsons KA (1999) Effect of oral androstenedione on serum testosterone and adaptations to resistance training in young men. *JAMA* 281:2020–2028

Kraemer RR, Kilgore JL, Kraemer GR, Castracane VD (1992) Growth hormone, IGF-1, and testosterone responses to resistive exercise. *Med Sci Sports Exerc* 24:1346–1352

Kraemer WJ, Gordon SE, Fleck SJ, Marchitelli LJ, Mello R, Dziados JE, Friedl K, Harman E, Maresh C, Fry AC (1991) Endogenous anabolic hormonal and growth factor responses to heavy resistance exercise in males and females. *Int J Sports Med* 12:228–235

Laron Z (2001) Insulin-like growth factor 1 (IGF-1): a growth hormone. *Mol Pathol* 54:311–316

Latunde-Dada GO (2012) Iron metabolism in athletes—achieving the gold standard. *Eur J Haematol* 90:10–15

Lippi G, Schena F, Salvagno GL, Aloe R, Banfi G, Guidi GC (2012) Foot-strike haemolysis after a 60-km ultramarathon. *Blood Tranfus* 10:377–383

Liu H, Bravata DM, Olkin I, Friedlander A, Liu V, Roberts B, Bendavid E, Saynina O, Salpeter SR, Garber AM, Hoffman AR (2008) Systematic review: the effects of growth hormone on athletic performance. *Annals Int Med* 148:747–758

Lu M, Flanagan JU, Langley RJ, Hay MP, Perry JK (2019) Targeting growth hormone function: strategies and therapeutic applications. *Signal Transduct Target Ther* 4:3

Nestler JE, Barlascini CO, Clore JN, Blackard WG (1988) Dehydroepiandrosterone reduces serum low density lipoprotein levels and body fat but does not alter insulin sensitivity in normal men. *J Clin Endocrinol Metab* 66:57–61

Nicklas BJ, Ryan AJ, Treuth MM, Harman SM, Blackman MR, Hurley BF, Rogers MA (1995) Testosterone, growth hormone and IGF-1 responses to acute and chronic restive exercise in men aged 55–70 years. *Int J Sports Med* 16:445–450

Pace N, Consolazio WV, Lozner EL (1945) The effect of transfusions of red blood cells on the hypoxia tolerance of normal men. *Science* 102(2658):589–591

Rabinovsky ED, Gelir E, Gelir S, Lui H, Kattash M, DeMayo FJ, Shenaq SM, Schwartz RJ (2003) Targeted expression of IGF-1 transgene to skeletal muscle accelerates muscle and motor neuron regeneration. *FASEB J* 17:53–55

Roberts D, Smith DJ (1999) Erythropoietin concentration and arterial haemoglobin saturation with supramaximal exercise. *J Sports Sci* 17:485–493

Robertson HT, Haley NR, Guthrie M, Cardenas D, Eschbach JW, Adamson JW (1990) Recombinant erythropoietin improves exercise capacity in anemic hemodialysis patients. *Am J Kidney Dis* 15:325–332

Tasaki I, Ohto H, Hashimoto C, Abe R, Saitoh A, Kikuchi S (1992) Recombinant human erythropoietin for autologous blood donation: effects on perioperative red-blood-cell and serum erythropoietin production. *Lancet* 339:773–775

Thomsen JJ, Rentsch RL, Robach P, Calbet JA, Boushel R, Rasmussen P, Juel C, Lundby C (2007) Prolonged administration of recombinant human erythropoietin increases submaximal performance more than maximal aerobic capacity. *Eur J Appl Physiol* 101:481–486

USADA (August 24, 2012) Lance Armstrong receives lifetime ban and disqualification of competitive results for doping violations stemming from his involvement in the United States Postal Service Pro-Cycling Team Doping Conspiracy. www.usada.org/lance-armstrong-receives-lifetime-ban-and-disqualification-of-competitive-results-for-doping-violations-stemming-from-his-involvement-in-the-united-states-postal-service-pro-cycling-team-doping-conspi/

Vlad RA, Hancu G, Popescu GC, Lungu IA (2018) Doping in sports, a never-ending story? *Adv Pharm Bull* 8:529–534

World Anti-doping Agency (February 5, 2013) WADA urges vigilance over deer antler velvet spray. www.wada-ama.org/en/media/news/2013-02/wada-urges-vigilance-over-deer-antler-velvet-spray#.VD7cLOevy60

Welle S, Jozefowicz R, Statt M (1990) Failure of dehydroepiandrosterone to influence energy and protein metabolism in humans. *J Clin Endrocrinol Metab* 71:1259–1264

Wu F, Li H, Jin L, Li X, Ma Y, You J, Li S, Xu Y (2013) Deer antler base as a traditional Chinese medicine: a review of its traditional uses, chemistry and pharmacology. *J Ethnopharmacol* 145:403–415

Yarasheski KE, Campbell JA, Smith K, Rennie MJ, Holloszy JO, Bier DM (1992) Effect of growth hormone and resistance exercise on muscle growth in young men. *Am J Physiol* 262:E268–E276

Yesalis CE, Kennedy NJ, Kopstein AN, Bahrke MS (1993) Anabolic-androgenic steroid use in the United States. *JAMA* 270:1217–1221

Glossary

1,25-dihydroxyvitamin D See *calcitriol.*

25-hydroxyvitamin D See *calcidiol.*

5-lipoxygenase An enzyme that produces eicosanoids such as leukotrienes.

absorption One of the major components of pharmacokinetics concerned with delivering the drug into the body via many possible routes, though oral administration is the most common.

acarbose A competitive inhibitor of intestinal glucosidases; it delays digestion and absorption of glucose derived from starch, oligosaccharides, and disaccharides.

acetaminophen An analgesic with antipyretic and analgesic activity but with little anti-inflammatory activity. It causes less stomach irritation than aspirin and is not considered an NSAID.

acetylcholine The neurotransmitter at muscarinic and nicotinic sites. It is rapidly metabolized by acetylcholinesterase.

acipimox A lipid-modifying drug related to niacin. It works through the same receptor as niacin but causes a longer sustained inhibition of lipase activity, interferes less with insulin control of sugar and lipid metabolism, and is effective at lower doses.

acromegaly A disease that results from overproduction of growth hormone, with symptoms that include increased size of the left ventricle and many other organs, as well as reduced exercise capacity.

acupuncture An alternative therapy for pain that involves inserting needles at specific locations (called acupoints) and twisting the needles in and out to stimulate afferent nerve fibers.

addiction The compulsive use of a drug despite the harmful effects. Addiction results from dependence, tolerance, and withdrawal.

adenosine triphosphate (ATP) The energy currency in cells; an energy-storing molecule that releases energy when it is hydrolyzed to adenosine diphosphate and stores energy from the oxidation of food.

adipocytes Cells that make up fat tissue and store triglycerides.

adipokines Hormone factors secreted by adipose tissue.

adiponectin An adipokine produced by adipocytes in visceral fat that protects against diabetes, atherosclerotic vascular disease, inflammation, and hypertension. Blood levels of adiponectin decrease as visceral fat accumulation increases.

adrenaline See *epinephrine.*

adrenergic Postganglionic sympathetic neurons, which release norepinephrine.

adrenocorticotropic hormone (ACTH) Hormone released by the pituitary that stimulates the adrenal cortex to release corticosteroids. Part of the HPA axis.

aerobic metabolism   The production of ATP by a process that requires oxygen.

afferent fiber   A nerve that transmits information from the body back to the cerebro-spinal axis.

affinity   Related to the force of attraction between two molecules such as a drug and its receptor, a hormone and its receptor, or between two proteins.

agonist   A drug that binds receptors with a certain affinity to initiate a response, producing intrinsic activity by mimicking the endogenous ligand and causing a similar response.

albumin   Serum protein involved in the transport of molecules in the blood, such as fatty acids and some drugs.

albuterol   A beta-2 agonist used in inhalers to relax smooth muscles in the lung during an asthmatic episode.

aldosterone   A potent hormone that stimulates the kidney to reabsorb sodium and retain water, contributing to a decrease in urine output and an increase in blood volume, which raises blood pressure.

aldosterone antagonists   A class of potassium-sparing drugs with aldosterone receptor antagonist activity that antagonize the increase in Na^+ reabsorption machinery.

alkaloids   Naturally occurring chemical compounds that are produced by a large variety of organisms, including plants, fungi, animals, and bacteria. Many alkaloids have potent biological activity.

allostatic load   Persistent (chronic) stress.

alpha-blockers   A class of drugs that are antagonists for the α-1 receptor; they are considered second-line agents for treating hypertension.

alpha cells   Cells that produce glucagon, somatostatin, and gastrin.

alpha-glucosidase inhibitors   A class of drugs for treating Type 2 diabetes, including acarbose and miglitol. They slow or decrease the uptake of glucose from the gut.

alveoli   Thin-walled sacs within the lungs that are highly vascularized with blood and lymph vessels and nerve input. Alveoli act as the end point for bronchioles and provide a large surface area for gas exchange.

Alzheimer's disease   Aging-related disease that decreases cognitive function and memory.

amlodipine   Long-acting calcium channel blocker.

amphetamines   Drugs that work by stimulating the sympathetic nervous system, particularly in the central nervous system.

amylin   A peptide containing 37 amino acids, released following nutrient stimulation. It suppresses glucagon release, slows gastric emptying, and reduces food intake and body weight, probably by affecting appetite.

anabolic   Tissue building, process of building larger macromolecules from smaller building block molecules.

anabolic steroids   Derivatives of the steroid hormone testosterone that produce both masculinizing and tissue-building effects. Sometimes called androgenic-anabolic steroids.

anaerobic metabolism   The production of ATP by a process that does not require oxygen; it includes fermentation.

analgesia   The deadening of pain while a person is conscious.

analgesics   Drugs distinguished by their antipyretic and anti-inflammatory activities, in addition to their effect on deadening of pain. Commonly referred to as painkillers.

anandamide An endogenous ligand for the endocannabinoid system that primarily works through the CB1 and CB2 receptors, involved in memory, pain relief, euphoria, and patterns of eating and sleeping behavior.

anaphylaxis A severe and sometimes life-threatening allergic reaction that results from the release of histamines and other factors that cause constriction of airways.

androgens Masculinizing hormones such as testosterone.

androstenedione A prohormone that is converted into testosterone in the circulation and can contribute to most circulating testosterone in females (but only a small percentage of testosterone in males).

anemia A condition of low mass of red blood cells (low hematocrit) or low concentration of hemoglobin.

angina Chest pain caused by inadequate blood flow and oxygen delivery to the heart muscle cells.

angioedema A condition similar to urticaria (hives), but with rapid swelling deeper in the dermis below the skin, often around the eyes and lips.

angiotensin I A peptide with little activity that is cleaved to an active peptide of only eight amino acids called angiotensin II.

angiotensin II A peptide of eight amino acids which is a very potent vasoconstrictor. Its actions can be separated into fast and slow responses.

angiotensin-converting enzyme (ACE) The predominant protease to cleave angiotensin I into angiotensin II.

angiotensin-converting enzyme (ACE) inhibitors A class of drugs used in treating hypertension and other types of cardiovascular disease; they decrease ACE activity, slow angiotensin II formation, suppress vasoconstriction, and limit excessive retention of salt and water.

angiotensin receptor blockers (ARBs) A class of drugs used in treating hypertension and other types of cardiovascular disease; they block the angiotensin II (AT_1) receptors that mediate most of the fast and slow responses caused by angiotensin II.

angiotensinogen The circulating protein that is a component of the hormone system that regulates blood pressure.

antagonist A drug that binds receptors with a certain affinity but does not initiate a response, acting as a blocker for the endogenous ligand.

anti-arrhythmic Drug action that helps return heart to normal rhythm.

anti-atherosclerotic Drug action that slows hardening of the arteries.

anti-coagulant Drug action that slows the blood clotting process.

anti-convulsant Drug action that decreases chance of seizures.

antidepressants Drugs used for the treatment of major depressive disorder. They increase the effective concentration of serotonin and norepinephrine and stimulate neurogenesis.

antidiuretic hormone Also known as arginine vasopressin. A hormone that activates vasopressin receptors in the collecting tubule system that leads to recruitment of aquaporin-2 to the apical membrane. The result is greater water uptake and a more concentrated urine.

antihistamines A class of drugs used for treating allergies; they are H_1-receptor antagonists.

anti-inflammatory drugs Drugs that reduce inflammation.

antimuscarinic anticholinergics A class of drugs used for treating respiratory disorders; they antagonize cholinergic receptors, causing relaxation with bronchodilation.

antipsychotics   Drugs that are effective in treating schizophrenia and other psychotic systems due to their calming effect. These drugs are thought to work by antagonizing dopamine receptors (D_2) in the brain. Also known as neuroleptics or major tranquilizers.

antipyretic   Fever reducing.

anti-thrombotic   Drug action that slows blood clotting.

anxiolytics   Drugs that effectively reduce anxiety. Anxiolytics function by binding to GABA receptors within the brain—formerly known as minor tranquilizers.

aquaporins   Water transporters that facilitate the movement of water along its concentration gradient.

arachidonic acid   A polyunsaturated omega-6 fatty acid, the source for many eicosanoids.

arginine vasopressin   See *antidiuretic hormone.*

arm-crank ergometer   Piece of exercise equipment that measures the force generated.

arrhythmias   Abnormal heart rhythms, resulting from congenital heart defects, coronary artery disease, or valvular heart disease.

arteriosclerosis   Hardening of the arteries.

ascorbate   Vitamin C, necessary for proline conversion into hydroxyproline in collagen. Ascorbate is needed to maintain a healthy extracellular matrix and a strong tissue structure.

asthma exacerbation   A narrowing of bronchial airways and associated inflammation of the bronchial mucosa.

atenolol   A common beta blocker.

atherogenesis   Formation of fatty plaques in arteries.

atherogenic profile   A triad of lipid abnormalities including elevated triglycerides, low HDL, and high LDL (particularly the smaller, denser subfraction of LDL).

atherosclerosis   The most common type of arteriosclerosis, caused by plaque building up in a blood vessel.

Atkins diet   Diet that is low in carbohydrates and high in fat and protein.

atomoxetine   Sympathomimetic drug used for ADHD.

ATP synthase   Mitochondrial enzyme that converts energy in the proton gradient to make ATP from ADP and Pi.

atrioventricular (AV) node   A structure of the heart that electrically connects the atria to the ventricles. The wave of contraction started in the SA node activates the AV node to cause contraction of the ventricles after the atria have emptied.

atrium Heart   chamber that collects blood from veins.

attention deficit hyperactivity disorder (ADHD)   A neurobehavioral disorder, usually diagnosed in childhood and sometimes lasting into adulthood, characterized by the inability to concentrate or maintain attention.

atypical antipsychotics   Second-generation antipsychotic drugs, which work by blocking dopamine receptors; some also block serotonin receptors (5-HT$_2$).

auditory hallucinations   The inability to distinguish real from imaginary sounds.

autacoids   Locally produced molecules that exert their effects locally. Also known as paracrine factors.

autoimmune disease   Disease where the immune system fails to recognize host tissue and mounts an attack against the body's own cells.

autologous transfusion   A reinfusion of blood or blood components into the same individual who originally donated them.

autonomic nervous system (ANS) See *involuntary nervous system.*

barbiturates Class of sedative-hypnotic drugs not used much anymore.

baseline The starting point or control level before a measurement is taken.

benzodiazepines A class of drugs with varying degrees of anxiolytic, anticonvulsant, muscle relaxant, and sedative properties, often used in medical procedures to reduce tension and induce sedation and amnesia.

beta-blockers Beta-receptor antagonists that treat problems associated with adrenergic-dependent responses such as blood pressure or arrythmias.

beta-blockers with ISA Beta-blockers with intrinsic sympathomimetic activity; they have low-level agonist activity at the receptor while blocking activity of endogenous epinephrine or norepinephrine to bind the receptor.

beta cells Pancreatic cells that secrete insulin. Stimuli include elevated blood levels of glucose, certain amino acids, and free fatty acids; beta-adrenergic input and incretins also increase insulin release.

biguanides A class of oral glucose-lowering agents that work primarily by preventing the liver from breaking down glycogen and increasing glucose utilization. They primarily lower blood glucose without involvement of pancreatic beta cells.

bile acid sequestrant A drug designed to bind components of bile in the gastrointestinal tract, preventing reabsorption from the gut.

bioavailability The portion of active drug that passes through bodily barriers to its site of action.

biomarker profiles Measurements of biological activities (e.g., drug metabolites) that can be made to create a unique set of results for individual members of a population.

biotransformation The chemical conversion of a drug in the body by enzymatic reactions, often changing the drug's biological activity, similar to drug metabolism.

bipolar disorder A disorder in which patients suffer from periods of high (manic) and low (depression) "poles." Referred to in the past as manic-depression.

blind study An experiment in which the participants do not know whether they are receiving the drug or placebo.

blood alcohol content (BAC) The percentage of alcohol in the blood in units of mass of alcohol per volume of blood.

blood–brain barrier Specialized capillary bed in the brain that restricts transport of drugs into the central nervous system.

blood sugar Glucose levels in the blood.

blood thinners Drugs that inhibit the clotting process.

body mass index (BMI) Calculation based on height and weight that approximates a person's percent body fat.

bone resorption Correction of serum calcium by the parathyroid hormone that promotes mobilization of calcium and phosphate from the bone.

Borg rating of perceived exertion (RPE) Relative measure of the level of exercise intensity perceived by the person exercising.

bradycardia A condition in which the resting heart rate becomes too low (less than 60 bpm) to pump sufficient oxygenated blood to the body.

brain-derived neurotrophic factor (BDNF) A polypeptide growth factor produced in the brain that mediates neurogenesis and neuronal plasticity.

bronchial hyperreactivity A condition observed in people who have asthma where bronchospasm is easily triggered.

bronchioles A set of branching tubes that extend from bronchi. Each terminal bronchiole divides into two respiratory bronchioles, which branch again, forming alveolar ducts.

bronchoconstriction The constriction of bronchioles.

bronchodilators Drugs that relax the smooth muscle in the airways to relieve or prevent bronchoconstriction.

bronchospasm Spasm of the muscle cells in the bronchioles, which induces fits of
coughing.

buccal administration Administration of a drug by placing it inside the mouth between the lining of the cheek and gums.

caffeine A xanthine alkaloid derived from the seeds, leaves, and fruits of certain
plants.

calcidiol The product of the reaction in the liver toward converting vitamin D_3 into
the precursor for hormonally active vitamin D. Also known as calcifediol.

calcitriol The hormonally active form of vitamin D, important in regulating calcium
and phosphate levels in the body and particularly in the mineralization of bone. It
is transformed from D_3 via enzymatic steps in the liver and kidney.

calcium antagonists See *calcium channel blockers.*

calcium channel blockers A class of drugs that slow calcium entry into cells; they are
used in treating hypertension and other types of cardiovascular diseases.

canagliflozin A drug used for Type 2 diabetes that increases loss of glucose during
urine formation.

cannabidiol (CBD) A nonpsychoactive component of cannabis that has therapeutic
benefits but does not produce feelings of euphoria.

cannabinoids A mixture of related compounds with differing biological activity extracted from cannabus.

cannabis A preparation of the cannabis plant. Usually, the term refers to the resin
(hashish) or the leaves and flowers (marijuana); these forms are usually smoked,
but they can also be consumed orally in baked goods.

captopril An older ACE inhibitor used in the past for hypertension.

carbonic anhydrase inhibitors A class of diuretics that are weak and are used for
high-altitude mountain sickness and glaucoma (as eye drops).

cardiac remodeling Adaption of the heart's anatomy in response to certain drugs or
exercise.

cardiomyopathy A thickening or enlarging of heart muscle.

cardiorespiratory fitness level Based on an individual's VO_2max, it provides a measure on an individual's health.

cardioselective beta-blockers Beta-blockers that are more selective toward the β-1
subtype of receptor than β-2.

cardiovascular disease A broad scope that includes disease associated with the heart
and the vasculature.

cardiovascular fitness The limiting factor to performing physical work, determined
by the ability of the heart to pump oxygen-rich blood to the tissues and the ability
of tissues to use oxygen to produce ATP.

carnitine A generic term for a number of compounds, including L-carnitine,
acetyl-L-carnitine, and propionyl-L-carnitine, that play an essential role in the
transfer of long-chain fatty acids into the mitochondria for beta-oxidation.

carvedilol A newer beta-blocker.

case-control study A study that compares patients who have a specific condition with people who do not and that uses a finding of statistical significance to confirm a difference between the groups.

case reports Collections of reports on the treatment of a single patient or a small group of patients.

catecholamines A group of chemicals including dopamine, norepinephrine, and epinephrine.

catechol-*O*-methyltransferase (COMT) An enzyme that inactivates neurotransmitters like dopamine and norepinephrine.

cathepsin B A protease with a wide variety of actions inside cells and with roles in hormone and immune function.

central nervous system (CNS) The part of the nervous system consisting of the brain and spinal cord.

cerebrospinal axis The brain and spinal cord together.

challenge stress The type of stress associated with an event like a race or a presentation.

cholecalciferol Vitamin D_3, generated in the skin when sunlight is absorbed by an inactive precursor. It is also found in certain dietary sources.

cholesterol biosynthesis A complex series of reactions that produce cholesterol, primarily in the liver.

cholinergic Postganglionic parasympathetic neurons, which release acetylcholine.

chondroitin sulfate An important component of the ground substance in the extracellular matrix. It is a common ingredient in joint care supplements, usually combined with glucosamine.

chronic obstructive pulmonary disease (COPD) A disease characterized by narrowing of the airways and low airflow; it is poorly reversible and generally worsens over time.

chronic stress Stress that persists and contributes to allostatic load.

chronotropic Affecting the rate of heart contractions.

chyme The gastric juices and partly digested food which passes from the stomach to the small intestine.

cilazapril An ACE inhibitor.

cimetidine A drug used to reduce acid in the stomach.

clearance One of the four components of pharmacokinetics concerned with elimination of drugs and metabolites from the body.

clenbuterol A beta-2 agonist not approved for human use that has PES potential and is on the WADA list of banned substances.

clozapine A drug used to treat schizophrenia.

cocaine A street drug that is a short-acting stimulant.

coenzyme Q Generated from an intermediate of cholesterol synthesis. It is involved in the electron transport chain in mitochondria and ATP production. Also called Q-10.

cohort study A study in which a large population of patients is observed over time and compared with a matched control group that does not have the condition or has not undergone the treatment being studied.

colesevelam A drug originally developed as a bile acid sequestrant to lower cholesterol; it also lowers HbA1c.

collagen The most abundant animal protein in the world and a component of the extracellular matrix. Each collagen protein contains three peptide chains that form a triple helix.

colonoscopy   Procedure using a camera to examine primarily the large bowel.

compensatory mechanisms   Processes that return the body back to homeostasis.

conditionally essential nutrients   Nutrients that the body normally produces but that some individuals cannot produce in sufficient quantity because of their age, genetics, or disease state, so these nutrients must be obtained from the diet.

Controlled Substances Act   Established federal drug policy regulating the manufacture, importation, possession, use, and distribution of certain substances.

coronary heart disease   Disease of the heart's major blood vessels.

corticotropin-releasing factor (CRF)   Peptide hormone produced in the hypothalamus that stimulates the pituitary to produce ACTH.

cortisol   A steroid hormone produced by the adrenal cortex as part of the HPA stress response.

COX-1   A version of COX that is widely distributed and has constitutive activity.

COX-2   A version of COX that is inducible and that plays a greater role in the inflammatory response than COX-1.

creatine kinase   An enzyme responsible for the phosphate transfer between ATP and creatine.

creatinine   The degradation product of creatine and phosphocreatine that is excreted in the urine.

cyclooxygenase (COX)   An enzyme that generates prostaglandins and thromboxanes from arachidonic acid as part of the inflammatory response.

cytochrome P450   A super family of heme-containing enzymes that function as monooxygenases that help the clearance of various compounds from the body.

cytokines   Molecules released by immune cells to communicate with other cells in the immune system to coordinate their activity.

dapagliflozin   Drug used for Type 2 diabetes that increases glucose loss during urine formation.

decongestant   A drug used to help keep airways open.

dehydration   A state of negative water balance or hypovolemia.

dehydroepiandrosterone (DHEA)   A prohormone that is converted into androstenedione, which can be converted into testosterone (or estrogen in females).

delayed onset muscle soreness (DOMS)   Muscle soreness that develops and peaks 24–72 hours following strenuous exercise.

dependence   Continued use of a drug to avoid the discomfort of withdrawal; in physical dependence, the drug is needed for everyday functioning.

derivative of fibric acid   See *fibrates*.

dextromethorphan   Opioid used for cough suppression.

diabetes   A chronic disease that results from elevated levels of glucose in the blood and defective insulin function.

diabetic ketoacidosis   A serious medical emergency that results when free fatty acids become the dominant energy source due to low levels of insulin, diminished glycogen stores, and low intracellular glucose. Ketone bodies, a product of fatty acid metabolism, build up to toxic levels that can result in vomiting, dehydration, breathing problems, confusion, and even coma.

diastole   Relaxation of heart muscle, in which the left and right ventricles fill with blood coming from the left and right atria.

dietary   approaches to stop hypertension [DASH diet] A diet recommended for people who want to prevent or treat hypertension and reduce their risk of heart disease.

Dietary Supplement Health and Education Act A 1994 statute of United States Federal legislation that defines and regulates dietary supplements.

dihydropyridine A class of calcium channel blockers that are more potent for vascular muscle cell relaxation than drugs in the phenylalkylamine and diltiazem classes.

dilated cardiomyopathy A condition in which the muscles of the left ventricle stretch, lengthen, and weaken over time, reducing the ventricle's ability to pump forcefully.

diltiazem A class of calcium channel blockers.

dipeptidyl peptidase-4 (DPP-4) Target enzyme for class of Type 2 diabetes drugs. Its inhibition extends the lifetime of hormones that help control blood glucose.

distribution One of the four major parameters for pharmacokinetics that helps describe how much drug gets to its site of action.

diuretics Drugs that inhibit sodium reabsorption in the kidneys, so that an increase in the rate of water and sodium loss occurs; they are used to treat hypertension.

diurnal rhythm Part of the internal clock that the body's processes follow on a daily basis.

dopamine A neurotransmitter found primarily in the brain that is implicated in the reward response and other critical brain activities.

dopamine hypothesis A hypothesis suggesting that hyperactivity of dopaminergic signaling in certain regions of the brain is associated with psychosis.

dose–response curve A plot of the measurable effect (response) of a drug on the Y-axis versus dose or concentration on the X-axis.

dosing The practice of getting the dose correct for patients.

double-blind study An experiment in which neither the administrator nor the subjects know whether a drug or placebo is being administered until the identity key is accessed.

downregulation The process that reduces the responses of a cell to a stimulus following repeated agonist stimulation by a drug.

doxazosin An alpha-adrenergic blocker that causes smooth muscle relaxation in the vasculature.

dromotropic Affecting conduction velocity in the heart.

drug A chemical used to prevent, treat, or cure disease.

drug receptor The protein to which a drug binds in order to modify biological processes.

duloxetine An SSNRI (selective serotonin and norepinephrine reuptake inhibitor) that is used as an antidepressant.

dynorphin A peptide with endogenous opioid activity, discovered after the endorphins.

dyrenium Diuretic that is potassium-sparing.

dysfunctional pain A type of pathological pain in which no clear nerve damage or inflammation is involved.

dyslipidemia A condition marked by an abnormal concentration of lipids or lipoproteins in the blood, such as elevated triglycerides.

ectoenzyme An enzyme that is attached to a cell's exterior, so that its activity is extracellular.

ectopic fat Fat that is abnormally distributed throughout tissues such as liver and skeletal muscle.

ED50 The dose that gives a therapeutic response in 50% of subjects.

efferent fiber A nerve that transmits output from the cerebrospinal axis.

efficacy   The maximum response for a drug's primary effect.

eicosanoids   Lipid mediators, such as prostaglandins, thromboxanes, and leukotrienes, that play a central role in inflammation and other processes.

electron transport chain   Located in the inner membrane of mitochondria, it uses oxidation-reduction reactions to generate the proton gradient.

electronic cigarette   An electronic device that simulates smoking; it contains synthetic nicotine and no tobacco products. Also known as e-cigarette.

elimination   Excretion of a drug from the body.

empagliflozin   A drug for Type 2 diabetes that increases glucose loss in the urine.

enalapril   An ACE inhibitor.

endocannabinoid   Natural molecules in the body that signal through receptors targeted by the active ingredients in marijuana.

endogenous ligand   The molecule that normally binds a target protein, for example, hormones and neurotransmitters.

endorphins   Endogenous opioid neuropeptides, from endogenous morphine.

enkephalin   A peptide with endogenous opioid activity, discovered after the endorphins.

enteral   Drugs or nutrients that pass through the intestines, usually taken by mouth.

ephedra   A naturally occurring plant alkaloid that has been used as part of herbal therapy for alleviating cold symptoms. Its active ingredient is ephedrine.

ephedrine   A prescription drug that has a weak central nervous system stimulatory effect and weak, nonselective agonist activity for α- and β-receptors.

epinephrine   The hormonal output of the adrenal medulla; formerly referred to as adrenaline.

epithelial Na$^+$ inhibitors   A class of potassium-sparing drugs that inhibit the epithelial Na$^+$ channels located on the apical membrane of principal cells, blocking Na$^+$ influx and lessening the lumen-negative electrical gradient, creating less pull on K$^+$ and H$^+$, and resulting in less K$^+$ loss and less acidic urine.

ergogenic drugs   Drugs that increase work capacity and are usually illegal for most sports and competitions.

ergolytic drugs   Drugs that decrease work capacity and are usually avoided by athletes and other physically active individuals.

ergosterol   Vitamin D$_2$, found primarily in plants and mushrooms and without significant biological activity.

ertugliflozin   A drug used for Type 2 diabetes that increases loss of glucose in the urine.

erythrocyte   Red blood cell.

erythropoietin   A naturally occurring hormone produced by the kidneys, a hematinic agent that stimulates red blood cell formation.

escitalopram   An anti-depressant that works as a selective serotonin reuptake inhibitor (SSRI).

essential nutrients   The nutrients required in the human diet; they must be consumed because the body cannot produce sufficient quantities of them. Nutrients that generally do not "cure" disease but rather prevent or cure the pathology associated with a deficiency.

ethanol   A byproduct of fermentation when yeasts have an ample supply of nutrients but have limited oxygen.

euglycemia   A normal concentration of glucose in the blood.

evaporative cooling   The cooling effect that occurs from sweat evaporating from the skin. This is the main mechanism by which heat is dissipated during exercise.

evidence pyramid A guideline to the hierarchy of evidence for researching and defending a hypothesis or developing a protocol.

exercise and sport pharmacology A branch of pharmacology that studies the interactions among the physiological changes caused by drugs and the physiological changes caused by physical activity.

exercise capacity The maximum amount of exertion an individual can sustain. Exercise capacity is based on an individual's VO_2max.

exercise-induced bronchoconstriction A condition were breathing is impaired following exercise. It probably results from loss of heat and water from airways and a greater possible intake of allergens and pollutants.

exercise-induced bronchoconstriction with asthma The term used when individuals with asthma experience exercise-induced bronchoconstriction.

exercise intensity The degree of physiological strain an individual experiences while exercising. It can be measured as a percentage VO_2max or in watts.

exercise prescription Exercise plan given to an individual who needs to improve cardiovascular health and fitness level, specifying the frequency, intensity, duration, and type of physical activities.

extracellular matrix A complex network of secreted proteins and carbohydrates that fills spaces between cells and that is important in cell attachment and tissue structure, providing a lattice through which nutrients diffuse and cells can move, especially during differentiation and development.

ezetimibe A drug that blocks dietary cholesterol uptake from the gut, sometimes used in conjunction with a statin.

facilitated diffusion Transport of materials along their concentration gradient by protein transporters within a cell's plasma membrane. Examples include glucose and amino acids.

Famotidine A histamine-2 receptor blocker used as an antacid.

fast angiotensin II responses Responses to angiotensin II that include direct vasoconstrictor activity. Total peripheral resistance increases due to angiotensin II receptors (AT_1 receptors) in blood vessels causing vasoconstriction.

fast-twitch glycolytic (FG) fibers Muscle fibers that have a fast contraction speed and low fatigue resistance and that favor glycolytic (anaerobic) methods of energy production. Also known as Type IIx fibers.

fast-twitch oxidative fibers Muscle fibers that are intermediate in their level of fatigue resistance, having available energy stored in glycogen, but in limited amounts. Also known as Type IIa fibers.

fenfluramine A drug used to decrease appetite and lose weight in the 1990s but was withdrawn due to heart-related issues.

fenofibric acid A drug (or fenofibrate) used to lower blood lipids.

fermentation A process in which pyruvate is reduced to lactate, maintaining glycolysis and ATP production.

fibrates A class of lipid-modifying drugs that effectively lower triglycerides by stimulating lipoprotein lipase activity in endothelial cells and decreasing triglyceride levels. Also referred to as fibric acid derivatives.

first-pass metabolism A metabolic process in which a certain percentage of the absorbed drug may be chemically altered in the liver before it enters the bloodstream and reaches its site of action.

flecainide An anti-arrhythmic drug that blocks sodium channels.

flow-limited   Describes drugs whose pharmacokinetic properties are influenced by exercise; usually, the redistribution of blood flow that accompanies physical exertion alters their blood levels during exercise.

fluoxymesterone   An anabolic steroid used in the treatment of low testosterone levels.

fluvastatin   A statin used to lower LDL.

forced expiratory volume in one second (FEV1)   A measurement of respiratory function: how much air an individual exhales during the first second of a forced breath.

free fatty acids (FFA)   The breakdown of stored triglycerides releases free fatty acids that can be burned for energy by oxidative metabolism in mitochondria.

furosemide   A loop diuretic.

gamma-aminobutyric acid (GABA)   The primary inhibitory neurotransmitter in the brain.

ganglion   A grouping of synapses between neurons.

gastric inhibitory polypeptide (GIP)   A peptide released during digestion that aids insulin in maintaining blood sugar levels.

generalized anxiety disorder (GAD)   Anxiety that is chronic and excessive; symptoms may include trouble concentrating, recurring headaches, very tense muscles, and sleep disorders.

ghrelin   A peptide hormone produced by cells in the fundus of the stomach and certain cells in the brain that increases appetite by decreasing leptin activity and stimulating neurons such as neuropeptide Y neurons.

GI-tract   A grouping of the organs from the stomach to the anus.

Glaucoma   Damage of the optic nerve, often caused by abnormally high pressure in the eye, causes vision problems.

glinides   A group of insulin secretagogues, including repaglinide; they can block the same K^+ channel as sulfonylureas, producing insulin release.

gliptins   Drugs that act as inhibitors of the enzyme dipeptidyl peptidase-4 (DPP-4), prolonging and enhancing activity of incretins.

glomerular filtration rate   The rate of flow of filtered fluid through the kidneys, controlled by arterial blood pressure and arteriole diameter.

glucagon   A peptide of 29 amino acids produced by pancreatic alpha cells. It raises the concentration of glucose in the bloodstream.

gluconeogenesis   The process in which glucose is made from lactate or breakdown products of amino acids, primarily in the fasting state. During longer states of fasting (over 8 to 12 hours), gluconeogenesis contributes more glucose than glycogenolysis as glycogen stores become depleted.

glucosamine   An important component of the ground substance in the extracellular matrix. It is a common ingredient in joint care supplements, usually combined with chondroitin sulfate.

glucose homeostasis   Complex process by which the body maintains blood glucose levels within a healthy range.

glucose intolerance   The inability to control blood sugar.

glucose transporters (GLUTs)   Members of a complex gene family with 14 members found in the human genome. Expression of different glucose transporters contributes to different glucose transport properties in different tissues.

glucose-6-phosphatase   An enzyme that removes phosphate from glucose, allowing the glucose to be transported out of cells and into the bloodstream.

glucosidases   Enzymes that break the bonds of sugars and release monosaccharides. They are produced in the pancreas and found on surfaces of cells lining the gut, mainly along the upper portion of the small intestine.

GLUTs   A family of many glucose transporters that play a critical role in glucose uptake and signaling.

glutamate   The most abundant excitatory neurotransmitter in vertebrate brains.

gluteal adipose tissue   Fat stored around the hips and thighs.

glyburide   A sulfonylurea used for diabetes that increases insulin secretion.

glycemic control   The maintenance of glucose levels.

glycemic index   A reference list of foods indicating their propensity to raise blood sugar levels, with white bread or pure glucose set at a level of 100.

glycemic response   Change in blood sugar levels.

glycogen   A large polymer containing thousands of glucose molecules.

glycogenolysis   The process by which glycogen is broken down and glucose is released. During short periods (8 to 12 hours) of fasting, glycogenolysis in the liver produces sufficient glucose to maintain blood sugar levels.

glycolytic pathway   Glycolysis is a fundamental pathway of enzymatic steps that converts glucose to pyruvic acid and makes a net of two ATP.

growth hormone   A peptide hormone of 191 amino acids long secreted from the anterior pituitary at about 0.4 to 1.0 mg per day in males, with higher values in women and adolescents. Also called somatotropin.

HbA1c test   A test capable of diagnosing prediabetes and metabolic syndrome, Type 1 diabetes, and Type 2 diabetes. It indicates the average level of glucose in the blood over the previous two to three months by monitoring the percentage of hemoglobin that is bound to sugar molecules. Also referred to as the A1c test.

hedonic eating   Consumption of food for pleasure rather than for maintenance of energy homeostasis.

hematinic agents   Agents that stimulate erythrocyte formation or increase the amount of hemoglobin in red blood cells.

hematocrit test   A test for the volume of whole blood composed of red blood cells. It can be used to help determine blood doping.

heme   The heme group contains iron and binds oxygen. They are found in oxygen-binding proteins hemoglobin and myoglobin, producing the red color.

hemoglobin   Oxygen-binding protein found in red blood cells that makes them red.

high-density lipoprotein (HDL)   A lipoprotein important in cholesterol transport and reverse cholesterol transport, formed from VLDL or chylomicron remnants. This is the "good" cholesterol.

high-intensity interval training (HIIT)   Alternating bouts of maximal effort and short periods of rest.

histamine   A chemical released from mast cells and basophils in response to allergens; it acts locally in the immune response and can be a trigger for inflammation.

HMG-CoA-reductase   The rate-limiting enzyme in the cholesterol synthetic pathway; it performs the first of a complex series of reactions responsible for producing cholesterol.

HMG-CoA-reductase inhibitors   See *statins*.

holiday heart syndrome   The increase in alcohol consumption added to the excitement and stress of the holidays often results in an uptick in the number of heart attack victims in emergency rooms.

homologous transfusion   A transfusion in which blood from a human donor is given to another person. Usually, the blood is stored for later transfusion.

HPA axis   The hypothalamus, pituitary gland, and adrenal cortex; it results in an increase in corticosteroids like cortisol during a stress event.

human growth hormone (HGH)   A bioengineered growth hormone that has limited clinical use; it is prescribed for individuals with a growth hormone insufficiency.

humulin N   An intermediate acting form of insulin.

hyaluronate   A large, charged polysaccharide of many thousands of disaccharides in length.

hydrochlorothiazide (HCTZ)   A thiazide diuretic.

hydroxyzine   An antihistamine.

hyperglycemia   Elevated blood sugar, which increases the risk for developing cardio-vascular disease, nephropathy, retinopathy, and neuropathy.

hyperlipidemia   Elevated levels of blood lipids, a positive risk factor for cardiovascular disease.

hyperplasia   The increase in the rate of cell reproduction, increasing the number of cells.

hyperresponsiveness   Increased responsiveness to inhaled stimuli, which can trigger recurrent bouts of shortness of breath, wheezing, and spasm of the muscle cells in the bronchioles.

hypertension   Chronic high blood pressure.

hyperthermia   Elevated body temperature.

hyperthyroidism   Overactive thyroid.

hypertrophic cardiomyopathy   A condition of abnormal growth and thickening of the ventricular wall, decreasing the ventricle's ability to deliver blood to the body.

hypoglycemia   The condition of having low blood sugar. Its dangers include a possibility of injuring the brain, as glucose is the brain's primary source of energy.

hypokalemia   Low blood potassium level.

hyponatremia   The condition of abnormally low levels of sodium in the blood.

hypovolemia   Decreased blood volume, often caused by dehydration.

ibuprofen A common OTC   (or prescription NSAID (nonsteroidal anti-inflammatory drug)).

IgE hypothesis   A hypothesis proposing that allergens bind IgE antibodies and cause mast cells to release various factors that trigger asthmatic attacks.

IM   Administration of a drug by injection into muscle; intramuscular.

imipramine   A tricyclic antidepressant.

immunoglobulin E (IgE)   A class of antibodies that bind and stimulate mast cells.

incretins   Gut peptides that increase insulin release in response to food intake. In the postprandial state, incretins enhance insulin secretion, suppress glucagon secretion, slow gastric emptying, and promote beta cell health.

inflammatory mediators   Chemical mediators released by cells at the onset of an infection or injury to produce acute inflammation. They include serotonin, histamine, heparin, prostaglandins, leukotrienes, monocytes, interleukins, interferon, bradykinin, and many others.

inflammatory pain   A type of pain related to recovery from damage, such as an inflamed joint, muscle sprain, or surgery. Inflammatory pain results from the inflammatory response in damaged or recovering areas and has a low threshold, in order to initiate an avoidance response.

inotropic   Affecting the force of contraction in the heart.

insomnia   A condition with impaired sleep.

insulin   A hormone produced in the pancreas consisting of two polypeptides; it stimulates cells to import glucose and helps regulate blood sugar.

insulin-like growth factor-1 (IGF-1)   A polypeptide hormone that stimulates different types of growth response. Expression can be induced by intense exercise, anabolic steroids, or growth hormone.

insulin resistance   A condition in which an individual's cells do not respond correctly to insulin and do not increase glucose uptake.

insulin secretagogues   Insulin-releasing drugs used to treat diabetes, including sulfonylureas and glinides.

integrins   Receptors on the surface of cells that bind multi-adhesive glycoproteins in the extracellular matrix and link to the cell's cytoskeleton, providing tissue strength.

intercalated cells   Cells in the collecting tubule system that help maintain acid/base balance, H^+, and bicarbonate transport.

intermediate-acting insulin   Insulin complexed with a small, positively charged protein called protamine. It has an expected onset of about 2 to 5 hours and a duration of 12 hours.

intramuscular fat   Fat used primarily for muscle function.

inverse agonist   A drug that binds receptors at the same site as an agonist, producing the opposite pharmacological response and decreasing receptor activity below basal level.

involuntary nervous system   The part of the nervous system that innervates smooth muscle, cardiac tissue, and secretory glands and works without our conscious control of its activities. It controls breathing, digestion, body temperature, sweating, blood pressure, and secretions from glands. Also called the autonomic nervous system.

ipragliflozin   A drug used for Type 2 diabetes that increases loss of glucose during urine formation.

iproniazid   An older antidepressant (monoamine oxidase inhibitor), no longer used.

irisin   A myokine with potential roles in fat metabolism and bone formation.

isosorbide mononitrate   Used for angina.

IV   Administration of a drug by injection into a vein; intravenous.

Januvia   Same as sitagliptin, used for regulating levels of insulin in diabetes.

kaliuresis   Excessive potassium (K^+) loss during urine formation.

ketogenic diet   A version of the low carb diet that encourages high fat and protein.

ketone bodies   Water-soluble breakdown products of fatty acids produced in the liver, used as a source of energy by the heart and brain during periods of fasting.

Krebs cycle   Central biochemical pathway in mitochondria that results in the complete oxidation of carbon from glucose, generating reducing equivalents that feed the electron transport chain.

LD50   The dose that kills 50% of test animals.

left ventricular hypertrophy (LVH)   A pathological condition that occurs when muscle cells in the left ventricle grow in size due to the increased load caused by prolonged elevated blood pressure.

leptin   A hormone produced by adipocytes that suppresses appetite and contributes to the sense of feeling full.

leukotriene modifiers   A class of drugs used for treating chronic asthma; they target leukotriene signaling, which plays a central role in inflammation.

levodopa   A precursor to dopamine used for the treatment of Parkinson disease.

librium   One of the earliest benzodiazepines used for anxiety.

lidocaine   A local anesthetic.

ligand   A molecule, such as a drug, hormone, or neurotransmitter, that binds to a protein.

lipase inhibitors   Drugs that slow the action of lipases and the breakdown of fat.

lipolysis   The enzymatic breakdown of triglycerides by lipases, releasing free fatty acids from glycerol to fuel ATP production.

lipoprotein complexes   Vesicles with a monolayer of phospholipids and a targeting protein used for lipid transport.

lipoprotein lipase (LPL)   An enzyme lining the surface of endothelial cells that releases free fatty acids from the triglycerides in VLDL.

lithium   The "gold standard" mood-stabilizing drug and one of the first effective treatments for mania.

long-acting insulin   Insulin with a slightly modified sequence that has a broad concentration plateau, keeping a relatively constant level in the blood that can last several hours.

loop diuretics   A class of diuretics that block the $Na^+/K^+/2Cl^-$ symporter in the thick ascending limb.

lorazepam   A benzodiazepines prescribed for anxiety and certain types of seizures.

lorcaserin   A selective serotonin receptor agonist designed to decrease appetite.

losartan   An angiotensin receptor blocker used for hypertension.

low-density lipoprotein (LDL)   A lipoprotein important in cholesterol transport, created from the remnants of VLDL. It is the "bad" cholesterol, associated with plaque formation, atherosclerosis, and cardiovascular disease.

L-type calcium channel   The prevalent voltage-activated (or gated) calcium channel in vascular smooth muscle, cardiac muscle, and the SA and AV nodes, which acts as a drug receptor for the calcium channel blockers.

lung ventilation rate   The volume of breathing per minute; it depends on frequency and tidal volume.

major depressive disorder (MDD)   A diagnosis based on symptoms of insomnia, depressed mood, diminished interest in day-to-day activities, significant weight loss or gain, psychomotor agitation or retardation, fatigue, feelings of worthlessness or guilt, diminished ability to concentrate or indecisiveness, and thoughts of death or suicide.

MAO inhibitors   Drugs developed and widely prescribed for depression in the 1960s and 1970s; their use is now limited because of their association with hepatotoxicity.

mast cells   Cells that release a wide range of factors, including histamine and eicosanoids, found in proximity to surfaces that interface with the external environment in association with blood vessels and nerves.

mast-cell stabilizers   A class of drugs used for treating asthma; they block membrane channels involved in the secretory response, resulting in a diminished response to allergens in mast cells and other responsive cells.

maximum heart rate   The highest target heart rate when a person is exercising: $MHR = 211 - 0.64 \times age$.

meta-analysis A quantitative approach for increasing the statistical power for specified end points or subgroups. A meta-analysis pools from many published studies that meet appropriate inclusion criteria.

metabolic cart A device used to measure VO_2max by determining oxygen levels in inspired and expired air.

metabolic equivalent of task (MET) A relative measure of exercise intensity that is independent of the subjects weight.

metabolic syndrome A cluster of risk factors associated with an increased risk for cardiovascular disease and Type 2 diabetes; it involves a complex interaction between genetic, metabolic, and environmental factors.

metered-dose inhaler An alternative to the nebulizer; it delivers the drug more quickly in a couple of puffs, usually at lower cost.

metformin A biguanide drug considered a first-line agent for Type 2 diabetes. Its primary effect is to lower blood glucose without involvement of pancreatic beta cells by activating AMP-activated protein kinase.

methamphetamine A powerful centrally acting stimulant (sympathomimetic) with abuse potential.

methylphenidate A centrally acting sympathomimetic prescribed for attention deficit and hyperactivity disorder.

methylsulfonylmethane (MSM) An additive to glucosamine supplements that provides a source of sulfur and methyl groups needed for the production of glycosaminoglycans, essential for a healthy extracellular matrix.

methylxanthines A class of drugs that includes theophylline and caffeine; theophylline has been used for long-term management of asthma and COPD.

metoprolol A common beta-blocker.

microsomal enzymes A preparation of enzymes from the endoplasmic reticulum and Golgi used by biochemists to study drug metabolism.

microvesicle A vesicle released by cells that can contain regulatory proteins and RNA. They have targeting proteins that attach and allow entry into target cells.

miglitol A competitive inhibitor of intestinal glucosidases; it delays digestion and absorption of glucose derived from starch, oligosaccharides, and disaccharides.

mineralocorticoids Steroid hormones produced and released by the adrenal cortex. They control salt and water balance, largely by affecting processes in the kidney.

miosis Contraction of the pupil.

modafinil A sympathomimetic use to treat sleep disorders like narcolepsy.

monoamine oxidase (MAO) An enzyme in the mitochondria that metabolizes neurotransmitters like norepinephrine, epinephrine, and dopamine.

monotherapy A patient is on only one drug (and presumably no OTCs or supplements).

mood-stabilizing drugs Drugs used to treat bipolar disorder, including lithium and drugs with anticonvulsant activity.

mu The predominant opioid receptor. It is widely distributed throughout the body and is involved in mediating the primary opioid effects, including spinal cord analgesia, respiratory depression, decreased GI-tract motility, and modification of hormone and neurotransmitter release.

muscarinic receptors Receptors that respond to acetyl choline at the target synapses of the parasympathetic nervous system.

myelin An electrically insulating layer in a nerve that dramatically speeds transmission allowing the brain to respond very quickly to stimulate skeletal muscle.

myocardial ischemia   Low oxygen levels in blood supply to heart tissue.

myoglobin   Protein that contains a heme group to bind oxygen in muscle cells, increasing oxidative capacity. It is a single polypeptide chain (monomer), unlike the closely related hemoglobin which is a tetramer.

nadolol   A non-selective beta-blocker.

NADP/NADPH   Coenzymes used primarily is synthetic reactions where they act as electron donors (NADPH) and acceptors (NADP).

naloxone   The prominent opioid antagonist useful in overdose cases.

narcolepsy   A neurological disorder characterized by overwhelming daytime drowsiness.

nateglinide   An insulin secretagogue used for diabetes.

natriuretic   Causing natriuresis, the process of excreting sodium in the urine, which results from inhibition of sodium (Na^+) reabsorption in the kidney.

nebivolol   A newer beta-blocker.

nebulizer   A device that turns a liquid solution into a fine mist and delivers the drug through a face mask or mouthpiece over the course of about 10 minutes.

nedocromil   A mast cell stabilizer that is a weak anti-inflammatory drug.

nephron   A fundamental unit of the kidney, containing the glomerulus and its associated capillary bed where filtration takes place, as well as a series of tubules where regulated reabsorption takes place.

neurogenesis theory   A current theory suggesting that depression results from low rates of neurogenesis in certain brain regions, impairing neuronal plasticity.

neuroleptic   An antipsychotic, previously called a major tranquilizer, typically used to manage psychosis.

neuropathic pain   A type of pathological pain in which nerve damage is the major cause.

neuropathy   Weakness caused by damage to the nerves outside of the brain and spinal cord.

neuropeptide Y   A peptide hormone that stimulates appetite and storage of fat.

neuroplasticity   The capacity of the brain to increase cell number, the number and strength of connections, cell survival, and maintain cognitive function as we age.

neurotransmitter hypothesis   An older hypothesis postulating that depression can result from defective neurotransmitter signaling in the brain.

neurotransmitters   Chemicals that transmit signals from one neuron to another neuron or a target cell.

niacin   A B-vitamin used as a drug to treat dyslipidemia by inhibiting lipolysis and release of fatty acids from adipose tissue.

niacin derivatives   A class of lipid-modifying drugs that work by inhibiting lipolysis in adipose tissue, decreasing the release of free fatty acids.

nicotine   A potent drug with complex pharmacological activities that is one of hundreds of chemicals present in cigarette smoke. It is used as a poison in pest control, as it acts as an acetylcholine receptor agonist.

nicotinic receptors   Acetyl choline receptors found in ganglia and neuromuscular junctions.

nifedipine   A calcium channel blocker.

nitric oxide (NO)   Produced by cells to cause vasodilation.

nociceptive pain   A type of pain that results from noxious stimuli, such as sharp objects, heat, or cold, acting as an early warning to immediately stop and withdraw. It has a high threshold, requiring an intense stimulus.

nonessential supplements Supplements used for putative gains in performance.

nonselective beta-blockers Beta-blockers that have similar affinity for β-1 and β-2 receptors.

nonsteroidal anti-inflammatory drugs (NSAIDs) Effective analgesics with antipyretic activity and anti-inflammatory action. They have anti-inflammatory activity due to their ability to inhibit the enzyme cyclooxygenase.

norepinephrine Neurotransmitter at the target site of the sympathetic nervous system and in the brain. Also make up about 20% of the adrenalin discharge from the adrenal medulla.

norepinephrine transporter (NET) Transporter that takes up norepinephrine in the presynaptic membrane.

novalin N Intermediate acting insulin preparation.

novocaine Local anesthetic.

nutraceuticals Nutritional or dietary supplements taken to benefit general health or athletic performance.

nutrigenomics Study of the genetic factors influencing the body's response to diet, examining how the bioactive constituents of food affect gene expression.

olanzapine An atypical antipsychotic prescribed for schizophrenia.

omega-3 fatty acids Essential fatty acids with a double bond three bonds from the methyl end of the molecule; important in many biological processes because of their length, the number and location of double bonds, and their unique structures. Also called n-3 fatty acids.

omega-6 fatty acids Essential fatty acids with a double bond six bonds from the methyl end of the molecule; they are precursors for the synthesis of arachidonic acid. Also called n-6.

onglyza Brand name for saxagliptin that helps regulate insulin in diabetes.

opiates Natural products processed from opium, including morphine and codeine.

opioid analgesics Natural and synthetic drugs that mimic the endogenous endorphins, generating similar responses through the opioid receptor system.

opioids Synthetic derivatives of opiates, including heroin and hydrocodone.

opium An extract from poppy plants.

orexin A peptide that has neurotransmitter-like activity that promotes wakefulness and appetite.

orlistat A gastric and pancreatic lipase inhibitor, stopping the release of fatty acids from triglycerides.

orosomucoid A plasma protein with many diverse roles, including anti-inflammatory activity.

orthostatic hypotension A type of hypotension that can occur when a person stands up after sitting or lying down for a while; it can cause dizziness or fainting.

osmotic agents A class of diuretics that pull water from various compartments of the body and increase the urinary excretion of all electrolytes.

osteoarthritis A form of arthritis that involves the deterioration over time of the connective tissue and cartilage that protects the ends of the bones, leading to inflammation, swelling, and pain.

osteomalacia The manifestation of vitamin D deficiency in adults, which leads to softening of the bones, bending of the spine, bowing of the legs, muscle weakness, bone fragility, and increased risk for fractures.

osteoporosis Lowered bone density.

OTC drugs   Drugs or drug combinations that can be purchased "over the counter" and do not require a prescription by a doctor or other appropriate healthcare practitioner.

overtraining syndrome   Decrease in performance due to inadequate recovery time.

oxidative phosphorylation   The process by which the enzyme ATP synthase uses the proton-motive force in the proton gradient to make ATP from ADP and Pi in mitochondria.

oxidative stress   Oxygen utilization generates free radicals that cause damage and stimulate recovery mechanisms. Exercise increase oxygen use and can increase oxidative stress.

P450 proteins   Family of heme-containing proteins involved in drug metabolism.

pacemaker   A structure composed of specialized heart cells that initiates contraction with a coordinated rhythm.

pain   Unpleasant adaptive and protective sensations resulting from noxious stimuli or inflammatory response. A disease state of the nervous system can cause pathological pain.

palpitations   An irregular, sometimes rapid heartbeat due to exertion, agitation, or illness.

panadol   Another name for acetaminophen or Tylenol.

papaverine   An alkaloid with weak vasodilator activity, originally isolated from the opium poppy plant.

paracetamol   Another name for acetaminophen or Tylenol.

parasympathetic nervous system (PSNS)   One of two branches of the ANS that is relatively limited in its range; the nerves extend preganglionic fibers from the cerebrospinal axis to ganglions relatively close to or even within their target tissues.

parathyroid hormone   Hormone secreted by the parathyroid glands that regulates the serum calcium. It helps regulate calcium by exerting effects on bone, kidney, and intestinal cells.

parenteral Drugs   administered that do pass through the mouth or alimentary canal.

Parkinson's disease   A progressive disorder of the nervous system that causes muscle stiffness or slowing of movement due to loss of neurons in the brain that produce dopamine.

paroxetine   A selective serotonin reuptake inhibitor used for depression.

pathological pain   A type of pain that is maladaptive, resulting from a disease state of the nervous system. Either the requirement for a noxious stimulus is uncoupled from the processing centers or the threshold for generating pain decreases to a point where it is easily reached.

performance-enhancing substances (PESs)   Drugs, supplements, and methods that are identified by the World Anti-doping Agency (WADA) and placed on its Prohibited List, including the substances and methods prohibited in and out of competition.

peripheral nervous system (PNS)   The part of the nervous system consisting of the nerves leading to and from the spinal cord.

peroxisome proliferator-activated receptors (PPARs)   A superfamily of nuclear receptors that includes steroid hormone and thyroid receptors. The PPAR family modulates genes involved in fat and sugar metabolism, mitochondrial activity, and insulin signal transduction.

personalized medicine   The concept that a person's genetic makeup, based on DNA sequencing, will allow individualized treatment.

pharmaceuticals   Prescription drugs.

pharmacodynamics   The study of what happens to the body in response to a drug at the physiological, cellular, metabolic, and receptor levels.

pharmacogenetics   The study of a patient's genetic makeup to provide a basis for predicting responses to drugs, choosing among different medications, optimizing dose, minimizing secondary effects, and determining preventive measures to support the patient's treatment regime.

pharmacogenomics   The use of DNA sequencing techniques to personalize treatment options.

pharmacokinetics   The study of what happens to a drug after it enters the body.

pharmacology   The study of drug action, including the chemistry, effects, and uses of drugs.

phenothiazine   A class of antipsychotic drugs, thought to work by antagonizing dopamine receptors (D_2) in the brain.

phentermine   A potent sympathomimetic that can help decrease appetite and encourage weight loss; it also increases heart rate and blood pressure. It is approved for use with topiramate.

phenylalkylamine   A class of calcium channel blockers that cause a mild decrease in heart rate and cardiac output, due to their depressive effect on cardiac muscle cells and the AV and SA nodes.

phenylephrine   Related to the sympathomimetic ephedra that works primarily in the periphery.

phenylpropanolamine   Related to the sympathomimetic ephedra that works primarily in the periphery.

phosphocreatine   A compound converted from creatine inside skeletal muscle cells that acts as a high-energy reservoir for ATP production. Also called creatine phosphate.

phosphodiesterase   The enzyme responsible for degradation of cyclic AMP, a very important intracellular messenger.

placental barrier   Specialized capillary bed that controls blood flow between the mother and her fetus.

plasma   The soluble portion of uncoagulated blood after centrifugation to remove blood cells.

platelet aggregation   Part of the clotting process.

platelet-derived factors   Signaling molecules released by platelets, often as part of the clotting process.

PO   Oral administration of a drug (from the Latin *per os,* meaning by mouth).

polypharmacy   Term for those individuals taking more than one drug.

postabsorptive state   A state in which the stomach is empty and no longer contributing energy by way of digestion and absorption. It can take 5 to 6 hours for the stomach to return to the postabsorptive state after eating, depending on what was eaten.

post-exercise hypotension   The drop in blood pressure that can occur during recovery.

postprandial state   The state the body enters immediately after eating, involving the uptake, storage, and utilization of glucose and other nutrients by tissues downstream of the liver.

postural hypotension   See *orthostatic hypotension.*

potassium-sparing drugs   A class of diuretics that either block an Na^+ channel or antagonize aldosterone in the collecting tubule system.

potency   The quantity of a drug required to produce a designated intensity of effect.

potentiation   When two or more drugs exert greater than additive effects.

PPAR-α (peroxisome proliferator-activated receptor-α) pathway   Pathway that responds to lipid metabolites and unsaturated fatty acids to upregulate lipid metabolism in liver and muscle. Fibrates activate this pathway, leading to an increase in the expression of genes involved in lipid metabolism. Niacin may also affect this pathway.

pramlinitide   A synthetic hormone that resembles human amylin.

prazosin   An alpha blocker that causes relaxion in blood vessels.

prehypertension   A stage of hypertension defined by blood pressure readings that range from 120 to 139 systolic and 80 to 89 diastolic.

primary hypertension   Hypertension where the cause of the elevated blood pressure is unclear.

principal cells   Cells in the collecting tubule system that regulate Na^+, K^+, and water transport.

procainamide   An antiarrhythmic drug that is a sodium channel blocker.

pro-inflammatory adipokines   Signaling molecules released by fat cells that increase inflammation.

prolactin   Pituitary hormone that stimulates milk production in female mammals.

propafenone   An anti-arrhythmic agent approved for ventricular tachycardia that is a sodium channel blocker.

propranolol   A common beta-blocker.

prostaglandins   A family of signaling molecules produced in response to a wide variety of stimuli.

proteoglycans   Large complexes of protein and carbohydrate that bind a lot of water to create gel-like properties associated with the ground substance of an extracellular matrix.

pseudoephedrine   A derivative of ephedrine, a sympathomimetic.

psychosis   A neurological condition that includes many types of mental disorders manifested by the loss of contact with reality.

psychotherapeutic drugs   Drugs that exert their primary effect on the central nervous system.

pyrogen   A type of cytokine that increases the thermoregulatory set point in the hypothalamus, so that the hypothalamus raises the body's temperature, causing a fever.

pyruvate   A metabolic intermediate of metabolism that can enter mitochondria to be oxidized or be reduced to lactate in the cytoplasm.

Qsymia   Combination of phentermine and topiramate used to treat obesity, along with dietary changes and exercise.

quinidine   Drug with antiarrhythmic agent activity also used for malaria.

radiant cooling   Cooling that occurs as circulation shunts blood to working muscle and to the skin where vessels are vasodilating and dissipating heat.

randomized controlled trial   Trial in which the subjects are randomly assigned to different treatment groups, often under a double-blind protocol for the treatment being analyzed.

reactive oxygen species (ROS)   Free radicals produced as a by-product of oxidative metabolism.

receptor-mediated endocytosis   The specific transport of matter into a cell, utilizing receptors in coated pits on the cell surface.

renin   A protease that when released into the bloodstream cleaves the circulating protein angiotensinogen to form angiotensin I.

renin-angiotensin system (loop)   A physiological system that regulates blood pressure, aldosterone levels, and electrolytes.

repaglinide   An insulin secretagogue used for Type 2 diabetes.

resolution   The series of events that return a tissue back to its original state from an inflammation.

resolvins   Important mediators produced from omega-3 fats that take part in the resolution phase after an inflammatory event and help return tissues back to their original state.

respiratory control center   A structure in the lower brain stem that is responsible for the automatic and rhythmic innervation of the muscles that control breathing.

restraint   The ability to stop eating when satiated.

restrictive cardiomyopathy   A condition that results from the heart losing elasticity and becoming unable to fill or eject properly.

retinopathy   Disease associated with the retina in the eye caused by elevated blood sugar in diabetics.

Reye syndrome   A condition that causes swelling in the liver and brain, most often affecting children and young adults. It is associated with aspirin but not acetaminophen.

rezulin   Drug used for Type 2 diabetes withdrawn from market due to liver damage.

rheumatoid arthritis   A form of arthritis that has an autoimmune basis.

rhinorrhea   Runny nose.

RICE formula   A commonly used method for the treatment of a muscle or joint injury: *Rest* the injured body part; *ice* the area four times a day, for approximately 10 to 15 minutes; *compress* the area by wrapping it with an elastic bandage; and *elevate* the injured area above the heart for a few hours a day.

rickets   The manifestation of vitamin D deficiency in children, resulting in bone deficiencies, including long, bowed legs.

Rimonabant   An anti-obesity drug with cannabinoid receptor activity withdrawn from the market due to psychiatric side effects.

risperidone   Antipsychotic drug used to treat schizophrenia and bipolar disorder.

salicylic acid   Used for skin issues, such as acne.

sarcopenia   Muscle wasting disease associated with aging.

satiation   A process that terminates food consumption.

saxagliptin   Drug used for Type 2 diabetes classified as a DPP-4 inhibitor.

SC   Administration of a drug by injection into the skin; subcutaneous.

schizophrenia   A severe chronic disorder characterized by abnormal perception and behavior.

scurvy   A disease caused by lack of vitamin C in the diet, characterized by saggy skin and the loss of teeth, nails, and hair.

secondary hypertension   Hypertension caused by a secondary disease etiology that leads to an elevation in blood pressure.

secondhand smoke   Environmental tobacco smoke.

sedative-hypnotics   Drugs that enhance GABA signaling. They help individuals with GAD or other phobias manage their day-to-day activities by lowering their anxiety level.

sedentary behavior   Too much sitting.

selective serotonin and norepinephrine reuptake inhibitors (SSNRIs)   A newer class of drugs, including Cymbalta, effective in treating major depressive disorder.

selective serotonin reuptake inhibitors (SSRIs)   A class of drugs, including Paxil, Zoloft, and Lexapro, that are now the first line of treatment for depression and certain anxiety or personality disorders.

sequestration   Some receptors or membrane proteins can be stored in vesicles and quickly recruited to membranes as needed.

serotonin   A chemical released by cells in the gut and central nervous system that has hormonal and neurotransmitter activity involved in many processes. It also suppresses appetite.

sertraline   Selective Serotonin Reuptake Inhibitor used for depression, obsessive-compulsive disorder, posttraumatic stress disorder, and panic disorder.

serum   The soluble portion of blood that remains after the blood is allowed to coagulate and the solid portion is removed by centrifugation.

SGLT2 inhibitors   Drugs that inhibit sodium glucose cotransporter 2, which is located in the proximal tubule of the kidneys and is responsible for 90% of glucose reabsorption during urine formation. Inhibition of SGLT2 leads to loss of glucose in the urine, lowering glucose levels.

sinoatrial (SA) node   The pacemaker located high in the right atrium that triggers cardiac contraction following input from the parasympathetic and sympathetic nervous systems.

sitagliptin   Used for Type 2 diabetes, where it increases insulin production by enhancing incretin levels. It is a DPP-4 inhibitor.

site of action   The location where a drug exerts its primary effect.

sleep apnea   Breathing issues during sleep.

slow angiotensin II   responses Responses to angiotensin II that include increasing sodium reabsorption in the kidney and stimulating the release of aldosterone from the adrenal cortex.

slow-twitch oxidative fibers   Fatigue-resistant muscle fibers that are efficient at aerobic methods of energy production. Also known as Type I fibers.

sodium-glucose cotransporter 2 Inhibitors   Drugs that block re-uptake of glucose during urine formation causing the loss of glucose. Used for Type 2 diabetes.

somatic nerves   Nerves that synapse in the cerebrospinal axis and extend myelinated fibers to skeletal muscles.

somatrem   A recombinant human growth hormone analog.

somatropin   A recombinant human growth hormone analog.

spillover   The effect of high levels of sympathetic activity increasing the amount of norepinephrine that diffuses away from a synapse and can reach additional targets.

spironolactone   A potassium-sparing diuretic.

sports anemia   Any pseudoanemic condition in athletes; usually, their hemoglobin concentration decreases due to plasma volume expansion.

stage 1 hypertension   A stage of hypertension defined by blood pressure readings that range from 140 to 159 systolic and 90 to 99 diastolic.

stage 2 hypertension A stage of hypertension defined by blood pressure readings that range from greater than or equal to 160 systolic and greater than or equal to 100 diastolic.

statins The most popular (and generally well-tolerated) class of lipid-modifying drugs. They act as competitive inhibitors for the rate-limiting enzyme in cholesterol biosynthesis, HMG-CoA-reductase.

stroke volume The volume of blood ejected each stroke by the heart.

subcutaneous fat Fat located just under the skin. Compared to other types of fat, it is less physiologically active in terms of immune response and adipokine production, instead acting primarily as an energy depot.

sublingual administration Administration of a drug by placing it under the tongue.

substrate-level phosphorylation The enzymatic transfer of high-energy phosphate intermediates to ADP, making ATP, primarily in the cytoplasm.

sulfonylureas Drugs used to treat Type 2 diabetes that release of insulin from pancreatic beta cells.

summation The additive effects of drugs taken together.

sympathetic nervous system (SNS) One of two branches of the ANS, the other being the PSNS. The nerves have relatively short preganglionic fibers that form ganglions close to the spinal cord and postganglionic fibers that are relatively long and can fork and form multiple connections with target tissues.

sympathomimetics Drugs with diverse mechanisms that have agonist activity or mimic the actions of norepinephrine, epinephrine, and dopamine and produce sympathetic-like responses.

symptomatic hypotension Blood pressure of less than 90/60 mmHg. Dizziness, vertigo, or fainting can occur. (not sure this is needed).

synapse The structure where a nerve cell (neuron) passes the signal to another neuron, muscle cell, or glandular cell.

synergism The property of one drug increasing the activity of another drug.

synthetic corticosteroids A class of drugs used for treating inflammation and chronic asthma; they suppress cytokine production to help decrease the level of inflammation and leukocyte infiltration in tissues such as the airways.

systematic review A summary of the conclusions supported by experimental evidence found in many published studies.

systole Contraction of heart muscle, in which the ventricles pump blood to the lungs or body.

T1/2 The half-life of a drug; the time necessary to decrease the drug's serum concentration by 50%.

teratogenesis Production of congenital malformations in an embryo or fetus.

tesofensine Originally prescribed as an antidepressant, it can cause weight loss; it inhibits norepinephrine, dopamine, and serotonin reuptake.

tetrahydrogestrinone (THG) The Clear - a synthetic, anabolic steroid that escaped detection for years before discovered as an illegal PES.

thalidomide Drug originally used for morning sickness in pregnant women during the 1950s until it was discovered to cause developmental defects. Now used for leprosy.

therapeutic index (TI) The ratio between the lethal dose for 50% of test animals and the effective dose for 50% of test animals ($TI = LD_{50}/ED_{50}$), or, in humans, the ratio between the toxic (unwanted side effect) dose (TD) in 1% of the subjects and the effective dose in 90% ($TI = TD_1/ED_{90}$).

therapeutic window   The interval and dosage of a drug that maintains its level in the body above the minimum effective concentration and below the minimum toxic concentration.

therapeutics   The medical aspects of drug treatment and care of patients, with the intent of relieving injury and pain or preventing and treating disease.

thiazide diuretics   A class of diuretics that block an Na^+/Cl^- symporter in the distal convoluted tubule.

thiazolidinediones   Drugs that decrease insulin resistance. They act as ligands for one of the peroxisome proliferator-activated receptors. The thiazolidinediones used for Type 2 diabetes likely target adipose tissue as their major site of action, modulating lipid synthesis and promoting glucose uptake and utilization.

third-generation beta-blockers   Newer beta-blockers that have additional properties, such as causing vasodilation.

thirdhand smoke   The oily residue that covers surface areas in places where people smoke.

threat stress   Type of stress from concerns about personal safety.

thyroid-stimulating hormone   A pituitary hormone that stimulates the thyroid gland to produce thyroxine.

tidal volume   Depth of respiration—the amount of air per breath.

tolerance   The need to increase drug dose over time to maintain the desired response.

topiramate   A drug originally prescribed as an antiepileptic, often combined with phentermine for weight loss.

tranquilizers   An older term that used to group together different anti-psychotic drugs.

tricyclic antidepressants   Drugs widely prescribed for depression in the 1970s, replacing the MAO inhibitors. They block reuptake of several different neurotransmitters, including norepinephrine, serotonin, and dopamine, and can antagonize acetylcholine and histamine receptors.

troglitazone   Drug used for diabetes that has been withdrawn from the market because of liver toxicity.

Tylenol   Brand name for acetaminophen.

Type 1 diabetes   Diabetes that results from the loss of pancreatic beta cells, requires insulin by injection or pump.

Type 2 diabetes   Diabetes that results from inadequate insulin production or loss of responsiveness to insulin's action; Associated with age, physical inactivity, race/ethnicity, family history, impaired glucose metabolism, and, most significantly, obesity.

Type 3 diabetes   A type of diabetes linked to Alzheimer's disease.

Type 4 diabetes   A type of diabetes including gestational diabetes.

Typical antipsychotics   Older, first-generation antipsychotic drugs, more effective at treating the active symptoms of the disease (delusions, hallucinations, and hyperactivity) than the negative symptoms (emotional blunting and social withdrawal).

upregulation   An increase in receptor number in a cell as it responds to the suppression of activity caused by drugs that act as antagonists.

valium   A benzodiazepine used for anxiety.

valsartan   An angiotensin receptor blocker used for hypertension.

vasoconstriction   Contraction of vascular smooth muscle increases blood pressure.

vasodilation   Relaxation of vascular smooth muscle decreases blood pressure.

Vaughan Williams classification   Five main classes of drugs for heart arrythmias.

ventilation equivalent for oxygen   The number of liters of air breathed for every 100 mL of oxygen consumed.

ventricle   Heart chamber that pumps blood into the arteries.

verapamil   A calcium channel blocker.

very low-density lipoprotein (VLDL)   A lipoprotein complex involved in cholesterol transport, secreted by the liver into the blood.

visceral fat   Fat that fills the abdominal cavity surrounding the major organs.

vitamin B$_3$ See *niacin*.

vitamin D   Members of a group of modified steroid molecules derived from cholesterol, but with one of the rings opened.

VO$_2$max   The maximal amount of oxygen that a person consumes per minute during maximal exercise measured in mL O$_2$/[kg · min].

volume of distribution   A theoretical measure or apparent volume of fluid into which an administered drug would need to be distributed to achieve the desired concentration in plasma.

voluntary nervous system   The part of the nervous system that is responsible for voluntary body movement and sensory information processing; it includes the somatic nerves. Also known as the somatic nervous system.

warfarin   Drug used as an anti-coagulant to prevent blood clots.

Wingate test   An exercise protocol that measures peak anaerobic power and capacity over 30 seconds.

withdrawal syndrome   The physiological response that occurs following the abrupt cessation of drug treatment.

xanthine alkaloids   A group of alkaloids that cross the blood–brain barrier, exerting a central effect in addition to systemic responses.

Z-line   Found on either end of a sarcomere, the primary structural and functional unit of muscle tissue.

Zyprexa   An antipsychotic used to treat schizophrenia and bipolar disorder.

Index

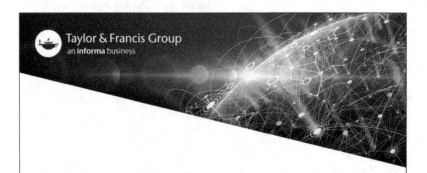

Printed in the United States
by Baker & Taylor Publisher Services